ATLAS OF
Clinical Urology

ATLAS OF Clinical Urology

VOLUME II
The Prostate

VOLUME EDITORS

NONCANCEROUS DISEASE SECTION

John D. McConnell, MD
Professor and Chairman
Department of Urology
University of Texas Southwestern Medical Center
Dallas, Texas

CANCEROUS DISEASE SECTION

Peter T. Scardino, MD
Chief, Urology Service
Department of Surgery
Murray F. Brennan Chair of Surgery
Head, Prostate Cancer Program
Memorial Sloan-Kettering Cancer Center
New York, New York

SERIES EDITORS

E. Darracott Vaughan, Jr., MD
Professor
Department of Urology
Joan and Sanford I. Weill Medical College and
 Graduate School of Medical Sciences of Cornell University
James J. Colt Professor and Chairman
Department of Urology
New York Presbyterian Hospital
New York, New York

Aaron P. Perlmutter, MD, PhD
Assistant Professor
Department of Urology
Joan and Sanford I. Weill Medical College and
 Graduate School of Medical Sciences of Cornell University
Assistant Attending Urologist
New York Presbyterian Hospital
New York, New York

With 28 Contributors

Developed by Current Medicine, Inc., Philadelphia

Current Medicine, Inc.

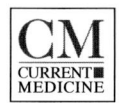

400 Market Street • Suite 700
Philadelphia, PA 19106
1-800-427-1796

Director of Product Development	Mary Kinsella
Editorial Supervisor	Susan L. Hunsberger
Senior Developmental Editor	Elise M. Paxson
Editorial Assistant	Forrest Perry
Art Director	Paul Fennessy
Associate Art Director	Jerilyn Bockorick
Design and Layout	Jerilyn Bockorick
Illustration Director	Birck Cox
Illustrators	Debra Wertz, Wiesia Langenfeld, Lisa Weischedel, Nicole Mock, Birck Cox, Paul Shiffmacher
Cover Design	Jerilyn Bockorick
Cover Illustration	Debra Wertz
Production	Lori Holland, Amy Giuffi, Constance Copeland
Indexing	Holly Lukens

The prostate.
    p. cm—(Atlas of clinical urology v. 2)
  Includes bibliographical references and index.
  Contents: Noncancerous disease section/[edited by] John McConnell—Cancerous disease section/
[edited by] Peter Scardino.
  ISBN 1-57340-123-64
  1. Prostate—Diseases Atlases. I. McConnell, John D. II. Scardino, Peter T. III. Series.
  [DNLM: 1. Prostatic Neoplasms—surgery Atlases. 2. Prostatectomy Atlases—therapy atlases.
3. Prostatic Hyperplasia—surgery Atlases. WJ 17 A8615 1999 v.2]
RC899.P6922 1999
616.6'5—dc21
DNLM/DLC   99-23135
  for Library of Congress   CIP

Library of Congress Cataloging-in-Publication Data

ISBN 1-57340-123-4

©1999 by Current Medicine, Inc. All rights reserved. No part of this publication may be reproduced, stored in a retrieval system, or transmitted in any form by any means electronic, mechanical, photocopying, recording, or otherwise, without prior consent of the publisher.

Although every effort has been made to ensure that drug doses and other information are presented accurately in this publication, the ultimate responsibility rests with the prescribing physician. Neither the publishers nor the author can be held responsible for errors or for any consequence arising from the use of the information contained therein. Any product mentioned in this publication should be used in accordance with the prescribing information prepared by the manufacturers. No claims or endorsements are made for any drug or compound at present under clinical investigation.

Printed in the United States by Quebecor
5 4 3 2 1

SERIES PREFACE

As urology enters the 21st century, it is appropriate that the *Atlas of Clinical Urology* series captures and explains the major areas of modern urologic practice using a unique combination of images, schematics, tables, and algorithms. It does so in a compelling fashion, by combining a multilevel approach that includes the individual volumes and the internet. Urology is a specialty of great breadth, and visual images provide much of the backbone of urologic diagnosis and endoscopy and are key to surgical technique. The increasingly complex diagnostic and treatment paths are best depicted and understood as visual algorithms.

The editors of this five-volume series have not only contributed their world-renowned expertise to the chapters but have also assembled an outstanding group of individual chapter authors. Together, they provide each volume with completeness, depth, and—most important in this age of rapidly expanding science and technology—*current* urologic thinking.

In Volume I, Tom Lue and his contributors cover the expanding area of impotence from anatomic considerations through many of the new treatment modalities. As our population ages, urologists are evaluating and treating an expanding number of impotent patients. This section provides an excellent understanding and practical approach. In the second half of Volume I, Marc Goldstein and his expert colleagues provide a beautiful series of images that depict the important aspects of reproductive anatomy and endocrinology, as well as detailed surgical schematics demonstrating the ever-evolving "standard" surgery for infertility in addition to new assisted-reproduction techniques.

It would be fair to say that the 1990s are the decade of the prostate, and Volume II captures the paradigm changes that occurred in the management of both prostate cancer and benign disease. Management of prostate cancer is challenging, and the section by Peter Scardino provides a clear, concise, factual background for understanding prostate cancer and the myriad of treatment options. John McConnell's section on noncancerous diseases provides the background for understanding the new treatment modalities available for benign prostatic hyperplasia (BPH). The choices of pharmacologic management and device therapies continue to challenge even the most seasoned urologist, and the diagnostic and treatment schematics provided in the section have been constructed by leaders in the field.

Renal carcinoma is covered in Volume III by section editor Andrew Novick. Radiologic images play an increasing role in our diagnosis and management of renal cancer, and the visual image format of the Atlas is ideal. The challenges of nephron sparing and vena caval surgery are clearly illustrated and are combined with an understanding of the appropriate patient populations for these procedures. This section also includes the management of benign and malignant adrenal disorders. Michael Marberger has assembled an extremely diverse and important set of noncancerous diseases of the kidney. Nephrolithiasis management is covered from medical therapy to endoscopy to incisional surgery. The important role that laparoscopy has established in both excisional and reconstructive renal surgery is visually depicted and explained. The evolution of the techniques illustrated in this section will likely provide the basis for renal intervention in the 21st century.

Volume IV covers the diversity of pediatric urology under the editorship of Dix Poppas and Alan Retik. This volume provides images illustrating the most important diseases that confront the pediatric urologist. In addition, the changes in management and thinking in classic conditions such as vesicoureteral reflux and neurogenic vesical dysfunction are illustrated. This volume will not only be of great value to the practicing pediatric urologist, but also to general urologists as well as pediatricians and pediatric nephrologists.

Bladder diseases cause many patients to seek urologic care. In Voume V, Donald Skinner and John Stein have assembled state-of-the-art contributions in the management of bladder and urethral cancer. The combination of a better understanding of bladder cancer and new options in surgical urinary diversions is changing the management of bladder cancer. The role of surgery and surgical approaches to bladder cancer are illustrated in this volume by the innovative surgeons who contributed chapters to the section. Voiding dysfunction and incontinence as well as inflammatory and infectious conditions of the bladder are covered by Alan Wein's section. The excellent contributions to this section provide an illustrated understanding of the neuromuscular function of the lower urinary tract, and the images reproduced in this volume allow an easy understanding of the diagnosis and management of incontinence, inflammatory conditions, and fistulae.

These section editors and authors deserve tremendous credit for this *Atlas of Clinical Urology*, which was initiated by Abe Krieger, President of Current Medicine. We thank Abe, the developmental editors, and the excellent illustrators of Current Medicine for their outstanding efforts.

E. Darracott Vaughan, Jr.
Aaron P. Perlmutter

CONTRIBUTORS

Edgar Ben-Josef, MD
Assistant Professor
Department of Radiation Oncology
Wayne State University;
Attending Radiation Oncologist
Barbara Ann Karmanos Cancer Institute, Harper Hospital
Detroit, Michigan

John C. Blasko, MD
Director of Clinical Research
Swedish Tumor Institute
Seattle, Washington

H. Ballentine Carter, MD
Professor
Department of Urology
Johns Hopkins Hospital
Baltimore, Maryland

Peter R. Carroll, MD
Professor and Chair
Department of Urology
University of California at San Francisco;
Urology Faculty Practice
University of California at San Francisco
San Francisco, California

William J. Ellis, MD
Associate Professor
Department of Urology
University of Washington
Seattle, Washington

William D. Figg, PhD
Senior Investigator
National Cancer Institute
Bethesda, Maryland

John N. Kabalin, MD, FACS
Scottsbluff Urology
Scottsbluff, Nebraska

Steven A. Kaplan, MD, FACS
Vice Chairman and Given Professor of Urology
Department of Urology
Columbia University
New York, New York

Michael W. Kattan, PhD
Assistant Attending
Department of Surgery;
Outcomes Research Scientist
Memorial Sloan-Kettering Cancer Center
New York, New York

Ira J. Kohn, MD
Clinical Assistant in Urology
Squier Urological Clinic
Columbia University
New York, New York;
Staff Urologist
Delta Medix
Scranton, Pennsylvania

John N. Krieger, MD
Professor
Department of Urology
University of Washington;
Chief, Urology
VA Puget Sound Health Care System
Seattle, Washington

John D. McConnell, MD
Professor and Chairman
Department of Urology
University of Texas Southwestern Medical Center
Dallas, Texas

Winston K. Mebust, MD
Professor of Urologic Surgery
Department of Urology
University of Kansas Medical Center
Kansas City, Kansas

Brian J. Miles, MD
Associate Professor
Scott Department of Urology
Baylor College of Medicine
Houston, Texas

Mark J. Noble, MD
Cleveland Clinic Hospital
Cleveland, Ohio

Alan W. Partin, MD, PhD
Associate Professor
Department of Urology
Johns Hopkins Medical School
Baltimore, Maryland

Aaron P. Perlmutter, MD
Assistant Professor
Department of Urology
Joan and Sanford I. Weill Medical College and
    Graduate School of Medical Sciences of Cornell University
Assistant Attending Urologist
New York Presbyterian Hospital
New York, New York

Arthur T. Porter, MD, MBA, FACR
Professor and Chairman
Department of Radiation Oncology
Wayne State University
Detroit, Michigan

Walter Rayford, MD, PhD
Assistant Professor
Department of Urology
Louisiana State University Medical Center
New Orleans, Louisiana

Claus G. Roehrborn, MD, FACS
Associate Professor
Department of Urology
The University of Texas Southwestern Medical Center
Dallas, Texas

Oliver Sartor, MD
Professor
Department of Medicine and Urology
Louisiana State University Medical School;
Director
Stanley S. Scott Cancer Center
New Orleans, Louisiana

Peter T. Scardino, MD
Chief, Urology Service
Department of Surgery;
Murray F. Brennan Chair of Surgery;
Head, Prostate Cancer Program;
Memorial Sloan-Kettering Cancer Center
New York, New York

Katsuto Shinohara, MD
Assistant Adjunct Professor
Department of Urology
University of California at San Francisco;
Attending Physician
University of California at San Francisco Medical Center
San Francisco, California

Alan M.F. Stapleton, FRACS, PhD
Senior Lecturer in Surgery
Department of Surgery
Flinders University of South Australia;
Director of Urology
Repatriation General Hospital and the Flinders Medical Center
Daw Park, Adelaide, SA Australia

Lorne D. Sullivan, MD, FRCS(S)
Professor
Department of Surgery
University of British Columbia;
Professor of Surgery
Division of Urology
Vancouver General Hospital
Vancouver, British Columbia, Canada

Maryrose P. Sullivan, PhD
Instructor
Department of Surgery
Harvard Medical School;
Biomedical Engineer
West Roxbury Veterans Affairs Medical Center
Boston, Massachusetts

Gregory M.M. Videtic, MD, CM, FRCPC
Assistant Professor
Department of Oncology
University of Western Ontario;
Consultant Radiation Oncologist
London Regional Cancer Centre
London, Ontario, Canada

Subbarao V. Yalla, MD
Associate Professor
Department of Urology and Surgery
Harvard Medical School;
Chief of Urology
West Roxbury Veterans Affairs Medical Center
Boston, Massachusetts

CONTENTS

NONCANCEROUS DISEASE SECTION

CHAPTER 1
The Epidemiology and Pathophysiology of Benign Prostatic Hyperplasia
John D. McConnell

CHAPTER 2
Clinical Evaluation of Lower Urinary Tract Symptoms Due to Benign Prostatic Hyperplasia
Subbarao V. Yalla and Maryrose P. Sullivan

The Relationships Among Lower Urinary Tract Symptoms,
    Benign Prostatic Hyperplasia, and Voiding Dysfunction 2.2
Urodynamic Evaluation 2.4
Radiologic Imaging of the Lower Urinary Tract 2.10
Cystourethroscopy 2.14
Clinical Approach for the Assessment of Lower Urinary Tract Symptoms 2.14

CHAPTER 3
Medical Management of Benign Prostatic Hyperplasia
Ira J. Kohn and Steven A. Kaplan

Selecting Patients for the Medical Management of Benign Prostatic Hyperplasia 3.2
Altering the Static Component of Benign Prostatic Hyperplasia
    Through Endocrine Therapy 3.3
Altering the Dynamic Component of Benign Prostatic Hyperplasia Through α-Blocker
Therapy 3.8

CHAPTER 4
Minimally Invasive Therapies for Benign Prostatic Hyperplasia
Claus G. Roehrborn

Microwave Hyperthermia 4.4
Transurethral Microwave Thermotherapy 4.6
High-intensity Focused Ultrasound 4.13
Transurethral Needle Ablation 4.16

CHAPTER 5
Laser Prostatectomy
Aaron P. Perlmutter and John N. Kabalin

Transurethral Ultrasound-guided Laser-induced Prostatectomy 5.2
ND:YAG Free-beam Laser Prostatectomy 5.3
HO:YAG Laser Resection of the Prostate 5.6
Interstitial Laser Prostatectomy 5.7

CHAPTER 6
Transurethral Resection of the Prostate, Transurethral Incision of the Prostate, and Open Prostatectomy for Benign Prostatic Hyperplasia
Winston K. Mebust & Mark J. Noble

Surgical Techniques 6.4
Transurethral Incision of the Prostate 6.9
Open Prostatectomy 6.10
Retropubic Prostatectomy 6.12

CHAPTER 7
Prostatitis: Definition and Clinical Approaches
John N. Krieger

CANCEROUS DISEASE SECTION

Introduction: Peter T. Scardino

CHAPTER 8
Clinical Aspects of Prostate Cancer
H. Ballentine Carter and Alan W. Partin

    Early Detection of Prostate Cancer 8.3
    Staging of Prostate Cancer. 8.7
    Pathologic Considerations. 8.12
    Conclusions 8.15

CHAPTER 9
The Patient's Choice of Surgery for Clinically Localized Prostate Cancer
Michael W. Kattan and Brian J. Miles

CHAPTER 10
Radical Perineal Prostatectomy
Lorne D. Sullivan

CHAPTER 11
Nerve-sparing Radical Retropubic Prostatectomy
Alan M.F. Stapleton and Peter T. Scardino

    Preoperative Considerations 11.2
    Operative Technique. 11.3
    Complications. 11.10

CHAPTER 12
External Beam Radiotherapy for Prostate Cancer
Gregory M.M. Videtic, Edgar Ben-Josef, and Arthur T. Porter

    Implications for EBRT Regarding Local Anatomy and
        Patterns of Disease Spread. 12.2
    Conventional Photon EBRT. 12.5
    Results of External Beam Radiotherapy for Prostate Cancer 12.7
    Advances in Treatment of Prostate Cancer Using External Beam Radiotherapy . . . 12.8
    External Beam Radiotherapy After Radical Prostatectomy. 12.12

CHAPTER 13
Interstitial Radiation Therapy
William J. Ellis and John C. Blasko

    Preoperative Evaluation. 13.2
    Therapy Selection 13.3
    Prostate Volume Study. 13.4
    Results. 13.8

CHAPTER 14

Cryoablation of Prostate Cancer
Katsuto Shinohara and Peter R. Carroll

- Cryobiology 14.2
- Equipment 14.3
- Patient Selection 14.4
- Procedure 14.5
- Complications 14.9
- Tumor Control 14.10
- Conclusions 14.12

CHAPTER 15

Management of Metastatic Prostate Cancer
Oliver Sartor, Walter Rayford, and William D. Figg

- Hormonal Therapy 15.5
- Hormone-refractory Prostate Cancer 15.7

Index I.1

Color Plates

The Epidemiology and Pathophysiology of Benign Prostatic Hyperplasia

NONCANCEROUS DISEASE SECTION

John D. McConnell

Although benign prostatic hyperplasia (BPH) is one of the most common disease processes affecting the aging man, surprisingly little is known about its pathophysiology [1]. Despite intense research efforts in the past four to five decades to find the underlying cause of prostatic growth in older men, cause and effect relationships have not been established. Previously held notions that the clinical symptoms of BPH (prostatism) are simply due to a mass-related increase in urethral resistance are too simplistic. It is now clear that a significant portion of the symptoms are caused by obstruction-induced detrusor dysfunction. Moreover, obstruction may induce a variety of neural alterations in the bladder and prostate that contribute to symptomatology. Undoubtedly, the constellation of cellular pathologies that give rise to the symptoms of BPH will be far more complex than we currently realize. Only by revealing these complexities, however, will we be able to successfully design alternative strategies to treat, and possibly prevent, BPH.

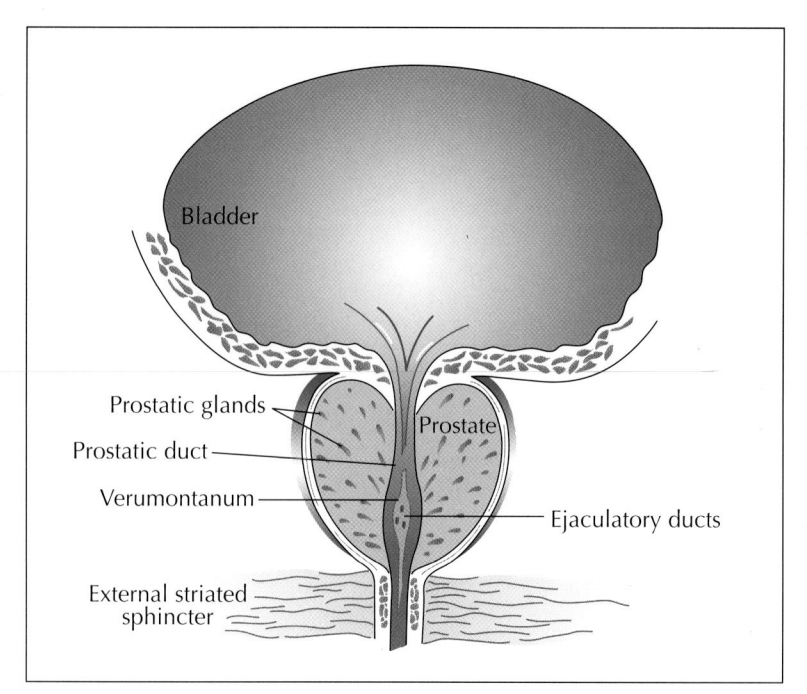

▶ **FIGURE 1-1.** Anatomy. Benign prostatic hyperplasia (BPH) begins as a histologic disease in the fifth or sixth decade of life. McNeal's [2] careful anatomic studies suggest that the hyperplasia starts first with mesenchymal nodule formation in the periurethral area of the prostate. This is followed by the development of epithelial nodules in the transition zone of the prostate. Outward growth of the prostate is somewhat contained by the presence of a fibrous capsule [1]. Because of the restraining influence of the capsule and the plastic elements present in the tissue, ongoing growth tends to increase urethral resistance. The only other animal species known to develop BPH, the dog, does not develop significant urinary difficulty. The canine prostate, which lacks a capsule, tends to grow away from the urethra, producing rectal obstruction.

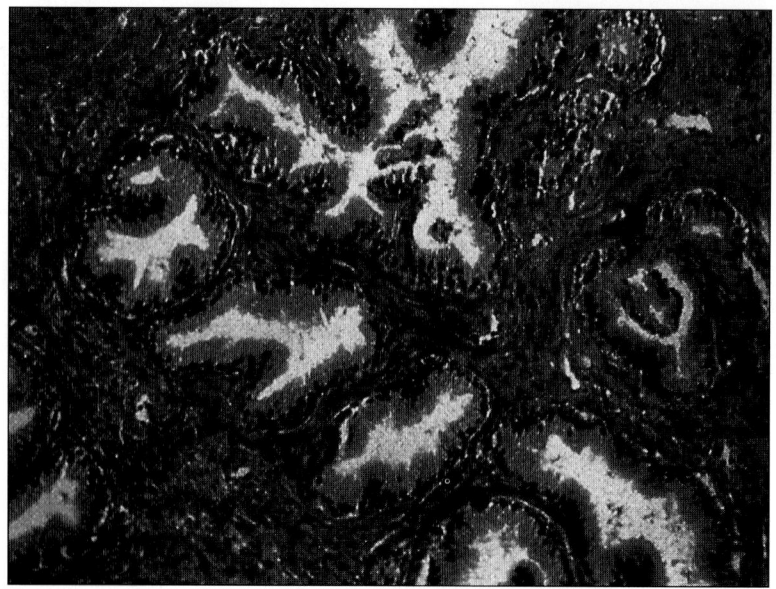

▶ **FIGURE 1-2.** Histology of benign prostatic hyperplasia (BPH). Histologically, BPH is characterized by a combination of epithelial and stromal hyperplasia of varying degrees. The majority of patients demonstrate a fibromyoadenomatosis pattern of hyperplasia [2]. However, the degree of stromal versus epithelial hyperplasia can be quite variable, with some patients demonstrating almost a pure smooth muscle proliferation pattern. Despite the increase in prostate epithelial mass, prostatic secretions actually decline with age, probably secondary to compressive ductal obstruction [1].

Definitions Useful for Increased Precision of Diagnosis and Treatment

Term	Definition
LUTS	Lower urinary tract *symptoms*
BPE	Benign prostatic *enlargement*
BOO	Bladder outlet *obstruction*
BPH	Benign prostatic *hyperplasia*

▶ **FIGURE 1-3.** Definitions useful for increased precision of diagnosis and treatment. Patients seek medical attention because of bothersome lower urinary tract symptoms (LUTS) [3]. Although 80% of men develop the histologic disease of benign prostatic hyperplasia (BPH) by the time they reach the eighth decade of life, only a subset of those men will develop bothersome urinary symptoms [4]. Although histologic hyperplasia is almost universal, not all men develop significant prostatic enlargement. Moreover, the degree of bladder outlet obstruction is only indirectly influenced by prostatic size. When studying the epidemiology and clinical course of BPH, it is important to precisely arrive at a *case definition* [4]. Are we studying enlargement, symptoms, obstruction, or a definition that combines all aspects of the disease? Moreover, the major benefit of treatment approaches should be defined according to these definitions. Does a given treatment target enlargement or symptoms?

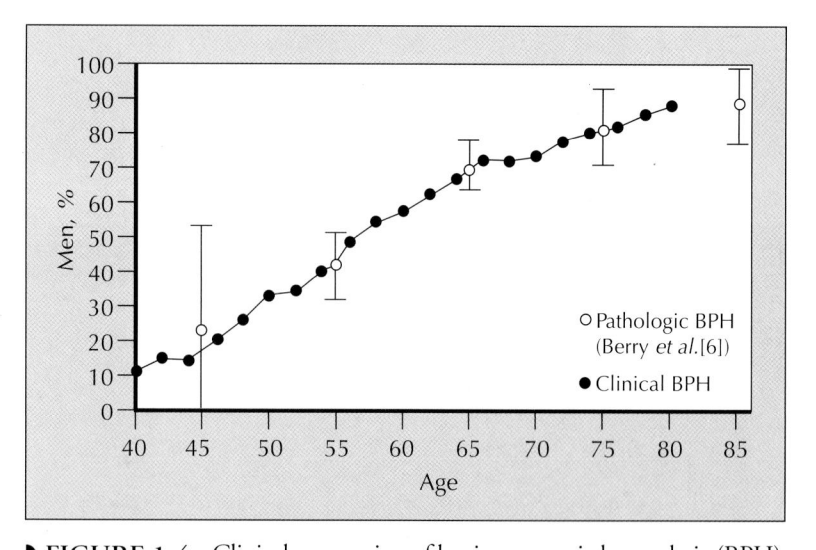

▶ **FIGURE 1-4.** Clinical progression of benign prostatic hyperplasia (BPH). Although the correlation between prostatic size and symptom severity is poor in individual patients, there is an interdependence that becomes apparent in analysis of large cohorts of men. Guess *et al.* [5] from the Baltimore Longitudinal Study of Aging (BLSA) demonstrated that a clinical definition of BPH (defined by symptoms and evidence of prostate enlargement on digital rectal examination) correlated closely with the histologic evidence of BPH at each decade of year (defined by the Hopkins autopsy study performed by Berry *et al.* [6].) Eighty percent of men in the BLSA study developed clinical evidence of BPH by the time they reached the eighth decade of life. Approximately 25% of these men have significant loss of quality of life and may be appropriate candidates for medical or surgical intervention [7].

Definitions of Benign Prostatic Hyperplasia Progression

Symptomatic deterioration
Increasing bothersomeness
Urinary retention
Progression to surgery
Renal insufficiency

▶ **FIGURE 1-5.** Definitions of benign prostatic hyperplasia (BPH) progression. The time course and severity of BPH in an individual patient is variable [7,8]. Moreover, the probability of specific adverse outcomes is variable. The most common adverse outcome is the development of bothersome urinary symptoms. In addition, a patient with a stable level of symptoms may develop increasing bothersomeness, *ie*, simply growing tired of the same level of symptoms. One to two percent of patients per year with significant prostatic enlargement may develop acute urinary retention [9]. Approximately one half of these cases will be precipitated by anesthesia or α-sympathomimetic medications, *eg*, decongestants. Because of symptom progression of the development of urinary retention, 10% to 25% of patients ultimately require BPH-related surgery [9]. The most unlikely complications are the development of obstruction-related renal insufficiency and recurrent urinary tract infection. "Silent prostatism" (*ie*, obstructive uropathy in the absence of symptoms) is an extremely rare outcome.

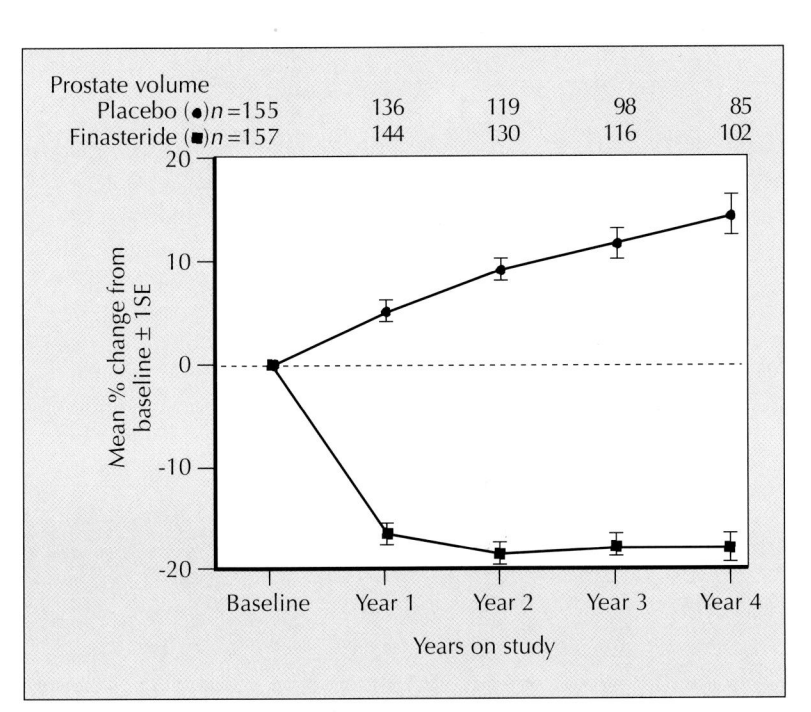

Biologic Progression of Benign Prostatic Hyperplasia

Prostate growth
Obstruction-related bladder dysfunction
Age-related bladder dysfunction
Medical comorbidity (diabetes, Parkinson's disease, stroke)

▶ **FIGURE 1-6.** Biologic progression of benign prostatic hyperplasia (BPH). The underlying biologic causes for clinical progression are complex. Ongoing growth of the prostate undoubtedly contributes significantly to clinical progression. However, nonprostatic causes are also important. Obstruction produces significant changes in bladder function, which may continue after relief of the obstruction [10]. Obstruction-related bladder dysfunction may also continue in patients who have partial relief of symptoms from medical therapy, but incomplete relief of obstruction. Often overlooked is the importance of age-related declines in bladder function, which occur in both men and women. The density of nerve fibers in the bladder decreases with age and extracellular matrix (ECM) formation (*eg*, collagen) increases [11]. Frequency, urgency, and incomplete emptying (often considered to be symptoms of prostatic enlargement) are also seen in women. Lastly, a patient may have symptomatic progression because of the development of medical comorbidities (*eg*, diabetes, Parkinson's disease, or stroke), which adversely affect bladder function [1].

▶ **FIGURE 1-7.** Changes in prostate volume over time according to the results of the Proscar Long-term Efficacy and Safety Study (PLESS). Once the benign prostatic hyperplasia (BPH) process has been set in motion, the prostate continues to grow in 80% to 90% of patients. PLESS, the longest term prospective trial to date, demonstrated a 2- to 3-cc increase in prostatic volume per year [9]. Community-based studies demonstrate a slower prostate growth rate of approximately 1- to 2-cc per year [12]. This finding suggests that men with significant prostate enlargement (*eg*, those enrolled in PLESS) may have more rapid rates of prostatic growth. Whether this is genetically determined or a result of feedback influences on prostate growth (*eg*, increased growth factor production in larger prostates leading to even more growth) is uncertain.

Controversy Regarding Prostate Size

Prostate size does not correlate with symptom severity
Weak correlation with urodynamic obstruction
Community-based studies demonstrate correlation between prostate size and risk

▶ **FIGURE 1-8.** Controversy regarding prostate size and future risk. Until recently, it was controversial whether ongoing growth of the prostate contributed significantly to the pathophysiology of lower urinary tract symptoms. This school of thought arose from clinical studies that demonstrated a very poor correlation between prostate size and symptom severity or the degree of urodynamic obstruction [13]. However, Jacobsen *et al.* [12] demonstrated in a community-based epidemiologic study that prostate size predicts the future risk of acute urinary retention and the need for prostate surgery.

The Epidemiology and Pathophysiology of Benign Prostatic Hyperplasia

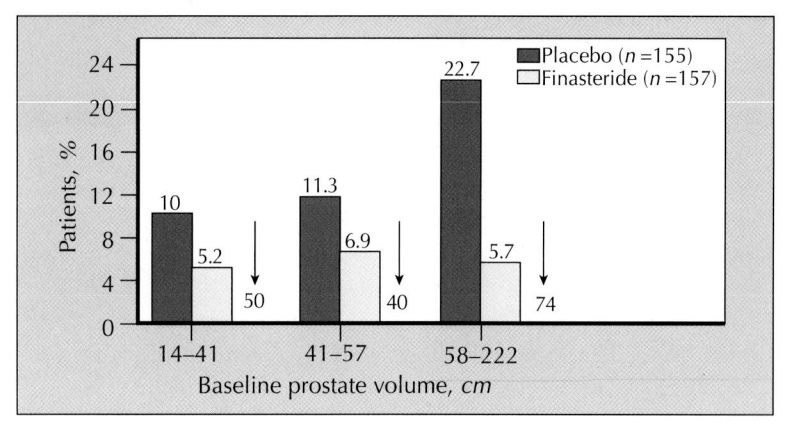

▶ **FIGURE 1-9.** Relationship between prostate size and the risk of benign prostatic hyperplasia (BPH) clinical progression. The Proscar Long-term Efficacy and Safety Study (PLESS) demonstrated a very clear relationship between prostate size and the risk of BPH clinical progression [9]. Men with prostate volumes greater than 58 cc were two times more likely to develop acute urinary retention or need BPH-related surgery than men with prostate volumes less than 40 cc. The androgen dependence of BPH progression was demonstrated by the ability of the 5α-reductase inhibitor finasteride to reduce the risk of future surgery or acute retention in men who had significant enlargement. Although these data strongly suggest that ongoing growth of the prostate is an important component of the disease process, the factors that contribute to symptom severity (bladder dysfunction and patient perception of difficulty) make it difficult to establish a correlation between symptoms and prostate size. In contrast, adverse outcomes, such as acute urinary retention, are clearly influenced by prostate size.

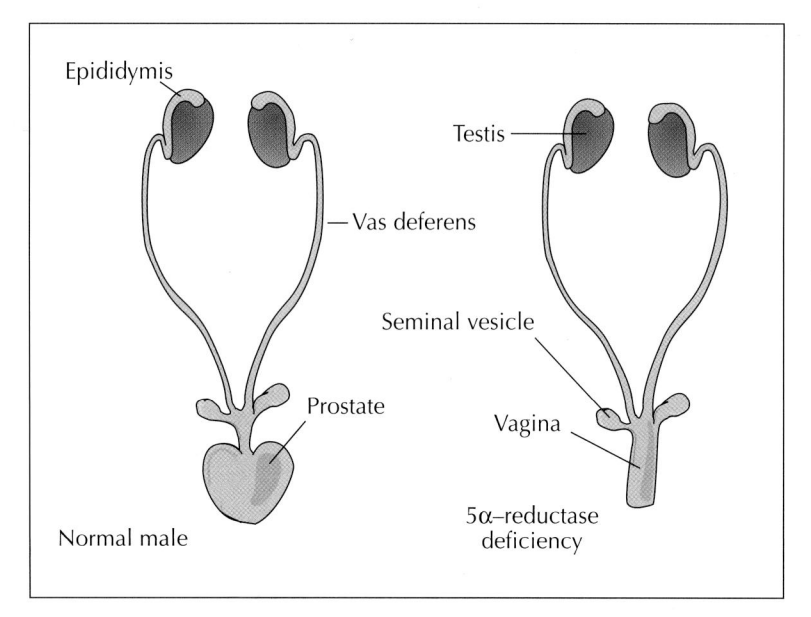

Pathophysiology of Benign Prostatic Hyperplasia

Prostate growth
Increased urethral resistance
Decreased force of stream and intermittency, primarily obstructive symptoms
Detrusor response to maintain flow
Frequency, urgency, and nocturia, primarily detrusor (failure to store) symptoms

▶ **FIGURE 1-10.** Pathophysiology of benign prostatic hyperplasia (BPH). The classic view of BPH pathophysiology is undoubtedly too simplistic. Nevertheless, this model still provides a rational framework for the diagnosis and treatment of the disease. Ongoing growth of the prostate leads to increases in urethral resistance. The symptoms of decreased force of stream and intermittency are primarily related to the increase in urethral resistance. The bladder responds to increased urethral resistance initially with smooth muscle hypertrophy, which permits the bladder to increase voiding pressures to maintain flow. However, the increased pressure occurs at the expense of bladder storage function, with symptoms such as frequency, urgency, and nocturia becoming the predominant aspects of the disease. This simple model ignores the important contribution of aging and central nervous system dysfunction, which may occur independent of prostatic obstruction.

▶ **FIGURE 1-11.** The syndrome of 5α-reductase deficiency. The development of benign prostatic hyperplasia requires testicular androgens and aging [14]. The importance of androgens in prostate development is demonstrated by the syndrome of 5α-reductase deficiency. Normally, the prostate develops from the urogenital sinus, under the influence of DHT (dihydrotestosterone), which is formed from testosterone by the enzyme 5α-reductase type 2. When 5α-reductase type 2 is genetically deficient, the prostate does not develop. The wolffian duct structures, which require testosterone for development, form normally. DHT is not only important for prostatic development, but is also required for growth of the prostate during puberty and adulthood.

II. The Prostate

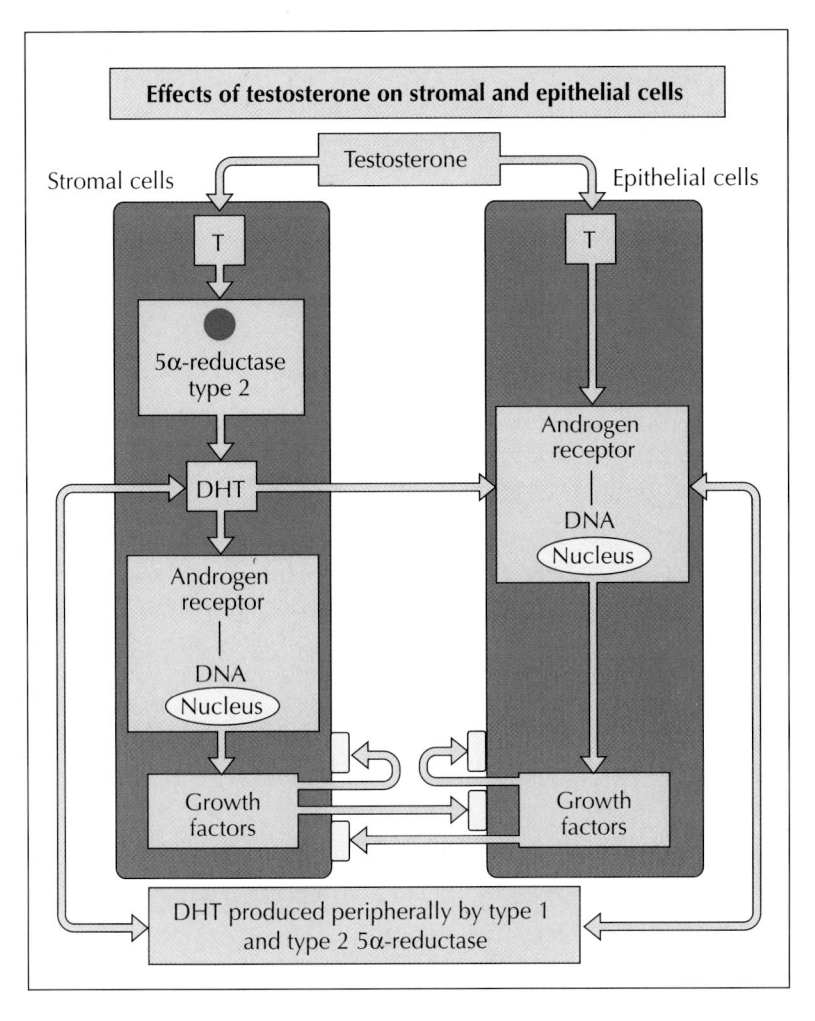

FIGURE 1-12. Effects of testosterone on stromal and epithelial cells. The primary androgen reaching the prostate is testosterone, which is produced in the Leydig cells of the testis [14]. Testosterone may have a direct effect on the epithelial cell of the prostate, but 90% of intraprostatic testosterone is converted to DHT (dihydrotestosterone) within the stromal cell by type 2 5α-reductase. The DHT made in the stromal cell then acts on the adjacent epithelial cells through a paracrine mechanism. Alternatively, DHT made in the stromal cell may promote the expression of growth factors that work secondarily on the epithelial cell. Significant levels of DHT are made in the skin and liver by type 1 and type 2 5α-reductase isoenzymes [15]. It is uncertain whether DHT made in the periphery can act on the prostate in a true endocrine fashion.

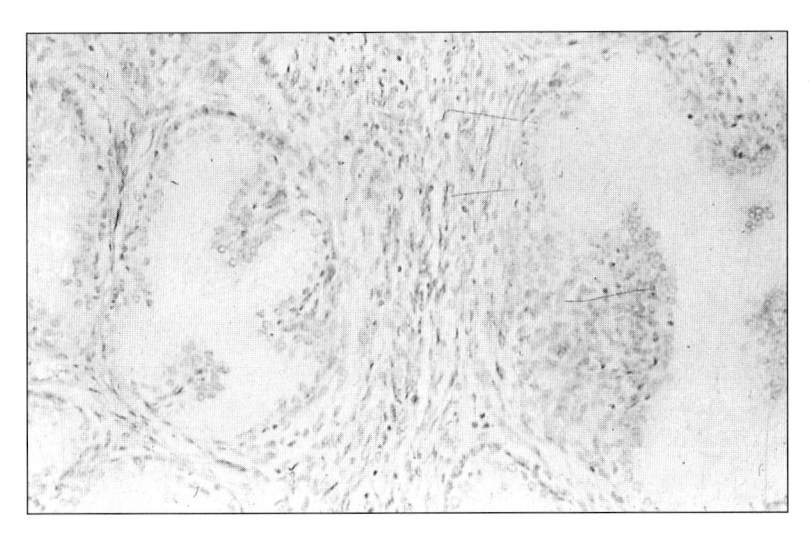

FIGURE 1-13. *(See Color Plate)* Prostate tissue sample. As demonstrated in this section stained with an antibody against type 2 5α-reductase, the enzyme is clearly located in the prostatic stroma [16,17]. Stroma immediately adjacent to hyperplastic epithelial nodules appear to express slightly higher levels of 5α-reductase, which may promote locally increased production of DHT (dihydrotestosterone). However, it appears that DHT production is necessary for the development of benign prostatic hyperplasia (BPH), but not causative. Analysis of prostate tissue samples from men with BPH demonstrates no higher levels of DHT [18].

The 5α-Reductase Isozymes

	Type 1	Type 2
pH optima	6.0–8.5	5.0
Ki finasteride	230–300 nM	3 to 5 nM
Activity in def. state	Normal	Reduced or abnormal
Homology, %	50	50

FIGURE 1-14. The 5α-reductase isoenzymes. Two 5α-reductase isoenzymes have been reported to date [15]. The type 2 isoenzyme is the predominant, if not exclusive, isoenzyme found in the prostate. It is the enzyme that is mutated in the 5α-reductase deficiency state and that is exquisitely sensitive to inhibition by finasteride. Type 1 5α-reductase is expressed mainly in skin and liver; it is not inhibited by finasteride. Pharmaceutical companies have developed drugs that inhibit both type 1 and type 2 5α-reductase isoenzymes. However, because the type 2 enzyme is the predominant form in the prostate, it is unclear whether combined inhibitors will have additional efficacy in the treatment of benign prostatic hyperplasia.

Stromal Hyperplasia in Benign Prostatic Hyperplasia

Primative mesenchymal nodules differentiated into stromal nodules containing mature smooth muscle cells

Ongoing growth of the prostate assumes ongoing stromal hyperplasia

FIGURE 1-15. Stromal hyperplasia in benign prostatic hyperplasia (BPH). Stromal hyperplasia is an important component of the disease process. Indeed, the normal ratio between stroma and epithelium in the prostate of a 20-year-old man is approximately 2:1. In prostate tissue obtained by transurethral resection, stromal-to-epithelial ratios are more commonly 5:1 [19]. Although the ratio between stroma and epithelium is variable, with more significant epithelial hyperplasia in larger prostates, it is clear that stromal proliferation is an important part of the disease process. Ongoing growth of the prostate cannot occur unless there is ongoing stromal hyperplasia.

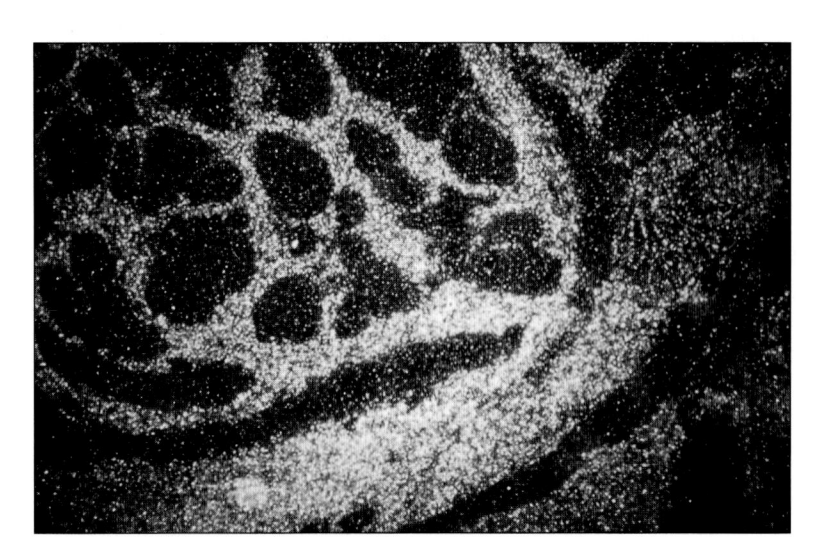

FIGURE 1-16. Prostatic stroma. A major component of the prostatic stroma is haphazardly arranged smooth muscle. This section demonstrates an *in situ* hybridization of a benign prostatic hyperplasia (BPH) nodule utilizing a probe that identifies the messenger RNA of a specific smooth muscle marker (myosin heavy chain). The dense bands of smooth muscle surrounding epithelial nodules, as well as significant smooth muscle between individual glands, is evident. Smooth muscle proliferation in other disease states (*eg*, atherosclerosis) is known to be regulated by growth factors. Some growth factors (*eg*, transforming growth factor-β) act as a "brake" on stromal cell proliferation [20]. Other growth factors (*eg*, basic fibroblast growth factor) produce stromal cell proliferation [22]. The role of growth factors in BPH remains to be elucidated.

Composition of Prostatic Stroma

Smooth muscle
Fibroblasts
Extracellular matrix
Vascular structures
Neural elements
Immune cells

FIGURE 1-17. Composition of prostatic stroma. Prostatic stroma has a complex composition. In addition to smooth muscle, there is significant volume of fiberblasts, extracellular matrix (collagen and elastin), vascular structures, neural elements, and immune cells. Indeed, morphometric measurements have demonstrated that the extracellular matrix on a volume basis is the most abundant component of the hyperplastic prostate [19]. Forty to fifty percent of benign prostatic hyperplasia (BPH) biopsy or surgical specimens demonstrate significant chronic and inflammatory infiltration. Because lymphocytes are known to elaborate cytokines that produce smooth muscle contraction and cell proliferation, the immune cells may well be part of the pathophysiology of BPH.

Force Generation of Prostate Tissue

A determinant of urethral resistance
Components of force include:
  Active (smooth muscle contraction)
  Passive (series elastic elements)

FIGURE 1-18. Force generation of prostate tissue. The importance of the extracellular matrix in benign prostatic hyperplasia (BPH) cannot be overestimated. Active contraction of the smooth muscle elements in the prostate (often referred to as the dynamic component of the disease) certainly influence urethral resistance. However, it has been estimated that only 50% of urethral resistance is determined by active smooth muscle contraction. The remainder of urethral resistance is determined by the so-called passive series elastic elements in the prostate [1]. These forces are caused by the intrinsic "rubberband" nature of the collagen and elastic tissue in the gland. The clinical importance of these passive forces is illustrated by the effectiveness of transurethral incision of the prostate, where simple incision through the prostatic tissue and capsule relieves outflow resistance without any debulking of prostatic tissue. This also explains why α-blockade (which does not affect the passive forces) fails to provide relief of urodynamic obstruction.

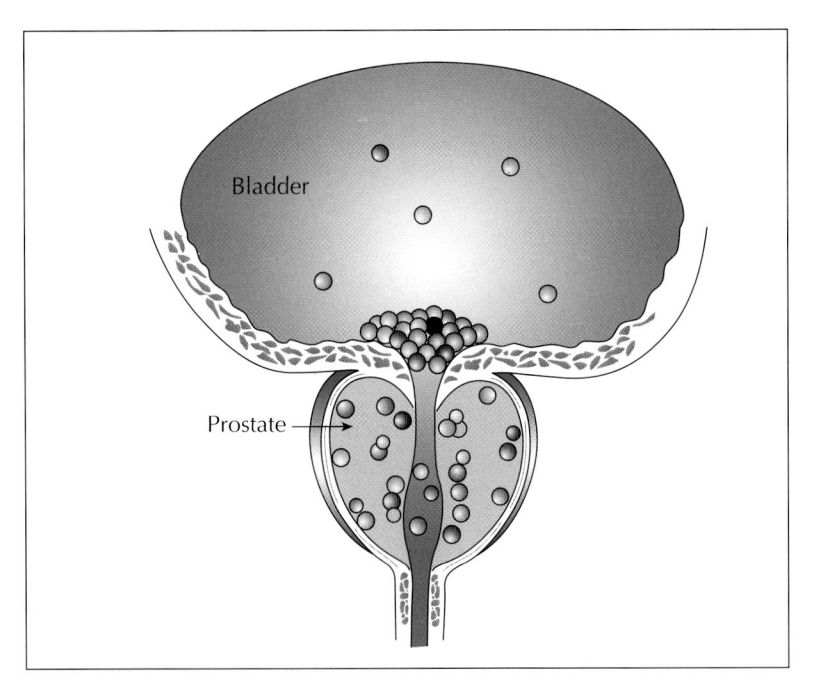

FIGURE 1-19. Distribution of α1 adrenoceptors in lower genitourinary tissues. The male lower urinary tract contains an abundance of $α_{1A}$-adrenoreceptors in the prostatic smooth muscle and bladder neck [22]. In contrast, the detrusor smooth muscle contains few, if any, α1 receptors. α-Adrenergic blockage, therefore, can produce selective relaxation of smooth muscle at the bladder outlet, without adversely affecting detrusor performance.

Active Force Generation in Prostate Smooth Muscle

Adrenergic neurotransmission
Purenergic neurotransmission
Endothelin
Nitric oxide inhibition
Cytokines

FIGURE 1-20. Active force generation of prostate smooth muscle. Although release of norepinephrine in adrenergic nerve terminals in the prostate is responsible for the majority of active smooth muscle contraction [23], other substances may modulate smooth muscle tone in the prostate. For example, endothelin, the most potent vasoconstrictor yet discovered, is present in fairly high levels in the prostate [24]. In addition, all the components of the nitric oxide pathway, which mediates smooth muscle relaxation, have been found in the prostate. As already mentioned, lymphocytes, commonly found in benign prostatic hyperplasia, may elaborate chemicals (cytokines) that produce smooth muscle contraction. It seems unlikely that adrenergic blockade will produce complete smooth muscle relaxation in the prostate. Some of the nonadrenergic pathways regulating smooth muscle contraction may be targeted for future drug development.

Aspects of the Adrenoreceptor Family

$α_{1a}$ is the most abundant adrenoreceptor messenger RNA in the prostate (60% to 85%)
The presence of another receptor subtype with low affinity to prazosin, $α_{1a'}$ is suggested

FIGURE 1-21. Aspects of the adrenoreceptor family of genes. This family encodes different receptor subtypes that vary in their tissue distribution. The most abundant adrenoreceptor messenger RNA in the prostate is the $α_{1A}$ subtype [25]. The $α_{1A}$ is clearly the subtype that mediates contraction of prostatic smooth muscle [22]. However, there are other adrenoceptor subtypes in the prostate and it is unclear whether the benefit of α-blocker therapy in benign prostatic hyperplasia resides purely with blockade of the $α_{1A}$ receptor.

α-Receptors in the Nervous System

Facilitatory α1 receptors tonically active in both the sympathetic and somatic control of the lower urinary tract
Doxazosin may have an action at the spinal cord and ganglia level to reduce activity in the parasympathetic nerves going to the bladder
Concept of prostate- versus uroselective

FIGURE 1-22. α-Receptors in the nervous system. There is increasing evidence that α-receptors in the central nervous system may be important modulators of urinary function. Facilitory α1 receptors are active in both the sympathetic and parasympathetic modulation of the lower urinary tract. The symptom improvement seen with α-blocker therapy may partially depend on central nervous system affects. Thus, drugs that are specifically designed to be "prostate selective" may have less than therapeutic benefit. Doxazosin, for example, has been shown in an animal model to have clear effects on the spinal cord to reduce the activity of parasymmetric nerves going to the bladder [25,26].

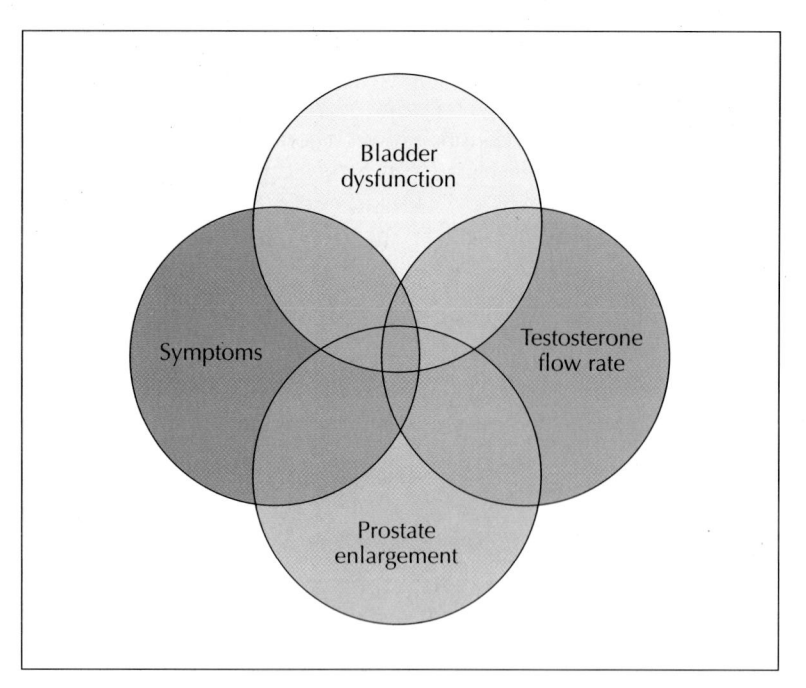

▶ **FIGURE 1-23.** Interrelated factors in prostate enlargement. Although ongoing growth of the prostate is clearly a major component of progressive symptoms and declining flow rate, the contribution of the bladder cannot be ignored [1]. Bladder dysfunction, in fact, may occur independent of obstruction and produce symptoms that are identical to those seen with prostatic enlargement.

Detrusor Response to Obstruction

Detrusor instability
Impaired contractility
Increased extracellular matrix
Decreased compliance
Alteration in neural pathways and modulation

▶ **FIGURE 1-24.** Detrusor response to obstruction. The bladder's response to obstruction is variable and incompletely defined. In animal models, bladder outlet obstruction initially leads to development of smooth muscle hypertrophy, which progresses over time to significant fibrosis [10]. Detrusor instability (uninhibited bladder contractions) occurs during this smooth muscle hypertrophy process, probably because of a disruption of coordinating signaling processes between individual smooth muscle cells. Paradoxically, instability is associated with impaired contractility. Increases in extracellular matrix (predominately collagen) become the predominant feature of the long-term obstructed bladder, ultimately leading to decreased compliance. There is also evidence that obstruction may lead to alteration of neural pathways in the sacral spinal cord, micturition center, and cerebral cortex [27].

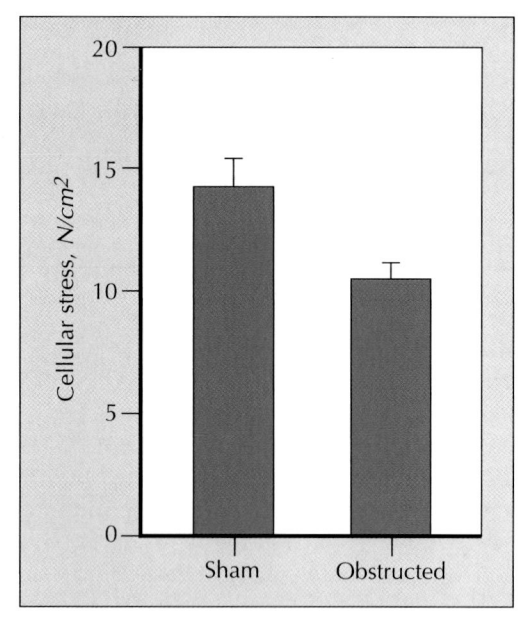

▶ **FIGURE 1-25.** Cellular stress study results. In our research laboratories at the University of Texas Southwestern Medical Center, we demonstrated that bladder outlet obstruction in an animal model (rabbit) produces significant smooth muscle hypertrophy in a period of 2 to 3 weeks [28]. Overall, there is a two- to fourfold increase in muscle mass in the bladder. However, the amount of force that individual muscle cells can produce per cross-sectional area declines significantly.

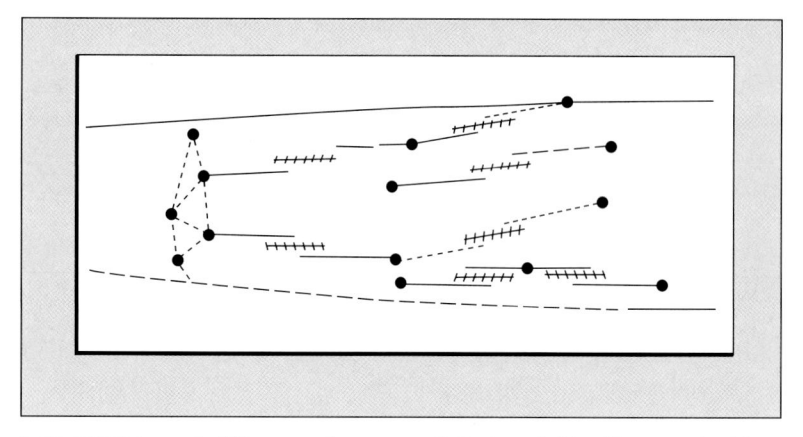

▶ **FIGURE 1-26.** The complex array of thick and thin filaments inside individual smooth muscle cells. The thin filaments consist of actin cables that provide structural support for the cell. The thick filaments consist of the protein myosin, which when stimulated produces movement along the actin cables. The movement along adjacent actin filaments produces shortening of the smooth muscle cells and thus bladder emptying. Studies of hypertrophied smooth muscle demonstrate that although the cells enlarge significantly, they tend not to increase their level of contractile filaments proportionately [28]. Hypertrophied smooth muscle does not behave like hypertrophied skeletal muscle (*eg*, in response to weight training), in which the number of contractile filaments keeps pace with overall growth of the cell.

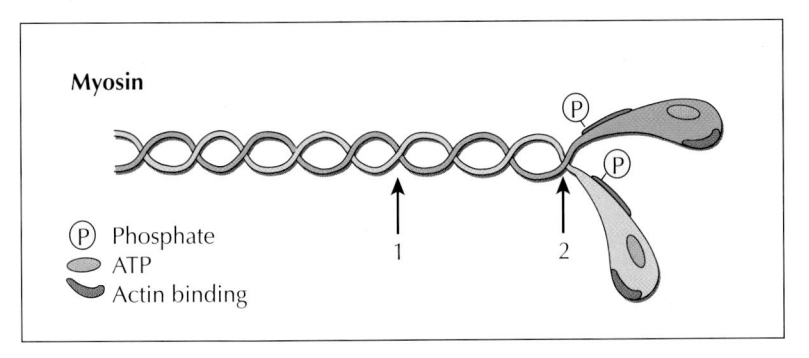

▶ **FIGURE 1-27.** Structure of myosin. The protein responsible for contraction of muscular tissue is myosin. Myosin is a complex hexometric molecule that consists of two heavy chains and four light chains. The myosin heavy chains catalyze the hydolysis of ATP, transforming the chemical energy of hydrolysis to the mechanical energy of myosin movement.

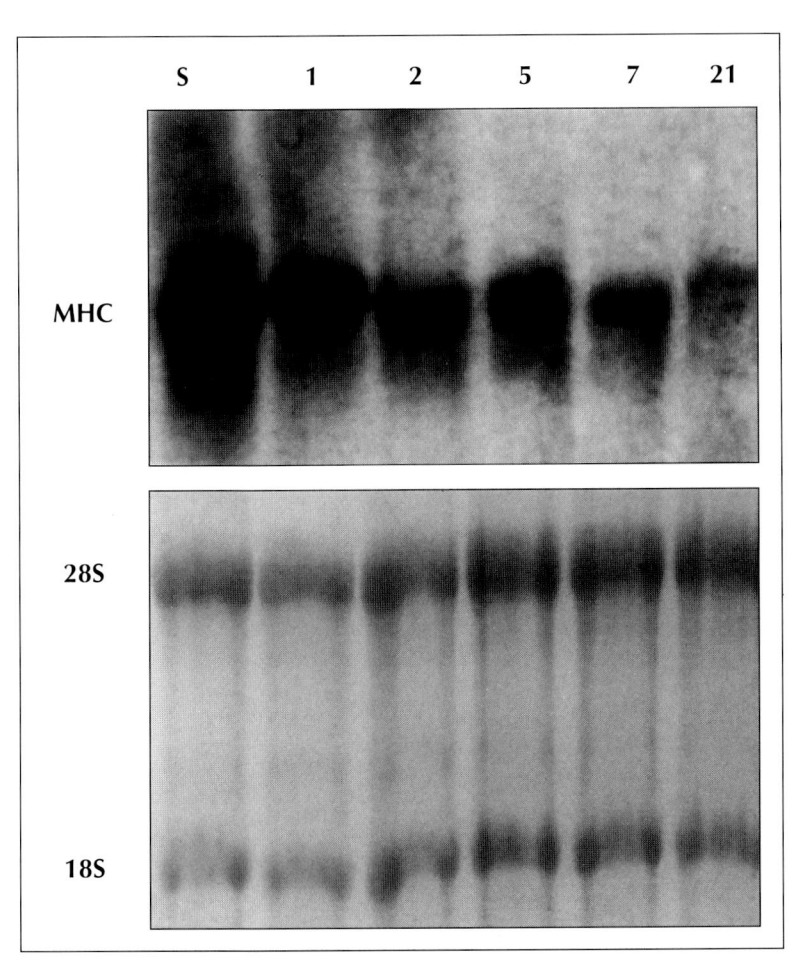

▶ **FIGURE 1-28.** Northern blot analysis of bladder obstruction in an animal model. We demonstrated that smooth muscle hypertrophy is associated with a significant decline in major histocompatibility complex (MHC) expression [28]. The amount of messenger RNA for MHC is evident as the dark band in the *upper panel*. The column labeled "S" is analysis of messenger RNA from sham-operated animals demonstrating a very high level of MHC expression. After only 1 day of obstruction, however, there is a significant decline in MHC expression, and by 21 days it is difficult to detect. Total RNA within the cell (*lower panel*) remains stable. The smooth muscle cells develop a significant increase in proteins that structurally support the cell (*eg*, desmin) but do not produce contraction.

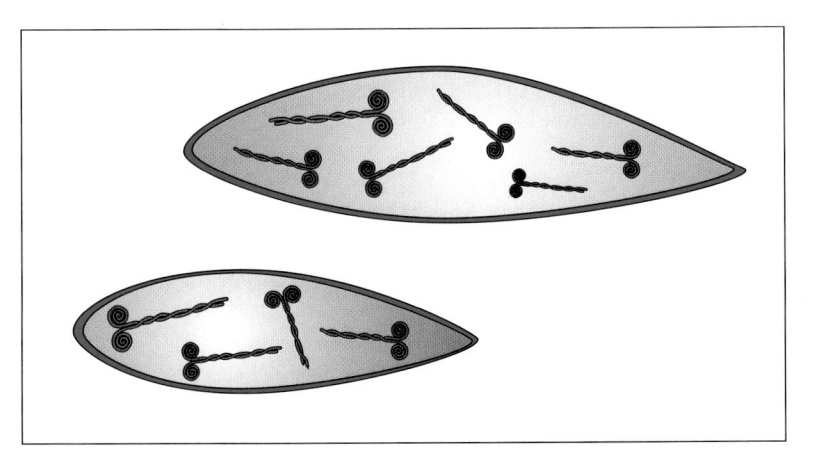

▶ **FIGURE 1-29.** Obstruction-induced smooth muscle cell hypertrophy. This is not an entirely adaptive process. Although the cell enlarges significantly, the number of contractile elements present in the cell do not increase proportionally. The overall increase in bladder muscle mass seen with obstruction permits the generation of higher pressures, but the decreased number of contractile elements adversely influences the performance of the bladder, leading to impaired emptying.

The Epidemiology and Pathophysiology of Benign Prostatic Hyperplasia

Smooth Muscle Proliferation and Dedifferentiation

Contractile phenotype
Secretory phenotype

FIGURE 1-30. Smooth muscle proliferation and dedifferentiation. Another important attribute of smooth muscle hypertrophy is the conversion from a muscle cell predominantly responsible for contraction (contractile phenotype) to a less differentiated type of smooth muscle cell that becomes more of a secretory cell [28]. The smooth muscle secretory phenotype is characterized by both a decline in smooth muscle contractile proteins and a significant increase in extracellular matrix production (predominantly collagen).

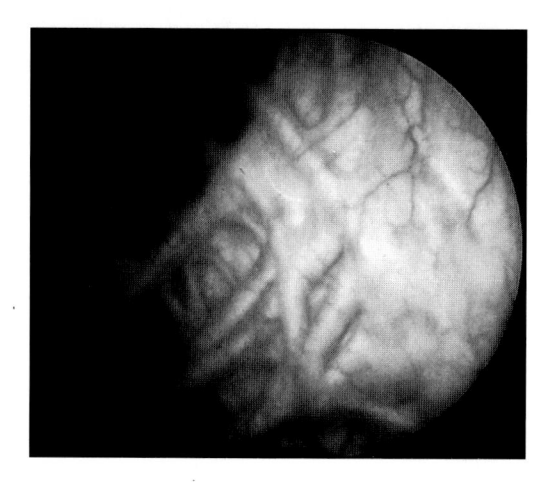

FIGURE 1-31. *(See Color Plate)* Endoscopic image of the obstructed bladder. The significant increase in collagen production seen in the obstructed bladder is responsible for the trabeculation seen endoscopically in men with bladder outlet obstruction. This is not the "rippling muscle" of an obstructed bladder, but rather a significant increase in extracellular matrix.

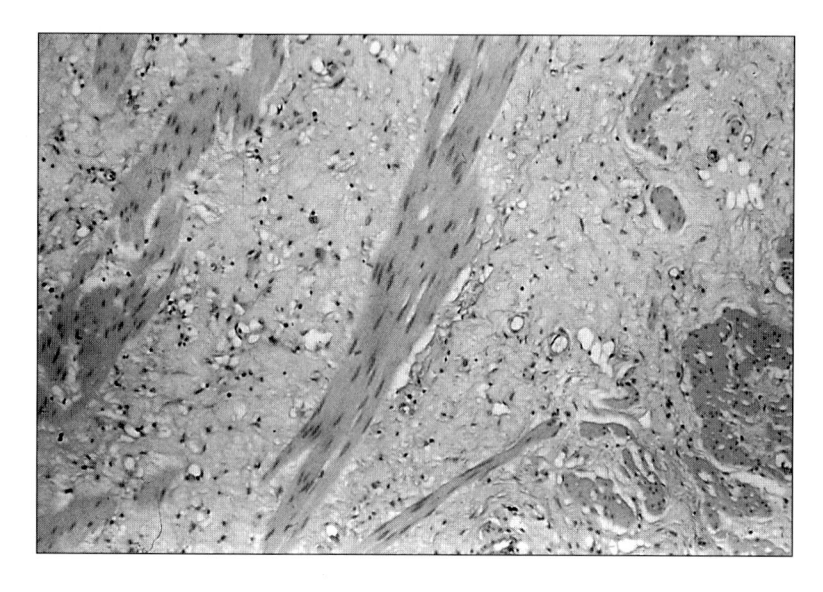

FIGURE 1-32. *(See Color Plate)* Biopsy specimen of a trabeculated bladder. This specimen demonstrates scarce smooth muscle fibers with a significant increase in collagen. This increase in extracellular matrix limits the compliance of the bladder, leading to higher pressures with bladder filling. Moreover, the collagen fibers limit shortening of adjacent smooth muscle cells. The increase in extracellular matrix in the bladder is the predominant cause of impaired emptying. Residual urine develops because the bladder wall cannot completely contract.

REFERENCES

1. McConnell JD: Epidemiology, etiology, pathophysiology and diagnosis of benign prostatic hyperplasia. In *Campbell's Urology*, edn 7. Edited by Walsh PC, Retik AB, Vaughan ED, *et al*. Philadelphia: WB Saunders; 1998:1429–1452.
2. McNeal J: Pathology of benign prostatic hyperplasia: insight into etiology. *Urol Clin North Am* 1990, 17:477–486.
3. Barry MJ, Boyle P, Garraway M, *et al*.: Epidemiology and natural history of BPH. In *Proceedings of the Second International Consultation on Benign Prostatic Hyperplasia (BPH)*. Channel Islands: Scientific Communications International; 1993:19.
4. Guess HA: Epidemiology and natural history of benign prostatic hyperplasia. *Urol Clin North Am* 1995, 22:247–261.
5. Guess HA, Arrighi HM, Metter AJ, *et al*.: Cumulative prevalence of prostatism matches the autopsy prevalence of benign prostatic hyperplasia. *Prostate* 1990, 17:241–246.
6. Berry SJ, Coffey DS, Walsh PC, *et al*.: The development of human benign prostatic hyperplasia with age. *J Urol* 1984, 132:474–479.
7. Girman CJ, Jacobsen SJ, Guess HA, *et al*.: Natural history of prostatism: relationship among symptoms, prostate volume and peak urinary flow. *J Urol* 1995, 153:1510–1515.
8. Girman CJ, Panser LA, Chute CG, *et al*.: Natural history of prostatism: urinary flow rates in a population-based study. *J Urol* 1993, 150:887–892.
9. McConnell JD, Bruskewitz R, Walsh P, *et al*. for the PLESS Group: The effect of finasteride on the risk of acute urinary retention and the need for surgical treatment among men with benign prostatic hyperplasia. *N Engl J Med* 1998, 338:557–563.
10. Levin RM, Monson FC, Haugaard N, *et al*.: Genetic and cellular characteristics of bladder outlet obstruction. *Urol Clin North Am* 1995, 22:263–283.
11. Gosling JA, Gilpin SA, Dixon JS, *et al*.: Decrease in the autonomic innervation of human detrusor muscle in outflow obstruction. *J Urol* 1986, 136:501–504.
12. Jacobsen SJ, Jacobsen DJ, Girman CJ, *et al*.: Natural history of prostatism: risk factors for acute urinary retention. *J Urol* 1997, 158:481–487.
13. Barry MJ, Cockett ATK, Holtgrewe HL, *et al*.: Relationship of symptoms of prostatism to commonly used physiological and anatomical measures of the severity of benign prostatic hyperplasia. *J Urol* 1993, 150:351–358.
14. McConnell JD: Prostate growth: new insights into hormonal regulation. *Br J Urol* 1995, 76 (suppl 1):5–10.
15. Russell DW, Wilson JD: Steroid 5α-reductase: two genes/two enzymes. *Annu Rev Biochem* 1994, 63:25–61.

16. Silver RI, Wiley EL, Thigpen AE, *et al.*: Cell type specific expression of steroid 5-α-reductase 2. *J Urol* 1994, 152:438–442.
17. Silver RI, Wiley EL, Davis DL, *et al.*: Expression and regulation of steroid 5α-reductase 2 in prostate disease. *J Urol* 1994, 152:433–437.
18. Walsh PC, Hutchins GM, Ewing LL: Tissue content of dihydrotestosterone in human prostatic hyperplasia is not supranormal. *J Clin Invest* 1983, 72:1772–1777.
19. Shapiro E, Hartanto V, Lepor H: Quantifying the smooth muscle content of the prostate using double-immuno-enzymatic staining and color assisted image analysis. *J Urol* 1992, 147:1167–1170.
20. Martikainen P, Kyprianou N, Isaacs JT: Effect of transforming growth factor-β on proliferation and death of rat prostatic cells. *Endocrinology* 1990, 127:2963–2968.
21. Story MT, Livingstone B, Baeten L, *et al.*: Cultured human prostate-derived fibroblasts produce a factor that stimulated their growth with properties indistinguishable from basic fibroblast growth factor. *Prostate* 1989, 15:355–365.
22. Lepor H, Tang R, Meretyk S, Shapiro E: Alpha$_1$ adrenoceptor subtypes in the human prostate. *J Urol* 1993, 149:640–642.
23. Lepor H, Tang R, Shapiro E: The alpha-adrenoceptor subtype mediating the tension of human prostatic smooth muscle. *Prostate* 1993, 22:301–307.
24. Kobayashi S, Tang R, Wang B, *et al.*: Binding and functional properties of endothelin receptor subtypes in the human prostate. *Mol Pharmacol* 1994, 45:306–311.
25. Steers WD, Ciambotti J, Erdman S, *et al.*: Morphological plasticity in efferent pathways to the urinary bladder of the rat following urethral obstruction. *J Neurosci* 1990, 19:1943.
26. Cher ML, Abernathy BB, McConnell JD, *et al.*: Smooth muscle myosin heavy chain isoform expression in bladder outlet obstruction. *World J Urol* 1996, 14:295–300.

Clinical Evaluation of Lower Urinary Tract Symptoms Due to Benign Prostatic Hyperplasia

2
NONCANCEROUS DISEASE SECTION

Subbarao V. Yalla & Maryrose P. Sullivan

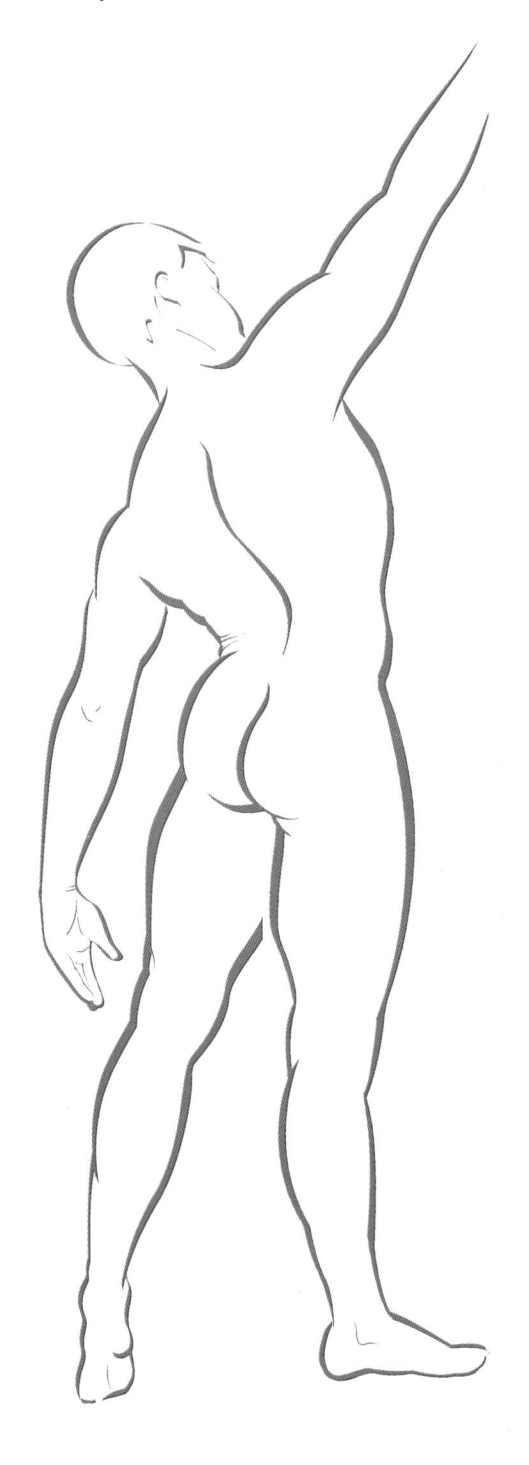

Benign prostatic hyperplasia (BPH), a highly prevalent condition in adult and elderly men, is a major cause of lower urinary tract symptoms (LUTS). This symptom complex, also known as prostatism, can be produced by other conditions that may be unrelated to BPH or other lower urinary tract diseases. Although BPH associated with bladder outlet obstruction (BOO) is a principal cause of LUTS, some patients with BPH, regardless of the degree of prostatic enlargement, may not be symptomatic and may not have urodynamically defined BOO [1]. Furthermore, a recent study of the effects of aging on the bladder found that many elderly volunteers with urodynamically confirmed BOO were, in fact, asymptomatic [2]. Although studies also have shown that patients presumed to have BPH but without urodynamically defined obstruction can have LUTS, it is not clear how BPH alone (*ie*, without BOO) can induce LUTS. It has been suggested that increased neural afferentation due to BPH may be responsible for the symptoms in this group [3].

Lower urinary tract symptoms can be precipitated by other factors such as detrusor dysfunction due to aging, subclinical autonomic neuropathies, myeloneuropathies, and extravesical causes [4,5]. Elderly men, who may have several comorbid diseases, often are treated with multiple pharmacologic agents that may directly or indirectly affect lower urinary tract function [6]. These agents include antihistaminics, diuretics, calcium channel blockers, tricyclic compounds, sedatives and cold remedies coupled with α-adrenergic agonists. This group of patients may complain of LUTS similar to those produced by obstructive BPH, although their symptoms may not be entirely related to BPH. Therefore, LUTS, regardless of the degree of prostatic enlargement, cannot always be equated with BPH, and vice versa. LUTS should be assessed using a multifactorial approach to rule out other factors responsible for the symptoms before therapies that are primarily directed at BPH are recommended.

Evaluation of LUTS requires a detailed history that includes a symptom questionnaire such as the American Urological Association Symptom Index or the International Prostate Symptom Score [7,8], and a targeted genitourinary and neurologic examination [9]. The central nervous system examination focuses on the pyramidal and extrapyramidal tracts and the sacral cord reflexes. Further objective assessment includes a rectal examination to determine abnormalities of the prostate in terms of degree of enlargement or presence of a discrete hard nodule that may prove to be prostatic carcinoma. During rectal examination of the prostate, anal sphincter tone also is assessed to determine the integrity of sacral cord reflexes. In elderly men with multiple comorbid diseases, a detailed pharmacologic history and a voiding diary are required. Laboratory investigations that are considered standard (*eg*, urinalysis and serum creatinine) as well as other tests (*eg*, cytology, blood area nitrogen [BUN], and prostate-specific antigen [PSA]) can be used to assess factors such as urinary tract infections, carcinoma in situ, renal dysfunction, and prostate cancer. Further evaluations such as urinary flowmetry, postvoid residual urine volume measurement, and comprehensive urodynamic evaluations should be performed as appropriate.

The precise role of urodynamic evaluation in men with LUTS has not been established. Early in the development of clinical urodynamics, one of the intentions was to develop a sensitive method of detecting minor degrees of BOO. The prevailing view was that early obstructions should be treated effectively to prevent morbidity that might be associated with undetected long-standing obstructions. Because recent studies on the epidemiology, natural history, and treatment outcomes of BPH suggest that morbidity rarely is associated with untreated BPH, LUTS due to BPH now is considered to be a quality-of-life issue [10]. Therefore, the use of comprehensive urodynamic studies in the routine work-up of patients with LUTS has been questioned. Regardless of the validity of such questions, functional evaluation of the lower urinary tract can be very helpful in establishing whether LUTS are caused primarily by significant prostatic obstruction or whether the symptoms are caused by other factors that are not related to the lower urinary tract [11–13]. These studies are particularly useful in the following situations: 1) younger men in whom other causes, such as primary bladder neck obstruction or chronic prostatitis, may play a predominant role in causing symptomatic dysfunction; 2) elderly men with multiple comorbidities (*eg*, spinal stenosis, parkinsonism, diabetes, stroke); 3) patients with chronic alcoholism or myelo- or autonomic neuropathies; 4) patients with previous failed surgical interventions; and 5) patients who are either prone to adverse reactions or refractory to pharmacologic management. Comprehensive urodynamic evaluations may not be required in patients with unusually large prostates combined with severe symptom scores, persistent low flow rates, and large postvoid residual volumes. Similarly, patients with large prostates and no relevant comorbidities who have episodes of urinary retention or urinary tract infections, bladder calculi, and imminent renal compromise may not require comprehensive functional evaluations. Patients in these categories usually respond well to interventional therapy that relieves outlet obstruction.

The goals of urodynamic evaluation are to confirm or exclude BOO, and, in the absence of BOO, identify other functional causes that may be responsible for LUTS. These studies also provide an opportunity to assess detrusor reflex activity, contractility, and compliance, which may be altered in patients with long-standing vesicourethral dysfunctions, and which together may lead to diminished renal function [14]. In many instances, however, no urodynamic abnormalities of either the detrusor or the outlet can be detected despite significant LUTS, suggesting that factors unrelated to the lower urinary tract may be responsible for the voiding symptoms. Because current strategies for management of BPH focus on reducing outlet resistance of the bladder neck and prostatic urethra, reliable objective evidence of BOO in patients with LUTS must be obtained before protracted pharmacologic management or interventional therapies are implemented. For successful management of elderly men with LUTS, the clinician must judiciously select appropriate methods of evaluation while keeping in mind the morbidity and cost effectiveness of these procedures. These factors must be weighed against the costs and morbidity of the unnecessary pharmacologic or surgical interventions that may result without objective functional assessment.

THE RELATIONSHIPS AMONG LOWER URINARY TRACT SYMPTOMS, BENIGN PROSTATIC HYPERPLASIA, AND VOIDING DYSFUNCTION

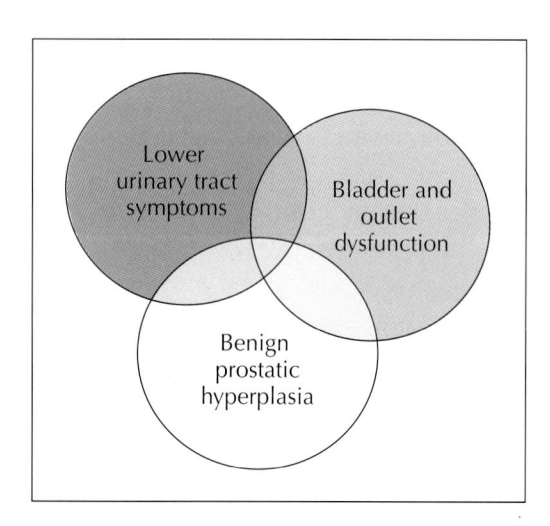

▶ **FIGURE 2-1.** The interrelationships among lower urinary tract symptoms, benign prostatic hyperplasia (BPH), and vesicourethral dysfunction are complex. As this Venn diagram shows, patients with BPH can have symptoms with or without bladder outlet obstruction. Furthermore, some patients with lower urinary tract symptoms do not have vesicourethral dysfunction. Other prostatic diseases, such as prostatitis with or without prostatic calculi or prostatic reflux and prostatic carcinoma, also can lead to lower urinary tract symptoms. Conversely, varying degrees of bladder outlet obstruction have been detected in some asymptomatic elderly men [2]. Although it may be that BPH without detectable bladder outlet obstruction can produce lower urinary tract symptoms via increased afferent neural input [3], no large-scale studies have been reported to support this hypothesis. (*Adapted from* Hald [1].)

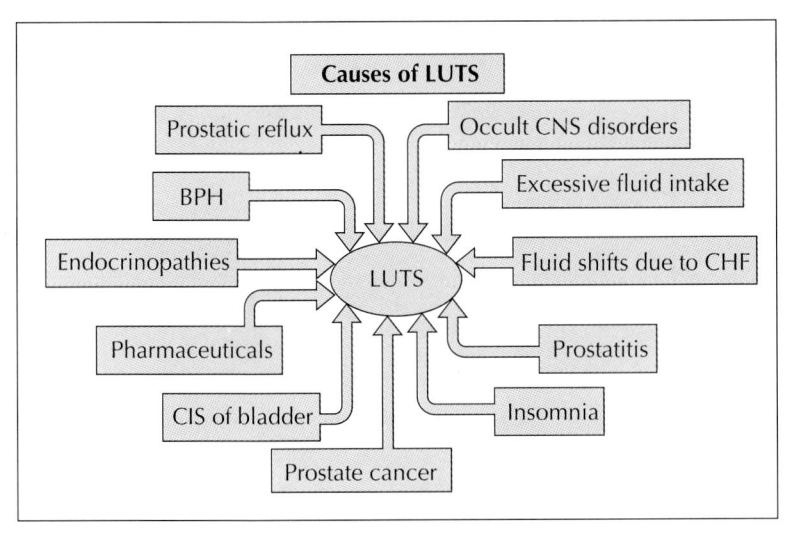

FIGURE 2-2. Lower urinary tract symptoms can be produced by several factors that are not related to benign prostatic hyperplasia. Several pharmacologic agents used to treat extragenitourinary conditions can affect lower urinary tract function. Some of these agents may have anticholinergic properties that may impair detrusor function. In addition, furosemide and hydrochlorothiazides, prescribed for cardiac conditions, lithium used to treat psychiatric disorders, and cold remedies consisting of adrenergic agonists and antihistaminics can lead to lower urinary tract symptoms. Endocrinopathies that result in hypermagnesemia and hypercalcemia are known to produce diuresis and consequently may promote lower urinary tract symptoms. Prostate pathologies unrelated to benign prostatic hyperplasia that produce lower urinary tract symptoms include prostatitis, calculi, reflux, and prostate cancer. Symptoms resulting from psychiatric disorders and insomnia can be mistaken for benign prostatic hyperplasia–induced symptoms if a proper history is not elicited. CIS—carcinoma in situ; CHF—congestive heart failure.

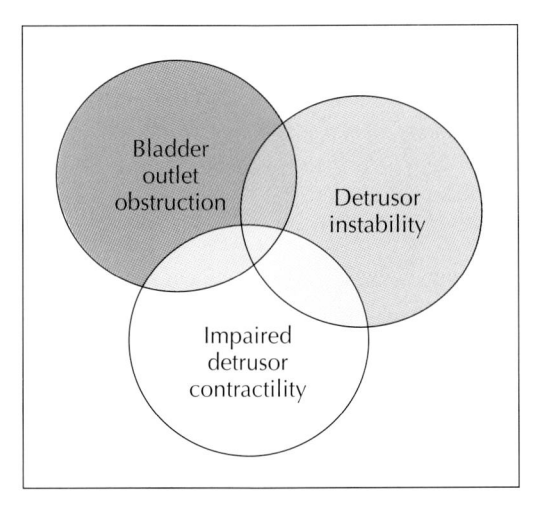

FIGURE 2-3. Functional abnormalities associated with benign prostatic hyperplasia (BPH) include bladder outlet obstruction, detrusor instability (DI), and impaired detrusor contractility (IC). A combination of BPH, bladder outlet obstruction, DI, and IC in an elderly patient is a typical setup for urinary retention when pharmacologic agents such as diuretics, cold remedies, and tranquilizers or sedatives are administered. Patients with prostatic enlargement presumed to be caused by BPH also can be asymptomatic and may not have urodynamic abnormalities.

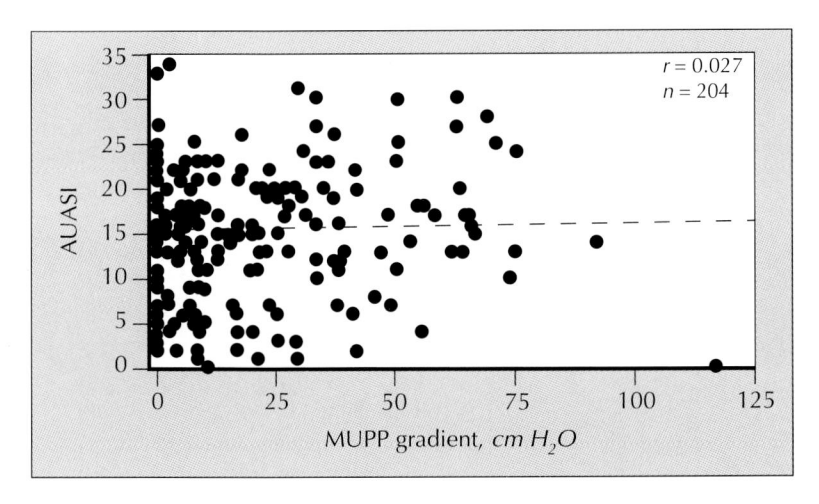

FIGURE 2-4. Several studies have shown that symptom scores correlate poorly with urodynamic evidence of bladder outlet obstruction (BOO) [15–17]. The relationship between the AUA Symptom Index (AUASI) and the severity of BOO as defined by voiding profilometry gradient is shown here. This lack of correlation indicates that AUASI is not representative of the nature or the degree of BOO.

Clinical Evaluation of Lower Urinary Tract Symptoms Due to Benign Prostatic Hyperplasia

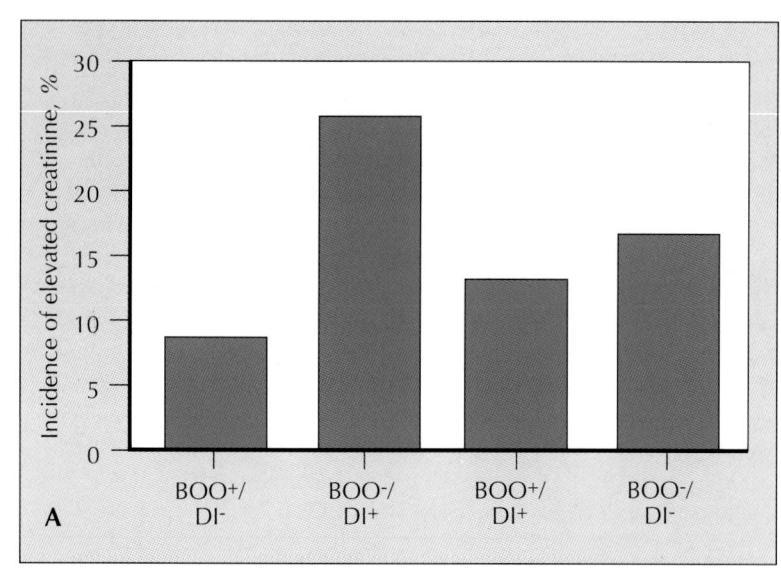

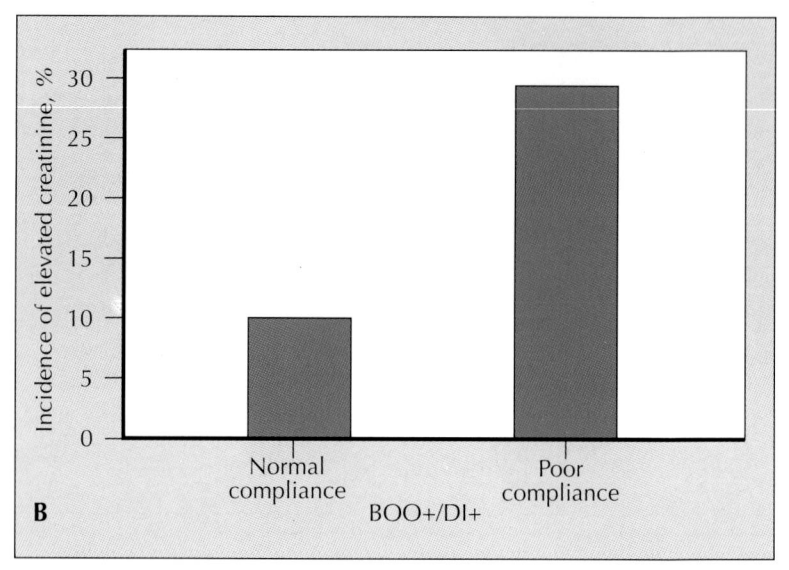

FIGURE 2-5. The theory that untreated chronic bladder outlet obstruction (BOO) caused by benign prostatic hyperplasia compromises renal function has been questioned. **A,** A recent study showed that the incidences of elevated creatinine in patients with BOO and detrusor instability (DI) (BOO+/DI+), with BOO only (BOO+), with DI only (DI+), and with neither bladder outlet obstruction nor DI (BOO−/DI−) are not statistically different [14]. **B,** However, among patients with both BOO and DI (BOO+/DI+), the incidence of elevated creatinine is higher in those with decreased bladder compliance (<30 mL/cmH$_2$O) than in those with normal compliance. These observations suggest that urodynamic evaluation can identify those patients with benign prostatic hyperplasia who may be at risk for compromise of renal function.

URODYNAMIC EVALUATION

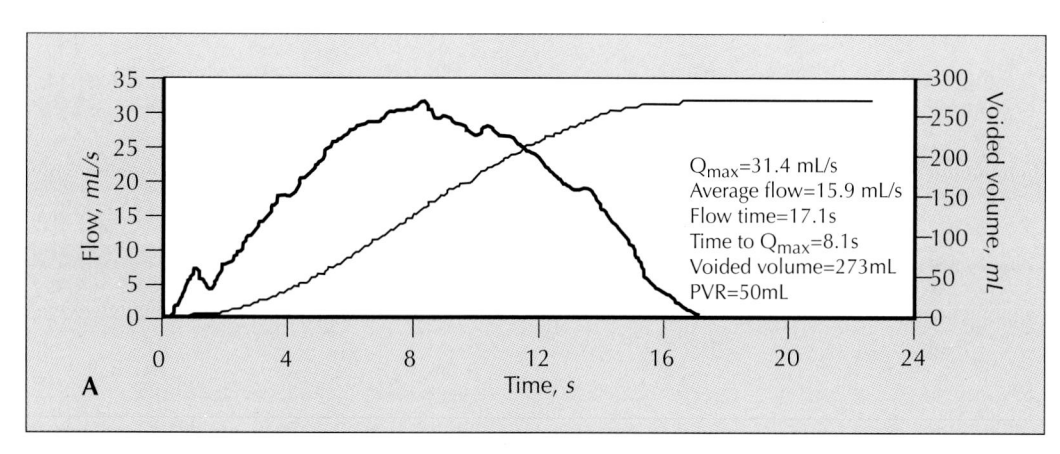

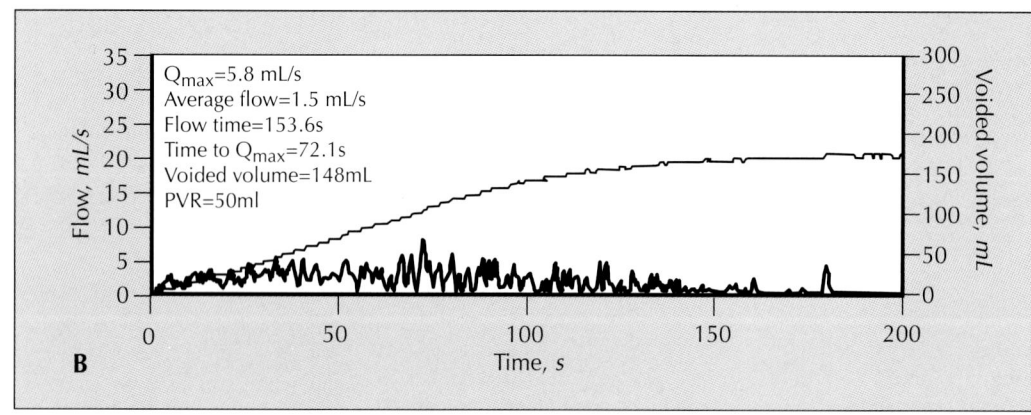

FIGURE 2-6. Uroflowmetry is a simple, noninvasive urodynamic test that can be an invaluable screening tool for identifying those patients who require more extensive urodynamic evaluation. Although uroflowmetry often can be used to exclude bladder outlet obstruction (BOO), low urinary flow rates typically cannot discriminate between poor detrusor contractility and BOO [19]. Various types of abnormal voiding can be recognized from uroflowmetry parameters, and from the flow pattern. In patients with normal bladder contractility, the maximum urinary flow rate (Q_{max}) provides a useful measure of the degree of bladder outlet obstruction and the response to treatment. However, the dependence of Q_{max} on age and bladder volume should be considered. **A,** A normal urinary flow pattern, obtained from an asymptomatic, urodynamically normal volunteer, is characterized by a bell-shaped curve with high Q_{max}. **B** Uroflowmetry in an obstructed patient is characterized by a sustained low maximum flow rate and a prolonged duration. A similar pattern can be seen with nonobstructed patients with large bladder capacity and impaired detrusor contractility. Therefore, more comprehensive urodynamic tests are required for a definitive diagnosis of BOO. PVR—postvoid residual.

II. The Prostate

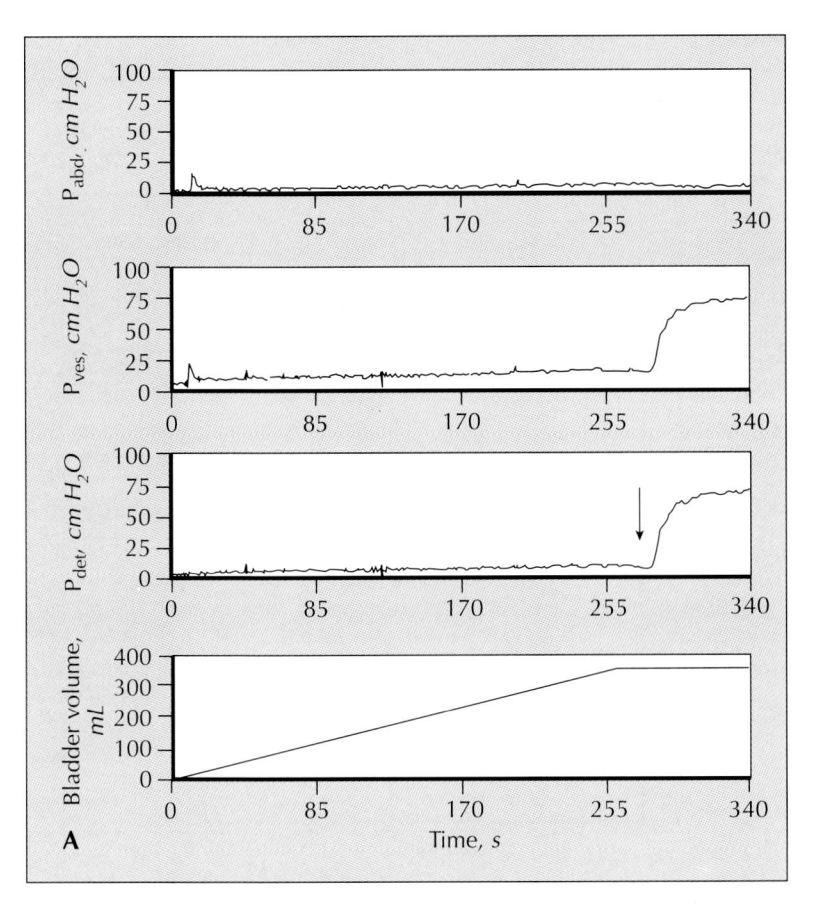

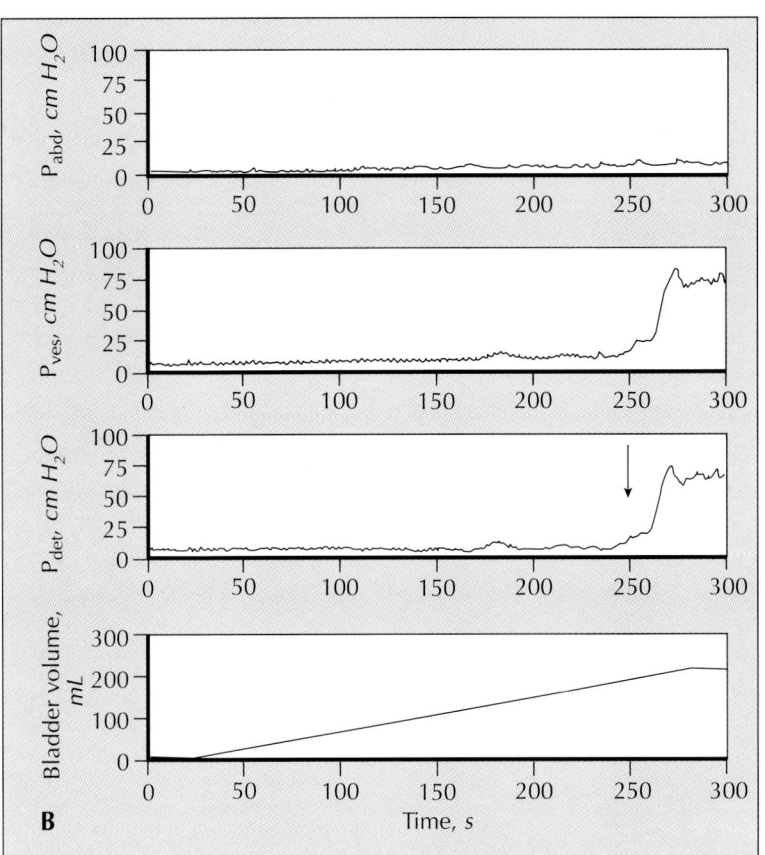

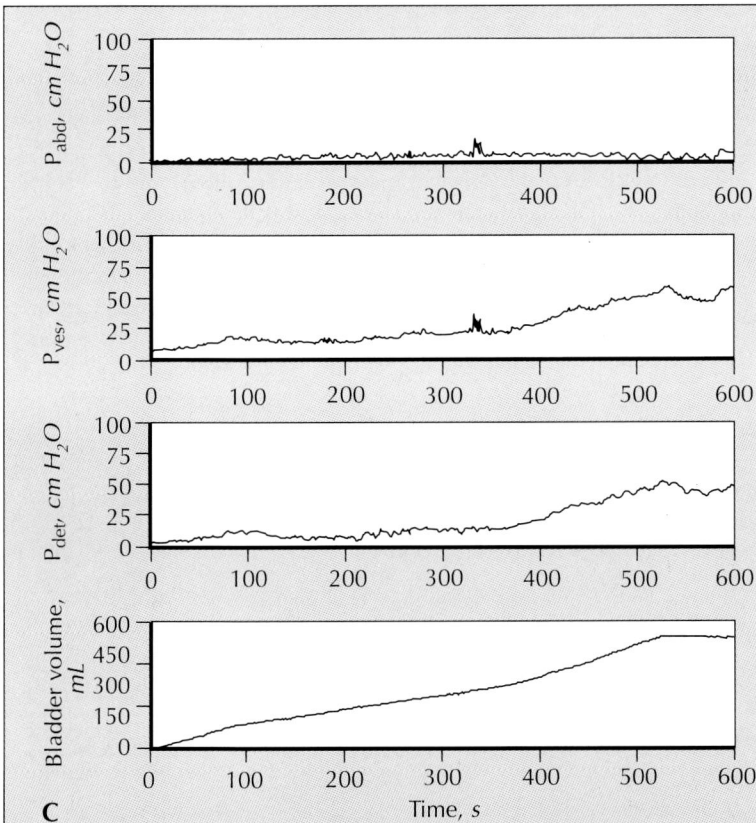

FIGURE 2-7. Cystometry in the evaluation of patients with LUTS is used to assess sensation of bladder filling and desire to void, detrusor capacity, detrusor compliance, and detrusor contractile activity. Slow or medium fill cystometry is recommended to avoid artifacts; low compliance or uninhibited detrusor activity can artifactually occur with rapid filling. Simultaneous rectal pressures that represent intra-abdominal pressures are recorded to determine detrusor pressures and prevent inaccurate interpretations of cystometry. However, failure to recognize spontaneous rectal contractions and their effect on subtracted detrusor pressure can lead to misdiagnosis. Detrusor compliance can be obtained from the cystometrogram by relating the change in the bladder volume to the rise in detrusor pressure. **A**, A normal filling cystometrogram in an adult man is characterized by a bladder capacity of 350 to 500 mL with low detrusor pressure and absence of involuntary contractions. In this 64-year-old asymptomatic man, bladder capacity was 360 mL with a bladder compliance of 60 mL/cm H_2O. *Arrow* indicates the onset of a voluntary bladder contraction. **B**, In patients with detrusor instability, a spectrum of abnormalities associated with urgency can be seen in the cystometrogram, varying from the presence of uninhibited detrusor contractions during filling to the inability to suppress a voiding contraction. This cystometrogram from an adult man with LUTS shows involuntary bladder contractions starting at 120 mL and a strong uninhibitable detrusor contraction at 190 mL. **C**, In the literature, diminished bladder compliance was arbitrarily defined as less than 20 to 30 mL/cm H_2O, although no definite numeric guidelines are provided by the International Continence Society. This filling cystometrogram demonstrates an increased slope of detrusor pressure in a patient with bladder outlet obstruction as the bladder was filled beyond 400 mL. This increased slope occurred in the later phase of bladder filling and could be mistaken for the onset of a detrusor contraction. Poor compliance can be differentiated from a detrusor contraction with poor velocity using various maneuvers. For example, if afferent pudendal nerve stimulation does not decrease bladder pressure, the rising pressure is due to poor compliance rather than a detrusor contraction. In addition, a continued increase in bladder pressure with cessation of bladder filling indicates a detrusor activation. In this patient, bladder compliance (10.9 mL/cm H_2O) was considered abnormal, since bladder pressure did not continue to rise after bladder filling was discontinued.

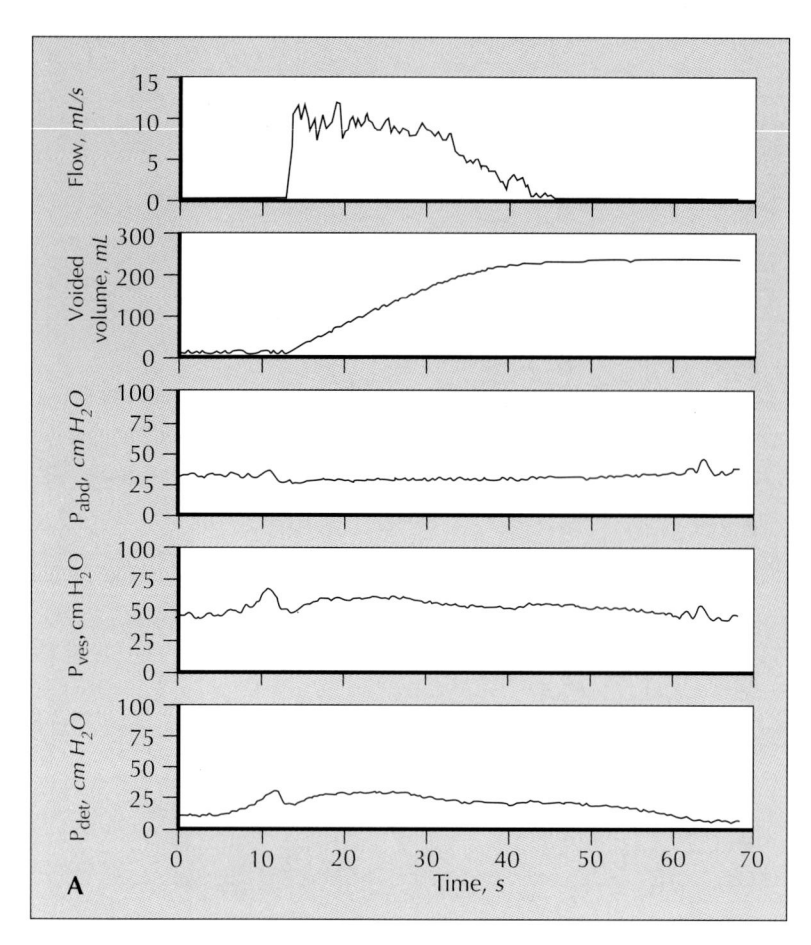

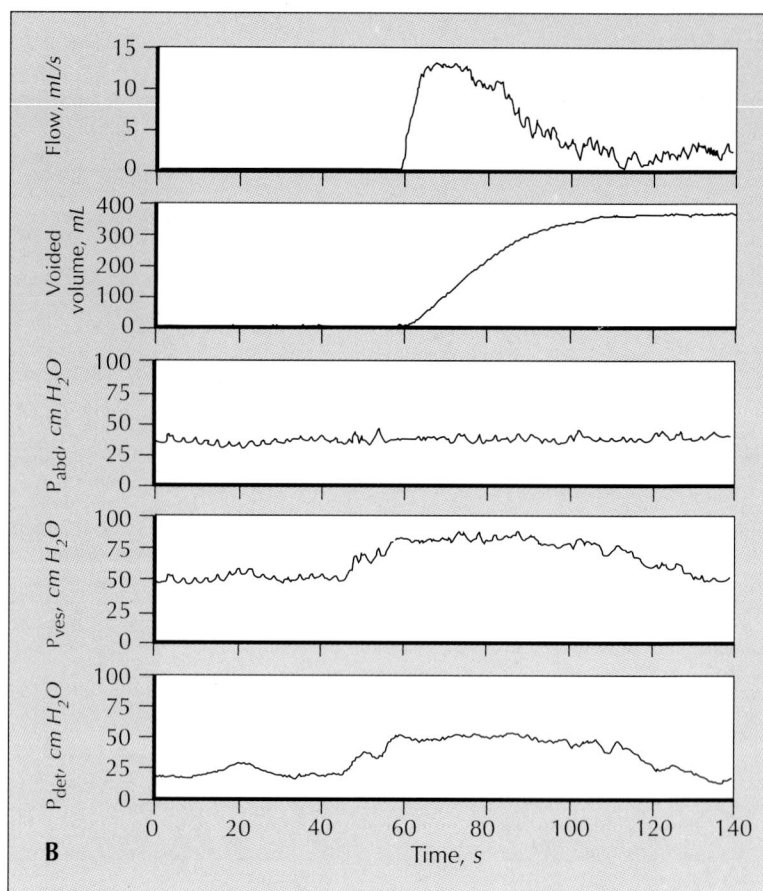

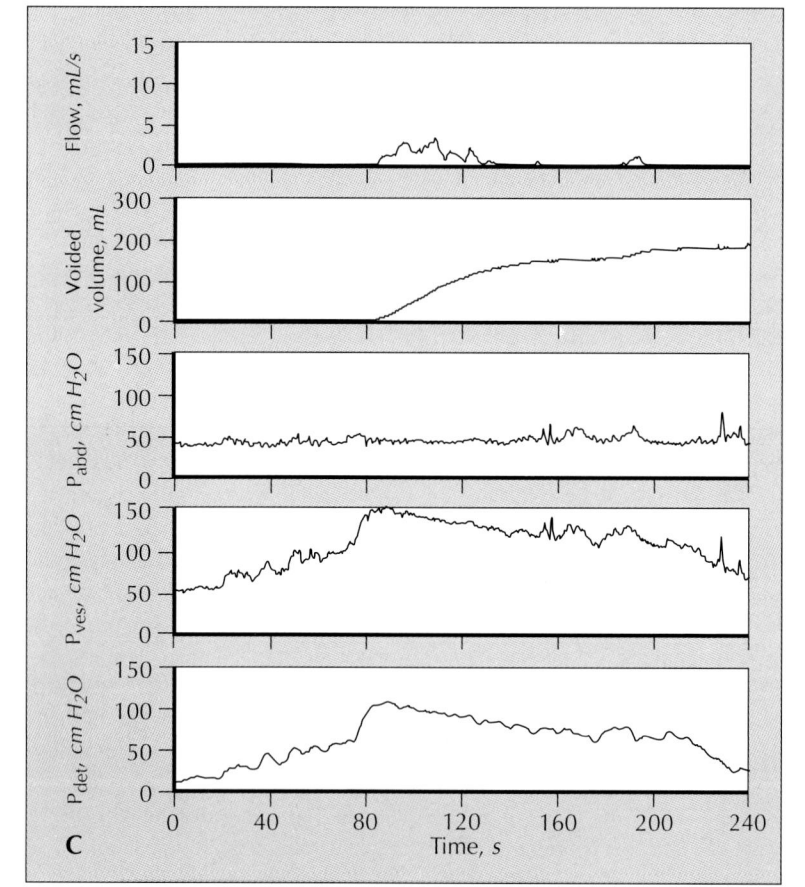

FIGURE 2-8. The pressure-flow (P-Q) study is widely accepted as an important urodynamic method of diagnosing bladder outlet obstruction [20]. Simultaneous intravesical, intrarectal pressures and urinary flow rates are recorded during voiding in either the sitting or standing position. These studies can be performed under fluoroscopy to detect any abnormal bladder morphology such as significant diverticula and vesicoureteral reflux. The pressure and flow tracings obtained from a nonobstructed (*panel A*), a mildly obstructed (*panel B*), and a severely obstructed (*panel C*) patient are shown. P_{abd}—abdominal pressure; P_{det}—detrusor pressure; P_{ves}—vesical pressure.

II. The Prostate

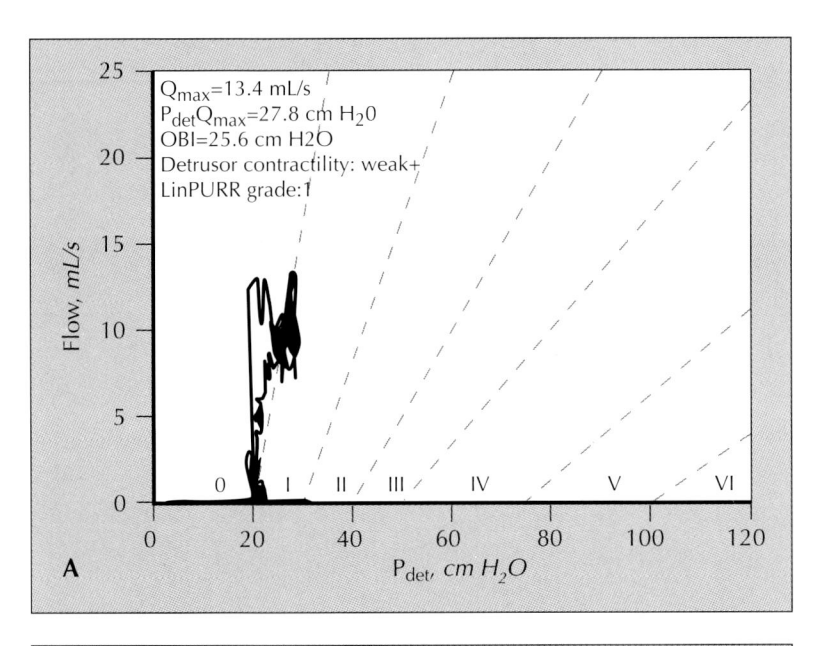

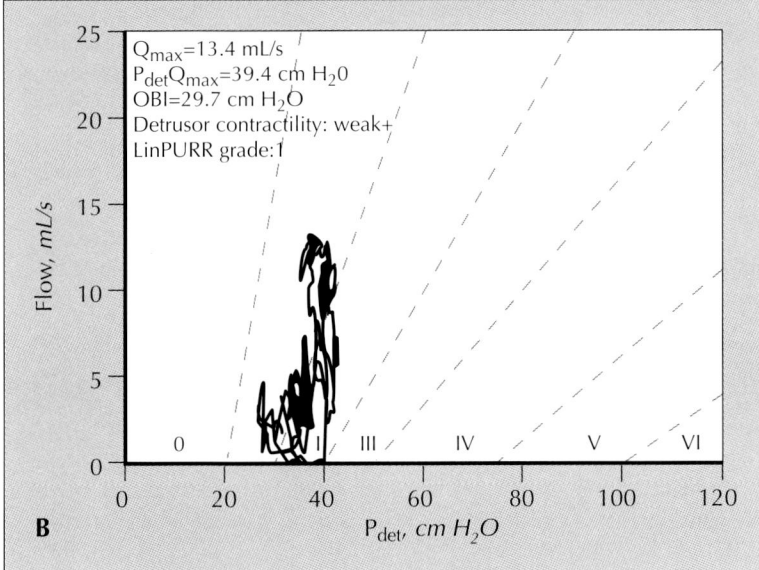

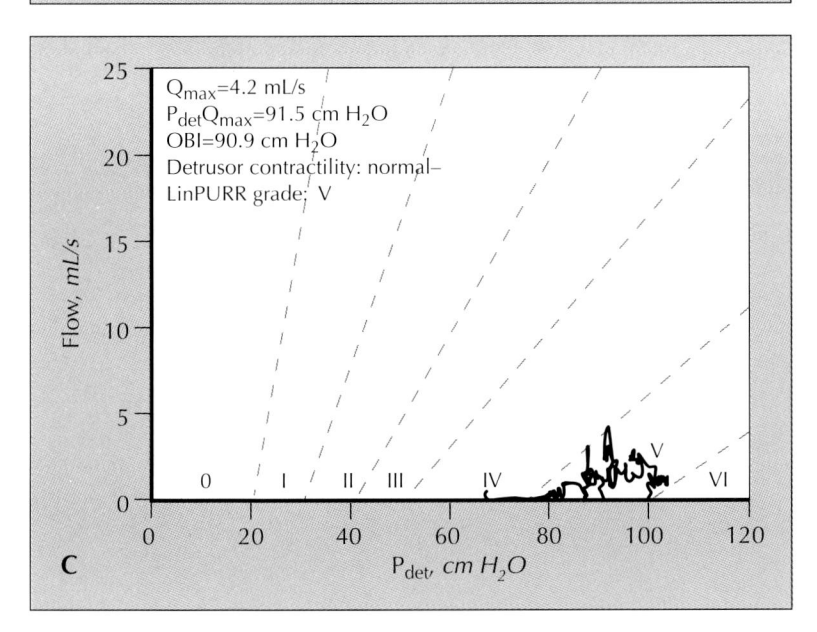

FIGURE 2-9. Pressure-flow (P-Q) studies can be analyzed using a number of methods of varying complexity that are based on similar concepts and thus produce comparable results [21]. Only a few of these are used by clinical urodynamicists, however. After eliminating artifacts and correcting the time lag between detrusor pressure and onset of flow, the urinary flow is plotted against the corresponding detrusor pressure during voiding. The nomogram proposed by Schafer for grading bladder outlet obstruction (BOO) is based on the concept of the passive urethral resistance relation (PURR) [22]. PURR represents the passive state of bladder outlet, which is presumed to be free from smooth muscle and striated sphincter influences during voiding. The resistance offered by the bladder outlet under these conditions is assumed to be entirely due to the mechanical properties of the posterior urethra, including the prostate gland. This analysis can be simplified by approximating the PURR with a straight line (LinPURR). LinPURR is graded into seven categories (0 through 6), with grade 2 and higher representing BOO. Bladder strength is classified in the nomogram as very weak, weak, normal, and strong. The obstruction index (OBI), derived from the height and slope of the PURR, is a less widely used parameter that provides a continuous grading of obstruction [23]. The P-Q plots, generated from the same patients studied in Figure 2-8, are superimposed on Schafer's nomogram to determine the severity of BOO and detrusor strength. Data from Figures 2-8*A* and 2-8*B* fall into grade 1 on Schafer's nomogram (Fig. 2-9*A* and *B*), whereas data from Figure 2-8*C* falls into grade 5, indicating severe obstruction (Fig. 2-9*C*). $P_{det}Q_{max}$—detrusor pressure at maximum flow.

Clinical Evaluation of Lower Urinary Tract Symptoms Due to Benign Prostatic Hyperplasia

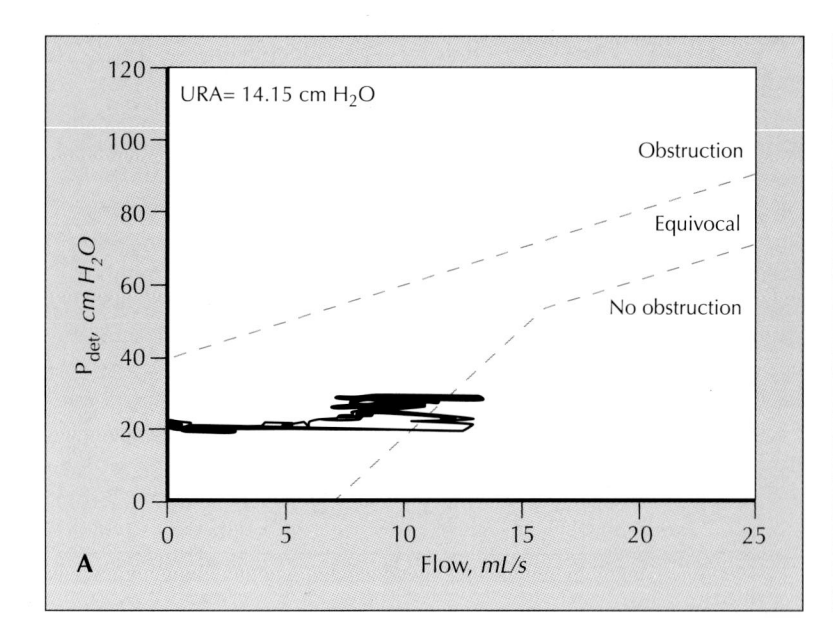

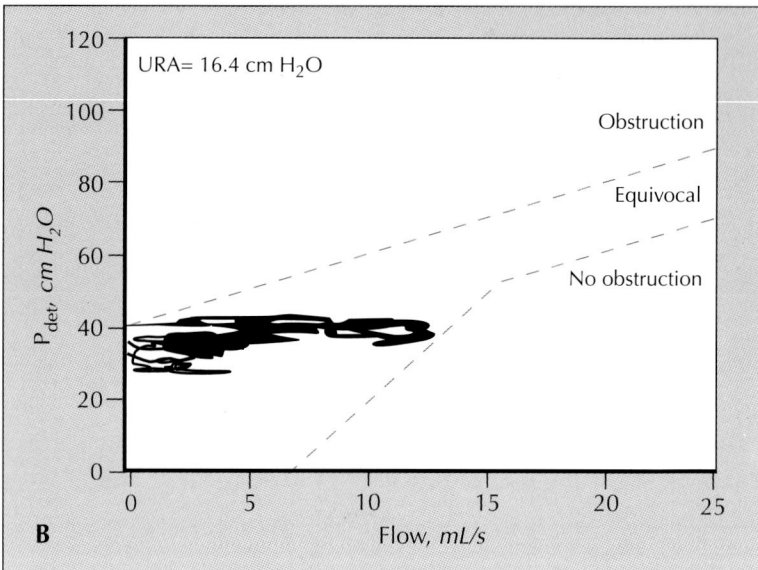

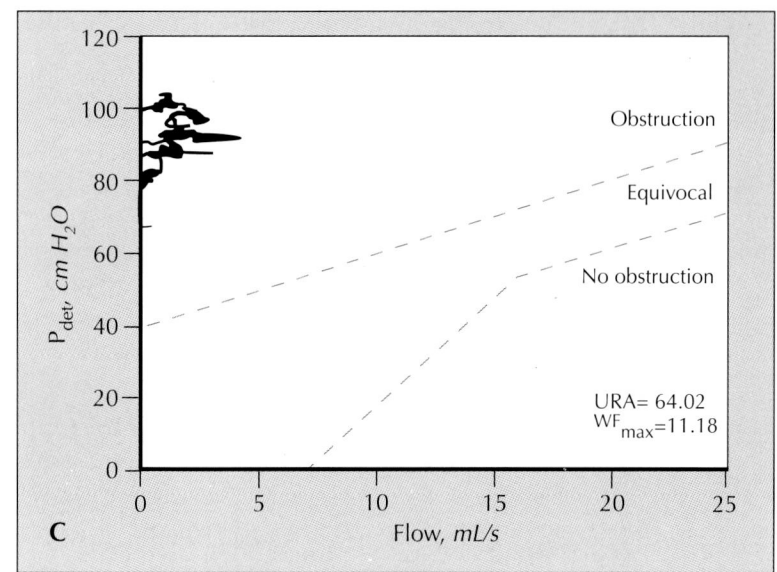

FIGURE 2-10. The Abrams-Griffiths (A-G) nomogram also can be used to characterize the bladder outlet as obstructed, nonobstructed, and equivocal based on the location of the point determined by the detrusor pressure at maximum flow ($P_{det}Q_{max}$) and the maximum flow rate (Q_{max}) [24]. The provisional standard of the International Continence Society (ICS) for P-Q analysis is a modified A-G nomogram in which the slope separating equivocal from unobstructed zones is constant [25]. The urethral resistance factor (URA), a BPH-specific parameter that approximates the passive urethral resistance relation (PURR), also can be used to diagnose bladder outlet obstruction on a continuous scale [26]. The P-Q plots generated from the data in Figure 2-8 are superimposed on the A-G nomogram. This analysis results in a diagnosis of no obstruction (*panel A*), equivocal obstruction (*panel B*), and obstruction (*panel C*) for the patients shown in Figure 2-8*A–C,* respectively. Detrusor contractility can be assessed by calculating the maximum Watts factor (WF_{max}) [27] or by generating the maximum isovolumetric detrusor pressure (Piso). The Watts factor has been shown to correlate well with Piso [28].

II. The Prostate

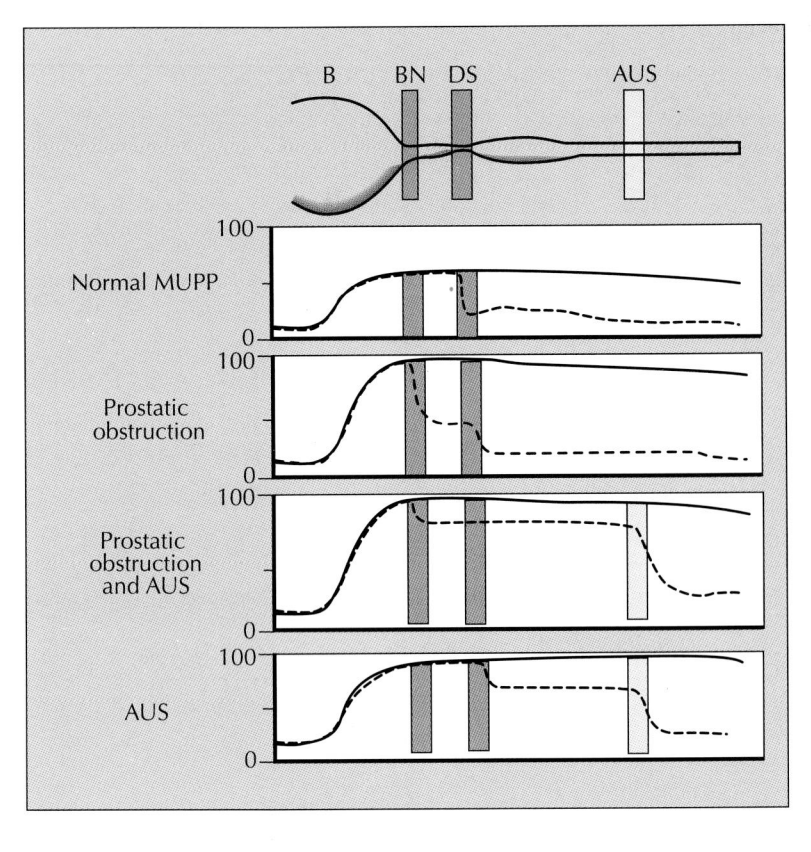

▶ **FIGURE 2-11.** Micturitional urethral pressure profilometry (MUPP), also known as voiding profilometry, also can be used to diagnose bladder outlet obstruction (BOO). Although voiding profilometry can identify the location and severity of BOO accurately, it is not widely used. The MUPP gradient correlates well with the passive urethral resistance relation (PURR) grade in the same patients, suggesting that voiding profilometry and pressure-flow studies are comparable for clinical diagnosis of BOO [29]. Voiding profilometry can be performed with the patient in any position using a small trilumen catheter (10 F) designed to record simultaneous intravesical and intraurethral pressures. During the steady state of micturition, the catheter is withdrawn gently from the bladder to the anterior urethra [30] while the catheter tip remains in the bladder. This figure illustrates the bladder (B), bladder neck (BN), distal or external sphincter zone (DS), and the site of an anterior urethral stricture (AUS). Normal and abnormal MUPP configurations are shown below these illustrations. During urination by the normal male, the bladder, the bladder neck, and most of the prostatic urethra are isobaric (*top panel*). Pressures in the bladder and prostatic urethra are in the range of 40 to 50 cm H_2O. In the vicinity of prostatic apex and the distal urethral sphincter or external sphincter zone (DS), where the urethra is relatively narrow, a pressure difference is seen with the intravesical pressures being higher than the intraurethral pressure. In patients with normal detrusor contractility, this pressure difference is about 20 to 25 cm H_2O. This disparity of pressures is not seen if a significant anterior urethral stenosis (AUS) exists distally. In patients with prostatic obstructions (*second tracing from top*), a significant pressure disparity is observed across the bladder neck and prostatic urethra, unless a distal obstruction is present (*third tracing from top*). The degree of pressure disparity at any location of the bladder outlet depends on the detrusor contractility, the degree of obstruction, and the conduit status of the distal urethra.

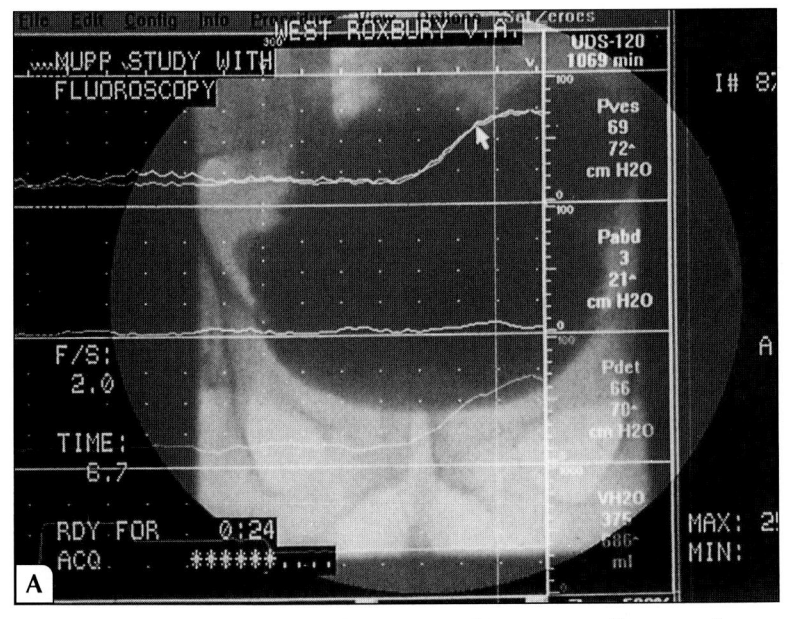

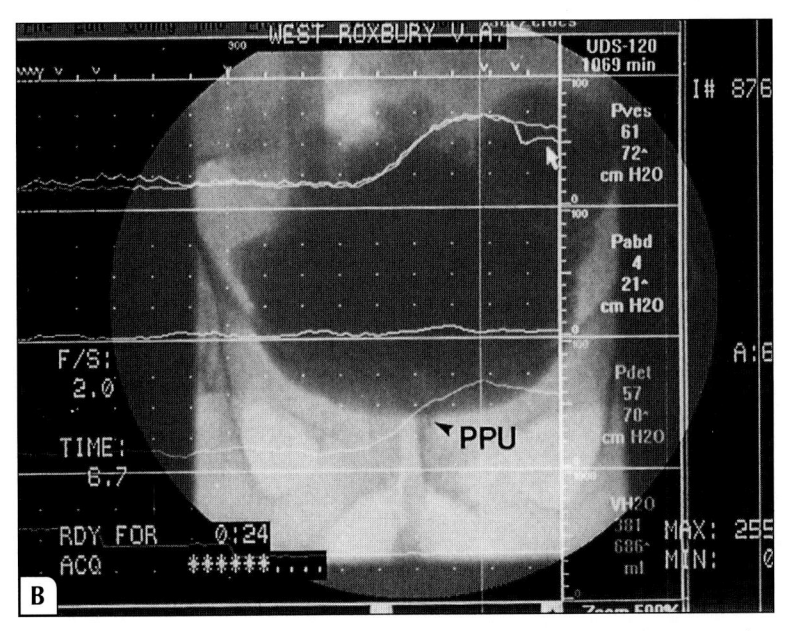

▶ **FIGURE 2-12.** Sequence of events in a fluoroscopically assisted micturitional urethral pressure profilometry (MUPP) study of a patient with a bladder outlet obstruction [31]. **A**, The superimposed intravesical pressures monitored by both the bladder pressure–sensing port at the catheter tip and the urethral pressure-sensing port of the catheter. At this time, the urethral pressure port of the catheter is proximal to the bladder neck and cannot be seen because of presence of the radiocontrast material in the bladder. The *white arrow* on the top tracings represents the time at which urination was first observed. **B**, The stage of voiding at which the urethral port enters the proximal prostatic urethra (PPU) during manual catheter withdrawal. The *white arrow* represents the corresponding pressure in the urethra.

(*Continued on next page*)

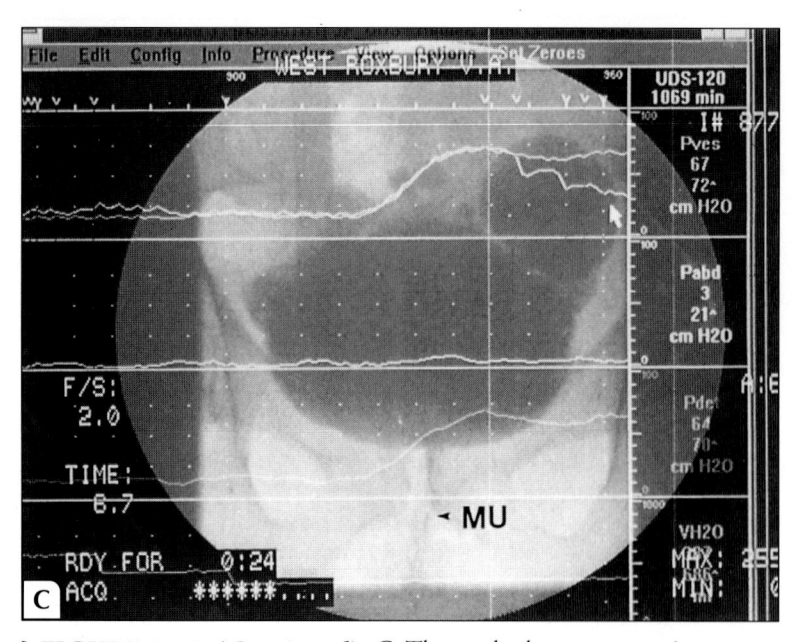

▶ **FIGURE 2-12.** (*Continued*) **C,** The urethral pressure–sensing port enters the narrow external sphincter zone or the membranous urethra (MU). Further drop of pressure (*white arrow*) occurs in this region. **D,** The stage of voiding at which the urethral pressure port enters the bulbous urethral (BU) region. The *white arrow* identifies the bulbous urethral pressure. In this patient, the entire prostatic urethra, including bladder neck, was obstructed.

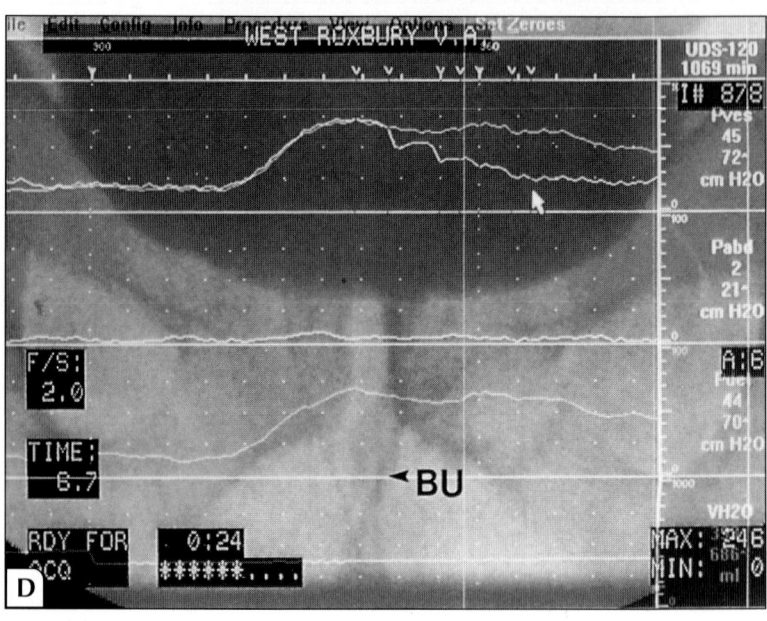

RADIOLOGIC IMAGING OF THE LOWER URINARY TRACT

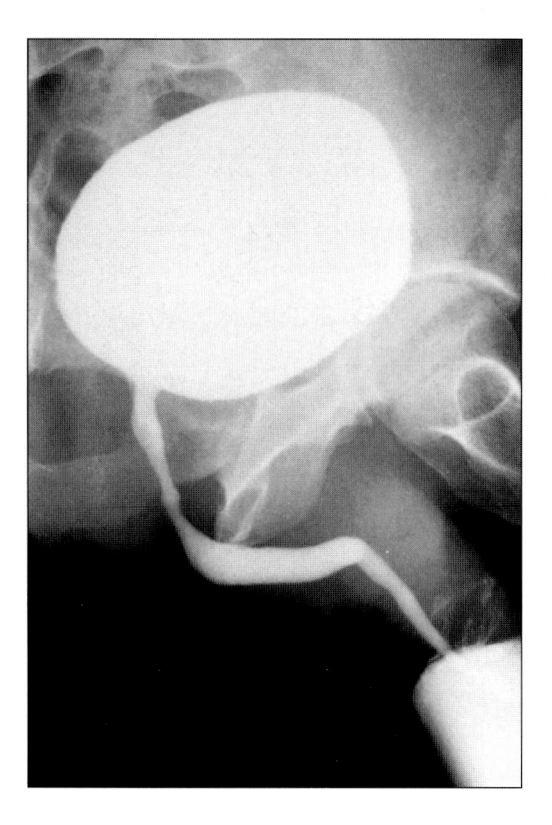

▶ **FIGURE 2-13.** Patients undergoing videourodynamics have the benefit of radiologic imaging of the lower urinary tract to identify significant structural abnormalities that may be associated with voiding dysfunctions. When fluoroscopic-assisted urodynamic evaluations are not feasible, voiding cystourethrography (VCUG) can be performed as an important adjunct to the functional evaluation. By observing the detrusor contour, the degree of bladder neck funneling, the degree of opacification of the prostatic fossa, and the degree of bulbous urethral filling, detrusor activity and bladder outlet characteristics can be reasonably determined [32]. VCUG thus complements urodynamic findings and reveals significant anatomic abnormalities that might not have been recognized without the radiologic complement to urodynamic studies. This normal VCUG of a 35-year-old asymptomatic volunteer with normal urodynamics is characterized by a smooth bladder contour, well-opened bladder neck and prostatic urethra, and well-distended bulbous urethra. The smooth filling defect in the middle of the prostatic urethra is the verumontanum.

II. The Prostate

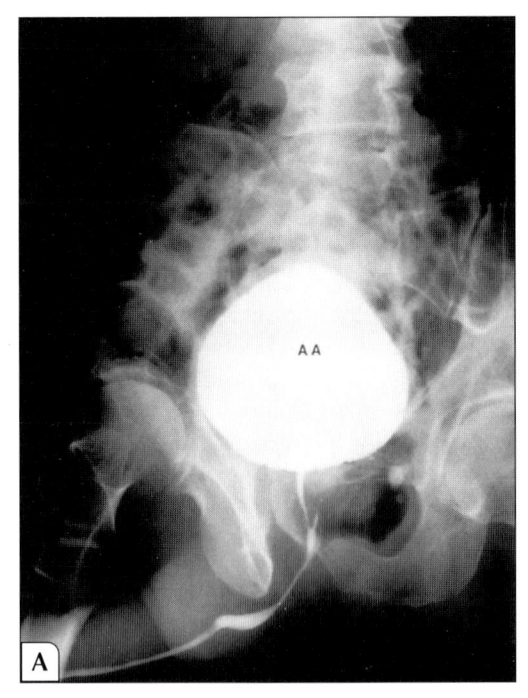

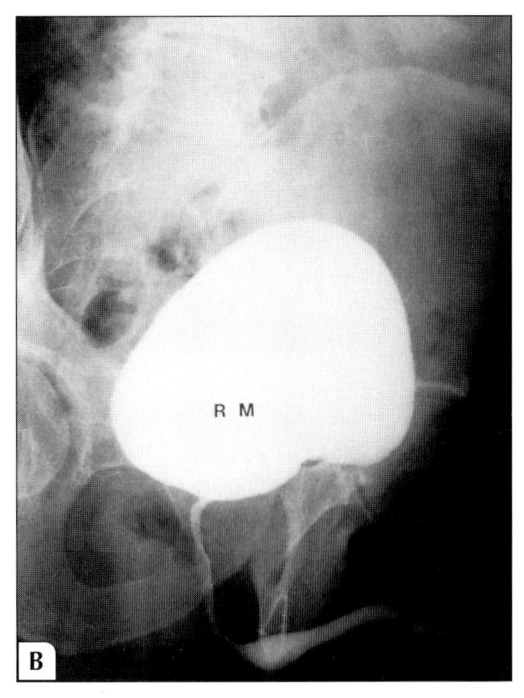

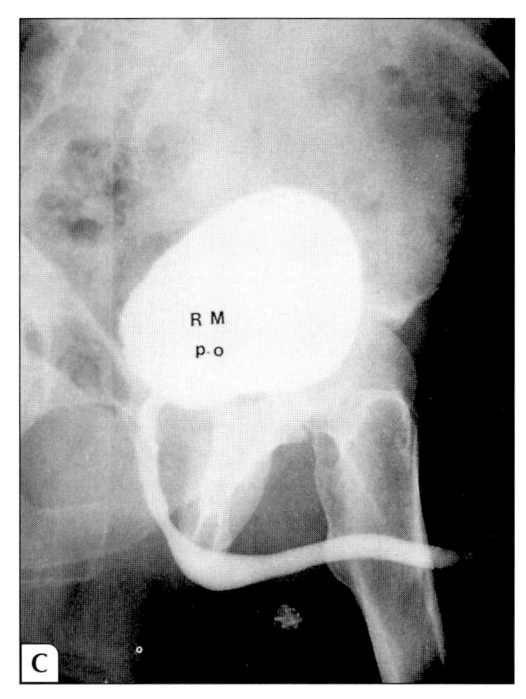

▶ **FIGURE 2-14.** Urodynamic evidence of bladder outlet obstruction (BOO) can be supported by the configuration of the bladder and the outlet in a voiding cystourethrogram (VCUG). **A,** VCUG of an elderly man with lower urinary tract symptoms and a large prostate on rectal examination shows a severely compressed and deviated bladder neck and prostatic urethra. The bulbous urethra was poorly filled. The urodynamic study showed severe BOO. **B,** In the VCUG of a 55-year-old symptomatic man, the partially opened bladder neck and prostatic urethra and poor filling of the bulbous urethra are consistent with urodynamic evidence of BOO. **C,** After bladder neck and prostatic incision in this patient, the VCUG shows a well-opened bladder neck and prostatic urethra and a well-filled and well-opacified bulbous urethra, indicating complete relief of BOO.

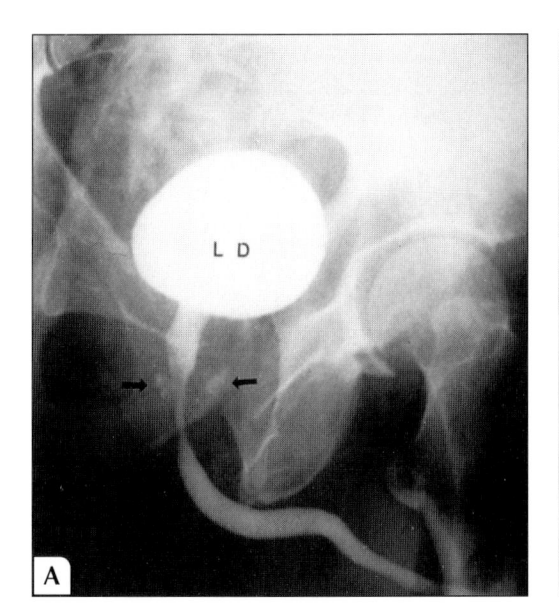

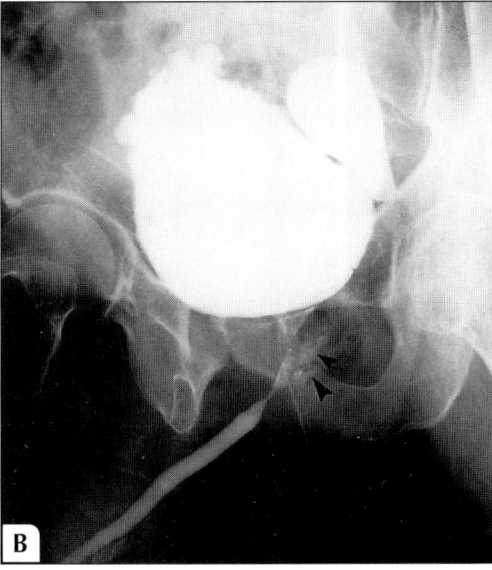

▶ **FIGURE 2-15.** The voiding cystourethrogram (VCUG) offers the advantage of identifying pathology in the prostate ducts that may be responsible for a patient's symptoms but is not revealed by urodynamic studies alone. **A,** VCUG of a 65-year-old symptomatic man shows prostatic reflux and calculi (*arrows*) at the apical region and a wide open bladder neck and prostatic urethra. No prostatic obstruction was demonstrated urodynamically. **B,** A patient with severe lower urinary tract symptoms shows reflux into the prostatic ducts and seminal vesicles (*arrows*) during voiding and a large, narrow-mouthed diverticulum on the left side of the bladder. Videourodynamics revealed severe prostatic obstruction. These types of pathology would be overlooked without such radiologic assistance.

Clinical Evaluation of Lower Urinary Tract Symptoms Due to Benign Prostatic Hyperplasia

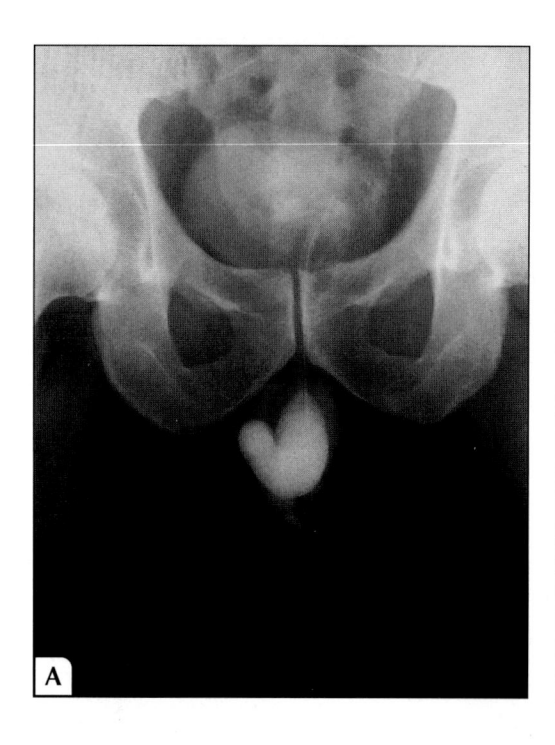

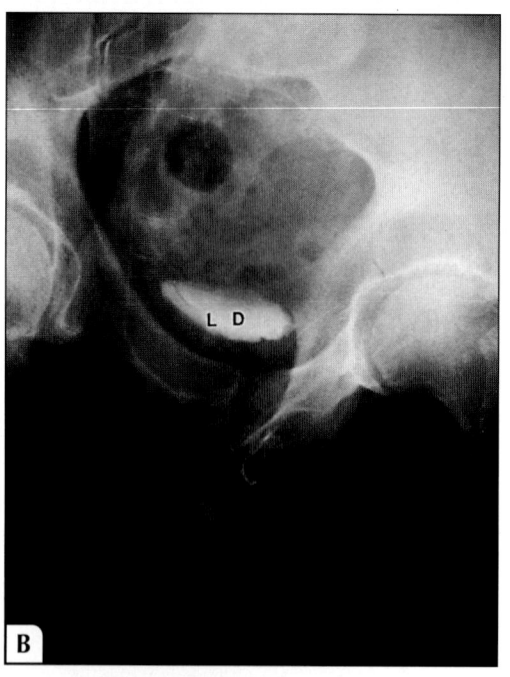

▶ **FIGURE 2-16.** Retrograde urethrography (RUG) may be beneficial in urodynamically normal patients suspected of having benign prostatic hyperplasia (BPH) with a predominant complaint of postvoid dribble. **A,** RUG of a patient with BPH shows a redundant bulbous urethra with more than 20 mL capacity with low pressure filling, which is responsible for his primary complaint of postvoid dribbling. The urodynamic evaluation is otherwise normal. Other possible causes of postvoid dribble are distal anterior urethral narrowing, urethral diverticulum, detrusor instability with after-contractions, and impaired detrusor contractility. **B,** In comparison, note the straight (nonsinuous) configuration of a normal bulbous urethra.

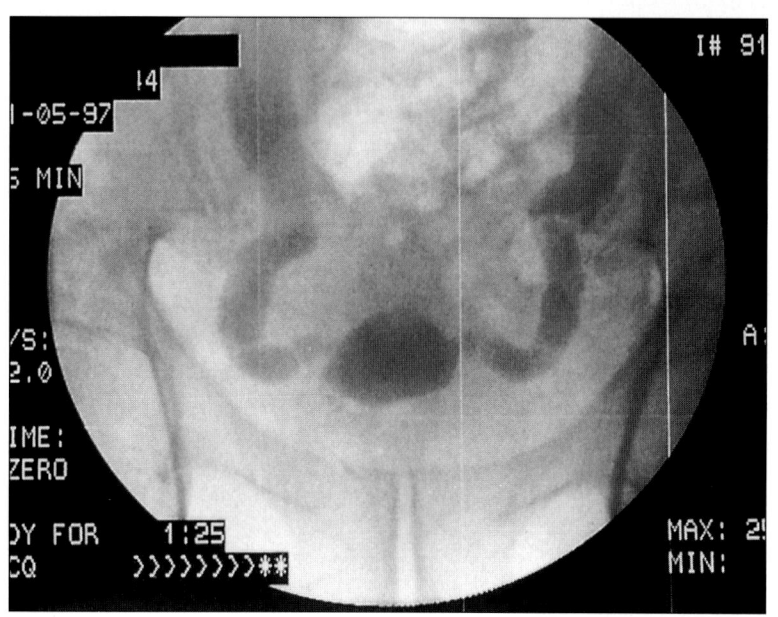

▶ **FIGURE 2-17.** Severe ureteral reflux can confound the urodynamic evaluation by distorting the true bladder capacity and compliance. Failure to radiologically recognize ureteral reflux can lead to misdiagnosis of detrusor function, and potentially cause complications such as acute pyelonephritis or acute renal shut-down. This radiologic information is vital in the accurate interpretation and proper management of patients with BPH. In this case, an 80-year-old man with severe lower urinary tract symptoms and a poorly compliant bladder showed high-grade bilateral ureteral reflux with most of the radiocontrast solution entering the renal pelvis and widely dilated ureters. Despite the marked redundancy in the upper urinary tract, the bladder pressures were elevated during filling. His renal function was impaired as demonstrated by elevated serum creatinine and blood urea nitrogen (BUN).

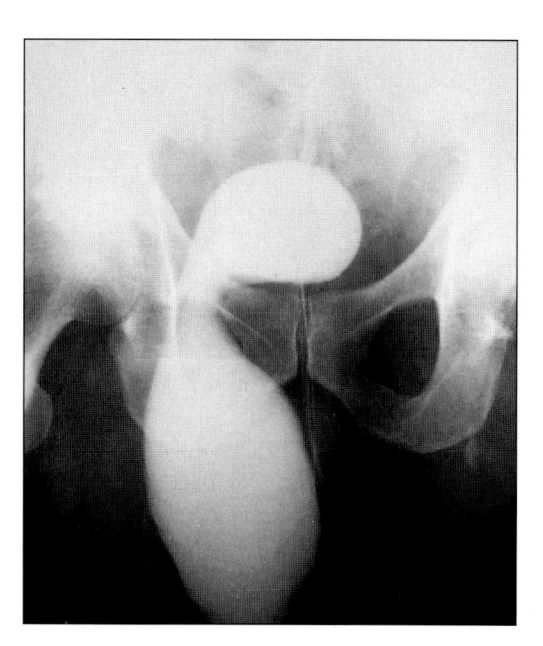

▶ **FIGURE 2-18.** In some cases, the structural abnormalities identified on voiding cystourethrogram (VCUG) can change the management strategy. The VCUG of a 65-year-old man with an AUA Symptom Index Score of 25 shows scrotal herniation of the urinary bladder. Urodynamic evidence of mild outlet obstruction with detrusor instability was seen. Cystoscopy and pressure-flow studies without radiologic assistance would have missed this severe structural abnormality. In fact, this patient had been treated for several months with an α-adrenergic blocker (terazosin) without relief of symptoms. The direct inguinal hernia was repaired following reduction of a wide-mouthed bladder diverticulum.

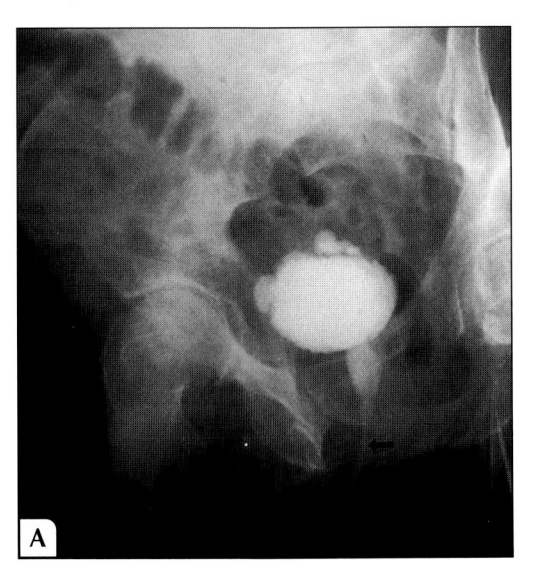

▶ **FIGURE 2-19.** In patients with bladder outlet obstruction, the site of obstruction cannot be determined by pressure-flow (P-Q) studies, although the prostate is the most likely location in elderly patients with nonneuropathic, nontraumatic lower urinary tract dysfunction. **A,** However, this voiding cystourethrogram in an elderly man with lower urinary tract symptoms shows a narrow membranous urethra with proximal dilation of the prostatic urethra, suggesting obstruction in the region of the membranous urethra but not in the prostatic urethra. Note the small diverticula in the bladder dome. **B,** The location of obstruction was confirmed by voiding profilometry. Intravesical and vesicourethral pressures are superimposed at the top. The dramatic drop in urethral pressure (*arrow*) corresponds with the location of the membranous urethra. Reliance on P-Q results without radiologic assistance would have led to inappropriate management in this case.

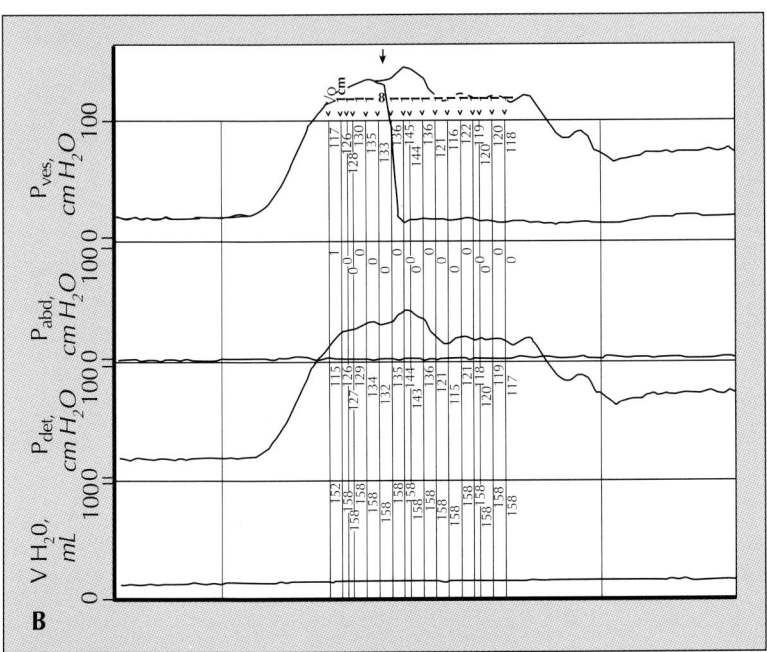

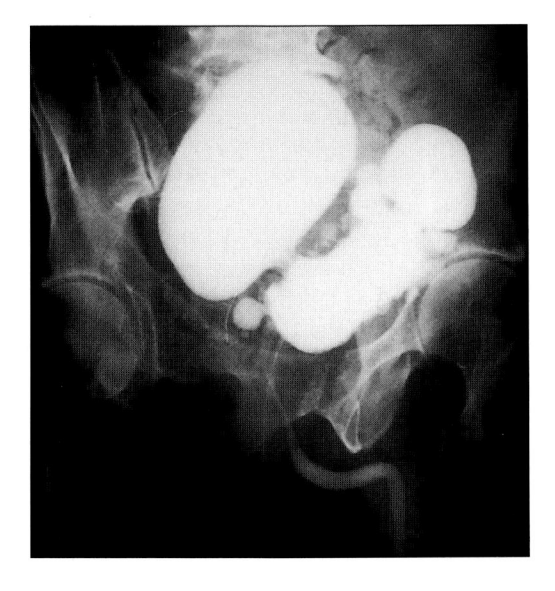

▶ **FIGURE 2-20.** Voiding cystourethrogram of an elderly man with lower urinary tract symptoms shows a large bladder diverticulum with a capacity greater than 50% of the total bladder capacity and multiple small diverticula. The prostatic urethra is compressed and distorted. Voiding profilometry confirmed severe prostatic obstruction. Urodynamic studies without radiologic support would have missed these gross morphologic changes in the detrusor, which resulted in persistent large postvoid residual volumes.

CYSTOURETHROSCOPY

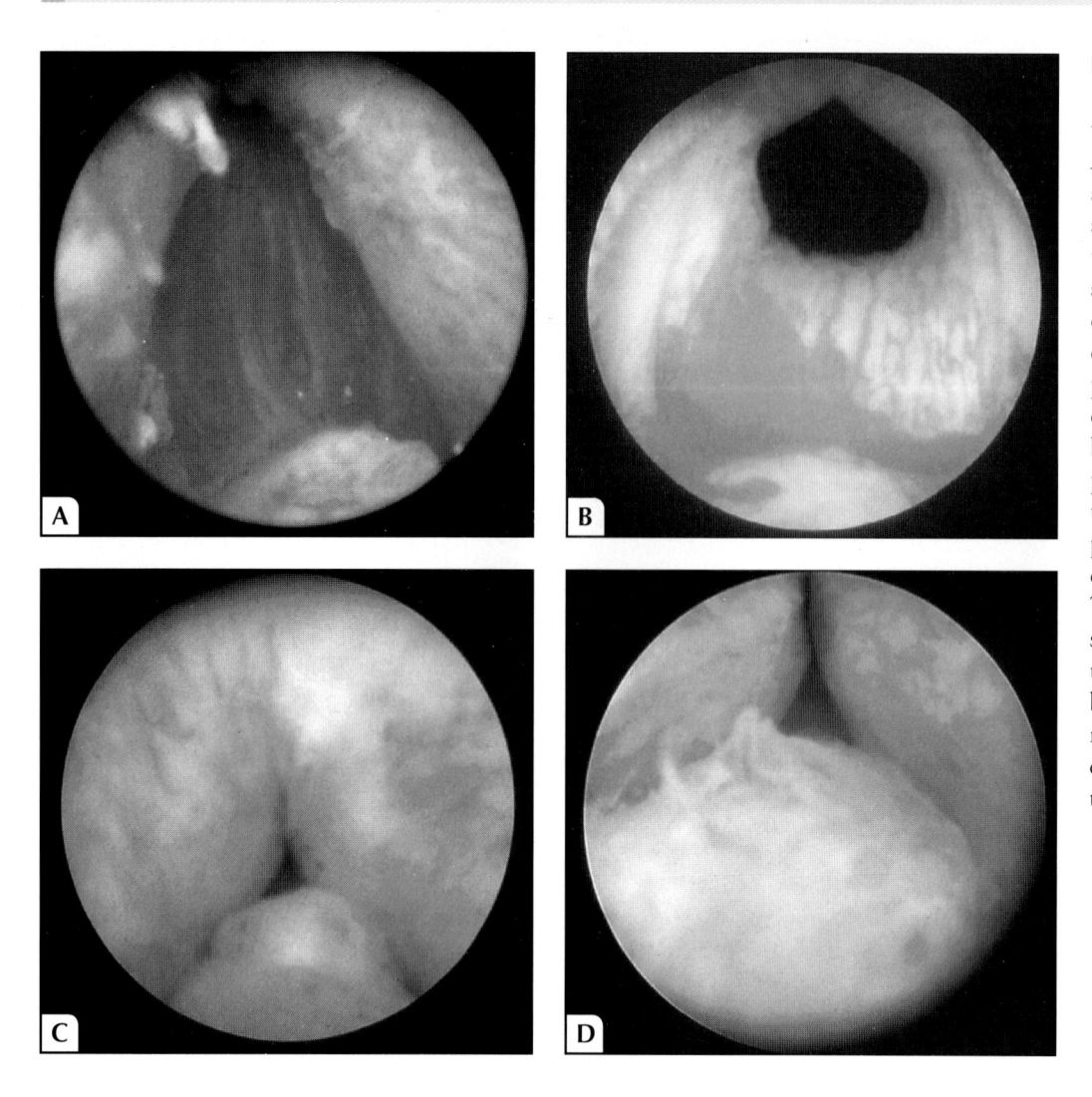

FIGURE 2-21. Endoscopic impressions of the prostatic urethra cannot reliably determine whether the bladder outlet is obstructed [33]. **A,** Cystoscopy of the bladder neck and midprostatic urethra shows minimal prostatic lobes and a closed bladder neck. No obstruction was found urodynamically as evidenced by isobaric detrusor and prostatic urethral pressures of 40 cm H_2O during steady state voiding. **B,** Endoscopic evidence of a partially open bladder neck without prostatic enlargement conflicts with the presence of bladder outlet obstruction, as demonstrated by urodynamics in this patient. **C,** In some patients with lower urinary tract symptoms, trilobar prostatic enlargement in the proximal prostatic urethra is consistent with urodynamically proven obstruction, as shown here. **D,** This endoscopic view of the prostatic apex showing an unusually prominent verumontanum and apical prostatic lobes suggests bladder outlet obstruction; however, a urodynamic study in this patient showed impaired detrusor contractility but not prostatic obstruction.

CLINICAL APPROACH FOR THE ASSESSMENT OF LOWER URINARY TRACT SYMPTOMS

Clinical Evaluation of LUTS

Thorough urologic history, including a voiding diary, pharmacologic history, and previous surgical procedures
AUA Symptom Index Score to determine patient's perception of and bother from LUTS
Details of other comorbidities
Physical examination of genitourinary system and focused neurologic examination
Digital rectal examination to assess prostate size, nodularity, and consistency
Urinalysis and serum creatinine

FIGURE 2-22. The diagnosis of benign prostatic hyperplasia (BPH) as a cause of lower urinary tract symptoms (LUTS) is an exclusion diagnosis because histologic BPH is highly prevalent in this aging population. Therefore, prior to initiating treatment, other factors that can provoke LUTS should be identified or excluded via a detailed clinical examination. In many patients, this method of thorough clinical assessment is adequate for the diagnosis of BPH.

Diagnostic Evaluation of LUTS

Relevant Tests	Tests with Limited Benefit
Uroflowmetry, to rule out bladder outlet obstruction by observing high flow rates	
Postvoid residual volume during follow-up of patients on watchful waiting	Ultrasonic or radiologic imaging of the upper urinary tract. Imaging is recommended, however, for patients with concomitant urinary tract abnormalities such as hematuria, urinary tract infection, renal insufficiency, and history of urinary stones and renal dysfunction
Urodynamic evaluation to characterize bladder and outlet function	Cystourethroscopy during initial evaluation
Radiologic imaging of the lower urinary tract to identify morphologic abnormalities	
Cystourethroscopy, if invasive treatment is planned	

FIGURE 2-23. Several diagnostic tests may be useful in accurately determining the cause of lower urinary tract symptoms (LUTS). Other tests add limited information to the evaluation or management of LUTS and thus are not recommended for routine use [9].

Indications for Urodynamic Evaluation

Obvious or suspicious myeloneuropathies
Failure of pharmacologic or surgical management
Geriatric population with comorbidities
Confirmation of bladder outlet obstruction before recommending invasive treatments, especially in the frail elderly patient
Patient's desire to objectively define the causes of his lower urinary tract symptoms
Pharmacologic or invasive treatment in an atypical younger patient
Assessment of functional and morphologic (with fluoroscopic support) deterioration due to long-standing, severe bladder outlet obstruction

FIGURE 2-24. The role of urodynamic studies in the management of lower urinary tract symptoms is continuously debated in terms of their cost-effectiveness and clinical outcomes. Since the introduction of the American Urological Assocation symptom index, 5α-reductase inhibitors (finasteride) and highly selective α-adrenergic blockers, most clinicians can successfully treat these patients without subjecting them to comprehensive urodynamics. However, in certain cases, urodynamic assessment can be particularly invaluable.

Advantages and Disadvantages of Videourodynamic Evaluation

Advantages	Disadvantages
Usually determines the pathogenesis of lower urinary tract symptoms	Invasive despite negligible morbidity
Confirms or excludes significant bladder outlet obstruction	Requires ability to recognize and interpret artifacts in the study
Changes in bladder wall compliance and structural abnormalities (eg, large diverticula, massive reflux) can be detected with radiologic assistance	Requires a good understanding of basic physical principles and experience with data interpretation
Often provides rational explanation to the patient of the causes of his lower urinary tract symptoms	Cost-effectiveness not established
Prevents unnecessary pharmacologic and invasive misadventures	Debatable influence on treatment outcomes
	Interpretation by computerized commercial systems may not be reliable

FIGURE 2-25. Advantages and disadvantages of videourodynamic evaluation.

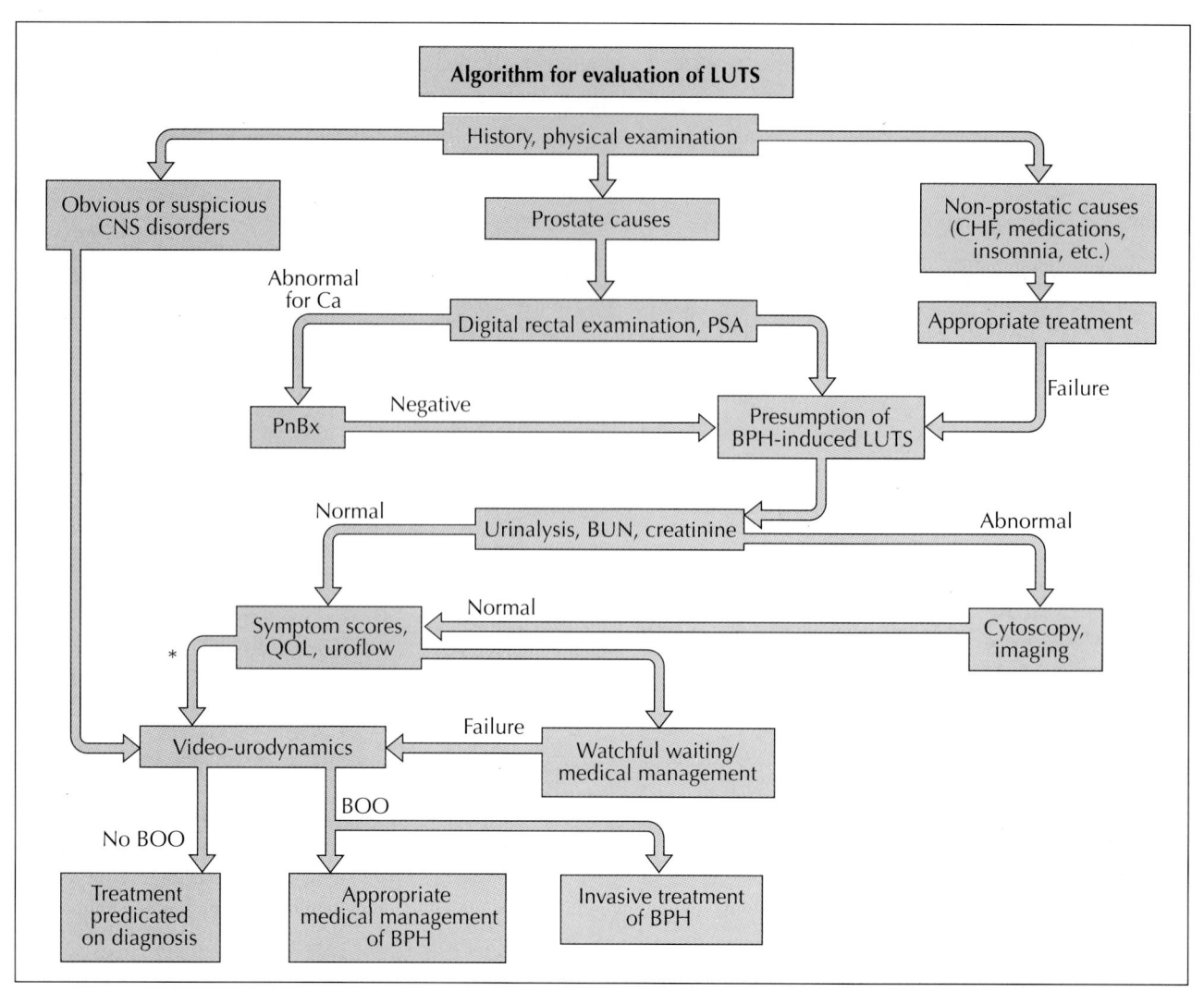

FIGURE 2-26. Algorithm for evaluating adult and elderly men with lower urinary tract symptoms (LUTS). Prostatic causes are separated from other factors that can produce symptoms. After deciding whether benign prostatic hyperplasia is presumed to be responsible for LUTS, the symptom scores decide the remaining part of the work-up of patients with lower urinary tract symptoms. The decision to perform cystoscopy, intravenous pyelogram (IVP), ultrasonic imaging, or other ancillary tests is prompted by abnormal urinalysis, BUN, and creatinine, but not by symptom scores alone. *Asterisk* denotes that urodynamic studies are indicated in patients with obvious or suspicious central nervous system disorders, in patients who may be candidates for invasive procedures, in younger patients in whom a more accurate diagnosis is required before pharmacologic or surgical intervention, and in frail, elderly patients who are prone to high morbidity with inappropriate management.

REFERENCES

1. Hald T: Urodynamics in benign prostatic hyperplasia: a survey. *Prostate* 1989, 2(suppl):69–77.
2. Resnick NM, Elbadawi A, Yalla SV: Age and the lower urinary tract: what is normal? *Neurourol Urodynam* 1995, 14:577–579.
3. Chalfin SA, Bradley WE: The etiology of detrusor hyperreflexia in patients with intravesical obstruction. *J Urol* 1982, 127:938–942.
4. Dyro FM, DuBeau CE, Sullivan MP, *et al.*: Covert comorbid neurologic abnormalities in patients presenting with symptoms of prostatism. *J Urol* 1992, 147:269A.
5. Resnick NM: Voiding dysfunction in the elderly. In *Neurourology and Urodynamics: Principles and Practice*. Edited by Yalla SV, McGuire EJ, Elbadawi A, Blaivas JG. New York: MacMillan; 1988:303–330.
6. Resnick NM, Yalla SV: Geriatric incontinence and voiding dysfunction. In *Campbell's Urology*. Edited by Walsh PC, Retik AB, Vaughan ED, Wein AJ. Philadelphia: WB Saunders 1997:1044–1058.
7. Barry MJ, Fowler FJ, O'Leary MP, *et al.*: The American Urological Association symptom index for benign prostatic hyperplasia. *J Urol* 1992, 148:1549–1557.
8. The International Prostate Symptom Score (I-PSS) and Quality-of-life Assessment. In *The 2nd International Consultation on Benign Prostatic Hyperplasia (BPH)*. Jersey, Channel Islands: Scientific Communication International; 1993:554–555.
9. McConnell JD, Barry MJ, Bruskewitz RC, *et al.*: Benign prostatic hyperplasia: diagnosis and treatment. Clinical practice guidelines. No. 8, AHCPR Publication No. 94-0582, Rockville, MD; Agency for Health Care Policy and Research, Public Health Service, United States Department of Health and Human Services; 1994.
10. McConnell JD: Epidemiology, etiology, pathophysiology, and diagnosis of benign prostatic hyperplasia. In *Campbell's Urology*. Edited by Walsh PC, Retik AB, Vaughan ED, Wein AJ. Philadelphia: WB Saunders; 1997:1429–1452.
11. Sullivan MP, Yalla SV: Urodynamic assessment of benign prostatic hypertrophy. In *Alternate Methods in the Treatment of Benign Prostatic Hyperplasia*. Edited by Romas NA, Vaughan ED. New York: Springer-Verlag; 1993:66–89.
12. Blaivas JG: Multichannel urodynamic studies in men with benign prostatic hyperplasia. *Urol Clin North Am* 1990, 17:543–552.
13. Sullivan MP, Yalla SV: Detrusor contractility and compliance characteristics in adult male patients with obstructive and nonobstructive voiding dysfunction. *J Urol* 1996, 155:1995–2000.
14. Comiter CV, Sullivan MP, Schacterle RS, *et al.*: Urodynamic risk factors for renal dysfunction in men with obstructive and nonobstructive voiding dysfunction. *J Urol* 1997, 158:181–185.
15. Barry MJ, Cockett ATK, Holtgrewe L, *et al.*: Relationship of symptoms of prostatism to commonly used physiologic and anatomic measures of the severity of benign prostatic hypertrophy. *J Urol* 1993, 150:351–358.
16. Sirls LT, Kirkemo AK, Jay J: Lack of correlation of the American Urological Association Symptom 7 Index with urodynamic bladder outlet obstruction. *Neurourol Urodynam* 1996, 15:447–457.
17. el Din KE, Kiemeney LA, de Wildt MJ, *et al.*: The correlation between bladder outlet obstruction and lower urinary tract symptoms as measured by the international prostate symptom score. *J Urol* 1996, 156:1020–1025.
18. Yalla SV, Sullivan MP, Lecamwasam HS, *et al.*: Correlation of American Urological Association Symptom Index with obstructive and nonobstructive prostatism. *J Urol* 1995, 153:674–680.
19. Chancellor MB, Blaivas JG, Kaplan SA, Axelrod S: Bladder outlet obstruction versus impaired detrusor contractility: the role of uroflow. *J Urol* 1991, 145:810–812.
20. Griffiths DJ: The mechanics of the urethra and of micturition. *Br J Urol* 1973, 45:497–507.
21. Abrams P, Blaivas J, Nordlin J, *et al.*: The objective evaluation of bladder outflow obstruction. In *The 2nd International Consultation on Benign Prostatic Hyperplasia*. Edited by Cockett ATK, Khoury S, Aso Y, *et al*. Channel Islands: Scientific Communication International; 1993:152–225.
22. Schafer W: Principles and clinical application of advanced urodynamic analysis of voiding function. *Urol Clin North Am* 1990, 17:553–566.
23. Kranse M, vanMastrigt R: The derivation of an obstruction index from a three parameter model fitted to the lowest part of the pressure flow plot [abstract]. *J Urol* 1991, 145:261.
24. Abrams P, Griffiths DJ: The assessment of prostatic obstruction from urodynamic measurements and from residual urine. *Br J Urol* 1979, 51:129–134.
25. Griffiths D, Hofner K, van Mastrigt R, *et al.*: Standardization of terminology of lower urinary tract function: pressure-flow studies of voiding, urethral resistance, and urethral obstruction. *Neurourol Urodynam* 1997, 16:1–18.
26. Griffiths DJ, VanMastrigt R, Bosch R: Quantification of urethral resistance and bladder function during voiding, with special reference to the effects of prostate size reduction on urethral obstruction due to benign prostatic hyperplasia. *Neurourol Urodynam* 1989, 8:17–27.
27. Griffiths DJ: Assessment of detrusor contraction strength or contractility. *Neurourol Urodynam* 1991, 10:1–18.
28. Sullivan MP, DuBeau CE, Resnick NM, *et al.*: Continuous occlusion test to determine detrusor contractile performance. *J Urol* 1995, 154:1834–1840.
29. DuBeau CE, Sullivan MP, Cravalho EG, *et al.*: Correlation between micturitional urethral pressure profile and pressure-flow criteria in bladder outlet obstruction. *J Urol* 1995, 154:498–503.
30. Yalla SV, Sharma GVRK, Barsamian EM: Micturitional static urethral pressure profile: a method of recording urethral pressure profile during voiding and the implications. *J Urol* 1980, 124:649–656.
31. Sullivan MP, Comiter CV, Yalla SV: Micturitional urethral pressure profilometry. *Urol Clin North Am* 1996, 23:263–278.
32. Yalla SV, Cravalho E, Resnick N, *et al.*: Elastic jump in male urethra during voiding: clinical observations in male subjects and experimental studies in dogs. *J Urol* 1985, 134:907–913.
33. Chapple C, Turner-Warwick R: Bladder outflow obstruction in the male. *Urodynamics: Principles, Practice and Application*. Edited by Mundy AR, Stephenson TP, Wein AJ. New York: Churchill Livingstone; 1994:233–262.

Medical Management of Benign Prostatic Hyperplasia

3
NONCANCEROUS DISEASE SECTION

Ira J. Kohn
Steven A. Kaplan

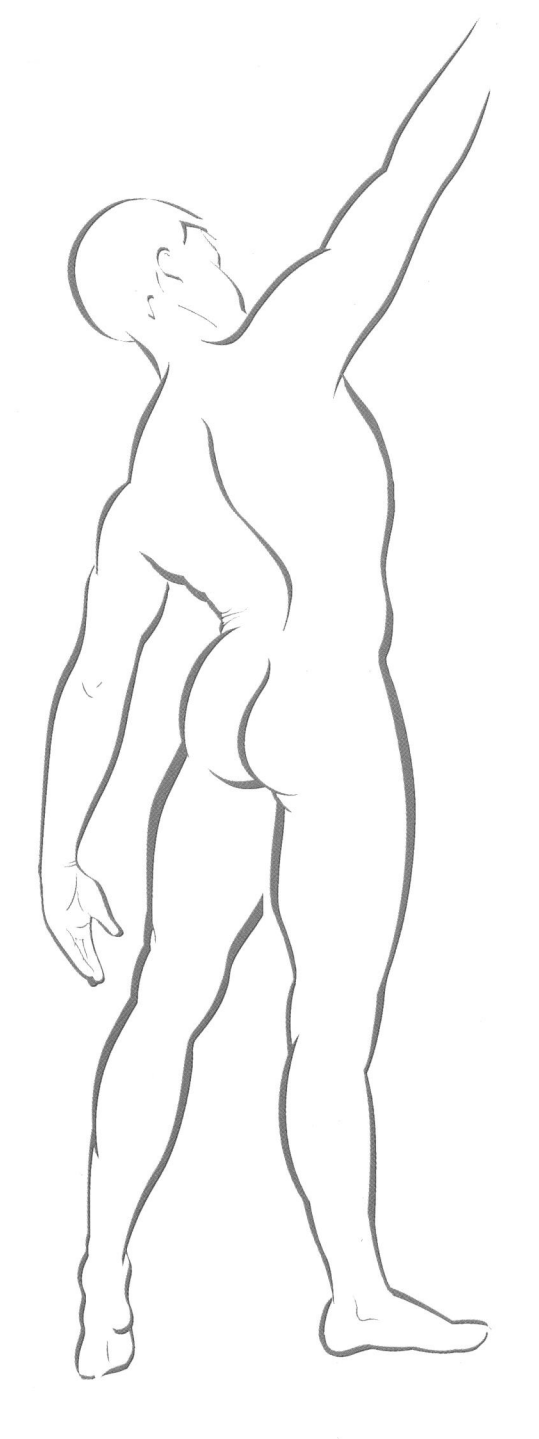

With histologic evidence of benign prostatic hyperplasia (BPH) in nearly 50% of men aged 50 years, and prevalence rates increasing with age, BPH is the most common benign neoplasm of elderly men [1]. Bladder outlet obstruction resulting from the hyperplastic prostate is believed to be secondary to two mechanisms: 1) the static component or bulk obstruction caused by the enlarged prostate encroaching on the prostatic urethra and 2) the dynamic component mediated by smooth muscle tone within the prostatic stroma. Traditionally, surgery has been the mainstay of treatment for symptomatic BPH. However, clinical practice guidelines developed by the Agency for Health Care Policy and Research and endorsed by the American Urological Association have recently been released to serve as a guide for the diagnosis and treatment of patients with BPH [2]. Treatment is recommended for the majority of patients with moderate to severe symptoms as defined by the American Urological Association symptom score. Medical therapy is among the recommended treatment options. The availability of medical therapy, which is less invasive and therefore more appealing to many patients, has been associated with huge increases in the total number of patients treated compared with the previous era, when surgery was the only option.

SELECTING PATIENTS FOR THE MEDICAL MANAGEMENT OF BENIGN PROSTATIC HYPERPLASIA

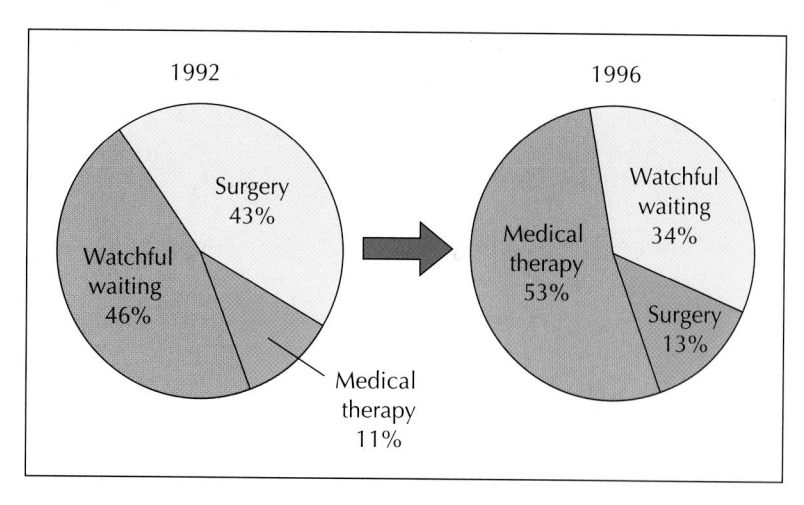

FIGURE 3-1. Impact of medical therapy on treatment trends, 1992 versus 1996. Despite an overall aging of the population and a progressively increasing number of men enrolled in the Medicare program, a recent review of the US Medicare data base reveals a continual decline in the annual number of prostatectomies performed for benign prostatic hyperplasia (BPH) [3]. This decline coincides with a progressive annual increase in the number of men choosing medical therapy for BPH. (*Data from* Miller [4].)

Candidates for Medical Therapy

Moderate to severe symptoms
Lack of absolute indications for surgery
   Recurrent urinary retention
   Recurrent or persistent gross hematuria
   Recurrent urinary tract infection
   Bladder stones
   Renal insufficiency

FIGURE 3-2. Candidates for medical therapy. Because the primary indication for intervention in the overwhelming majority of patients with benign prostatic hyperplasia is to improve quality of life by relieving symptoms, the ideal candidate for medical therapy should have symptoms bothersome enough to have a negative impact on his quality of life. This patient should also be motivated to be compliant with a potentially life-long commitment to taking medication, provided that the medication is effective and the side effects are minimal. Individuals presenting with any of the absolute indications for surgery listed in the Agency for Health Care Policy and Research guidelines should be treated with prostatectomy [2].

Natural History of Benign Prostatic Hyperplasia

Cross-sectional longitudinal studies of aging reveal
   Age-dependent prevalence of macroscopic BPH
   Age-dependent prevalence of symptomatic BPH
Clinical studies of watchful waiting for symptomatic BPH reveal
   50%   Patients with symptoms unchanged
   30%–50% Patients with spontaneous resolution of symptoms
   10%–20% Patients with progressive symptoms

FIGURE 3-3. Natural history of benign prostatic hyperplasia (BPH). Because no prospective long-term study of untreated symptomatic prostatism has ever been reported, the natural history of benign prostatic hyperplasia (BPH) remains poorly defined. Several large-scale longitudinal population-based studies of aging men reveal increasing age-dependent prevalence rates for detection of macroscopic and symptomatic BPH [5–7]. Symptomatic BPH is often presumed to be a progressive process resulting in urinary retention if left untreated. However, several clinical studies of a watchful waiting strategy for monitoring symptomatic BPH patients reveal that only approximately 20% of the patients have progressive symptoms or resort to surgery during a 5-year follow-up period [8–11]. In fact, urinary symptoms for the great majority of men observed remain unchanged or actually improve over time [8–11].

Placebo Effect in Benign Prostatic Hyperplasia Studies

↓ Symptom scores
↑ Qmax
↑ Prostate volume

FIGURE 3-4. Placebo effect in benign prostatic hyperplasia (BPH) studies. Prospective, randomized, double-blind, placebo-controlled studies are the ideal method to evaluate the clinical efficacy of various treatments for BPH. Analysis of several trials of BPH medical therapy reveals that placebo treatment results in modest but statistically significant improvements in symptom scores and peak flow rates [12,13]. The maximum placebo effect is likely to be noted within the first 6 months of treatment, but beneficial effects of placebo have been noted up to 2 years after starting therapy. Placebo response tends to be greater in patients who are less symptomatic and in those with smaller prostate glands (<40 g) [12]. Prostate volume continues to increase with time despite placebo therapy [12]. This placebo effect must be kept in mind when judging the efficacy of treatment medication. Qmax—maximum urine flow.

ALTERING THE STATIC COMPONENT OF BENIGN PROSTATIC HYPERPLASIA THROUGH ENDOCRINE THERAPY

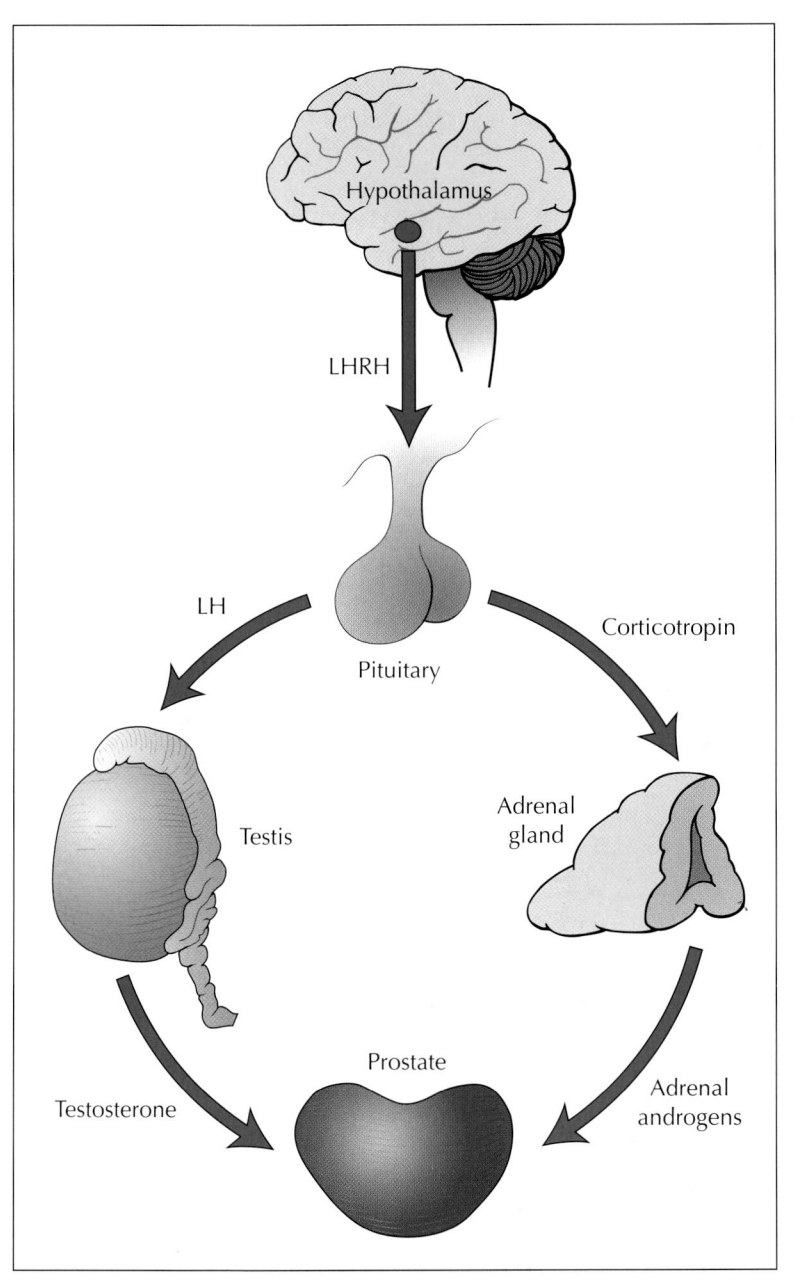

FIGURE 3-5. The hypothalamic-gonadal axis. Adequate levels of circulating testosterone are necessary for the prostate to develop and grow. Luteinizing hormone–releasing hormone (LHRH) is released in a pulsatile fashion by the hypothalamus into the portal circulation, stimulating the anterior pituitary to secrete luteinizing hormone (LH). LH enters the systemic circulation and then stimulates the Leydig cells of the testes to release testosterone. Of circulating androgens, 95% are composed of testosterone released by the testes, and the other 5% are composed of adrenal androgens, such as dehydroepiandrosterone sulfate. Ninety-eight percent of circulating androgens are bound to plasma proteins, primarily albumin and sex hormone binding globulin [14]. Only free testosterone is biologically active and available to enter prostatic cells by a process of simple diffusion.

Clinical Studies of Luteinizing Hormone–Releasing Hormone Agonists for the Treatment of Benign Prostatic Hyperplasia

Study	LHRH Agonist	Patients, n	Treatment Time, mo	Decrease in Prostate Volume, %	Qmax	Symptom Score
Peters and Walsh [15]	Nafarelin acetate	9	6	24	↑	↓
Gabrilove et al. [16]	Leuprolide acetate	15	6	46	↑	↓
Eri and Tveter [17]	Leuprolide acetate	50	6	35	↑	↓

FIGURE 3-6. Clinical studies of luteinizing hormone–releasing hormone (LHRH) agonists for the treatment of benign prostatic hyperplasia (BPH). By continuous rather than pulsatile stimulation, LHRH agonists inhibit pituitary release of luteinizing hormone, resulting in decreased release of testosterone by Leydig cells. Several short-term, nonrandomized clinical studies have documented the effects of using LHRH agonists for treating patients with BPH [15–17]. Serum testosterone levels are decreased to castrate levels during treatment. After 6 months of treatment with an LHRH agonist, prostate volume decreases an average of 36%, and plasma levels of prostate specific antigen decrease accordingly. Peak urinary flow rates have been noted to increase an average of 15% to 25%, and symptom scores have decreased accordingly an average of 30% to 40% following 6 months of treatment. Side effects of sexual dysfunction associated with decreased levels of circulating testosterone have limited the widespread use of LHRH agonists for treating BPH. Prostate volumes return to approximately pretreatment values 3 to 6 months following withdrawal of LHRH agonist treatment. Qmax—maximum urine flow.

Clinical Studies of Antiandrogens for the Treatment of Benign Prostatic Hyperplasia

Study	Antiandrogen	Patients, n	Treatment Time, mo	Decrease in Prostate Volume, %	Qmax	Symptom Score
Stone et al. [18]	Flutamide	84	6	41	↑	↓
Eri and Tveter [17]	Bicalutamide	30	6	26	↑	↓

FIGURE 3-7. Clinical studies of antiandrogens for the treatment of benign prostatic hyperplasia (BPH). Antiandrogens are competitive inhibitors, thereby blocking the action of testosterone at the androgen receptor without decreasing plasma levels of testosterone. Several clinical trials have evaluated the short-term effectiveness of antiandrogens for treating symptomatic BPH [18,19]. After 6 months of treatment, prostate volume significantly decreases on the order of 30%. In addition, symptom scores and flow rates have been noted to improve. However, despite normal circulating levels of testosterone, the side effects of decreased libido and painful gynecomastia have limited the use of antiandrogens. Qmax—maximum urine flow.

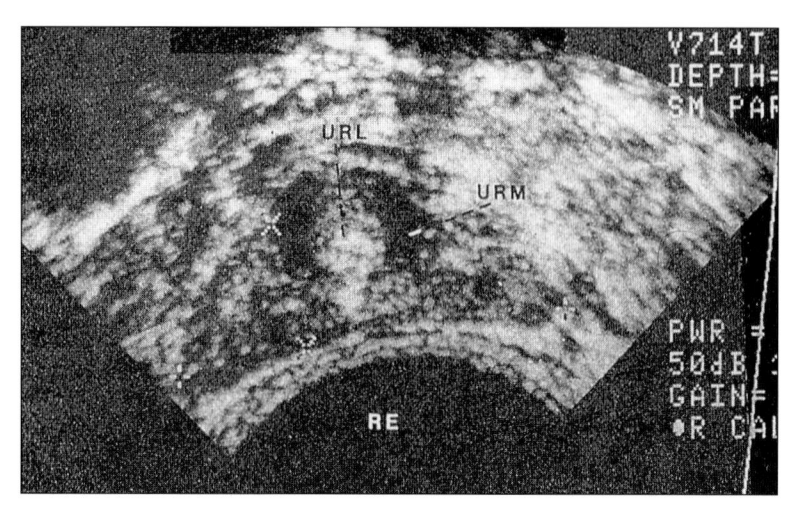

FIGURE 3-8. Clinical support of the dihydrotestosterone (DHT) hypothesis. Transrectal ultrasound of rudimentary prostate (cursors) in male pseudohermaphrodite with 5α-reductase deficiency. Benign prostatic hyperplasia (BPH) does not occur or rarely occurs in men castrated prior to puberty [20]. Numerous clinical studies have documented the regression of BPH and improved voiding symptomatology in men with prostatism following bilateral orchiectomy [21–23]. Male human pseudohermaphrodites resulting from a congenital deficiency of the enzyme 5α-reductase have vestigial prostates, consisting only of a central zone, despite normal serum testosterone levels and no defect in the androgen receptor [24–26]. Administration of DHT results in prostatic growth, indicating that DHT is the primary mediator of prostate growth and that testosterone cannot act alone to support growth and development of the prostate [27]. RE—rectal lumen; URL—urethral lumen; URM—urethromuscular wall. (*Courtesy of* Journal of Clinical Endocrinology.)

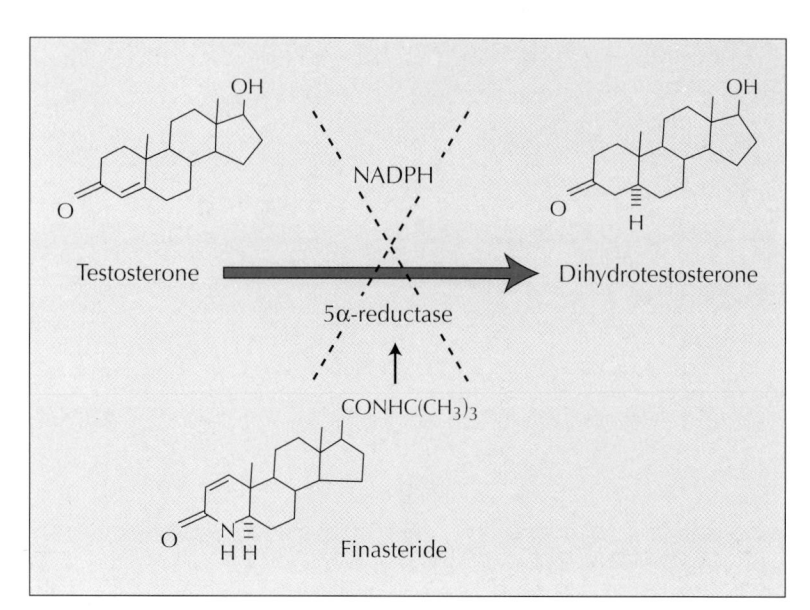

FIGURE 3-9. The mechanism of action of finasteride. This mechanism is based on blocking the conversion of testosterone to dihydrotestosterone (DHT) by inhibiting the action of 5α-reductase within cells of the prostate. Two isotypes of 5α-reductase exist, but only 5α-reductase type 2 is detectable within the prostate [28]. Finasteride is a pure 5α-reductase type 2 inhibitor that does not bind the androgen receptor or inhibit the formation or action of other steroid hormones [29]. Administration of finasteride results in an 80% to 90% decrease in the concentration of DHT within both the prostate and the general circulation [30,31]. Accompanying this response is a 560% increase in the local concentration of testosterone within the prostate, without a significant change in the serum concentration of testosterone [32–34]. NADPH—ferrihemoprotein reductase.

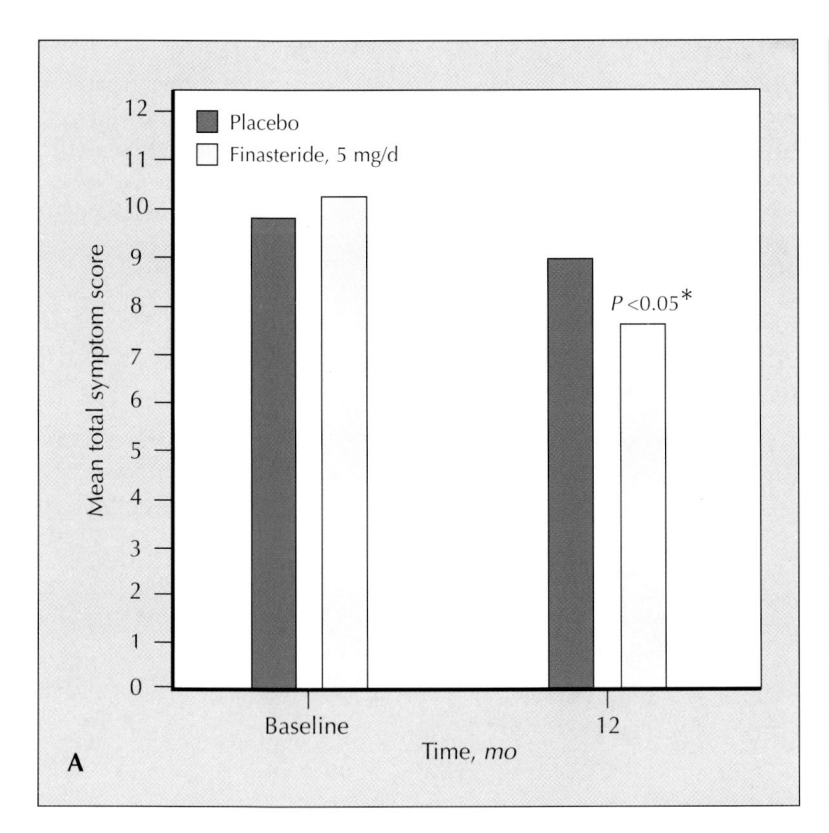

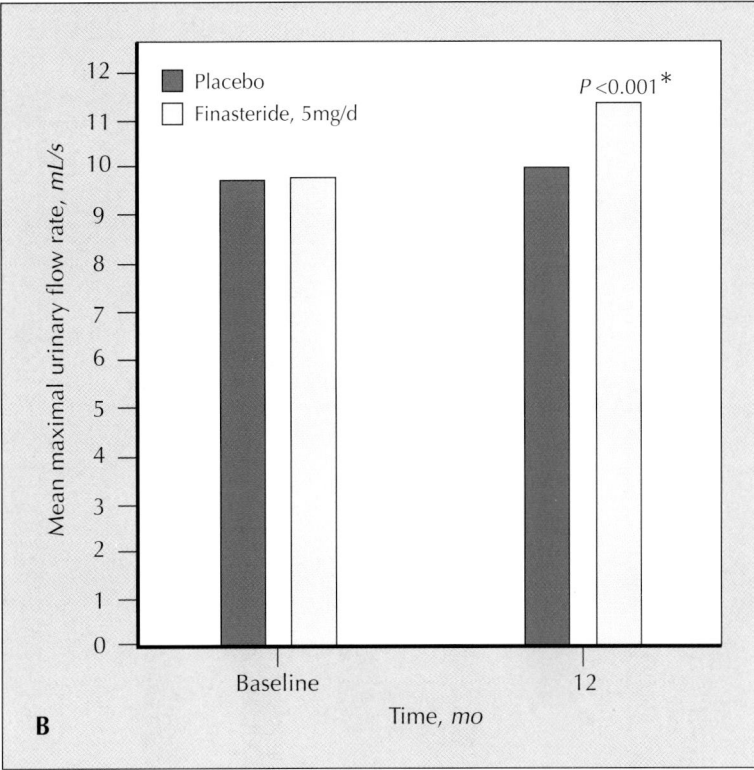

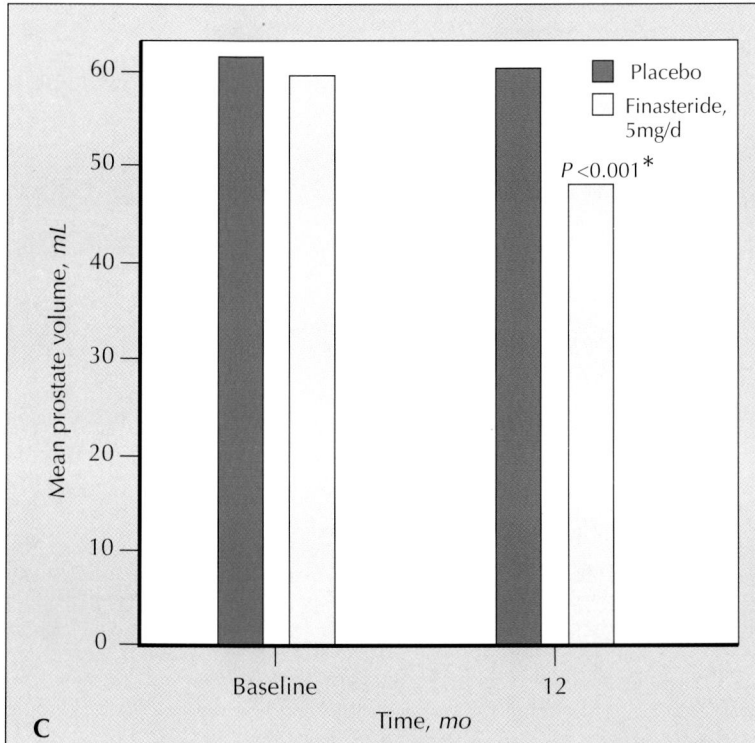

FIGURE 3-10. Results of 1-year clinical trials with finasteride. Entry criteria for initial multicenter, randomized, double-blind, placebo-controlled studies with finasteride included men with lower urinary tract symptoms, a maximum urinary flow rate of less 15 mL/s, and an enlarged prostate on digital rectal examinations. The data revealed a mean decrease in circulating dihydrotestosterone levels of 80% that was sustained without escape during 12 months of treatment and without significant change in circulating serum testosterone levels [35,36]. **A,** Total symptom scores decreased by approximately 20%, or 2 to 3 points. **B,** Improvements in maximum and mean urinary flow rates were on the order of 1.6 and 0.6 mL/s, respectively, after 12 months of treatment. **C,** Prostate volume decreased by approximately 20% to 30% [36–38] after 6 months of treatment and remained at that level after 1 year of treatment with finasteride. Side effects of decreased libido, impotence, and ejaculatory disorder were noted in 3% to 5% of patients. All of these changes were statistically significant compared with findings of the placebo group. *Asterisk* indicates that the *P* value is versus placebo.

Medical Management of Benign Prostatic Hyperplasia

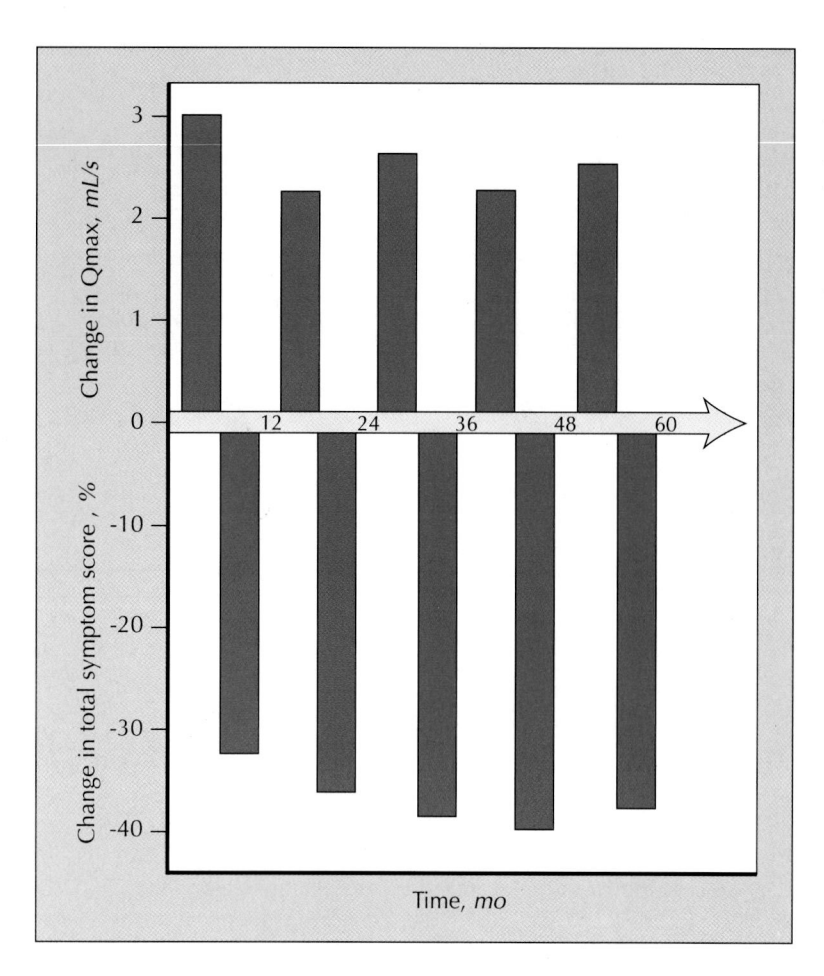

FIGURE 3-11. Long-term clinical results with finasteride. Longer-term multicenter placebo-controlled studies, up to 36 months of treatment with finasteride, reveal continued statistically significant improvement in symptom scores, maximum urinary flow rates, and decrease in prostate size when compared with placebo [38–41]. Men with larger prostates and lower urinary flow rates appear to benefit most from treatment with finasteride [42]. Results of 5-year treatment with finasteride are shown. Qmax—maximum urine flow.

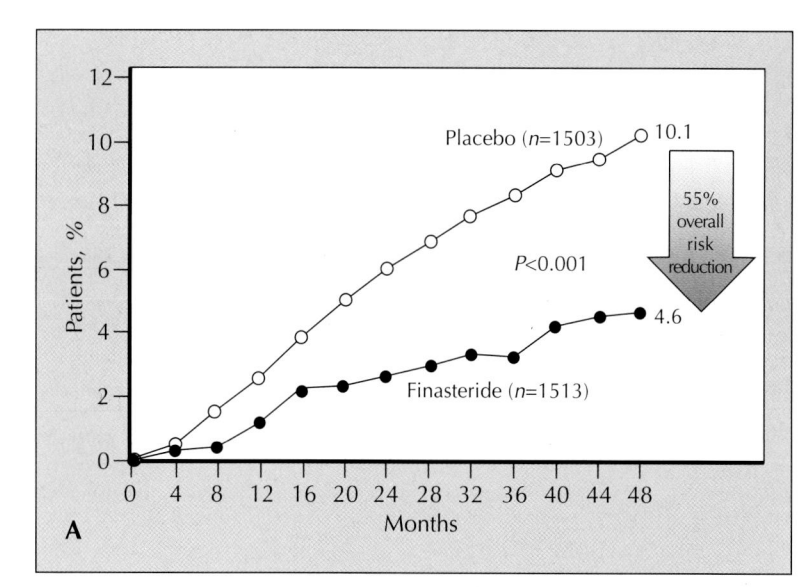

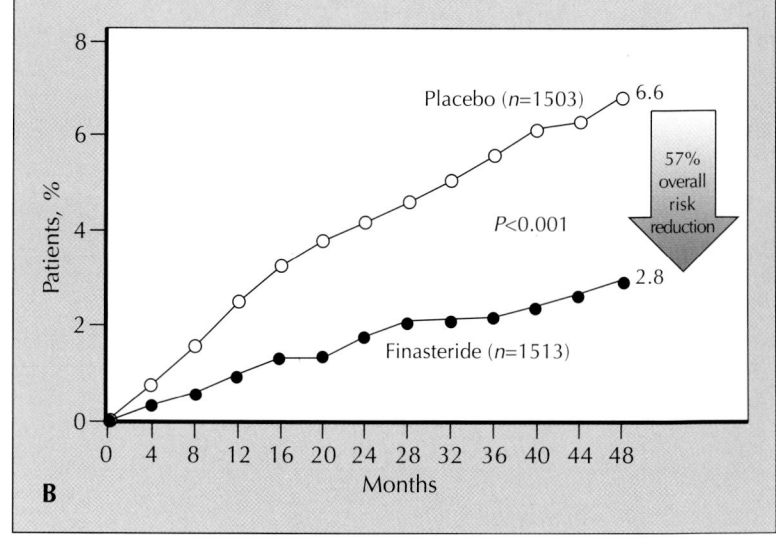

FIGURE 3-12. Effect of finasteride on the risk of acute urinary retention (**A**) and benign prostatic hyperplasia (BPH)-related surgery (**B**). Several large-scale population-based longitudinal epidemiologic studies of aging reveal an increased risk of acute urinary retention and BPH-related surgery (*eg,* transurethral resection of the prostate) over time for men with obstructive urinary symptoms and enlarged prostates [43,44]. Finasteride reduced the risk of acute urinary retention by 57% and the need for BPH-related surgery by 55% compared with placebo during the 4-year study period of a randomized, double-blind, multicenter trial that enrolled over 3000 men. (*Adapted from* McConnell *et al.* [41].)

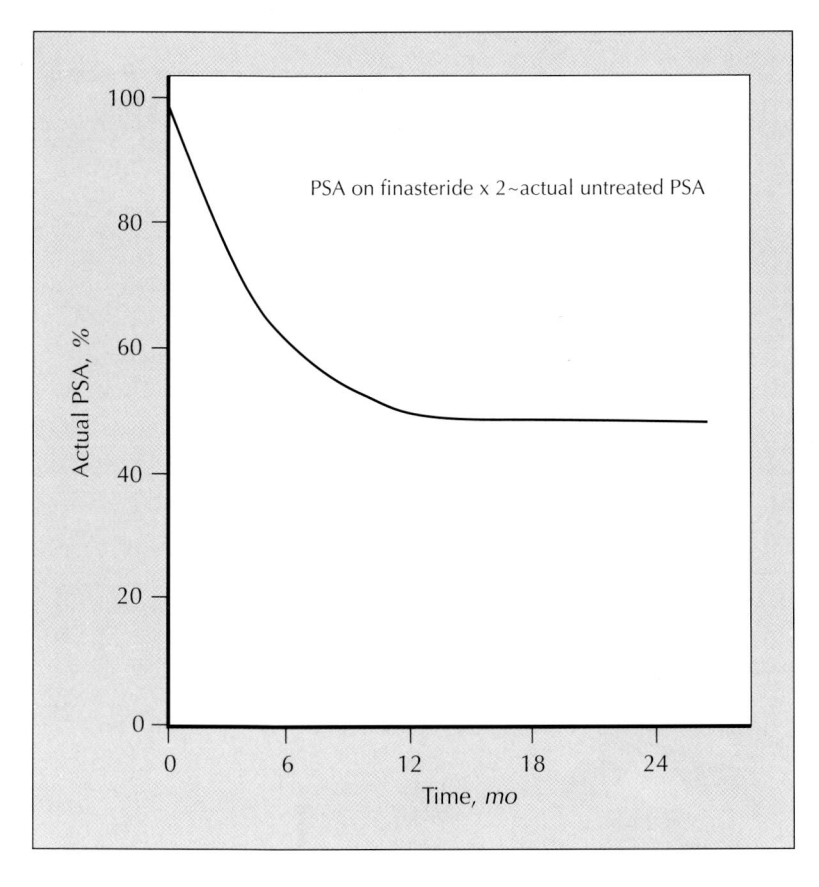

FIGURE 3-13. Effect of treatment with finasteride on prostate-specific antigen (PSA) levels over time. Prostate cancer is the most common non-skin cancer affecting men and the third most common cause of cancer death in American men. Early detection of prostate cancer has been enhanced since the introduction of the PSA screening assay. PSA is an enzyme produced by the prostate and is usually only detectable at low levels in the blood. Most men with prostate cancer have elevated serum levels of PSA. Other variables that can increase PSA levels include prostatitis, prostate infarction, and recent ejaculation. In addition, as prostate volume increases secondary to benign prostatic hyperplasia, PSA values tend to rise. Treatment with finasteride decreases serum PSA levels by approximately 50% [36,46]. Because benign prostatic hyperplasia and prostate cancer can coexist in the same patient, there has been some concern regarding the detection of prostate cancer in patients taking finasteride [47]. Stoner et al. [47] showed that despite a 560% decrease in intraprostatic concentrations of testosterone, there appears to be no increased risk of prostate cancer for patients taking finasteride. Doubling the serum PSA for patients taking finasteride and then interpreting the resulting PSA value as in untreated men has been recommended [46]. A recent study by Oesterling et al. [48] seems to indicate that doubling PSA levels in finasteride-treated patients allows for appropriate interpretation of PSA and does not mask the detection of prostate cancer. Any sustained increases in PSA levels during finasteride treatment should be carefully evaluated, including consideration of noncompliance with therapy. To date, no clinical benefit has been demonstrated in prostate cancer patients treated with finasteride.

Adverse Effects of Hormonal Therapy

Effect	LHRH Agonists, %	Antiandrogens, %	5α-Reductase Inhibitors, %
Impotence	95–100	10–20	3–4
Loss of libido	95–100	10–20	4–5
Ejaculatory disorder	—	—	4–5
Hot flashes	95–100	—	—
Gynecomastia	0–5	50–100	—
Diarrhea	—	50	—

FIGURE 3-14. Adverse effects of hormonal therapy. The most deleterious effects of agents that alter the hypothalamic-gonadal axis at different levels along the pathway are related to varying degrees of sexual dysfunction. Interventions that markedly lower serum testosterone levels are associated with greater degrees of sexual dysfunction (eg, loss of libido) than are agents that block the effect of testosterone on target organs. LHRH—luteinizing hormone–releasing hormone. (*Data from* Physician's Desk Reference [49].)

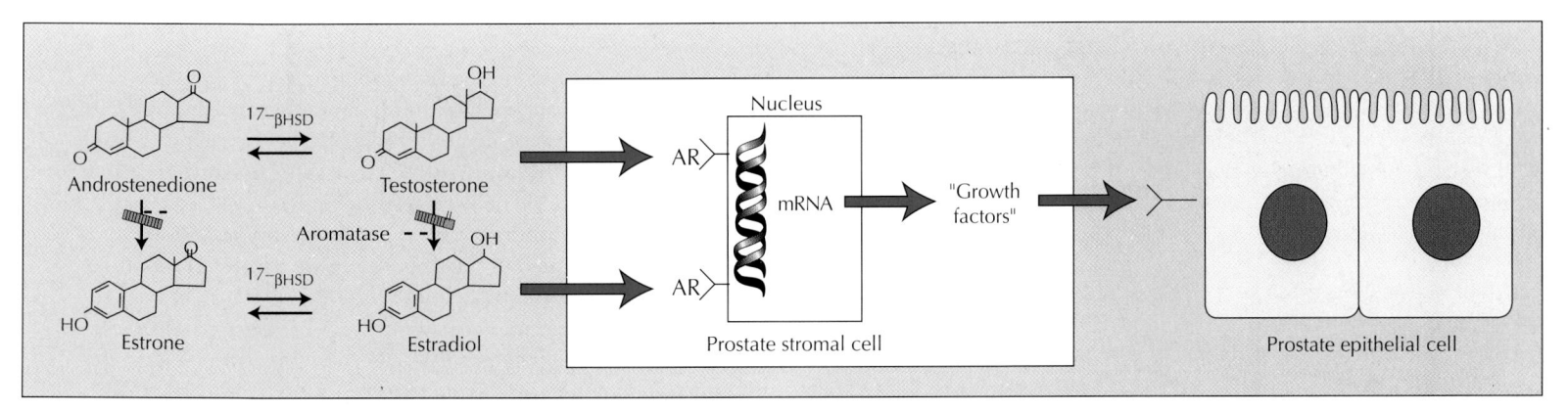

FIGURE 3-15. Effects of estrogens on the pathophysiology of benign prostatic hyperplasia (BPH). As men age, there is a direct correlation between prostate volume and increased serum levels of free testosterone, estradiol, and estriol [50]. In a canine model of BPH, experiments have shown estrogens to act synergistically with androgens in the formation of BPH by inducing the androgen receptor, promoting increased prostatic concentrations of dihydrotestosterone, and reducing the rate of prostate cell death [51–53]. BPH can be induced in castrated dogs via supplementation with aromatizable androgens, and this effect can be blocked by concomitant administration of aromatase inhibitors that prevent conversion of testosterone to estrogen [54]. Clinical studies using aromatase inhibitors, such as atamestane or testolactone, as monotherapy for the treatment of BPH have failed to yield encouraging results [55–57]. Failure of aromatase inhibitors to improve BPH symptomatology may be related to a simultaneous rise in testosterone concentration that leads to glandular epithelial hyperplasia of the prostate [55]. AR—androgen receptor; β-HSD—β-hydroxysteroid dehydrogenase; ER—estrogen receptor.

Medical Management of Benign Prostatic Hyperplasia

ALTERING THE DYNAMIC COMPONENT OF BENIGN PROSTATIC HYPERPLASIA THROUGH α-BLOCKER THERAPY

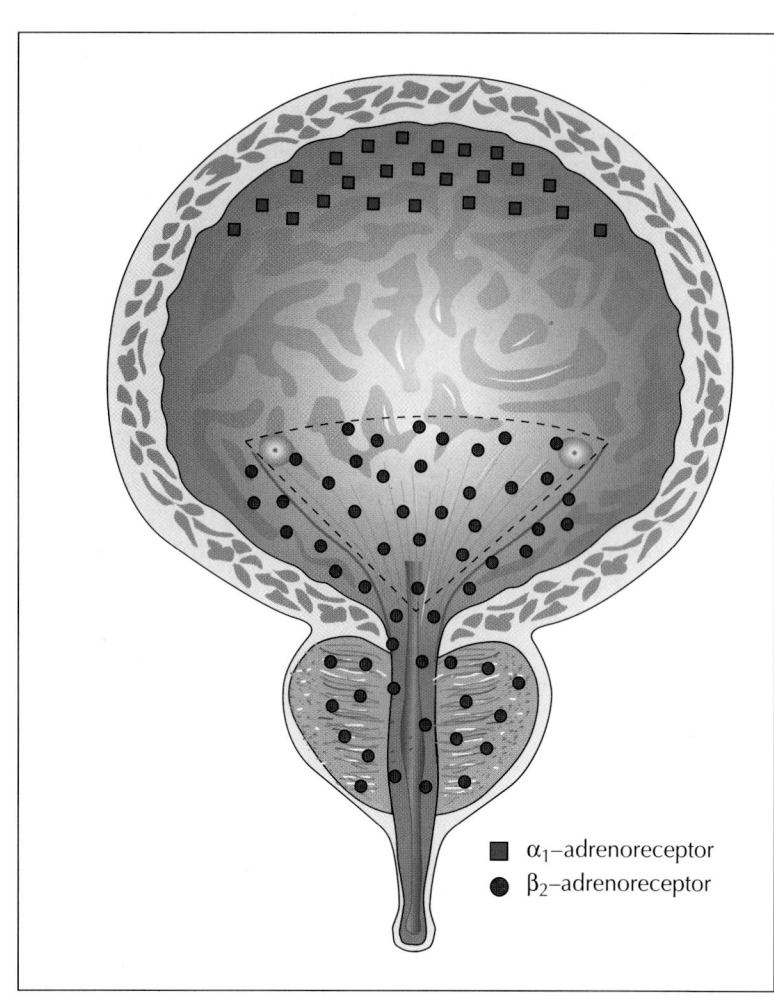

FIGURE 3-16. Distribution of α-andrenoreceptor subtypes in the lower urinary tract. α_1-Adrenoreceptors are abundant within the trigone, bladder neck, smooth muscle of the prostatic stroma, and prostate capsule [56]. Experiments have shown that in the presence of norepinephrine, mediated by the α_1-receptor, the human prostate adenoma and capsule contract [56–58]. In fact, experimental evidence suggests that approximately 40% of urethral pressure in patients with benign prostatic hyperplasia (BPH) is believed to be secondary to sympathetic innervation via α-adrenergic receptors [59]. Therefore, although the mass of obstructing BPH tissue is not reduced, α_1 blockers are believed to improve micturition parameters and symptoms by decreasing the dynamic resting tone of the prostate, thereby decreasing bladder outlet obstruction.

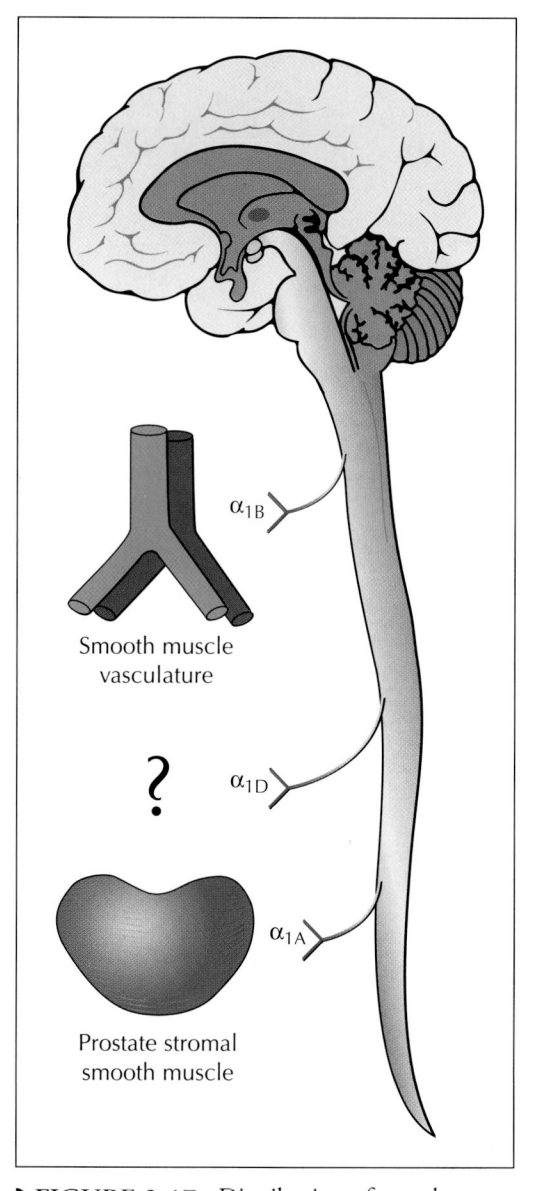

FIGURE 3-17. Distribution of α_1-adrenoreceptor subtypes. α-Receptors are distributed ubiquitously throughout the human body [60]. There are two different subtypes of the α-receptor [61,62]. α_2-Receptors are located presynaptically and cause downregulation of norepinephrine release via negative feedback [60,61]. α_1-Adrenoreceptors are further categorized into α_{1A}, α_{1B}, and α_{1D} subtypes [60,61]. α_{1B}-Receptors are located in the smooth muscle of arteries and veins. Blockade of these α_{1B}-receptors in the cardiovascular system leads to a decreased total peripheral resistance via veno- and arterial dilatation. The function of the α_{1D}-receptors is currently unknown. Within the prostate, α_{1A}-receptors are the predominant subtype, with a smaller proportion of α_{1B}-receptors located in the prostate microvasculature [62]. Contraction of prostate smooth muscle is believed to be mediated via the α_{1A}-receptor [63].

Randomized, Placebo-Controlled, Double-Blind Studies of Phenoxybenzamine

Study	Year	Patients, n	Dose, mg	Follow-up, wk	↑ Qmax, mL/s	↓ PVR, %
Caine et al. [64]	1978	50	20	2	6.2*	NR
Abrams et al. [65]	1982	41	20	4	3.1*	60*
Ferrie and Paterson [66]	1987	45	10	5	1.7	36

Statistically significant compared with placebo-based values.

▶ **FIGURE 3-18.** Randomized, placebo-controlled, double-blind studies of phenoxybenzamine. Phenoxybenzamine, a nonselective α-blocker that competitively inhibits both α_1- and α_2-adrenoreceptors, was the first α-blocker used for the treatment of benign prostatic hyperplasia [65]. In several short-term, randomized, placebo-controlled clinical studies, phenoxybenzamine, at a dose of 20 mg daily, increased maximum urinary flow rates on the order of 3 to 6 mL/s [64,65]. However, adverse effects in more than 40% of patients treated, including tiredness, dizziness, impaired ejaculation, nasal stuffiness, and difficulty with visual accommodation, have limited its clinical usefulness [64,66]. In addition, phenoxybenzamine has been withdrawn from the market in several countries after in vitro testing revealed increased rates of mutagenicity [67]. NR—not reported; Qmax—maximum volume of blood; PVR—peripheral vascular resistance.

Randomized, Placebo-Controlled, Double-Blind Studies of Prazosin

Study	Year	Patients, n	Dose, mg	Follow-up, wk	↑ Qmax, mL/s	↓ PVR, %
Hedlund et al. [68]	1983	20	4	4	2.2*	NR
Kirby et al. [69]	1987	80	4	4	4.3*	21
Chapple et al. [70]	1990	58	4	12	2.4	↑39
Le Duc et al. [71]	1990	39	4	4	3.2	31
Chapple et al. [72]	1992	93	4	12	2.4*	56

Statistically significant compared with placebo-based values.

▶ **FIGURE 3-19.** Randomized, placebo-controlled, double-blind studies of prazosin. Prazosin, a short-acting α_1-selective blocker, at a dose of 2 mg twice daily, has been documented to increase maximum urinary flow rates on the order of 2 to 4 mL/s in several short-term placebo-controlled clinical trials [68–72]. Unfortunately, these studies lack specific qualitative assessment of symptomatic outcome with treatment as compared with placebo. NR—not reported; PVR—postvoid residual volume; Qmax—maximum volume of blood.

Randomized, Placebo-Controlled, Double-Blind Phase-III Clinical Trials of Terazosin

Study	Year	Patients, n	Dose, mg	Follow-up, wk	↑ Qmax, mL/s	↓ Symptom Score, %
Fabricius and MacHannaford [73]	1990	30	10	12	2.3*	NR
Lepor et al. [74]	1992	285	2–10	12	0.7–1.3*	23–44*
Lepor et al. [75]	1992	199	2–20	24	1.5*	33*
Brawer et al. [76]	1993	160	1–10	24	1.4*	31*
Debruyne et al. [77]	1995	427	5–10	26	3.2*	55*
Roehrborn et al. [78]	1996	2084	2–10	52	2.2*	38*

Statistically significant compared with placebo-based values.

▶ **FIGURE 3-20.** Randomized, placebo-controlled, double-blind phase-III clinical trials of terazosin. The efficacy of terazosin, a long-acting selective α_1-blocker that allows for once-daily dosing, has been documented in numerous clinical trials [73–78]. The largest of these clinical trials, The Hytrin Community Assessment Trial, is representative of results obtained in patients treated with terazosin [78]. This study enrolled 2084 men at least 55 years of age with moderate to severe symptoms of benign prostatic hyperplasia and peak urinary flow rates less than 15 mL/s. Patients were randomly assigned to treatment with either placebo or terazosin in a titrate to effect dosing. After 1 year of treatment, peak flow increased an average of 2.2 mL/s, and symptom scores decreased a mean of 38% compared with baseline. Both changes were statistically significant compared with the findings from placebo. In addition, a quality of life score was significantly improved in the terazosin-treated group versus the placebo-treated group. Treatment failure occurred in 11% of the terazosin group. Withdrawal from the study due to adverse effect of treatment occurred in 20% of the terazosin group. NR—not reported; Qmax—maximum urine flow.

Randomized, Placebo-Controlled, Double-Blind Phase-III Clinical Trials of Doxazosin

Study	Year	Patients, n	Dose, mg	Follow-up, wk	↑ Qmax, mL/s	↓ Symptom Score, %
Gillenwater and Mobley [79]	1993	100	8	6	2.9*	56*
Janknegt and Chapple [80]	1993	456	1–16	4–29	1.2–3.9*	NR
Chapple et al. [81]	1994	135	4	12	1.0	NR
Holme et al. [82]	1994	100	4	29	1.7*	NR
Fawzy et al. [83]	1995	100	2–8	16	2.9*	40*
Gillenwater et al. [84]	1995	216	2–12	16	2.3–3.6*	NR
Kirby [85]	1995	232	4	9–12	2–2.4*	NR

*Statistically significant compared with placebo-based values.

▶ **FIGURE 3-21.** Randomized, placebo-controlled, double-blind phase-III clinical trials of doxazosin. Doxazosin is also a long-acting selective α_1-blocker allowing for once-daily dosing. Short-term clinical trials have shown doxazosin to increase peak flow rates by about 1 to 4 mL/s and decrease symptom scores by 30% to 50% in men with symptomatic benign prostatic hyperplasia (BPH) [79–85]. The clinical response to α-blockers in terms of decreased symptomatology and increased flow rates in men with symptomatic BPH is dose dependent; however, the side effect profile is also dose dependent. Studies attempting to determine variables, such as patient's age, prostate size, total symptom score, and flow rate, that are predictive of the clinical response to α-blockers have failed to delineate a significant association between baseline factors and treatment effect. NR—not reported; Qmax—maximum urine flow.

Randomized, Placebo-Controlled, Double-Blind Phase-III Clinical Trials of Tamsulosin

Study	Year	Patients, n	Dose, mg	Follow-up, wk	↑ Qmax, mL/s	↓ Symptom Score, %	PVR, %
Abrams et al. [87]	1995	296	0.4	12	1.4*	36*	21*
Lepor et al. [88]	1995	1488	0.4	13	1.8*	42*	NR
Chapple et al. [89]	1996	575	0.4	12	1.6*	35*	23*

*Statistically significant compared with placebo-based values.

▶ **FIGURE 3-22.** Randomized, placebo-controlled, double-blind phase-III clinical trials of tamsulosin. Pharmacokinetic studies have demonstrated tamsulosin to be a long-acting α-blocker with selectivity for the α_{1A}-adrenoreceptor [86]. Theoretically, a prostate-specific α-blocker would maximize clinical efficacy while minimizing side effects. Short-term clinical studies to date have shown tamsulosin to increase peak flow rates approximately 1.5 mL/s and to decrease symptom scores by about 35% [88–90]. The side effect profile appears similar to that of other long-acting agents such as terazosin or doxazosin. Longer term clinical trials are pending. NR—not reported; PVR—postvoid residual volume; Qmax—maximum urine flow.

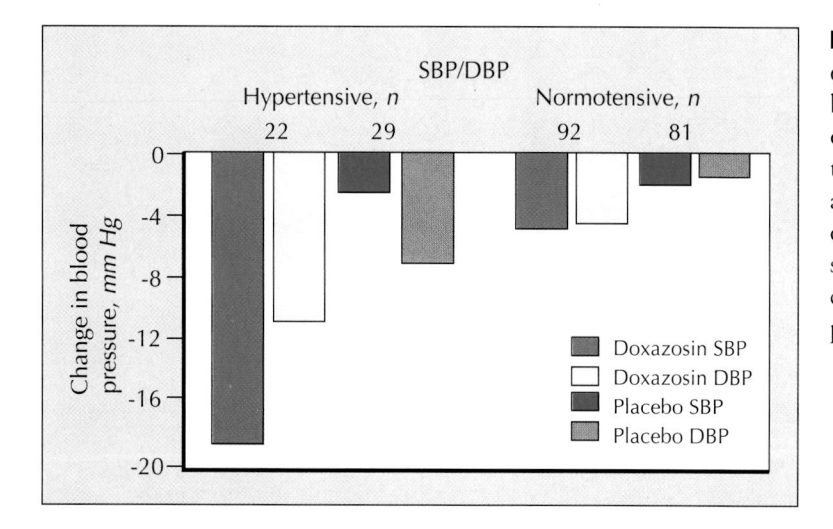

▶ **FIGURE 3-23.** Cardiovascular effects of α-blockers. Long-acting α-blockers in doses used to treat benign prostatic hyperplasia (BPH) have been shown to cause clinically insignificant decreases in the blood pressure of normotensive patients [90–92]. However, these same doses used for the treatment of BPH in hypertensive men have been noted to cause larger and clinically significant decreases in blood pressure [90–92]. The effect of doxazosin on blood pressure in hypertensive and normotensive men is shown. In addition, α-blockers have been shown to lower serum lipid and cholesterol levels. DBP—diastolic blood pressure; SBP—systolic blood pressure. (*Adapted from* Kirby [85].)

Adverse Effects of α-Blockers

Effect	Prazosin, %	Phenoxybenzamine, %	Terazosin, %	Doxazosin, %	Tamsulosin, %
Hypotension	10–15	15–20	2–8	1–2	<1
Dizziness	15–17	10–14	7–14	10–15	15
Headache	13–15	4–15	4–10	9–10	19
Sexual dysfunction	NI	5–8	2–7	NI	8
Fatigue	10	10–15	4–8	1–2	8
Syncope	NI	NI	<1	<1	<1
Nasal congestion	NI	8	2	NI	13

▶ **FIGURE 3-24.** Adverse effects of α-blockers. Dizziness, lightheadedness, and asthenia are the most common side effects noted with selective long-acting α-blockers. The incidence of hypotension decreases with the use of longer- compared with shorter-acting agents. Dizziness and hypotension appear to be slightly more common in men over 65 years of age. The mechanism of orthostatic hypotension is most probably secondary to α-agonist–induced vasodilation of arteriolar smooth muscle. Most of these side effects are mild and usually do not require dose reduction. Bedtime dosing of α-blockers appears to reduce the incidence and severity of these side effects. (*Data from* Physician's Desk Reference [49].)

Combination Therapy for the Treatment of Benign Prostatic Hyperplasia

Agent	Patients, n	Qmax, mL/s	Symptom Score, units	Prostate Volume, mL
Placebo	254	1.4	-2.6	0.5
Terazosin	256	2.7	-6.1	0.5
Finasteride	243	1.6	-3.2	-6.1
Terazosin + finasteride	254	3.2	-6.2	-7.0

▶ **FIGURE 3-25.** Combination therapy for the treatment of benign prostatic hyperplasia (BPH). The Veterans Affairs Cooperative Study [94] attempted to determine whether terazosin, finasteride, or a combination of the two resulted in clinically superior results for the treatment of BPH. In this multicenter, double-blind trial, patients were randomly assigned to treatment with placebo, terazosin, finasteride, or a combination of terazosin and finasteride. After 1 year of treatment, the investigators concluded that terazosin alone produced superior results in terms of improvement in symptom score and peak urinary flow rates. The applicability of this study's conclusion to the general population of men with symptomatic BPH has been challenged because of the relatively small percentage of men with larger prostates included in this study [94]. Qmax—maximum urine flow.

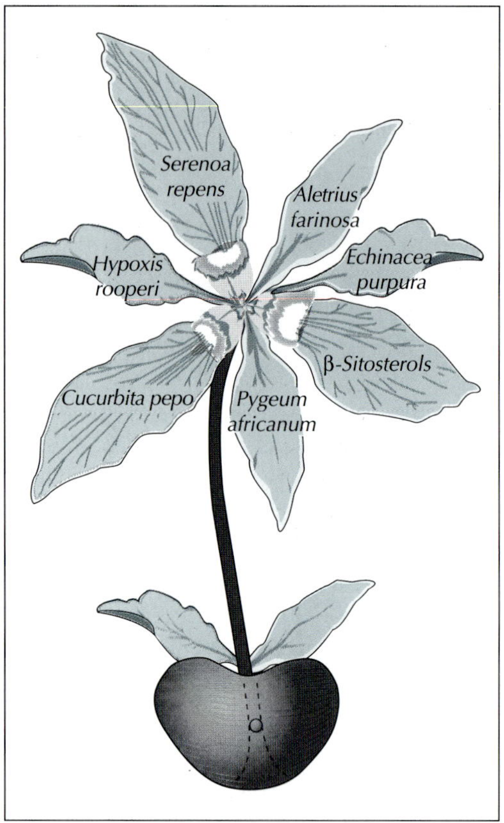

FIGURE 3-26. Phytotherapy. Phytotherapy refers to the use of plants or plant extracts for medicinal purposes. Since ancient times, a variety of phytotherapeutic agents have been used for the treatment of benign prostatic hyperplasia (BPH). Unfortunately, few of these agents have undergone formal scientific testing to determine clinical efficacy. The reported effect of phytotherapeutic agents used to treat BPH is believed to be mediated by phytosterols. Phytosterols are compounds chemically related to cholesterol, of which sitosterol is purported to be the most important [95]. Proposed mechanisms of sitosterol in alleviating the symptoms of BPH include 1) anti-inflammatory effects via interference with prostaglandin synthesis, 2) alteration of cholesterol metabolism, 3) direct inhibition of prostate growth, 4) antiandrogenic or antiestrogenic effects or both, and 5) decrease in available sex hormone binding globulin [95].

Double-Blind Studies of *Serenoa repens* for the Treatment of Benign Prostatic Hyperplasia

Study	Year	Dose, mg	Patients, n	Follow-up, mo	Symptom Score	↑ Qmax, mL/s
Boccafoschi and Annoscia [96]	1983	320	22	2	↓	4.1*
Emili *et al.* [97]	1983	320	30	1	↓	3.4*
Champault *et al.* [98]	1984	320	110	1	↓	3.0*
Tasca *et al.* [99]	1985	320	30	1–3	↓	3.3*
Reece Smith *et al.* [100]	1986	320	70	3	-	2.5
Carbin *et al.* [101]	1990	480	53	3	↓	3.0*

*Statistically significant compared with placebo-based values.

FIGURE 3-27. Double-blind studies of *Serenoa repens* for the treatment of benign prostate hyperplasia (BPH). *S. repens*, more commonly known as the saw palmetto berry, is the most widely used phytotherapeutic agent and serves as an example of the shortcomings of research regarding the use of phytomedicinals for treating BPH. Several clinical trials [96–99,101] have documented statistically significant decreased symptom scores and increased flow rates in men using *S. repens*; however, this finding has not been universally validated [101]. The shortcomings of clinical research on the use of phytotherapeutic agents for the symptomatic treatment of BPH include 1) lack of uniform inclusion and exclusion criteria for study patients, 2) lack of standardized symptom score analysis, 3) varying purity of different phytotherapeutic preparations, and 4) short-term duration of reported studies. Because of the increasingly prevalent use of phytotherapeutic agents among symptomatic BPH patients and because of associated costs, well-designed, placebo-controlled, long-term clinical trials of various phytotherapeutic agents would be beneficial to assess clinical efficacy. Qmax—maximum urine flow.

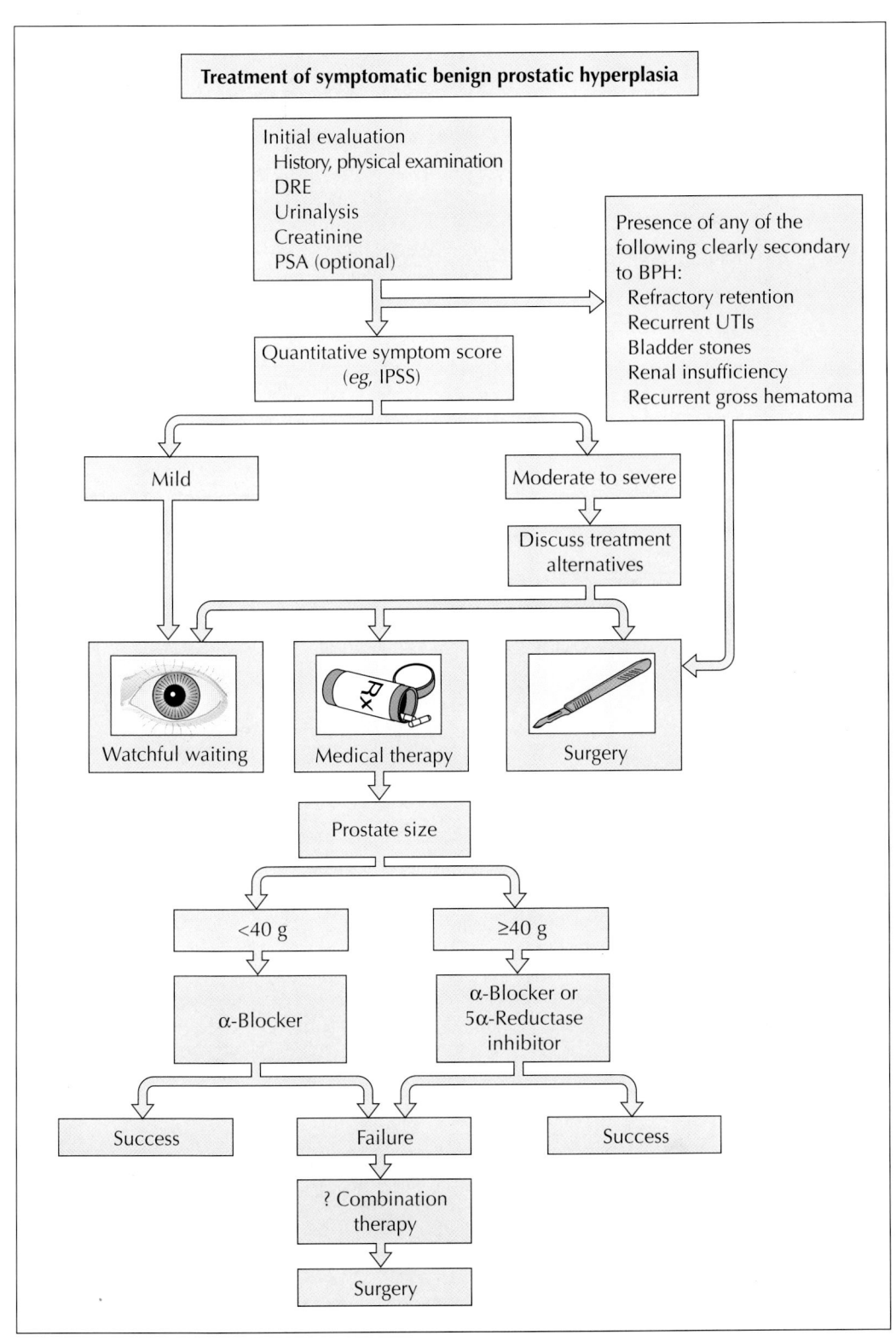

FIGURE 3-28. Treatment algorithm for symptomatic benign prostatic hyperplasia (BPH). In general, highly symptomatic patients or patients suffering from acute urinary retention tend to respond more rapidly to treatment with α-blockers than to other currently available agents. Therefore, when prompt symptomatic relief is of utmost importance, α-blockers are a logical first-line treatment choice in men with moderate to severe symptoms, seeking medical treatment. For men with prostate glands 40 g or larger, finasteride should be given consideration as either monotherapy or combination therapy with an α-blocker. DRE—digital rectal examination; IPSS—International Prostate Symptom Score; PSA—prostate specific antigen; UTI—urinary tract infection.

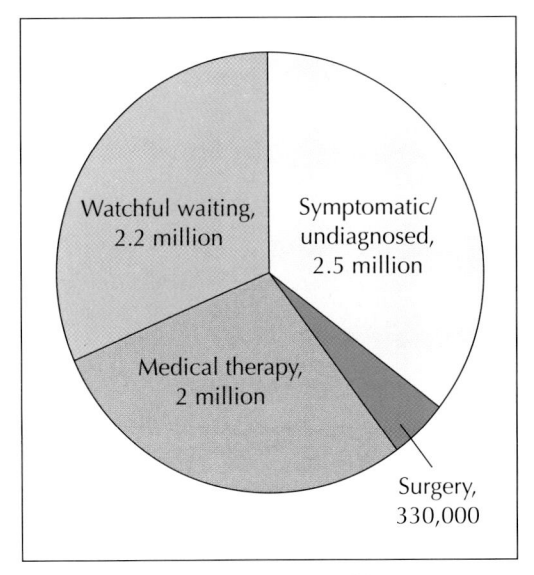

FIGURE 3-29. Prevalence of benign prostatic hyperplasia (BPH) and treatment trends. BPH will remain the predominant disease that urologists treat. As the average life span continues to increase, the number of potential patients with symptomatic BPH will continue to rise. Most recent statistics show that, currently, 7 million men suffer from clinical BPH. Due to its noninvasiveness, medical therapy will most likely be the most commonly used initial treatment.

Medical Management of Benign Prostatic Hyperplasia

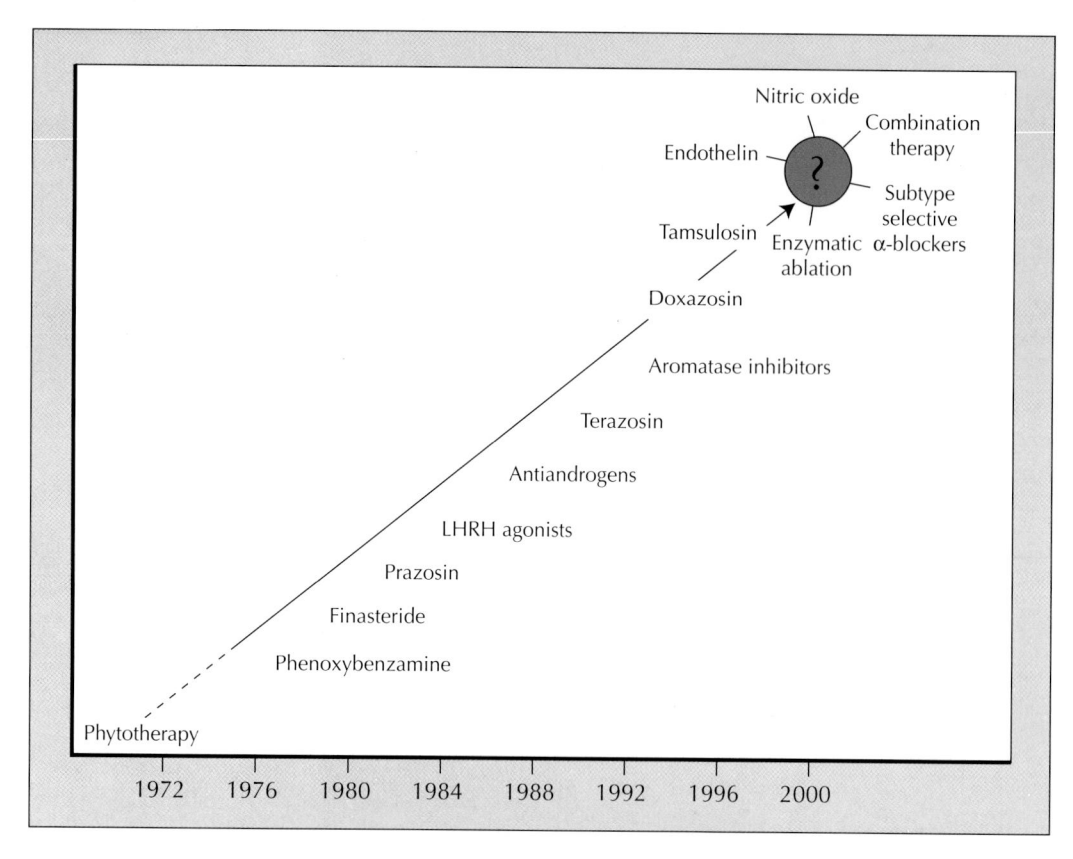

FIGURE 30. Timeline for the medical management of benign prostatic hyperplasia (BPH). Although medical therapy will continue to be the most commonly used treatment for symptomatic BPH, future strategies for the medical management of BPH are evolving. The ideal agent will produce symptomatic relief of both irritative and obstructive voiding symptoms of long duration without tachyphylaxis; allow for once daily dosing to increase compliance; have a rapid onset of action; be prostate specific and have minimal side effects; increase maximum flow rates while lowering voiding pressures; and halt the progression of BPH. As we learn more about the pathophysiology of BPH, it is hoped that more specific treatments will emerge. LHRH—luteinizing hormone–releasing hormone.

REFERENCES

1. Berry SJ, Coffey DS, Walsh PC: The development of human prostatic hyperplasia with age. *J Urol* 1984, 132:474–479.
2. Benign Prostatic Hyperplasia Guideline Panel: *Benign Prostatic Hyperplasia: Diagnosis and Treatment. Clinical Practice Guideline, Number 8.* Rockville, MD: US Department of Health and Human Services; 1994. [AHCPR publication no. 94-0582, February, 1994.]
3. Holtgrewe HL: Economic issues and the management of benign prostatic hyperplasia. *Urology* 1995, 46(suppl):23–25.
4. Miller TA: BPH Survey.
5. Glynn RJ, Campion EW, Bouchard GR, et al.: The development of benign prostatic hyperplasia among volunteers in the Normative Aging Study. *Am J Epidemiol* 1985, 121:78–90.
6. Guess HA, Chute CG, Garraway WM, et al.: The cumulative prevalence of prostatism matches the autopsy prevalence of benign prostatic hyperplasia. *Prostate* 1990, 17:241–246.
7. Chute CG, Panser LA, Girman CJ, et al.: The prevalence of prostatism: a population based survey of urinary symptoms. *J Urol* 1993, 150:85–89.
8. Clark R: The prostate and the endocrines: a control series. *Br J Urol* 1937, 9:254–271.
9. Craigen AA, Hickling JB, Saunders CRG, et al.: Natural history of prostatic obstruction: a prospective survey. *J R Coll Gen Pract* 1969, 18:226–232.
10. Birkhoff JD, Wiederhorn AR, Hamilton ML, et al.: Natural history of benign prostatic hypertrophy and acute urinary retention. *Urology* 1976, 7:48–52.
11. Ball AJ, Fenely RCL, Abrams PH: The natural history of untreated "prostatism." *Br J Urol* 1981, 53:613–616.
12. Nickel JC: The Canadian PROSPECT Study Group: placebo therapy in benign prostatic hyperplasia [abstract]. *Br J Urol* 1997, 80(suppl):194.
13. Hansen BJ, Meyerhoff HH, Nordling J, et al.: Placebo effects in the pharmacological treatment of uncomplicated benign prostatic hyperplasia. *Scand J Urol Nephrol* 1996, 30:373–377.
14. Isaacs JT, Coffey DS: Changes in DHT metabolism associated with the development of canine benign prostatic hyperplasia. *Endocrinology* 1981, 108:445–453.
15. Peters CA, Walsh PC: The effect of nafarelin acetate, a luteinizing-hormone-releasing agonist, on benign prostatic hyperplasia. *N Engl J Med* 1987, 317:599–604.
16. Gabrilove JL, Levine AC, Kirschenbaum A, Droller M: Effect of long-acting gonadotropin-releasing hormone (leuprolide) therapy on prostatic size and symptoms in 15 men with benign prostatic hyperplasia. *J Clin Endocrinol Metab* 1989, 69:629–632.
17. Eri LM, Tveter KJ: A prospective, placebo-controlled study of luteinizing hormone–releasing hormone agonist leuprolide as treatment for patients with benign prostatic hyperplasia. *J Urol* 1993, 150:359–364.
18. Stone NN, Ray PS, Smith JA, et al.: A double-blind randomized controlled study of the effect of flutamide on benign prostatic hypertrophy: clinical efficacy [abstract]. *J Urol* 1989, 141:240A.
19. Eri LM, Tveter KJ: A prospective, placebo-controlled study of the antiandrogen Casodex as treatment for patients with benign prostatic hyperplasia. *J Urol* 1993, 150:90–94.
20. Coffey D: The molecular biology, endocrinology and physiology of the prostate and seminal vesicles. In *Campbell's Urology*, edn 6. Edited by Walsh PC et al. Philadelphia: WB Saunders; 1992:221–266.
21. Cabot AT: The question of castration for enlarged prostate. *Ann Surg* 1896, 24:265–309.
22. White JW: The results of double castration in hypertrophy of the prostate. *Ann Surg* 1895, 22:1–80.
23. Schroder FH, Westerhof M, Bosch RJL, Kurth KH: Benign prostatic hyperplasia treated by castration or the LH-RH analogue Buserelin: a report of 6 cases. *Eur Urol* 1986, 12:318–321.
24. Imperato-McGinley J, Guevro L, Gauteri T, Petersen RE: Steroid 5-α-reductase deficiency in a man: an inherited form of pseudohermaphroditism. *Science* 1974, 186:1213–1215.
25. Imperato-Mcginley J, Gauteri T, Zirinsky K, et al.: Prostate visualization studies in males, homozygous and heterozygous with 5α-reductase deficiency. *J Clin Endocrinol Metab* 1992, 75:1022–1026.
26. Walsh PC, Madden JD, Harrod MJ, et al.: Familial incomplete male pseudohermaphroditism type II. Decreased dihydrotestosterone formation in pseudovaginal perineoscrotal hypospadias. *N Engl J Med* 1974, 291:944–949.
27. Coffey DS: The endocrine control of normal and abnormal growth of the prostate. In *Urologic Endocrinology.* Edited by Jacob Rajfer Philadelphia: WB Saunders; 1986:170–193.

28. Thigpen AE, Davis DL, Milatovitch A, et al.: Molecular genetics of steroid 5α-reductase-2 deficiency. *J Clin Invest* 1992, 90:799–809.

29. Liang T, Cascieri MA, Cheung AH, et al.: Species differences in prostatic steroid 5α-reductases of rat, dog and human. *Endocrinology* 1985, 117:571–579.

30. Brooks JR, Berman D, Glitzer MS, et al.: Effect of a new 5α-reductase inhibitor on size, histologic characteristics, and androgen concentrations of the canine prostate. *Prostate* 1982, 3:35–44.

31. McConnell J, Akakura K, Bartsch G, et al.: Hormonal treatment of benign prostatic hyperplasia. In *The 2nd International Consultation on Benign Prostatic Hyperplasia (BPH)*, Proceedings 2. Edited by Cocket ATK, Khourg S, Aso Y, et al. Paris: Scientific Communications International; 1993:417.

32. Vermeulen A, Giagulli VA, Schepper PD, et al.: Hormonal effects of an orally active 4-azosteroid inhibitor of 5-α reductase in humans. *Eur Urol* 1991, 20(suppl 2):82–86.

33. McConnell JD, Wilson JD, George FW, et al.: Finasteride, an inhibitor of 5α-reductase, suppresses prostatic dihydrotestosterone in men with benign prostatic hyperplasia. *J Clin Endocrinol Metab* 1992, 74:505–508.

34. Geller J: Effect of finasteride, a 5α-reductase inhibitor on prostatic tissue androgens and prostatic specific antigen. *J Clin Endocrinol Metab* 1990, 71:1552–1555.

35. The MK406 (Finasteride) Study Group: A one year experience in the treatment of benign prostatic hyperplasia with finasteride. *J Androl* 1991, 12:372.

36. Gormley GJ, Stoner E, Bruskewitz RC, et al.: The effect of finasteride in men with benign prostatic hyperplasia. *N Engl J Med* 1992, 327:1185–1191.

37. Stoner E and The Finasteride Study Group: The clinical effects of a 5α-reductase inhibitor, finasteride, on benign prostatic hyperplasia. *J Urol* 1992, 147:1298–1302.

38. The Finasteride Study Group: Finasteride (MK-406) in the treatment of benign prostatic hyperplasia. *Prostate* 1993, 22:291–299.

39. Anderson JT, Ekman P, Wolf H, et al.: Can finasteride reverse the progress of benign prostatic hyperplasia? A two-year placebo controlled study. *Urology* 1995, 46:631–637.

40. Anderson JT, Nickel JC, Marshall VR, et al.: Finasteride significantly reduces acute urinary retention and need for surgery in patients with symptomatic benign prostatic hyperplasia. *Urology* 1997, 49:839–845.

41. McConnell JD, Bruskewitz R, Walsh P, et al.: The effect of finasteride on the risk of acute urinary retention and the need for surgical treatment among men with benign prostatic hyperplasia. *N Engl J Med* 1998, 338:557–563.

42. Boyle P, Gould AL, Roehrborn C: Prostate volume predicts outcome of treatment of benign prostatic hyperplasia with finasteride: meta-analysis of randomized clinical trials. *Urology* 1996, 48:398–405.

43. Jacobsen SJ, Jacobson DJ, Girman CJ, et al.: Natural history of prostatism: risk factors for acute urinary retention. *J Urol* 1997, 158:481–487.

44. Arrighi HM, Metter EJ, Guess HA, Fozzard JL: Natural history of benign prostatic hyperplasia and risk of prostatectomy: the Baltimore longitudinal study of aging. *Urology* 1991, 38(suppl):4–8.

45. Guess HA, Heyse JF, Gormley GJ, et al.: Effect of finasteride on serum PSA concentration in men with benign prostatic hyperplasia. Results from the North American phase II clinical trial. *Urol Clin North Am* 1993, 20:627–636.

46. Lange PH: Is the prostate pill finally here? *N Engl J Med* 1992, 327:1234–1236.

47. Stoner E and the Finasteride Study Group: Three year safety and efficacy data on the use of finasteride in the treatment of benign prostatic hyperplasia. *Urology* 1994, 43:284–292.

48. Oesterling JE, Roy J, Agha A, et al.: Biologic variability of prostate-specific antigen and its usefulness as a marker for prostate cancer: effects of finasteride. *Urology* 1997, 50:13–18.

49. *Physicians' Desk Reference*, edn 52. Montvale, NJ: Medical Economics Company; 1998:447–3198.

50. Coffey DS, Walsh PC: Clinical and experimental studies of benign prostatic hyperplasia. *Urol Clin North Am* 1990, 17:461–475.

51. Moore RJ, Gazak JM, Wilson JD: Regulation of cytoplasmic dihydrotestosterone binding in dog prostate by 17β-estradiol. *J Clin Invest* 1979, 63:351–357.

52. Berry SJ, Strandberg JD, Saunders WJ, et al.: The development of canine benign prostatic hyperplasia with age. *Prostate* 1986, 9:363.

53. Barrack ER, Berry SJ: DNA synthesis in the canine prostate: effects of androgen and estrogen treatment. *Prostate* 1987, 10:45–56.

54. Habenicht UF, Tunn UW, Senge TH, et al.: Management of benign prostatic hyperplasia with particular emphasis on aromatase inhibitors. *J Steroid Biochem Mol Biol* 1993, 44:557–563.

55. Gingell JC, Knonagel H, Kurth KH, et al.: Placebo-controlled, double-blind study to test the efficacy of the aromatase inhibitor atamestane in patients with benign prostatic hyperplasia not requiring operation. *J Urol* 1995, 154:399–401.

56. Caine M, Raz S, Ziegler M: Adrenergic and cholinergic receptors in the human prostate, prostatic capsule and bladder neck. *Br J Urol* 1975, 47:193–202.

57. Gup DI, Shapiro E, Baumann M, Lepor H: The contractile properties of human prostatic adenomas and the development of infravesical obstruction. *Prostate* 1989, 15:105–114.

58. Hieble JP, Caine M, Zalaznik E: In vitro characterization of the alpha-adrenoreceptors in human prostate. *Eur J Pharmacol* 1985, 134:1291–1298.

59. Furuya S, Kumamoto Y, Yokoyama E, et al.: Alpha-adrenergic activity and urethral pressure in prostatic zone in benign prostatic hypertrophy. *J Urol* 1982, 128:836–839.

60. Ruffolo RR, Hieble JP: α-Adrenoreceptors. *Pharmacol Ther* 1994, 61:1–64.

61. Ruffolo R, Nichols A, Stadel J, Hieble J: Structure and function of the alpha-adrenoreceptors. *Pharmacol Rev* 1991, 43:475–505.

62. Lepor H, Tang R, Meretyk S, Shapiro E: The alpha-adrenoreceptor subtypes in the human prostate. *J Urol* 1993, 149:640–642.

63. Lepor H, Tang R, Shapiro E: The α-adrenoreceptor subtype mediating the tension in human prostatic smooth muscle. *Prostate* 1993, 22:301–307.

64. Caine M, Perlberg S, Meretyk S: A placebo-controlled double-blind study of the effect of phenoxybenzamine in benign prostatic obstruction. *Br J Urol* 1978, 50:551–554.

65. Abrams P, Shah PJR, Stone R, Choa RG: Bladder outflow obstruction treated with phenoxybenzamine. *Br J Urol* 1982, 54:527–530.

66. Ferrie BG, Paterson PJ: Phenoxybenzamine in prostatic hypertrophy. *Br J Urol* 1987, 59:63–65.

67. Kane MM, Fields WD, Vaughan ED: Medical management of benign prostatic hyperplasia. *Urology* 1990, 36(suppl):5–12.

68. Hedlund H, Andersson KE, Ek A: Effects of prazosin in patients with benign prostatic obstruction. *J Urol* 1983, 130:275–278.

69. Kirby RS, Coppinger SWC, Corcoran MO, et al.: Prazosin in the treatment of prostatic obstruction. A placebo-controlled study. *Br J Urol* 1987, 60:136–142.

70. Chapple CR, Christmas TJ, Milroy EJG: A twelve-week placebo-controlled study of prazosin in the treatment of prostatic obstruction. *Urol Int* 1990, 45(suppl 1):47–55.

71. Le Duc A, Cariou G, Baron C, et al.: A multicenter, double-blind, placebo-controlled trial of the efficacy of prazosin in the treatment of dysuria associated with benign prostatic hypertrophy. *Urol Int* 1990, 45(suppl):56–62.

72. Chapple CR, Stott M, Abrams PH, et al.: A 12-week placebo-controlled double blind study of prazosin in the treatment of prostatic obstruction due to benign prostatic hyperplasia. *Br J Urol* 1992, 70:285–294.

73. Fabricius PG, MacHannaford HM: Placebo-controlled study of terazosin in the treatment of benign prostatic hyperplasia with 2-year follow-up. *Br J Urol* 1992, 70(suppl):10.

74. Lepor H, Auerbach S, Puras-Baez A, et al.: A randomized, placebo-controlled multicenter study of the efficacy and safety of terazosin in the treatment of benign prostatic hyperplasia. *J Urol* 1992, 148:1467–1474.

75. Lepor H, Soloway M, Appell R, et al.: A double-blind randomized multicenter trial involving comparison of terazosin and placebo in patients with benign prostatic hyperplasia [abstract 215]. *Proceedings of the 10th Congress of the European Association of Urologists*. Genoa: European Association of Urologists; 1992:309.

76. Brawer MK, Adams G, Epstein H: Terazosin in the treatment of benign prostatic hyperplasia. Terazosin Benign Prostatic Hyperplasia Study Group. *Arch Fam Med* 1993, 2:929–935.

77. Debruyne FMJ, Lodewijk D, Arocena F, Kirk D: Efficacy of terazosin in benign prostatic hyperplasia from a randomized withdrawal International Terazosin Trial (ITT) [abstract 177]. *J Urol* 1995, 153(suppl):273A.

78. Roehrborn C, Oesterling JE, Auerbach S, et al.: The Hytrin Community Assessment Trial Study: A one-year study of terazosin versus placebo in the treatment of men with symptomatic benign prostatic hyperplasia. *Urology* 1996, 47:159–168.

79. Gillenwater JY, Mobley DL: A sixteen week, double-blind, placebo-controlled, dose-titration study using doxazosin tablets for the treatment of benign prostatic hyperplasia (BPH) in normotensive males. A multicenter study group [abstract 447]. *J Urol* 1993, 149:324A.

80. Janknegt RA, Chapple CR: Efficacy and safety of the α_1-blocker doxazosin in the treatment of benign prostatic hyperplasia: analysis of 5 studies. Doxazosin study groups. *Eur Urol* 1993, 24:319–326.

81. Chapple CR, Carter P, Christmas TJ, *et al.*: A three month double-blind study of doxazosin as treatment for benign prostatic outlet obstruction. *Br J Urol* 1994, 74:50.

82. Holme BJ, Christensen MM, Rasmussen PC, *et al.*: 29-Week doxazosin treatment in patients with symptomatic benign prostatic hyperplasia. A double-blind, placebo-controlled study. *Scand J Urol Nephrol* 1994, 28:77–82.

83. Fawzy A, Braun K, Lewis GP, *et al.*: Doxazosin in the treatment of benign prostatic hyperplasia in normotensive patients: a multicenter study. *J Urol* 1995, 154:129–130.

84. Gillenwater JY, Conn RL, Chrysant SG, *et al.*: Doxazosin for the treatment of benign prostatic hyperplasia in patients with mild to moderate essential hypertension: a double-blind, placebo-controlled, dose-response multicenter trial. *J Urol* 1995, 154:110–115.

85. Kirby RS: Doxazosin in benign prostatic hyperplasia: effects on blood pressure and urinary flow in normotensive and hypertensive men. *Urology* 1995, 46:182–186.

86. Wilde MI, McTavish D: Tamsulosin: a review of it pharmacological properties and therapeutic potential in the management of symptomatic benign prostatic hyperplasia. *Drugs* 1996, 52:883–898.

87. Abrams P, Schulman CC, Vaage S: Tamsulosin, a selective α_{1c}-adrenoreceptor antagonist: a randomized, controlled trial in patients with benign prostatic "obstruction" (symptomatic BPH). The European Tamsulosin Study Group. *Br J Urol* 1995; 76:325–336.

88. Lepor H, Tamsulosin Investigator Group: Clinical evaluation of tamsulosin, a prostate selective α_{1c}-antagonist. *J Urol* 1995; 153(suppl):274A.

89. Chapple CR, Wyndaele JJ, Nordling J, *et al.*: Tamsulosin, the first prostate-selective α_{1a}-adrenoreceptor antagonist. *Eur Urol* 1996, 29:155–167.

90. Lowe FC, Tuttle J, Marks S, for the HYCAT Investigator Group: Blood pressure effects of men with prostatism concurrently treated with antihypertensives and terazosin. *J Urol* 1995, 153:272A.

91. Kaplan SA, Meade-D'Alisera P, Quinones S, Soldo KA: Doxazosin in physiologically and pharmacologically normotensive men with benign prostatic hyperplasia. *Urology* 1995, 46:512–517.

92. Cohen J: Long term efficacy and safety of terazosin. *J Clin Pharmacol* 1993, 33:272–278.

93. Lepor H, Williford WO, Barry MJ, *et al.*: The Veterans Affairs Cooperative Studies Benign Prostatic Hyperplasia Study Group: the efficacy of terazosin, finasteride, or both in benign prostatic hyperplasia. *N Engl J Med* 1996, 335:533–539.

94. Walsh PC: Treatment of benign prostatic hyperplasia. *N Engl J Med* 1996, 335:586–587.

95. Lowe FC, Ku JC: Phytotherapy in treatment of benign prostatic hyperplasia: a critical review. *Urology* 1996, 48:12–20.

96. Boccafoschi C, Annoscia S: Confronto fra estratto di *Serenoa repens* e placebo mediate prova clinica controllata in pazienti con adenomatosi prostatica. *Urologia* 1983, 50:1257–1267.

97. Emili E, LoCigno M, Petrone U: Risulati clinici su un nuovo farmaco nella terapia dell'ipertrofia della prostata (Permixon). *Urologia* 1983, 50:1042–1068.

98. Champault G, Patel JC, Bonnard AM: A double-blind trial of an extract of the plant *Serenoa repens* in benign prostatic hyperplasia. *Br J Clin Pharmacol* 1984, 18:461.

99. Tasca A, Barulla M, Cavazzana A, *et al.*: Trattamento della sintomatologia ostruttiva da adenoma prostatico conestratto di *Serenoa repens*. *Minerva Urol Nefrol* 1985, 37:87–91.

100. Reece Smith H, Memon A, Smart CJ, Dewbury K: The value of permixon in benign prostatic hypertrophy. *Br J Urol* 1986, 58:36–40.

101. Carbin BE, Larsson B, Lindahl O: Treatment of benign prostatic hyperplasia with phytosterols. *Br J Urol* 1990, 66:639–641.

Minimally Invasive Therapies for Benign Prostatic Hyperplasia

Claus G. Roehrborn

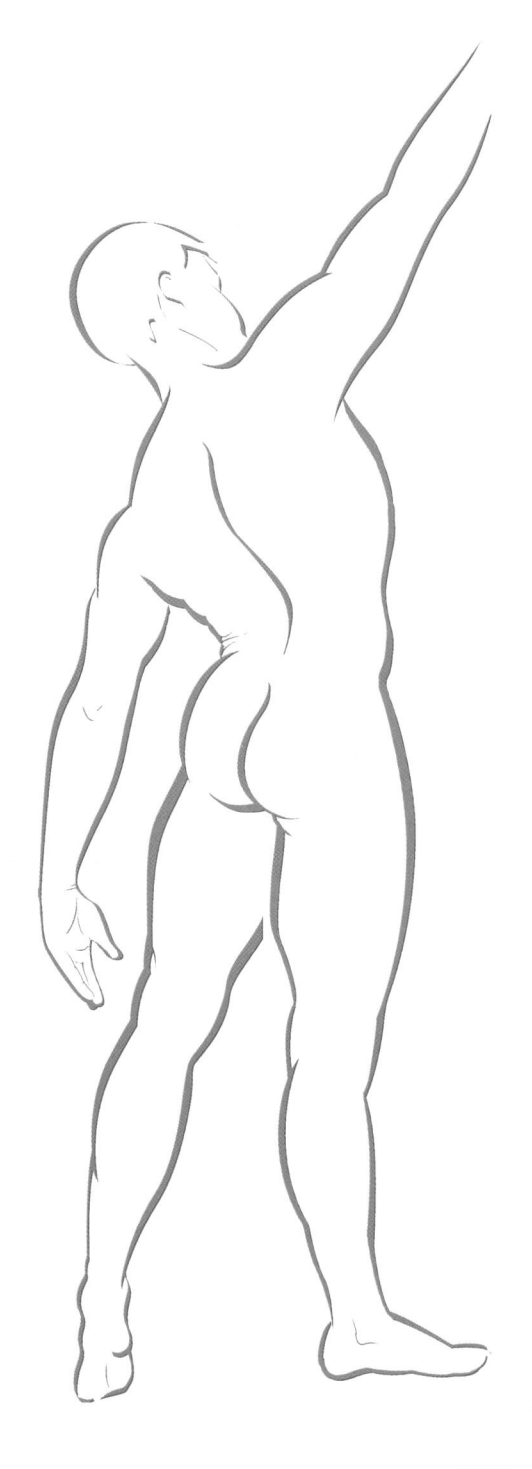

NONCANCEROUS DISEASE SECTION

Approximately 50% of all men will eventually develop lower urinary tract symptoms (LUTS), the clinical hallmark of benign prostatic hyperplasia (BPH), and will require some form of medical or surgical intervention during their lifetime [1,2]. Transurethral resection of the prostate (TURP), introduced more than 50 years ago, is still the standard treatment of BPH against which other treatments are compared [3]. However, many medical and minimally invasive treatments for LUTS and BPH have been developed and investigated in the past 10 years, effectively competing with TURP in the treatment of men with BPH. There are many reasons for the desire on the part of both patients and physicians to develop therapeutic alternatives to TURP. Aside from the obvious hesitation on the part of patients to undergo a surgical procedure in general, there are well known and described risks associated with a TURP, which are summarized in the Agency for Health Care Policy and Research guidelines for the diagnosis and treatment of BPH [4]. A careful analysis of long-term outcome data further revealed that even the presumably definite TURP procedure has a sizable re-treatment rate over time, for which various estimates are available. The best estimate reports a rate of approximately 10% over 5 years of follow-up (2% per year) compared with a significantly lower rate of 2% over 5 years following open enucleation of the prostate [4]. An additional incentive for the development of treatment alternatives is the aging of the population, with more and more older men seeking therapy who have more comorbidities and higher anesthetic risks, making them an ideal target for medical and less or minimally invasive therapies.

The use of heat to treat diseases is a very old method originally described in Egyptian papyrus scrolls. The application of heat to the prostate has been described in the form of hot water perfusion of the urethra, galvanocautery (Newman, 1886), heat-induced shrinkage (Kirwin, 1932), and prostatic desiccation (Mebust, 1977). The modern era of heat treatment for benign enlargement of the prostate was ushered in by the use of first rigid [5] and then flexible [6] microwave antennae placed in proximity of the prostatic adenoma.

Since then, at least four distinct heat-based therapies for BPH have undergone preclinical development and been tested in clinical trials: microwave hyperthermia administered either transurethrally or transrectally [7], transurethral microwave thermotherapy (TUMT) [8], high-intensity focused ultrasound (HIFU) [9], and transurethral needle ablation of the prostate (TUNA) [10–14]. The available basic science and clinical assumptions underlying heat therapy for BPH are reviewed, as well as the physical principles of the different technologies and their clinical results as they are known to date.

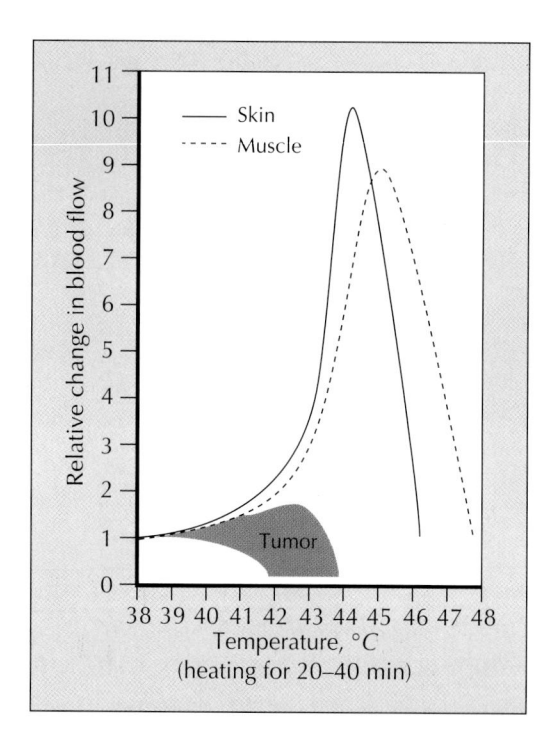

▶ **FIGURE 4-1.** Comparison of blood flow due to vasodilation in normal tissue versus that in tumor tissue. It had long been recognized that malignant cells are more susceptible to heat than normal tissue. Part of this reaction is due to the type of vascularity found in malignant tissue, which provides high resistance to blood flow and poor response to heat with vasodilation as is the case in normal tissue. In addition, hypoxic cells, often found in tumor cells, are particularly sensitive to heat destruction. Lastly, it was theorized that the use of local hyperthermia to cancers may enhance the immunologic response to a tumor. This figure illustrates how skin and muscle tissue exhibit a tremendous increase in blood flow due to vasodilation, while tumor tissue demonstrates little to no change in blood flow. For this reason, early efforts at hyperthermia were directed toward prostate malignancies, and many reports have been published using transurethral microwave hyperthermia for the treatment of prostate cancer [15].

Effect of Heat on Normal Prostate Tissue

Temperature	Tissue Effect	Therapy
37°	None	Fever
42° to 44°	No histologic changes	Hyperthermia
45° to 50°	Minimal changes	Thermotherapy
60°	Protein denaturization	Thermocoagulation
100° +	Coagulation and vaporization	Thermoablation

▶ **FIGURE 4-2.** Effect of heat on normal prostate tissue. By convention, hyperthermia is defined as raising tissue temperature from 42° to 44°C. Whereas at this temperature normal tissue does not exhibit any histologic changes, malignant tissues are susceptible to this level of heat. At temperatures above 45°C, both malignant and normal cells are affected by heat, and cell death may occur. Temperatures of higher than 60°C induce protein denaturation (thermocoagulation), and temperatures higher than 100°C induce coagulation and ultimately vaporization of tissue (thermoablation). It is thus apparent that any treatment aiming at tissue ablation in the prostate should strive to achieve temperatures higher than 45°C—a theoretical observation that was proven correct by the ineffectiveness of those treatments that achieved temperatures of lower than 45°C.

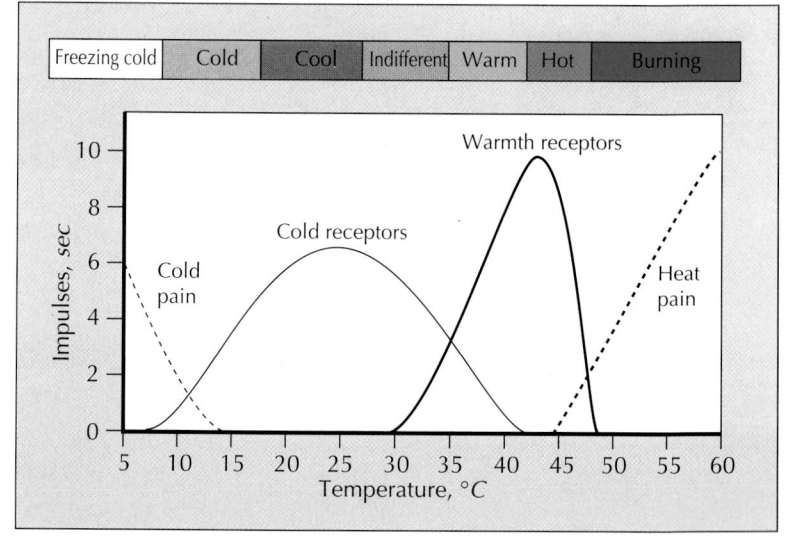

▶ **FIGURE 4-3.** Frequencies of discharge of various fibers. One problem with the theoretic observation described in Figure 4-2 is the normal body response to temperature changes. While the peak discharge of cold fibers occurs at temperatures between 20°C and 30°C, warm fibers start discharging at 30°C up to approximately 50°C, and at 45°C, heat–pain fibers start discharging.

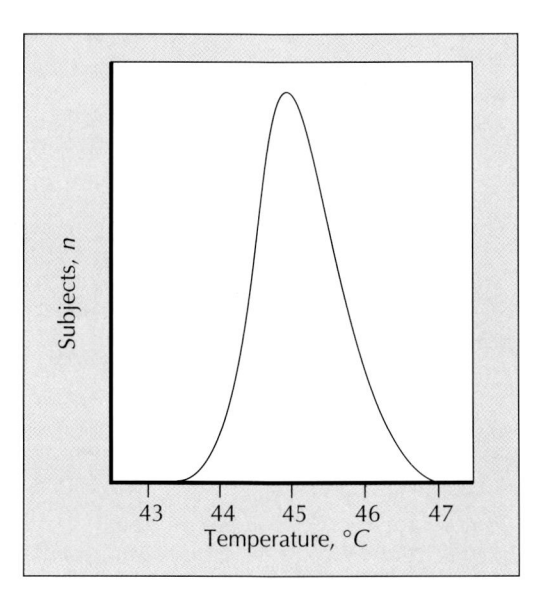

▶ **FIGURE 4-4.** Distribution curve of the minimal skin temperature that causes pain. Accordingly, most normal subjects perceive pain at skin temperatures between 44°C and 46°C. Although most physiologic research done on heat receptors and pain fibers is done on tissues other than prostate and urethra, it appears logical to conclude that at about the temperature threshold needed for effective damaging of tissue, pain and heat fibers will start discharging, thus limiting the ability of administering temperature without appropriate preventive and corrective measures.

Biologic Effects of Various Wave Frequencies

Frequency, Hz	Spectrum	Biologic Effects
$10^2 / 10^4$	Audio frequency	Ventricular fibrillation
	Power transmission	Convulsions
	Telephone	
$10^6 / 10^8$	Commercial and short-wave radio waves	No effect except by direct contact
$10^{10} / 10^{12}$	Microwave	Molecular excitation
	Radar	Tissue heating
	Diathermy	
10^{14}	Infrared, cooking, heating, lasers, photography	
$10^{14} / 10^{16}$		Molecular disruption
		Sunburn, tanning, cancer
		Photoreactions
10^{16}	Light: ultraviolet, spectroscopy	
$10^{16} / 10^{18}$		Atomic and molecular ionization
$10^{18} / 10^{20} / 10^{22}$	Ionizing radiation	Nuclear interactions
	Therapy	
	Diagnosis	
	Radiography	

▶ **FIGURE 4-5.** Biologic effects of various wave frequencies. Waves with a frequency of less than 10^8 Hz or 100 MHz (*eg*, telephone, commercial, and short-wave radio waves) do not cause any biologic effects. Microwave energy, radar, and diathermy cause molecular excitation and radiative tissue heating. Waves with frequencies above this level cause various biologic effects, ranging from molecular disruption (sunburn, photo reactions, cancer) to atomic and molecular ionization, and, ultimately, nuclear interactions (ionizing radiation for diagnostic and therapeutic purposes).

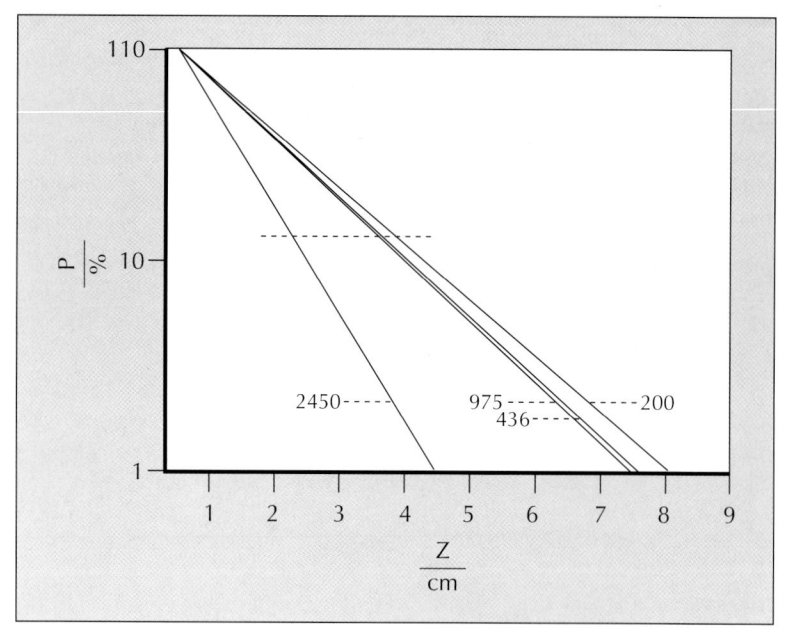

▶ **FIGURE 4-6.** Frequency dependence of penetration into muscle from 10 cm × 10 cm aperture. Radiative heating by microwave energy can be conducted with a number of applicators ranging in frequency from 434 to 2450 MHz. However, the depth of tissue penetration is inversely correlated to the frequency of the wave length: the higher the wave length, the less penetration can be achieved. Individual variations in the anatomies, such as blood supply of the urethra, the rectum, the prostate, and variations in prostate morphology affect radiative heatings. Energies are delivered to the tissue by conductive, convective, and absorptive mechanisms; the exact mechanisms of microwave energy treatment of the prostate is, however, extrapolated from oncology data.

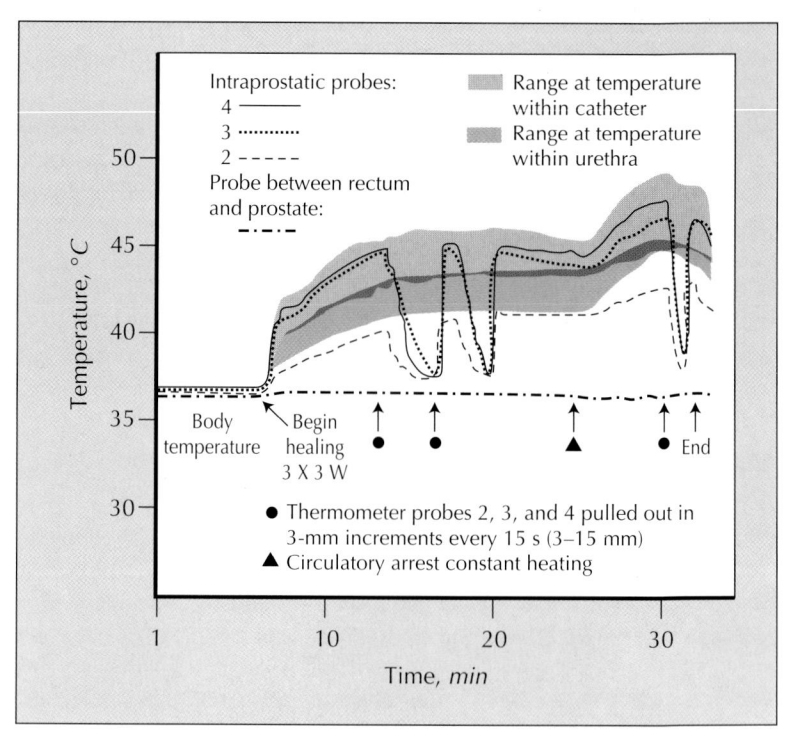

▶ **FIGURE 4-7.** Temperature readings during a microwave hyperthermia session in a dog prostate with a 950-MHz microwave power generator (Prostek 3000; CliniTherm Corp., Dallas, TX) [16]. Interstitial thermometry experiments have been performed in both animal and human studies. Several important observations can be made from this experiment. On withdrawal of the thermometry probes (two, three, and four, in 3-mm increments), the intraprostatic temperature decreases by approximately 1°C per 3-mm increment. This figure illustrates the relatively steep radial temperature drop-off in the prostate of about 1°C per 3-mm distance from the catheter, limiting the zone of potential effectiveness of microwave hyperthermia. The impact of blood flow is evident from the induction of circulatory arrest with constant heating. As soon as circulatory arrest is induced, the convection of heat by blood-flowing blood is eliminated, and the temperature begins to rise steadily despite constant energy supply. Despite this effect, the sharp temperature drop-off on withdrawal of the temperature probes is again noted. Similar observations of nearly exponential temperature drop-off radially to the microwave antennae have been made by others.

MICROWAVE HYPERTHERMIA

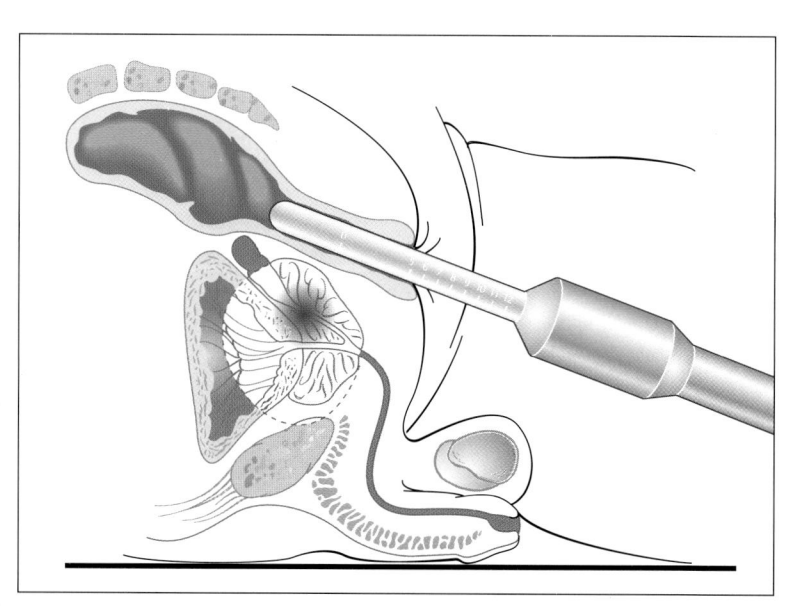

▶ **FIGURE 4-8.** The transrectal route of microwave hyperthermia. Microwave hyperthermia has been administered by both a transrectal and transurethral (see Fig. 4-9) route. The transrectal route has the advantage of comfortable positioning and good patient acceptance. However, even under ideal circumstances, maximal penetration of the microwave energy is limited to less than 2 cm; thus the maximum position of energy is in the peripheral zone of the prostate and not the periurethral glands.

II. The Prostate

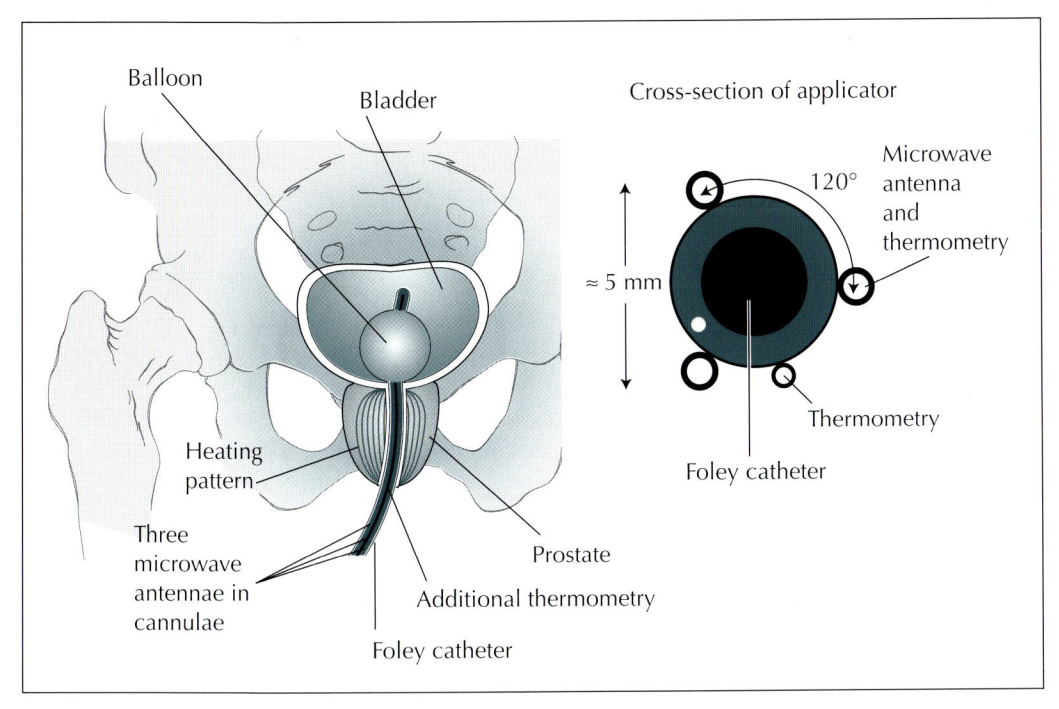

FIGURE 4-9. The transurethral route of microwave hyperthermia. The transurethral route appears to be a better approach in terms of proximity to the transition zone of the prostate or the periurethral glands. Transurethral hyperthermia systems were designed to operate without urethral cooling: thus the urethral tissue in closest proximity to the applicator received the highest output of energy, with a resulting steep grading of temperature decrease away from the applicator. Both transrectal and transurethral hyperthermia devices therefore required multiple treatment sessions.

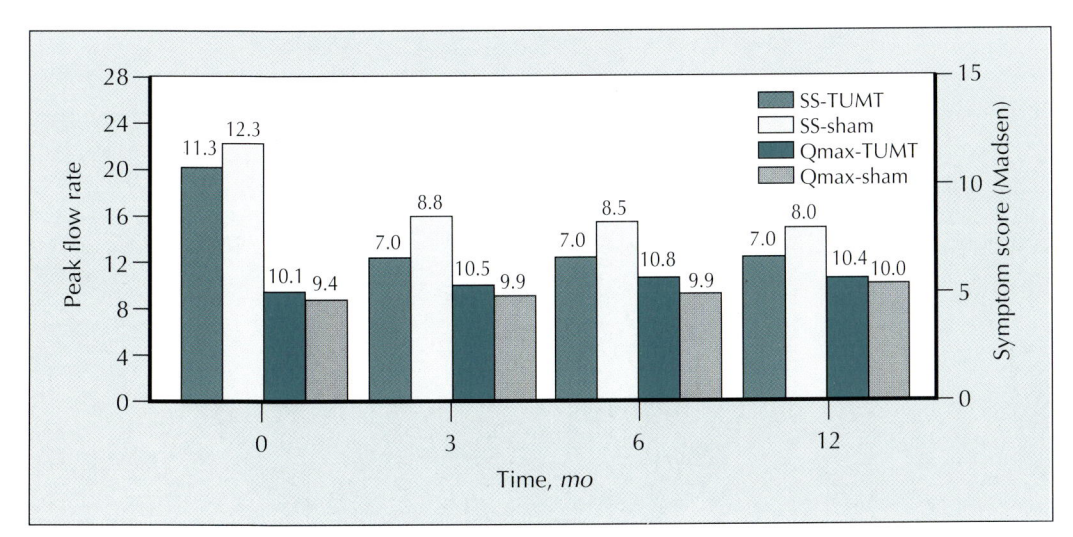

FIGURE 4-10. Data from a multicenter French trial of hyperthermia versus sham ($n = 200$). Although at one time almost 12 transrectal and transurethral hyperthermia devices were commercially available in various countries, the randomized, sham-controlled trial performed in the Paris Public Hospital System proved conclusively that this form of treatment is not associated with measurable changes in either symptoms or flow rate different from sham-treated patients. In this study, 200 patients over 50 years of age with a peak flow rate of less than 15 mL/s, a prostate-specific antigen level of less than 10 mL, and prostates from 30 to 80 mL in size were randomly assigned in seven public hospitals in Paris, France into three transrectal treatment groups, or to receive a sham treatment using the same device without actually turning on the energy source. The randomization was done at a 2:1 ratio (active versus sham patients). Twenty-five percent of patients dropped out in both groups, and 19% of patients in the active treatment group required complementary medical or surgical treatment during the 12-month duration of the study. Twenty minor complications were noted exclusively in the active treatment group. Because no major differences between transurethral and transrectal approaches could be found, the active groups were combined and compared with the sham group. In both groups, a moderate decrease in the Madsen symptom severity and frequency score was noted, but this was not different between the active and the sham-treated groups. Similarly, the observed changes in the peak urinary flow rate were not different between the active (0.25 mL/s change) and the sham (0.01 mL/s) treated patients. Subjective response at 12 months was noted in 25% of the active transrectal–treated patients versus 29% of the sham transrectal-treated patients (not significant), whereas subjective responses were found in 50% of the active transurethrally treated patients versus only in 17% of the actively sham-treated patients. Following the conclusion of this study—that hyperthermia, either transrectally or transurethrally administered, cannot be considered as a genuine alternative to surgery—the procedure is no longer listed as an acceptable treatment recommendation by the Fourth International Consultation on Benign Prostatic Hyperplasia [17].

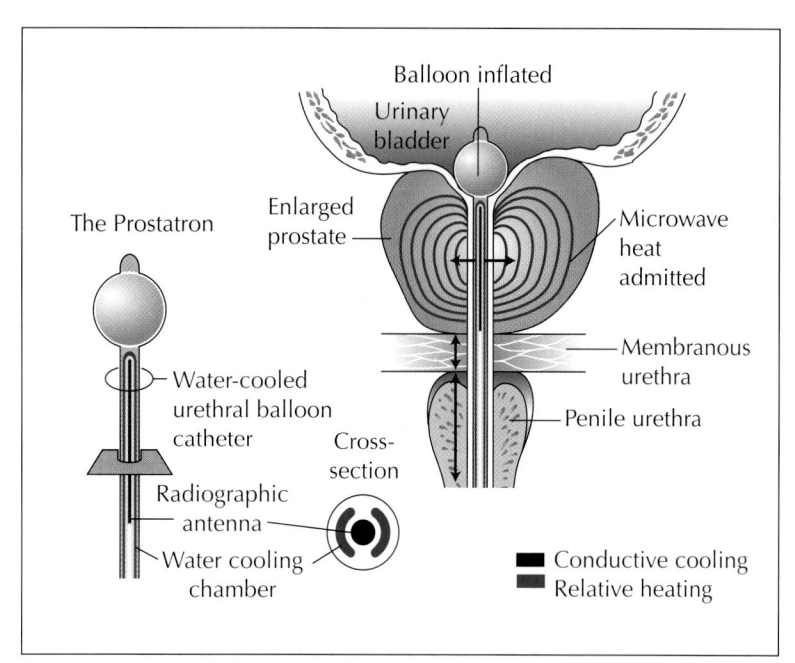

TRANSURETHRAL MICROWAVE THERMOTHERAPY

FIGURE 4-11. Transurethral microwave thermotherapy (TUMT). In contrast to microwave hyperthermia, TUMT refers to the heating of the prostate in excess of 45°C, thus inducing noticeable histologic changes. The increase in the energy and temperature associated with TUMT as compared with hyperthermia incurs two problems: 1) the increased temperature has the potential of inducing necrosis of the urethral lining, which would result in tissue sloughing with unpleasant and bothersome irritative symptoms following treatment; and 2) temperatures in excess of 45°C in most patients induce pain sensation (see Figs. 4-3 and 4-4) and, accordingly, would require anesthetic provisions.

A cooling system has been developed (Edap Technomed, Cambridge, MA) that is currently in use in commercially available TUMT devices. The microwave antennae placed in the prostatic urethra is surrounded by a second chamber that is perfused with prechilled water. The configuration of the balloon (*eg*, completely circumferential, only lateral, mostly posterior) as well as the temperature of the prechilled fluid with which the system is perfused varies from device to device. The fundamental principal, however, is the same: the cooling of the immediate urethral lining and the first few millimeters of periurethral tissue prevents both necrosis and tissue sloughing as well as pain sensation in the patient.

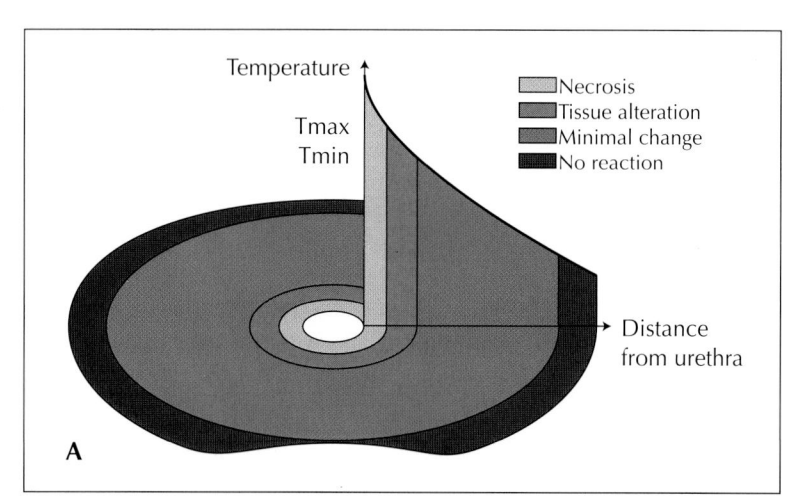

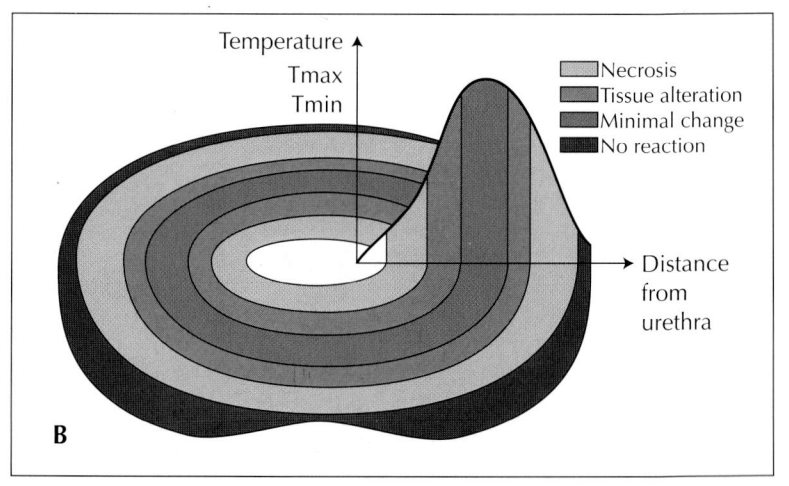

FIGURE 4-12. Urethral heating with and without cooling. **A,** Urethral heating without cooling leads in the peak temperature being measurable in the immediate periurethral tissue with a sharp radial temperature drop-off away from the energy source. **B,** Urethral heating with cooling protects the urethral lining and the immediate periurethral tissue. The peak temperature is achieved deeper within the prostate, namely in the periurethral glandular tissue, which is the primary target on any minimally invasive treatment modality.

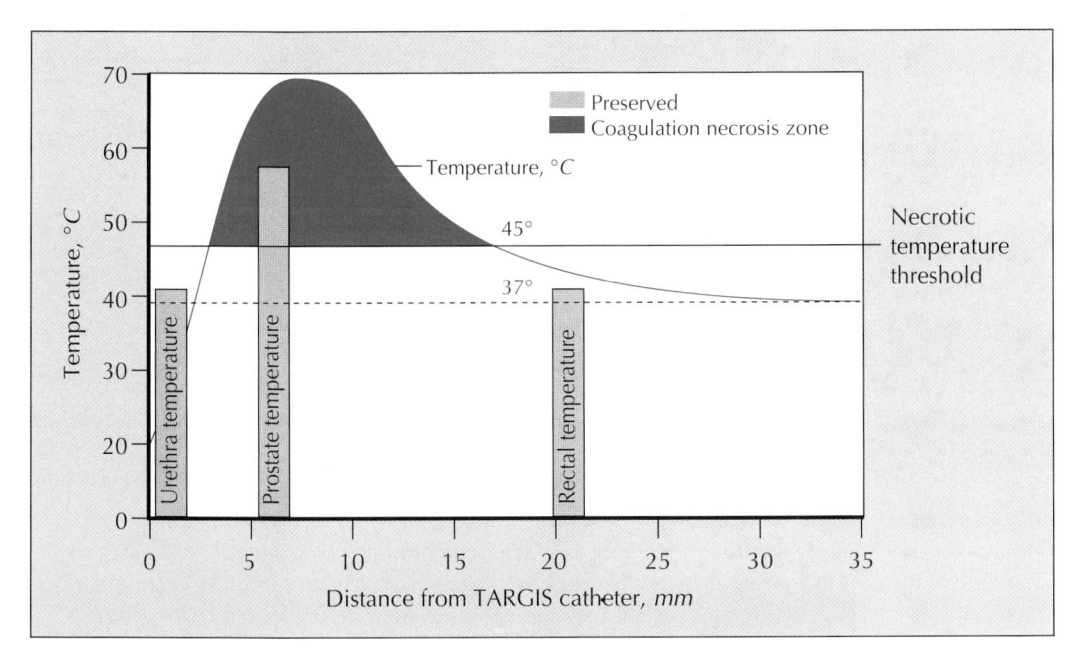

▶ **FIGURE 4-13.** Microwave treatment of the prostate. While using different frequencies ranging from 95 to 1296 MHz, extensive interstitial temperature mapping studies performed with all commercially available devices have demonstrated that temperature in excess of 45°C can be achieved in the actual advance. The actual distribution of temperatures differs considerably, presumably depending on anatomy and histologic composition. Careful mapping studies with the TARGIS (Urologix, Minneapolis, MN) device demonstrates effective temperatures within the prostate from about 3 to 15 mm away from the urethra. Cooling provides adequate protection of the urethral lining, and peripheral prostate tissue, rectal wall, and tissue outside the prostate remains at body temperature.

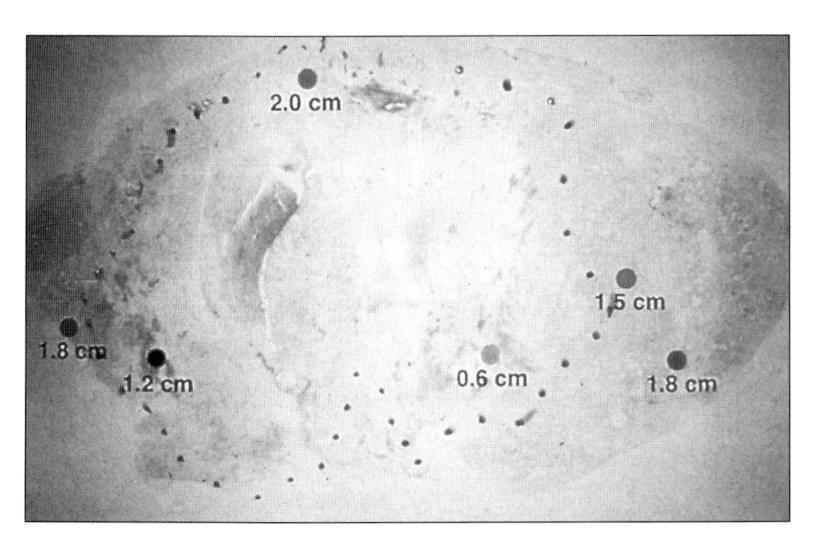

▶ **FIGURE 4-14.** *(See Color Plate)* Interstitial pathology specimen following TARGIS (Urologix, Minneapolis, MN) therapy. In this whole-mount histologic section, the interstitial thermometry measurements are indicated by their distance from the antennae in the urethra. The *dotted line* indicates the area of necrosis induced, which is roughly an area 1.5 to 2.0 cm circumferentially around the urethra.

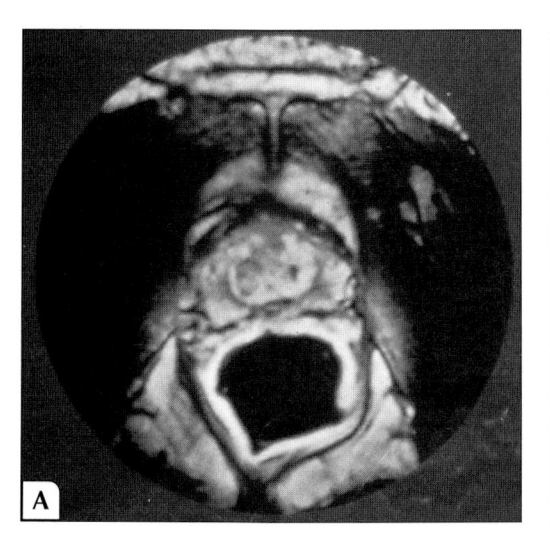

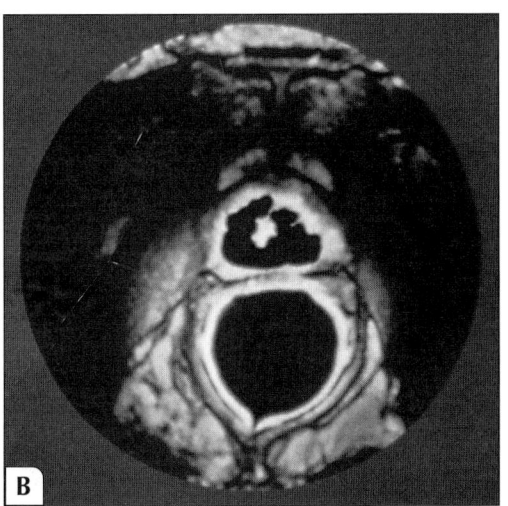

▶ **FIGURE 4-15.** Prostatic tissue necrosis. T_2-weighted, fat-suppressed, gadolinium-enhanced pelvic magnetic resonance imaging (MRI) has provided visual evidence of necrosis induced in the prostate. These MRI images obtained before (*A*) and after (*B*) transurethral microwave thermotherapy (TARGIS; Urologix, Minneapolis, MN) therapy indicates a necrotic area in the prostate circumferentially surrounding the urethra.

Minimally Invasive Therapies for Benign Prostatic Hyperplasia

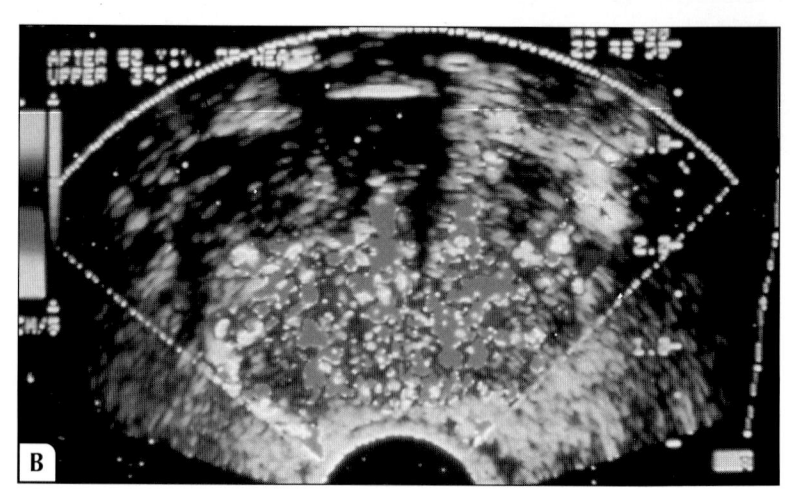

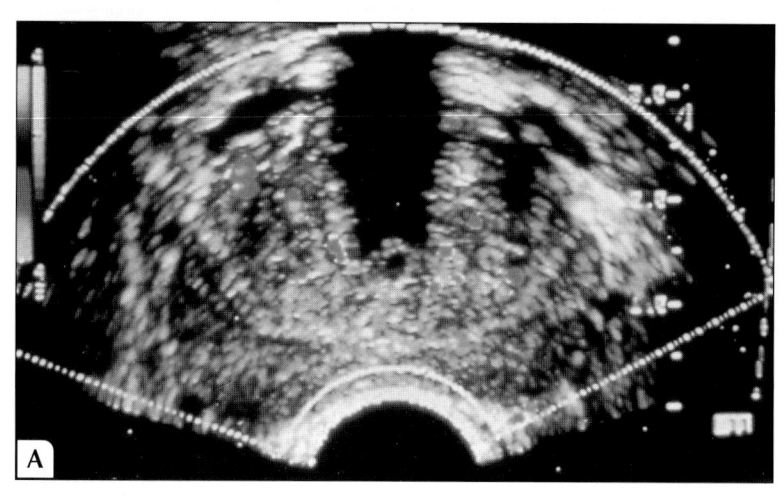

▶ **FIGURE 4-16.** *(See Color Plate)* Color Doppler–enhanced transrectal ultrasonography has also proven useful in the assessment of the treatment efficacy of transurethral microwave thermotherapy. **A,** Prior to therapy, there is very little blood flow in the peripheral and transition zone of the prostate. **B,** However, after approximately 40 minutes of treatment, an enormous increase in blood flow pattern in the peripheral and transition zone of the prostate is noted. This blood flow is mostly due to heat-induced vasodilation (see earlier discussion). Initially, the heat-induced vasodilation distributes the heat in the prostate by convection and, ultimately, causes a loss of energy by carrying the heat away via venous outflow from the prostate. Later in the treatment, however, small blood vessels become obliterated, making the prostate in essence a "heat sink." It is at those time points that in general the requirement of additional energy input to maintain therapeutic temperature decreases, while ongoing tissue damage occurs.

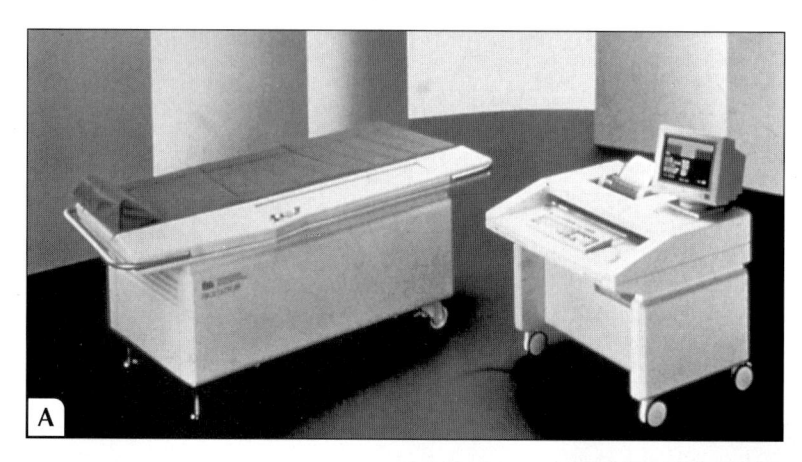

▶ **FIGURE 4-17.** Devices used for transurethral microwave thermotherapy. Although the available equipment differs in the external appearance, all devices have a microwave power generator, a keyboard for pertinent data entry, and a computer screen to display in real-time treatment parameters, adjust temperatures, energies, coolant flow, and so on. **A,** The Prostatron (EDAP Technomed, Cambridge, MA). **B,** The TARGIS T3 (Urologix, Minneapolis, MN). **C,** The Dornier Urowave (Dornier Med Tech, Kennesaw, GA).

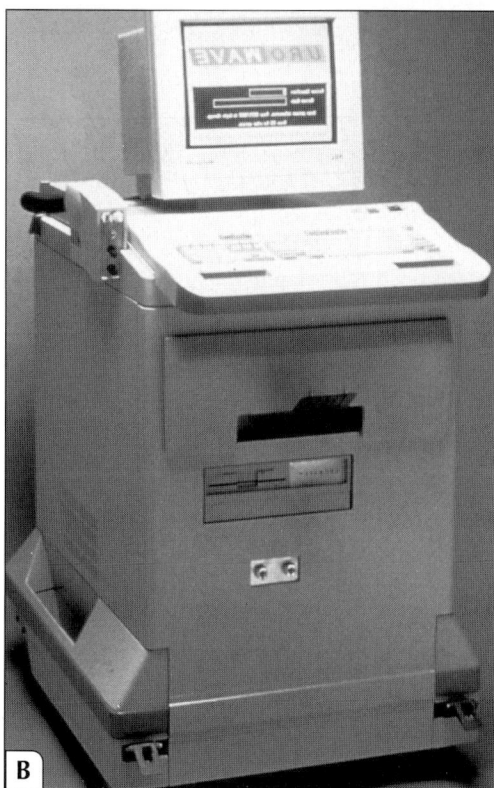

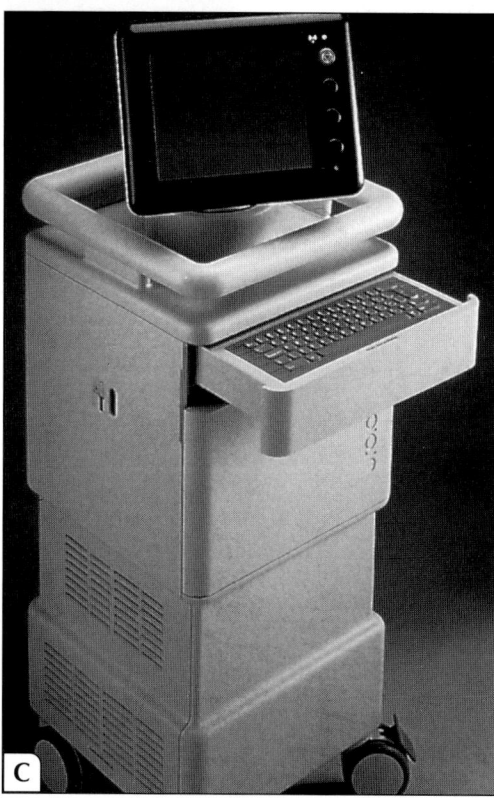

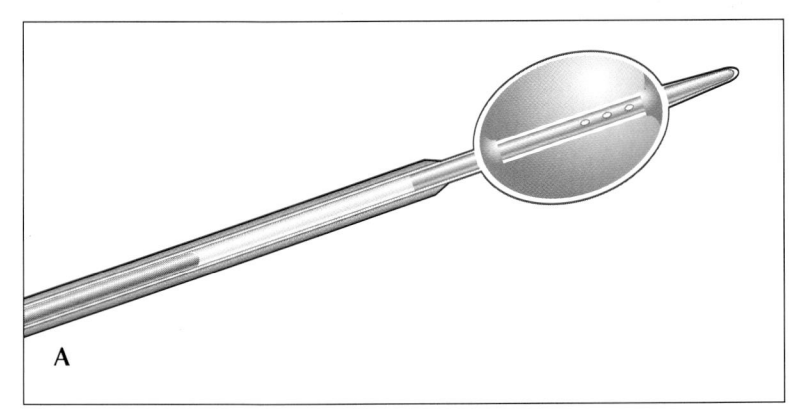

▶ **FIGURE 4-18.** Treatment catheters. The disposable part of the system, the treatment catheter, also varies from device to device. Fundamentally, however, all commercially available and currently used devices employ a catheter featuring an anchoring balloon (*panel A*) to secure the catheter firmly at the bladder neck, usually verified by transabdominal or transrectal ultrasonography. Furthermore, they feature an antennae that is surrounded by a chamber allowing perfusion with prechilled water for urethral cooling (*panel B*). The configuration of the cooling chamber, the temperature of the water, and the intensity of water flow during treatment varies from device to device. In addition to these elements, most catheters also feature a central channel to drain the urine during the actual treatment. (Courtesy of Dornier Med Tech, Kennesaw, GA.)

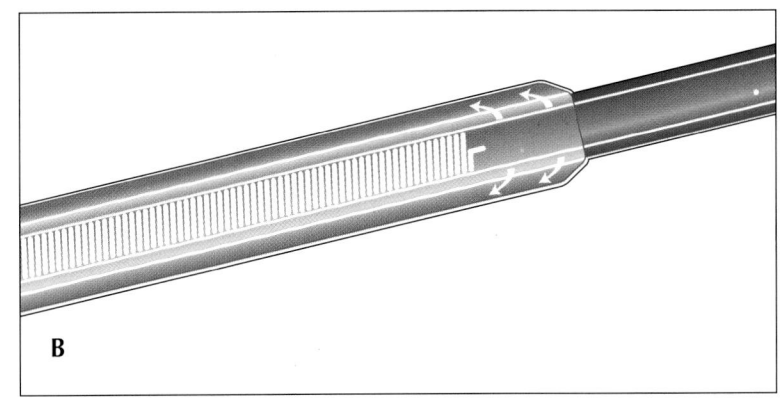

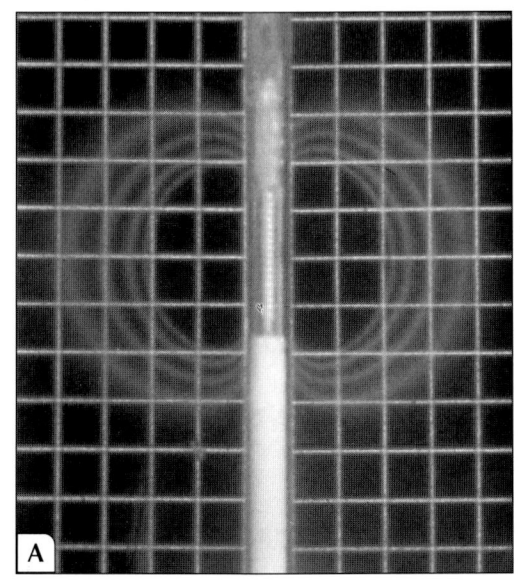

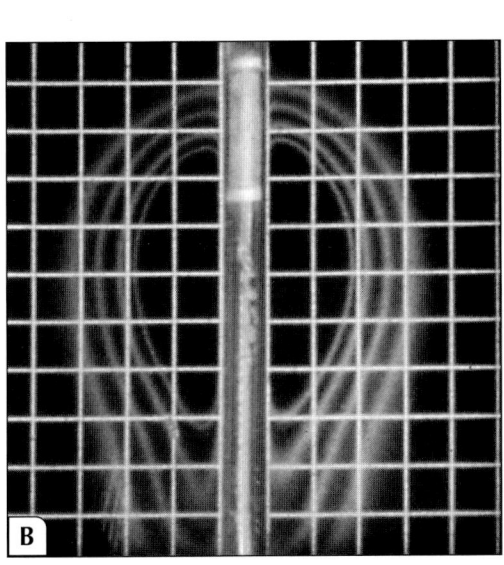

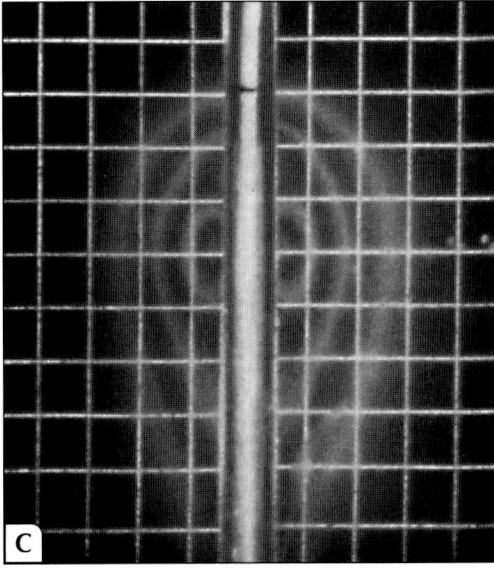

▶ **FIGURE 4-19.** Energy transmission patterns. **A,** TARGIS (Urologix, Minneapolis, MN). **B,** Prostatron (EDAP Technomed, Cambridge, MA). **C,** Urowave (Dornier Med Tech, Kennesaw, GA). The most complex part of the energy delivery unit is the microwave antennae. The problem with delivering microwave energy into the prostate is that of the appropriate and optimized configuration of the antennae. Impedance (see previous discussion) often leads to a significant amount of the energy being reflected rather than entering the prostate. Thus, calculation of delivered energy by the treatment console often overestimates the actual energy and heat transmitted into the prostate proper. These antennae demonstrate different energy transmission patterns in heat-sensitive materials. The TARGIS antennae feature a strict dipole configuration with a circular heating pattern around the antennae. The other two antennae feature a monopole design with "leakage" of energy along the shaft of the catheter into the area of the external urinary sphincter. Whether these design differences translate into actual clinical differences in terms of patient outcomes remains to be seen. However, it is noticeable that despite the apparent energy leak proximal to the antenna with the theoretical risk of external sphincter damage, no cases of urinary incontinence induced by any one of the machines have been reported to date.

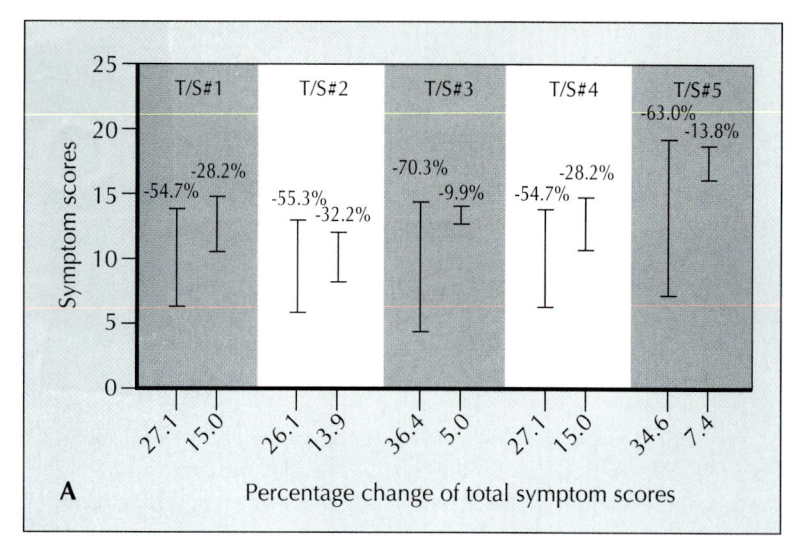

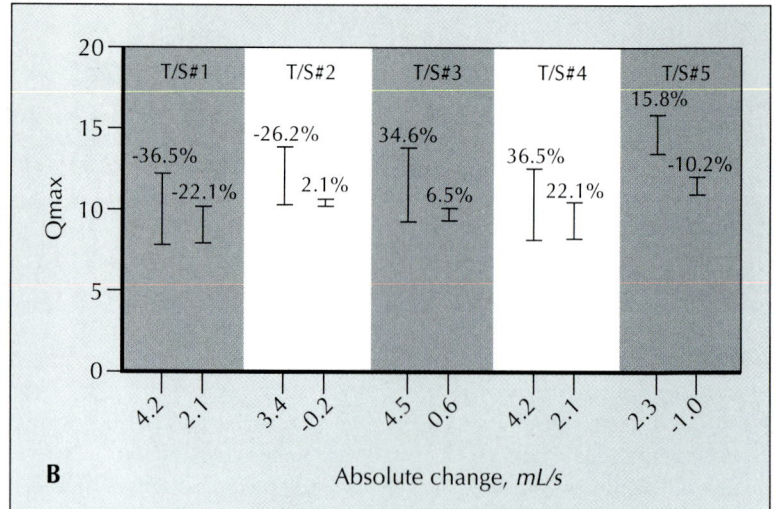

FIGURE 4-20. Pre- and posttreatment symptom scores (*panel A*) and peak urinary flow rate (*panel B*) for five sham-controlled transurethral microwave thermotherapy trials. The *top of the bar* indicates the pretreatment symptom score; the *bottom of the bar* indicates the posttreatment symptom score (vice versa for the peak urinary flow rate). The *first vertical bar* for each trial indicates the active treatment group; the *second vertical bar* indicates the sham treatment group. Percentage reduction is indicated on top (bottom for peak flow rate) of the bars and the percent change of the total symptom score and the absolute change (in milliliters per second) along the X axis. Two observations are pertinent. In all trials, the active treatment group was significantly superior in terms of symptom and reduction in flow rate improvement compared with the sham treatment group arm. Secondly, in all studies there was a response to the sham treatment both in terms of symptom and peak urinary flow rate with the exception of the fifth trial, in which a 10% decrease in peak flow rate occurred (*panel B*). Thus, it appears that transurethral microwave thermotherapy provides symptomatic and flow rate improvement above and beyond that achieved by simple placebo or sham treatment, or by the 1 hour catheterization associated with the sham therapy [18].

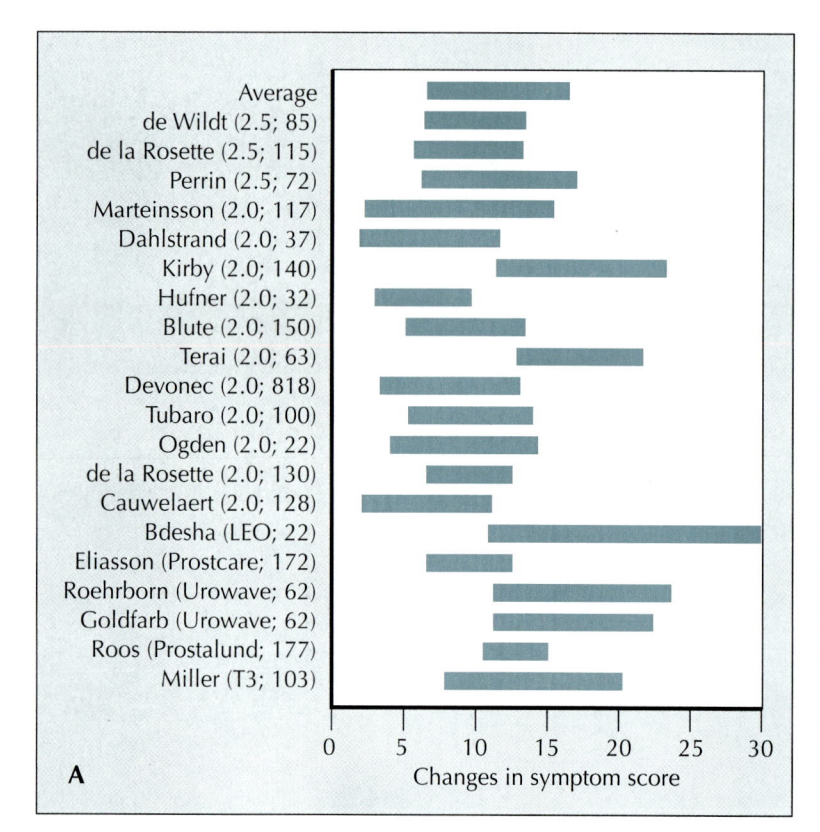

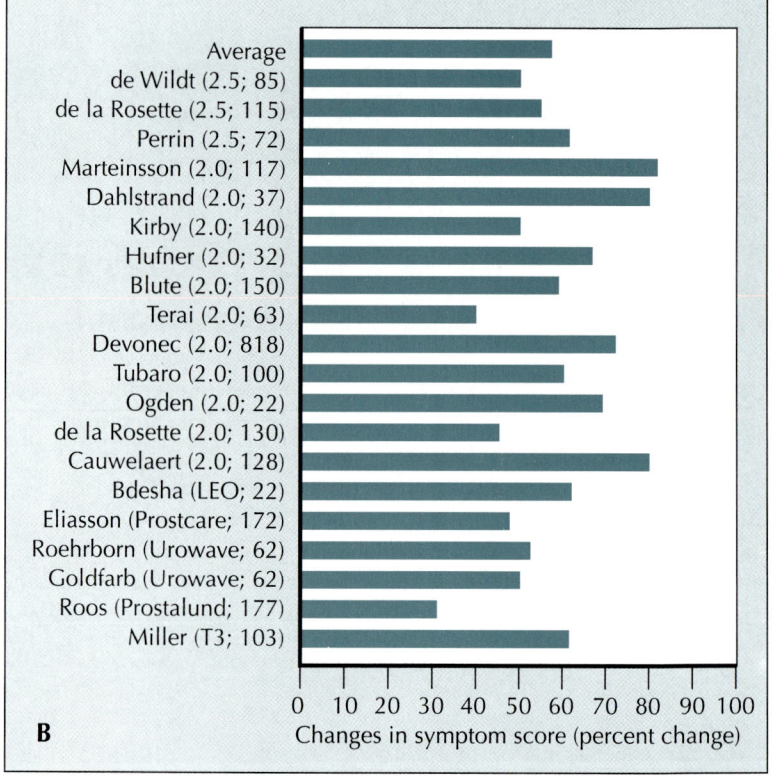

FIGURE 4-21. A summary of studies conducted with either the Prostatron (EDAP Technomed, Cambridge, MA) 2.0 software, the Prostatron 2.5 software, or other devices such as the Leo Prostatherma, the ProstaCare device, the Urowave (Dornier Med Tech, Kennesaw, GA), or the TARGIS T3 (Urologix, Minneapolis, MN) device. The numbers in parentheses indicate the number of patients in the study. The abundance of clinical data published in the peer-reviewed literature has recently been summarized by de la Rosette *et al.* [8]. **A,** The changes in symptom score are shown along the X axis. The *right side* of the bar illustrates the pretreatment symptom score; the *left side* of the bar, the posttreatment symptom score. It is evident that all devices reduce the symptom score considerably; however, the pretreatment symptom severity was very different from trial to trial. **B,** The same trials, but the symptom score improvement is expressed as a percent change. It is evident that on average, a 60% symptom score reduction was achieved (*first row*), whereas the percent improvement ranges from 30% to 80%.

Morbidity After Treatment

Study*	Patients, n	Catheterization	Retention, %	Hematuria, %	UTIs, %	Ejaculation Problem, %	Stricture, %	Incontinence, %	Re-treated, %
Miller et al.	103	—	—	—	—	—	—	—	—
Roos and Pedersen	177	—	3.3	2.2	2.3	—	0.0	0.0	9.0
Goldfarb et al.	62	—	4.8	12.9	0.0	3.2	0.0	0.0	—
Eliasson et al.	172	—	6.0	62.0	2.3	0.0	—	0.0	1.1
Bdesha et al.	22	—	—	31.8	—	0.0	—	—	—
Van Cauweaert et al.	128	3.1 d	33.0	2.6	—	0.0	—	—	0.6
de la Rosette et al.	130	—	26.0	4.5	—	0.8	0.0	0.0	10.7
Ogden et al.	22	—	22.0	—	—	—	—	—	4.5
Tubaro et al.	100	—	—	—	—	—	—	—	—
Devonec et al.	818	—	10 to 40	—	—	0.0	—	—	7.0
Terai et al.	63	3.9 d	36.0	1.5	1.5	1.5	—	—	—
Blute et al.	150	—	36.0	40.0	—	0.6	—	—	—
Hofner et al.	32	—	—	—	—	—	—	—	—
Kirby et al.	140	—	25.0	†	15.0[†]	—	—	—	3.0
Dahlstrand et al.	37	1 to 7 d	13.5	0.0	13.5	—	—	—	10.8
Marteinsson and Due	115	14.8 d	28.6	—	6.9	1.7	—	—	—
Netto et al.	100	—	—	—	—	11.0	—	—	—
Perrin et al.	72	> 2 wk	80.0	—	—	—	—	—	—
de la Rosette et al.	116	16 d	100.0	76.0	7.0	44.0	0.0	0.0	5.9
de Wildt et al.	85	14.3 d	100.0	—	—	33.0	—	—	2.6

*For complete reference information, see Gibbons et al. [19].
[†]Hematuria and infections.

FIGURE 4-22. Morbidity after treatment. Adverse events in general have been temporary, mild, and comparable between the different treatment modalities. Urinary incontinence and erectile dysfunction have not been a significant problem with any of the devices; hemospermia and other ejaculatory problems have occurred with varying frequency. The higher intensity devices appear to induce more hemospermia and occasionally other ejaculatory dysfunctions. Since the publication of this table, several individual cases of urethral stricture formation in the prostatic urethra have been reported. These, however, have remained isolated cases. Intermittent hematuria is reported by a significant number of patients, but it is of no clinical consequence because it is not associated with clot formation or clot retention. A considerable problem in the analysis and comparison of data is the issue of retention following treatment. In most research protocols, the protocol specifically instructed physicians to place a Foley catheter or a suprapubic catheter for a specified period of time. Thus, if every patient in a given trial by protocol has to have an indwelling catheter for at least 5 days, the average duration of catheterization can only be 5 days or greater. In other studies, voiding trials were allowed as early as on the first postoperative day. Thus, because the days of catheter requirement vary greatly, caution is advised when interpreting such data. The only way to determine whether or not differences exist between different modalities would be to have a direct comparison of different devices in which each patient is given a voiding trial every 24 hours until he is able to empty his bladder with reasonable residual urines. The issue of re-treatments is of great concern. Treatment failure and subsequent re-treatment with another invasive modality incurs considerable cost and is a disadvantage for any minimally invasive treatment. In this context, it is relevant to note that re-treatment dates have been reported very inconsistently. (*From* Gibbons *et al.* [19]; with permission.)

Prostratron 2.0 Long-term Follow-up

	1 y	2 y	3 y	Total, n(%)
TUMT only	233	112	133	133 (52)
Medication	18	11	16	45 (17)
Medication followed by surgery	2	9	5	16 (6)
Surgery	22	23	19	64 (25)
Death	1	2	3	6 (2)
Lost to follow-up	18	21	8	47 (15)
Missed visit	12	69	—	—

FIGURE 4-23. Prostratron 2.0 (EDAP Technomed, Cambridge, MA) long-term follow-up. de Wildt *et al.* [20] analyzed the long-term follow-up of 305 patients treated with the Prostatron 2.0 software. At the end of 3 years, 52% of patients had only received a single transurethral microwave thermotherapy (TUMT) treatment and no subsequent therapy. Seventeen percent of patients had received additional medication and 6% had advanced from medication to other forms of surgery. Twenty-five percent of patients underwent post-TUMT surgery and 15% of patients were lost to follow-up. This relatively high re-treatment rate is the source of great concern to those involved in analyzing the cost-effectiveness and cost-benefit ratio of minimally invasive treatments. (*Data from* de Wildt *et al.* [20].)

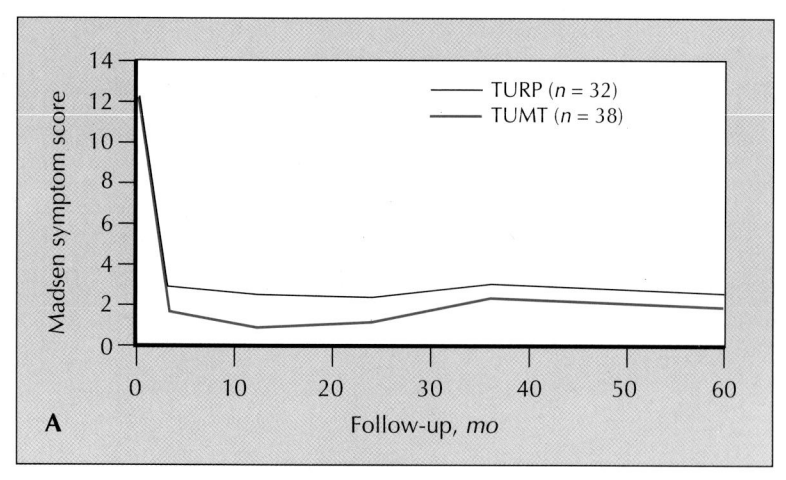

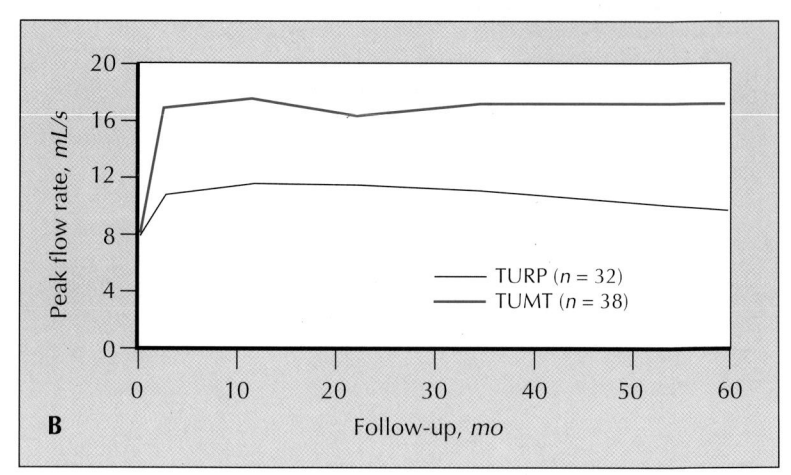

FIGURE 4-24. Long-term transurethral microwave thermotherapy (TUMT) versus transurethral resection of the prostate (TURP). Long-term follow-up studies with the Prostatron 2.0 (EDAP Technomed, Cambridge, MA) software has demonstrated that the improvement in Madsen symptom score (*panel A*) and in peak urinary flow rate (*panel B*) is maintained over at least 5 years in a study conducted in Scandinavia. In this unique study, patients were randomly assigned to TURP versus TUMT and were followed for up to 5 years. The degree of symptom improvement was nearly identical between the TUMT and TURP group. Although the improvement in peak flow rate was considerably less with TUMT than TURP, the magnitude of improvement was maintained in those patients followed over the entire study duration, with very little appreciable attenuation [21].

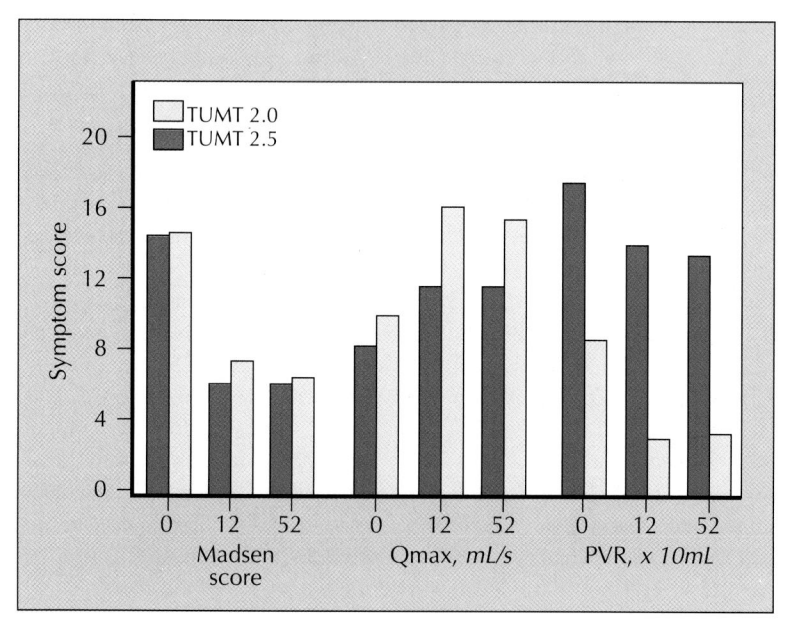

FIGURE 4-25. Improvement in efficacy parameters of the Prostatron (EDAP Technomed, Cambridge, MA) versions 2.0 versus 2.5. Recently, an updated version of the Prostatron 2.0 software has become available. This new high-energy software allows energy output up to 70 W. More significant improvements in urodynamic parameters, such as peak urinary flow rate, have been observed [22].

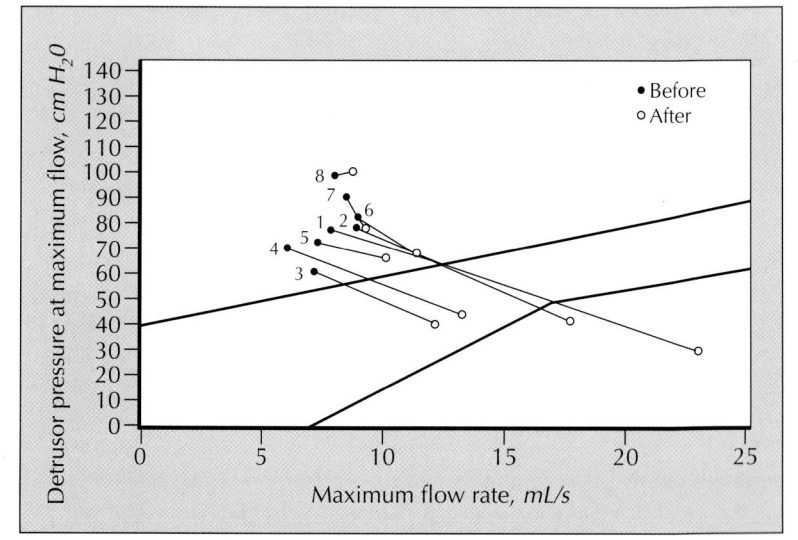

FIGURE 4-26. The urodynamic effects of various treatment modalities for benign prostatic hyperplasia [23]. The figure shows the average effect of open prostatectomy (line 1), transurethral resection (TURP) (line 2), transurethral incision (TUIP) (line 3), laser prostatectomy (line 4), transurethral microwave thermotherapy (TUMT) (line 5), α-blocker treatment (line 6), androgen deprivation (line 7), and placebo (line 8) on the P_{det} (detrusor pressure) at Qmax and the peak urinary flow rate plotted on the Abrams-Griffith nomogram. Whereas all surgical modalities (lines 1 through 4) on average transfer the patient population from an obstructed to an unobstructed or at least equivocal state, none of the other treatment modalities does so. Specific to TUMT, there is improvement in peak urinary flow rate with only a minor reduction in the P_{det} at Qmax. Further research with the high-energy software (ProstaSoft 2.5) may prove that greater effects regarding urodynamic parameters can be achieved [23]. Without doubt, one of the most important research agenda items in the area of TUMT is currently to determine which patients are ideally suited candidates for this form of therapy. It is very evident that there are some patients who have an excellent symptomatic and occasionally also flow rate improvement, whereas there are other patients who have no improvement at all or actually worsening of their symptoms. Ability to predict such response prior to treatment discussion would greatly help in reducing the number of re-treatments [25].

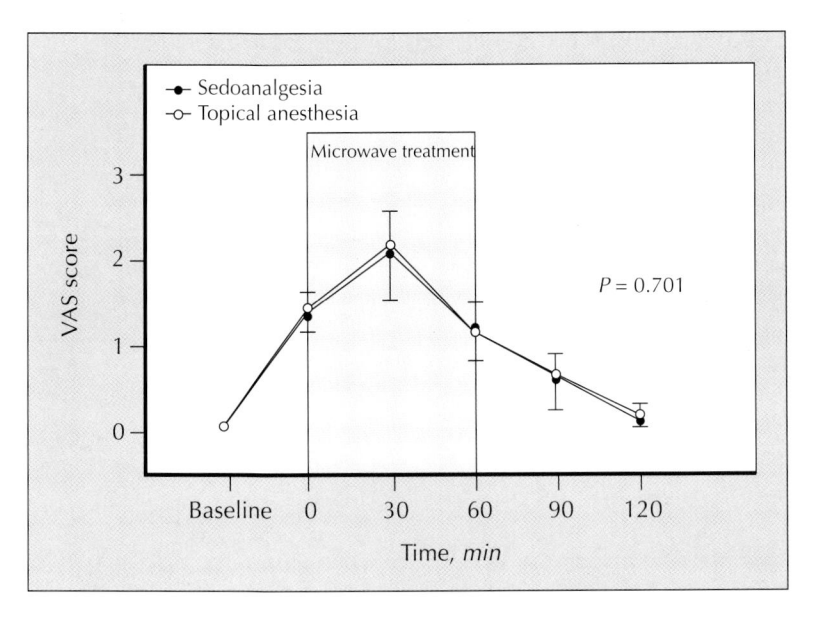

FIGURE 4-27. Mean visual analog scale (VAS) scores with 95% CI before, during, and after transurethral microwave thermotherapy (TUMT). Although anesthetic requirements reported differ from trial to trial, it is evident that all TUMT treatments may be performed in an office setting. In most cases, topical intraurethral anesthesia is used, augmented with a variety of analgesic or anesthetic medications, given either orally, intramuscularly, or intravenously. In this context, a recent study by Djavan *et al.* [26] is of considerable interest. Forty-five patients were treated with high-energy TUMT and randomly assigned to receive either topical intraurethral anesthesia alone or topical anesthesia with adjunctive intravenous sedoanalgesia. The treatment was delivered with the TARGIS T3 (Urologix, Minneapolis, MN) device. Patients were given a VAS before, during, and after treatment, and as is evident from the figure shown, the perception of pain was very similar between the two groups with no significant differences occurring at any time point either during or after the treatment. Although individual patients may vary in their perception of pain, overall the principal of urethral cooling has resulted in the TUMT treatment being fundamentally an outpatient, office-based therapy with no need for anesthesia services. What is currently needed is longer follow-up with more precise definition of re-treatment rates, and further research into predictors of response.

HIGH-INTENSITY FOCUSED ULTRASOUND

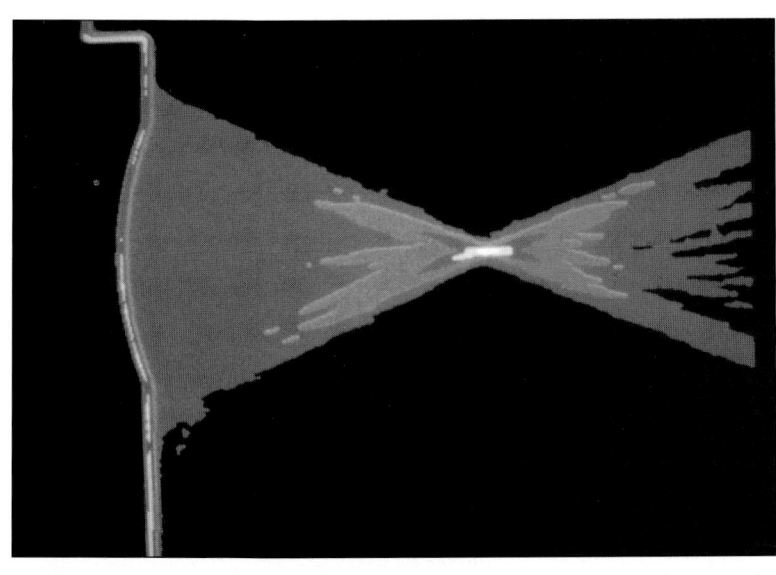

FIGURE 4-28. *(See Color Plate)* High-intensity focused ultrasound (HIFU) is the only currently available means permitting contact- and radiation-free thermoablation [27]. A beam of ultrasound waves can be brought to a tight focus at a selected depth within the body, producing a region of high-energy density. Biologic tissues, like all media, transform the mechanical energy of the ultrasound in part into heat. In this fashion, temperatures in the range of 80°C to 200°C are induced. This sharp heat impulse leads to the immediate death of all cellular elements within the beam focus. As the HIFU beam is focused, thermal damage to intervening tissue can be avoided.

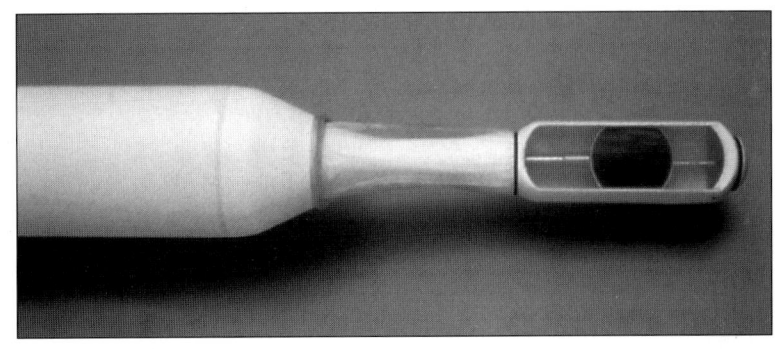

FIGURE 4-29. Piezoceramic transducer. The source of high-intensity focused ultrasound (HIFU) is a piezoceramic transducer, which has the property of changing its thickness and response to an applied voltage, generating an ultrasound wave with a frequency equal to that to the voltage applied. Frequencies used for HIFU therapy range between 0.5 and 10 MHz. Focusing of the beam is achieved by using a transducer that in itself has the shape of a part of a spherical bowl. The intensity at the site has to be above the temperature threshold, yet below the threshold for tissue cavitation, which results in uncontrollable tissue destruction. In most experimental designs and clinical trials to date, the respective site intensities are between 1000 and 3000 W/cm^2 [28,29]. To obtain a clinically useful treatment volume, a series of laterally or axially displaced lesions can be generated by physical movement of the sound head or by electronically sweeping the focused beam.

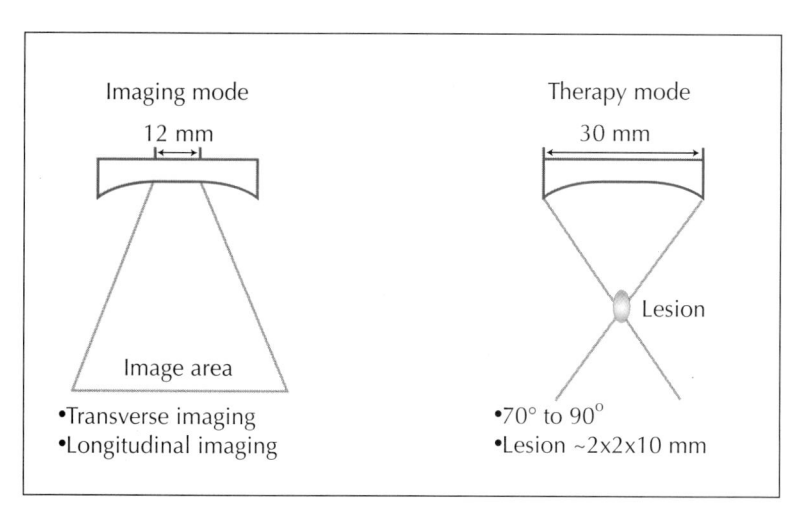

FIGURE 4-30. Imaging and high-intensity focused ultrasound (HIFU) modes of a transrectal HIFU transducer. To ablate prostate tissue by HIFU, the transrectal approach is most suitable. The device with which clinical experience has been gathered (Sonablate; Focus Surgery, Fremont, CA) uses the same 4.0-MHz transducer for imaging and therapy. The focal length depends on the transducer used and, at present, focal length of 2.5, 3.0, 3.5, and 4.0 cm are available, with the site intensity variable from 1260 to 2200 W/cm^2. (*Adapted from* Kirby *et al.* [30]; with permission.)

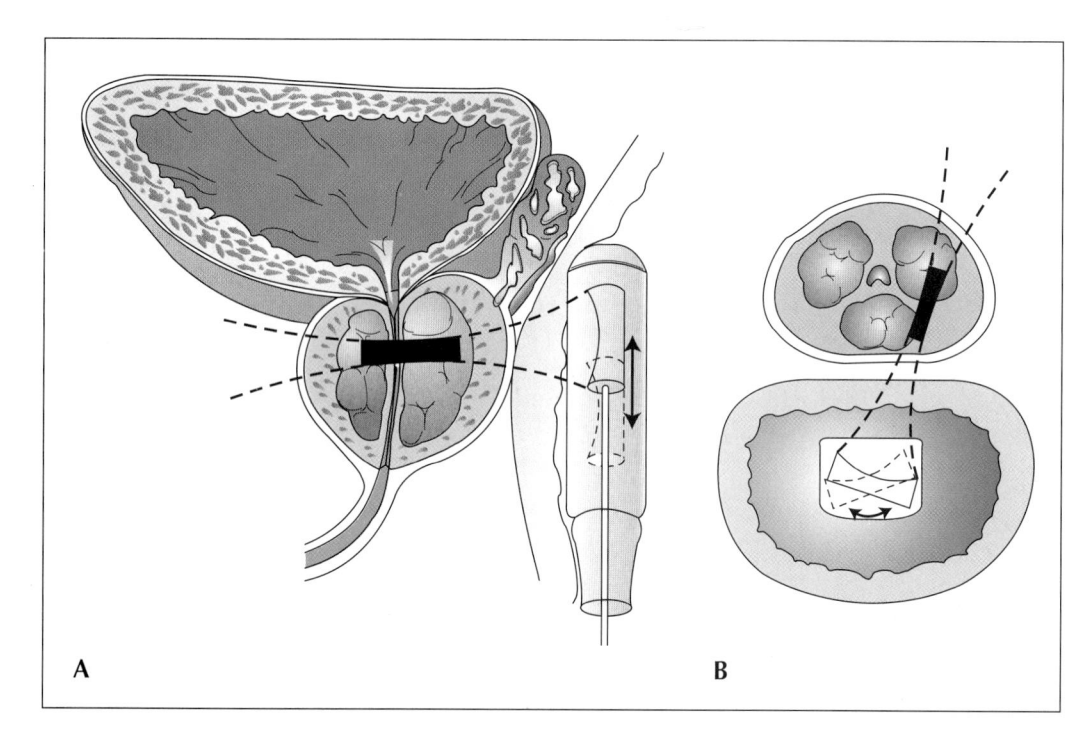

FIGURE 4-31. Volume lesion generation by transrectal high-intensity focused ultrasound (HIFU). The probe is covered by a condom filled with degassed water after insertion into the rectum to provide air-free coupling of the beam to tissue. Although the single focal lesion is very distinct and comprises only a few millimeters, moving the focal zone under computer control in a longitudinal (*panel A*) and a transverse (*panel B*) mode generates a lesion of clinically significant size. (*Adapted from* Kirby *et al.* [30]; with permission.)

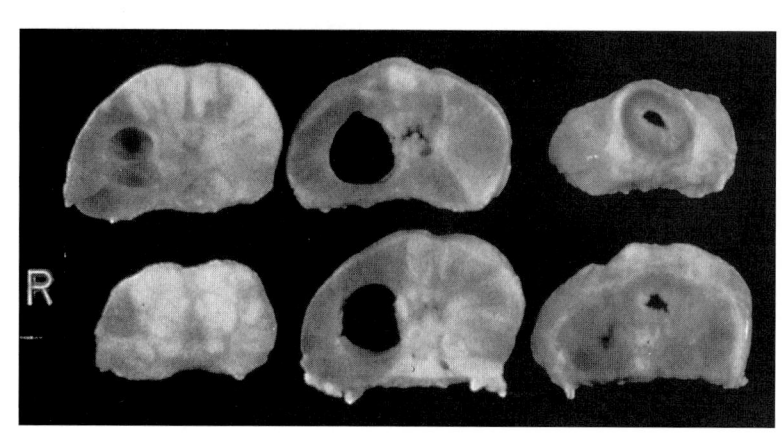

FIGURE 4-32. *(See Color Plate)* In animal experiments, it was possible to create distinct prostatic lesions in dog prostates using transrectally administered high-intensity focused ultrasound [28]. The preciseness of the lesion and the distinct margins beyond which the tissue is completely normal are remarkable and unique to this technology.

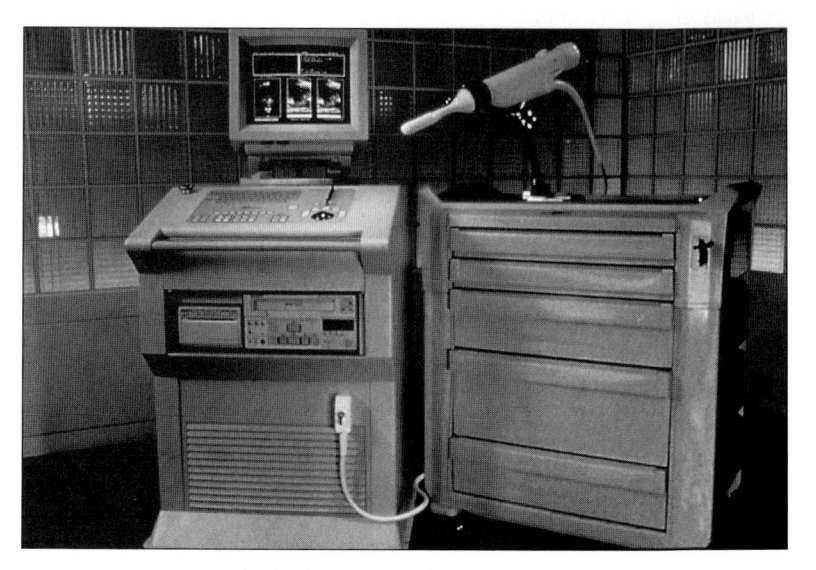

FIGURE 4-33. The high-intensity focused ultrasound (HIFU) device (Sonablate; Focus Surgery, Fremont, CA) used for human trials consists of a treatment console, a keyboard for entering of data, a computer display (see Fig. 4-34), and the actual treatment transducer, which is mounted and secured on the table with the patient in the lithotomy position.

II. The Prostate

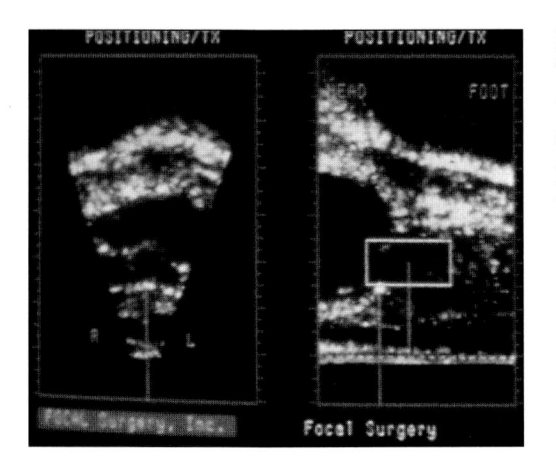

FIGURE 4-34. Computer display from the high-intensity focused ultrasound device. The display on the computer shows the ultrasound image of the bladder and the prostate with the area of planned tissue destruction highlighted in the rectangular box. Depending on the focal depth of the chosen transducer, the area of destruction can be moved to incorporate the periurethral glands or the bladder neck area. Additional treatment parameters are displayed on the computer screen.

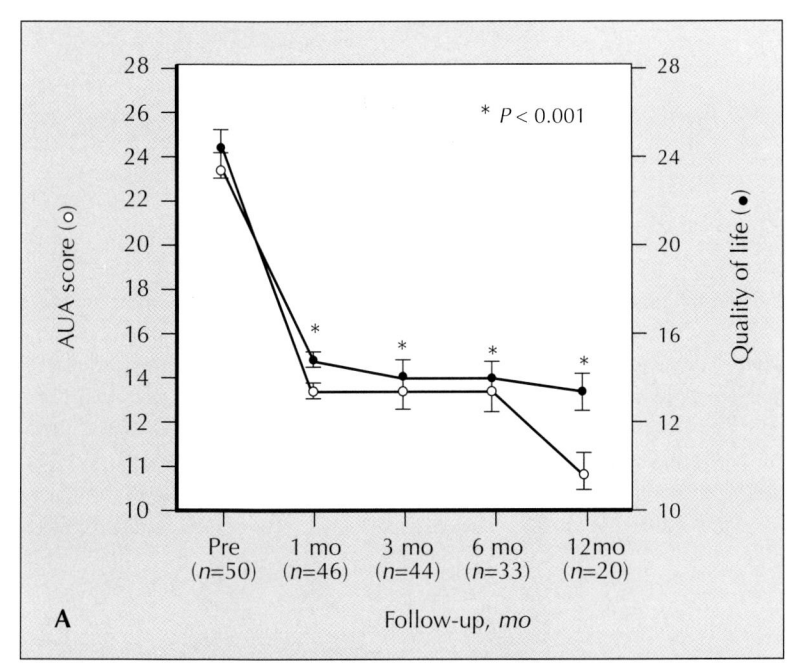

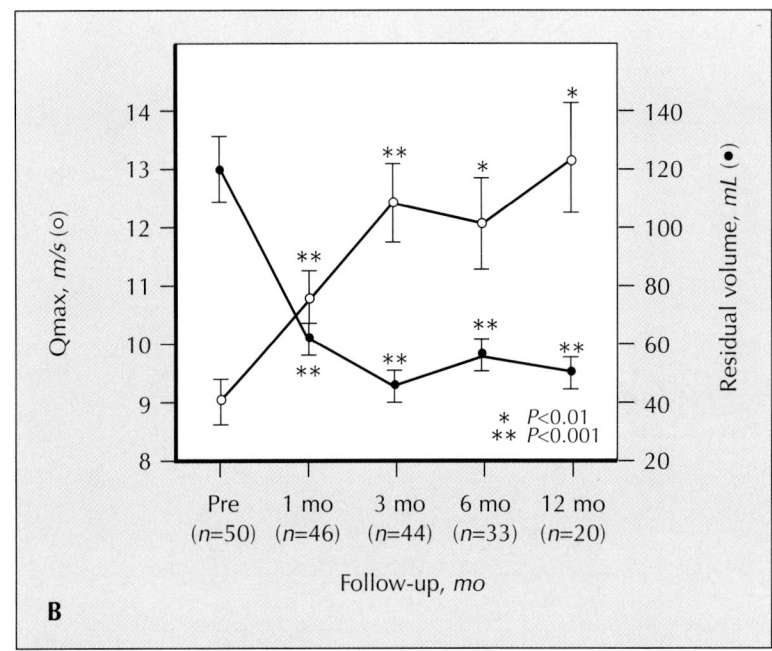

FIGURE 4-35. Worldwide, approximately 250 patients with lower urinary tract symptoms (LUTS) and benign prostatic hyperplasia (BPH), a peak flow rate of less than 15 mL/s, a prostate-specific antigen (PSA) level of less than 10 ng/mL, and a prostate volume by transurethral ultrasound of less than 75 mL have been treated and results up to 12 months have been published on a subset of these patients. Eighty-six patients treated at the University of Vienna required a treatment time of 40.2 ± 14 minutes. At 12 months, the American Urological Association (AUA) symptom score was reduced by a mean of 55% with a similar decrease in the quality of life score (*panel A*). At the same time, peak urinary flow rate improved by 47% and residual urine decreased from approximately a mean of 120 mL to a mean of 50 mL. All changes from baseline were highly significant (*panel B*) [31]. Very similar results were reported by US investigators [32]. Subset analyses have demonstrated that the effect of peak urinary flow rate and pressure-flow urodynamic parameters was better in patients in whom the bladder neck area was incorporated into the treatment zone (see Fig. 4-34). Although the technology itself is remarkable in terms of the position with which tissue can be ablated, some caveats should be noted: first, the intensely high pressure in temperatures induced in the prostate require the use of either a periprostatic bloc or intravenous sedation as a minimum. Second, the instrumentation present is quite cumbersome to operate. High-intensity focused ultrasound may have a major impact in the field of minimally invasive surgery for treatments of other non–prostate-related malignant tumors, because all organs that are accessible for ultrasound are potentially suitable for this kind of therapy.

TRANSURETHRAL NEEDLE ABLATION

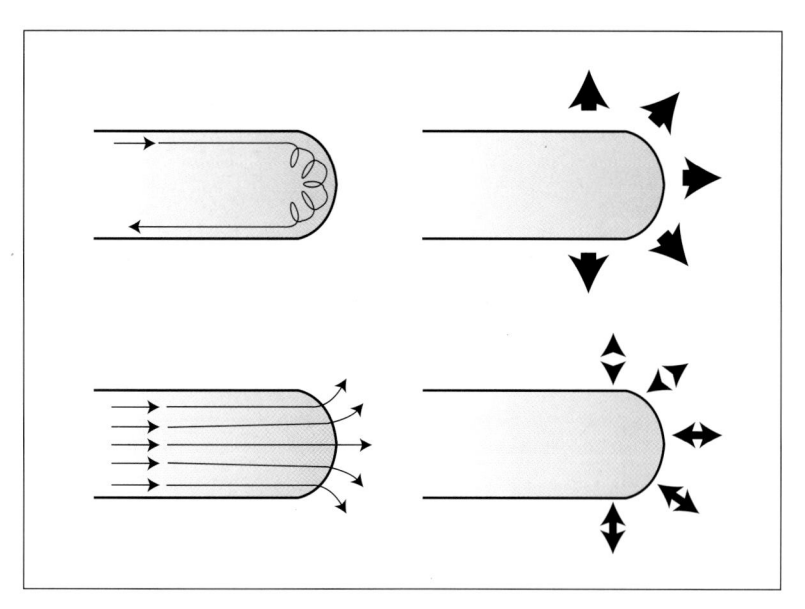

FIGURE 4-36. Principles of radiofrequency (RF) energy. Transurethral needle ablation (TUNA) uses low-level RF generator operating frequency of 415 KHz, which is delivered under visual control into specific prostatic areas by means of endoscopic needle placements. In contrast to resistive heating (*top*), RF is delivered to the tissue without the needles actually getting hot themselves. The frequency of the RF waves causes this agitation of the tissue particles and ions. This produces friction and creates heating of tissue. The tissue itself then becomes the conductor of the heat, not the needles.

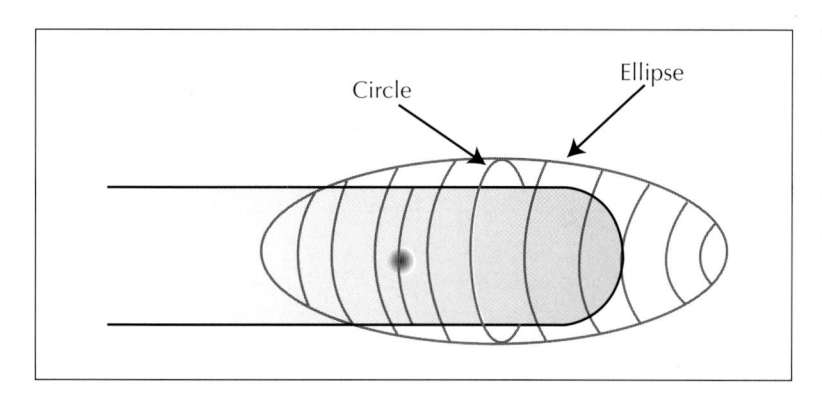

FIGURE 4-37. The radiofrequency (RF) lesion. As with other sources of energy, a feature of RF energy is a steep thermal gradient that is created when RF waves are delivered interstitially. The tissue immediately adjacent to the needle tip is heated to temperatures as high as 100°C, and then the temperature falls off, quickly reaching body temperature within 1 to 2 cm. The resulting lesion size is elliptic in shape, centered around the exposed needle electrode.

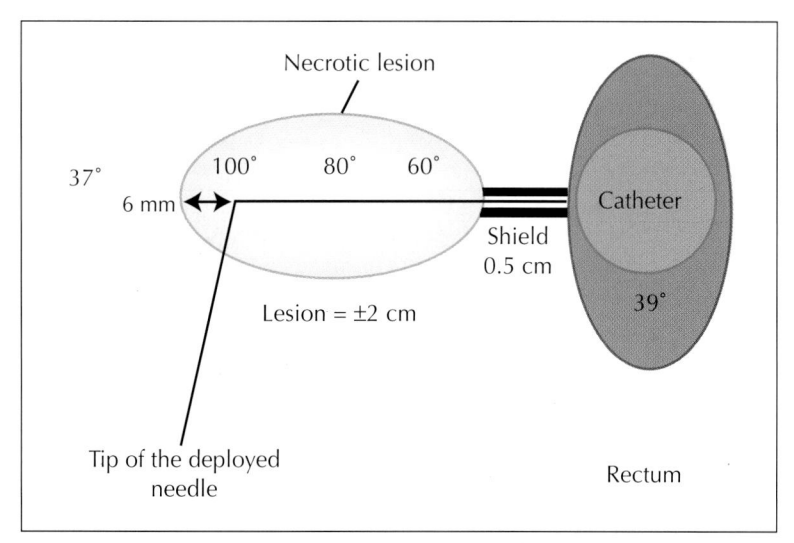

FIGURE 4-38. Temperature distribution and lesion size with transurethral needle ablation. By shielding the exposed needle immediately adjacent to the urethra with a polytef sheath, the elliptical shape necrotic lesion is positioned in the periurethral gland with the urethral lining itself remaining at body temperatures without need for water cooling, and thereby eliminating tissue sloughing.

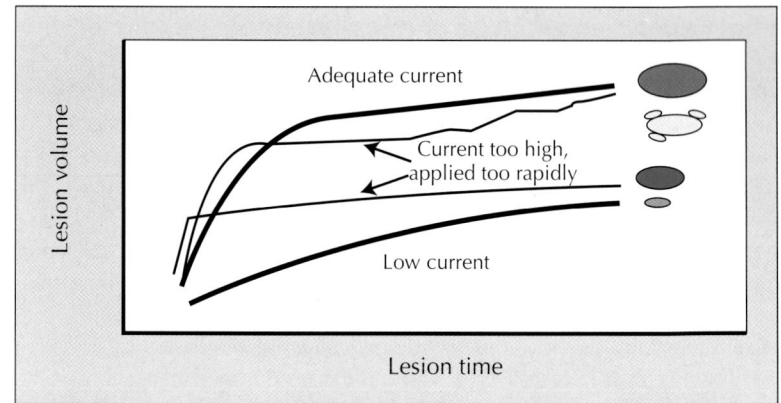

FIGURE 4-39. The resulting lesion size is a function of the energy delivered over time. The automated radiofrequency generator is programmed to achieve the best possible result. This is partially done by monitoring impedance in the tissue. Impedance is the resistance to the flow of current in the tissue that increases as tissue is desiccated and current flow is restricted. By continually monitoring impedance, optimization of the lesion volume is achieved.

II. The Prostate

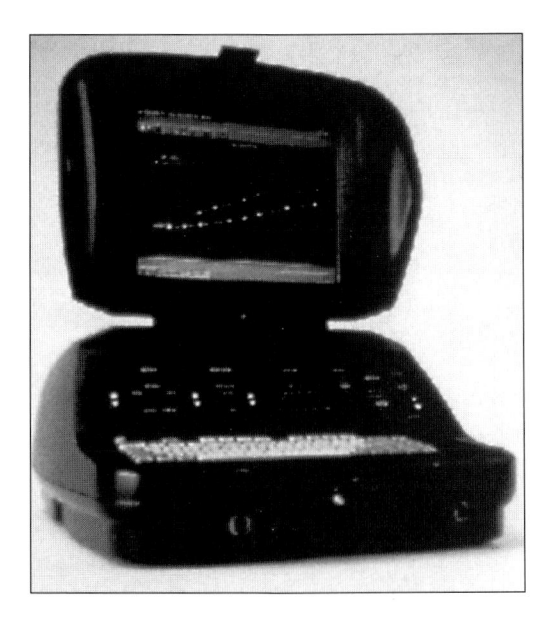

● **FIGURE 4-40.** The transurethral needle ablation (TUNA) system. The TUNA system consists of a radiofrequency generator with an integrated keyboard for data entry, which allows for simultaneous monitoring of urethral, prostatic, and rectal temperatures in real time.

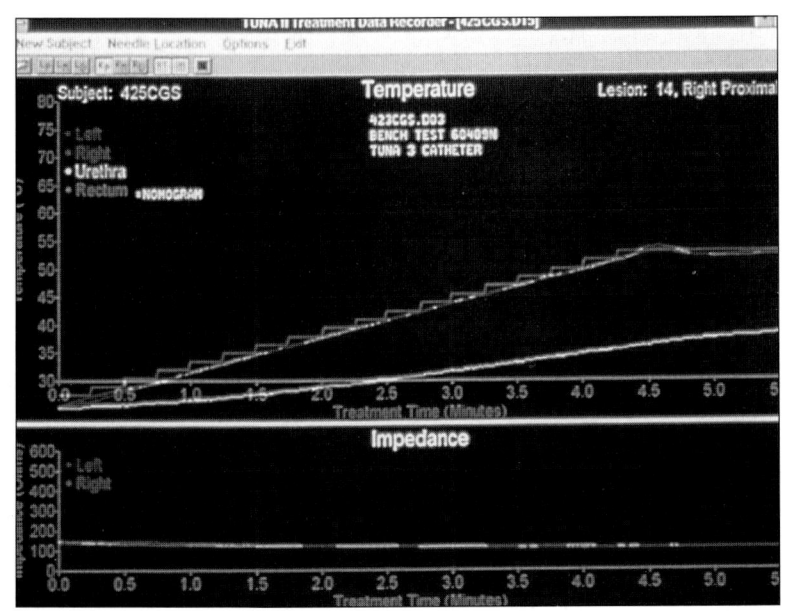

● **FIGURE 4-41.** Additional capabilities of the transurethral needle ablation (TUNA) system. The TUNA system also automatically calculates impedance and energy output to achieve ideal treatment levels with each application. A standard automated treatment consists of a 4-minute temperature rise time and a hold time of approximately 1.5 minutes at a target temperature of 53°C at the end of the shielding.

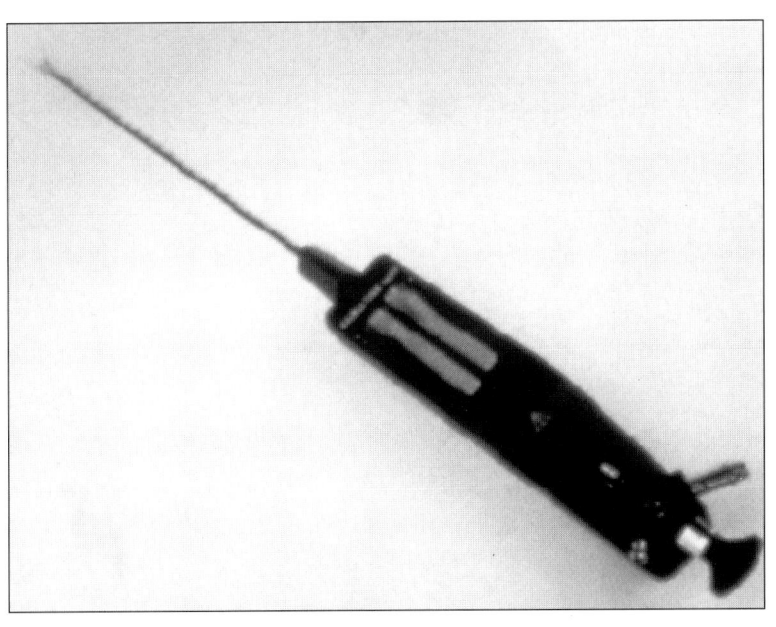

● **FIGURE 4-42.** Hand piece of the transurethral needle ablation system. The hand piece consists of the treatment catheter with the needles, and accepts a 0° optical lens. Integrated thermocouples monitor urethral temperature to prevent urethral damage.

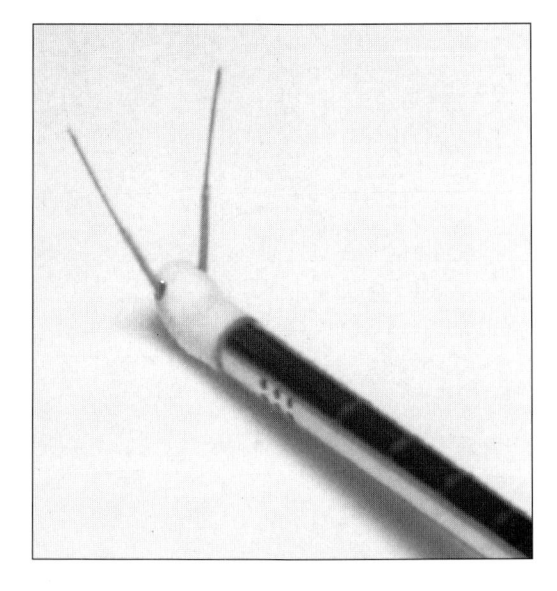

● **FIGURE 4-43.** The catheter tip. The tip of the catheter is clear, allowing visualization for accurate needle placement. The needle tips and the polytef shields are advanced according to the transverse diameter of the prostate assessed by transrectal ultrasonography. If the transverse measurements range from 34 to 46 mm, the exposed needle length should range from 11 to 18 mm and the shield should be advanced by 5 mm. If the transverse measurement ranges from 47 to 64 mm, the needle length should range from 18 to 22 mm with 6 mm of shielding.

Minimally Invasive Therapies for Benign Prostatic Hyperplasia

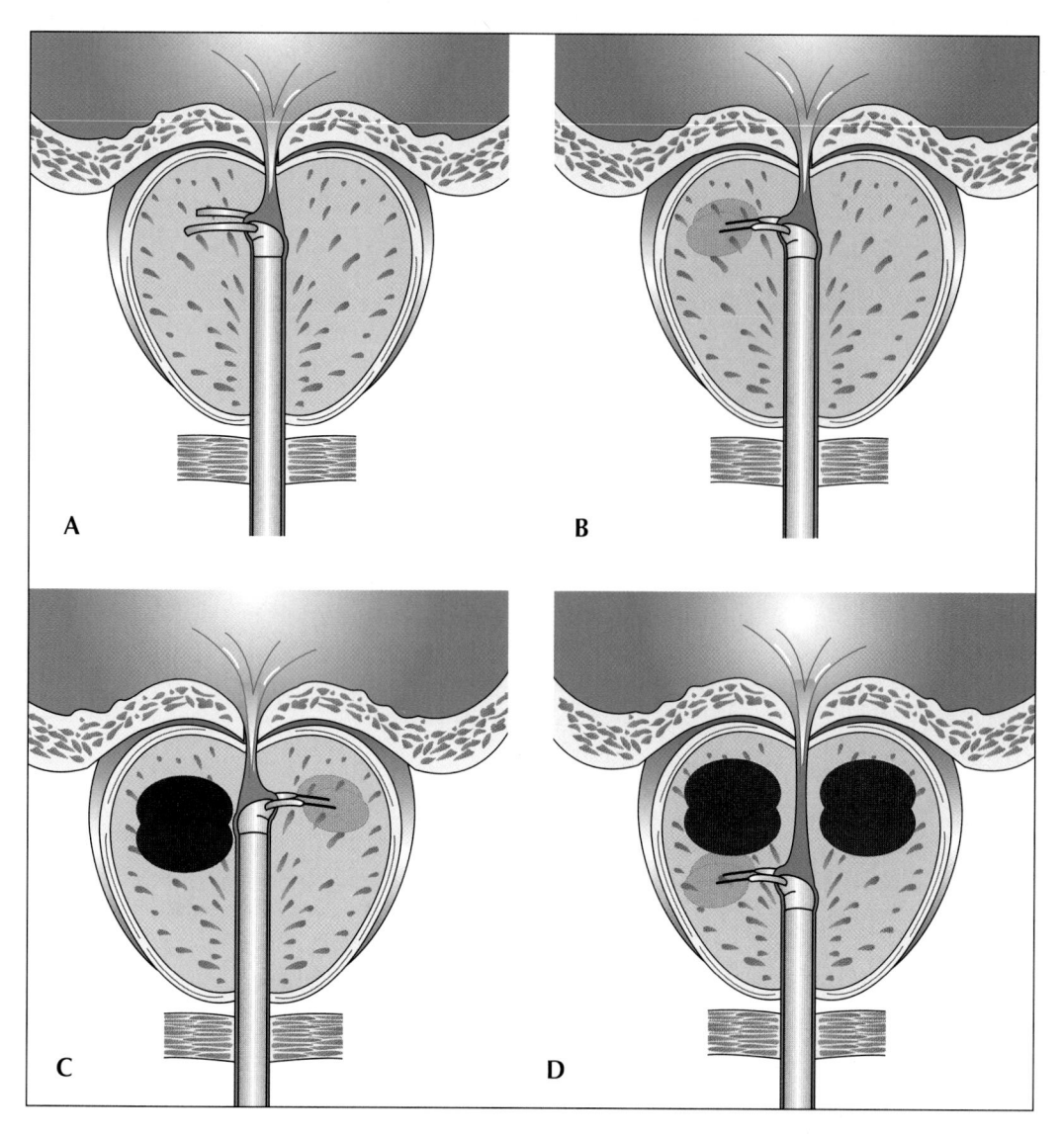

FIGURE 4-44. Sequence of the transurethral needle ablation procedure. The number of treatment planes depends on the length of the prostatic urethra as determined by transrectal ultrasonography or cystoscopy. If the distance from the bladder neck to the verumontanum is less than 4 cm, right and left treatments are administered in two planes. If the distance is 4 to 5 cm, three planes are treated, and if the distance is over 5 cm, four planes are treated. After the first treatment is administered at the bladder neck plane on the right-hand side (*panels A and B*), the orientation of the needle is changed and the contralateral site is treated (*panel C*). Thereafter, the next tissue plane is treated in the same fashion (*panel D*).

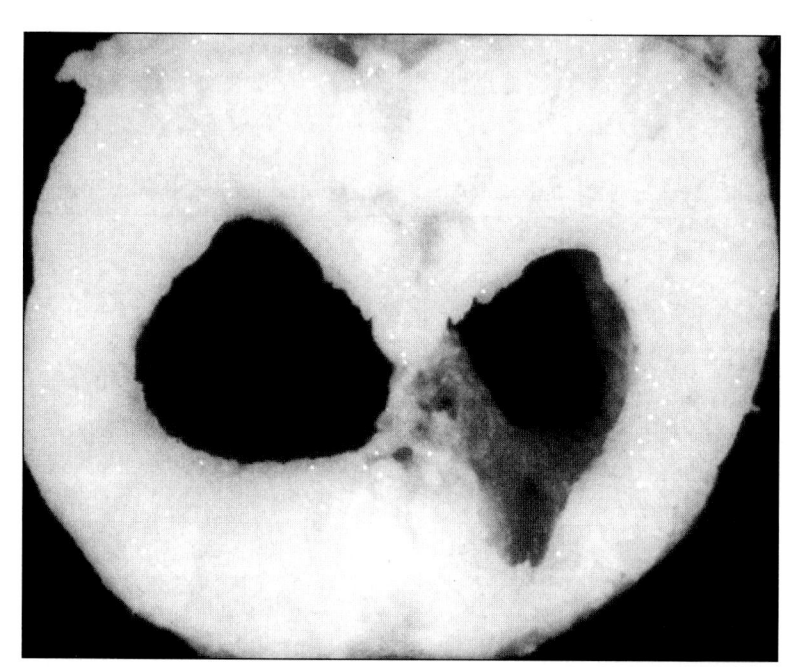

FIGURE 4-45. Prior to human treatments, animal experiments were conducted demonstrating that necrotic lesions could be created in the dog prostate using the transurethral needle ablation with no resultant damage to the rectum, bladder, external sphincter, or distal prostatic urethra [34].

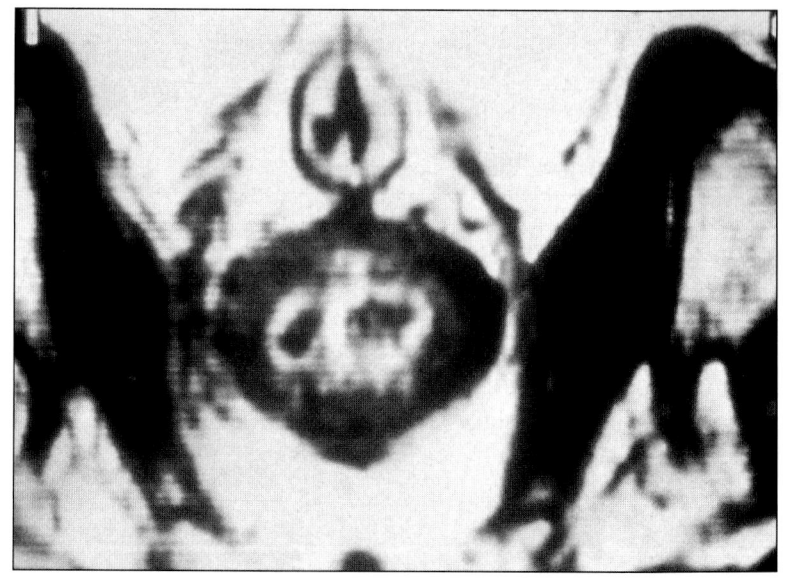

FIGURE 4-46. Gadolinium-enhanced magnetic resonance images of the pelvis demonstrate symmetrically placed necrotic lesions within the prostate following transurethral needle ablation treatment corresponding to areas of necrosis demonstrated on a cross-section of the surgically removed prostate (see Fig. 4-47) [11–13].

II. The Prostate

FIGURE 4-47. Cross-section of the surgically removed prostate.

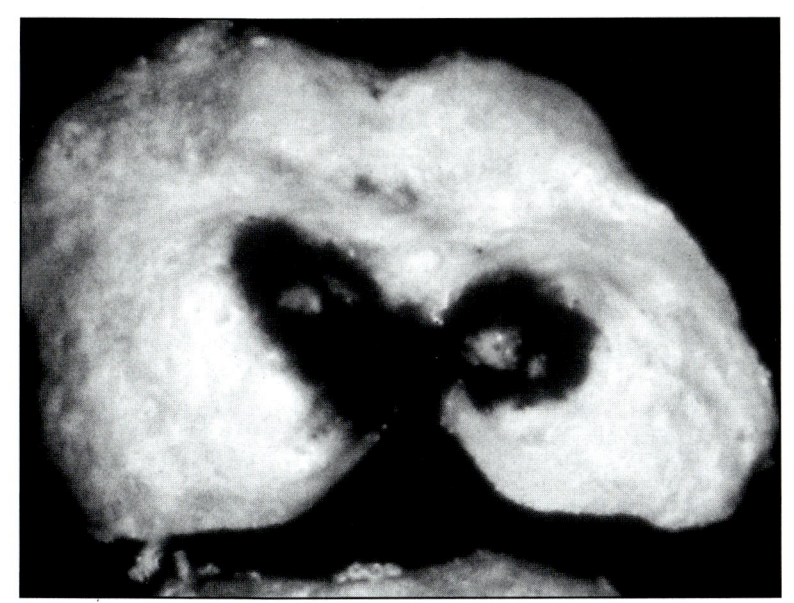

Wordwide Results of Transurethral Ablation of the Prostate

Study Group*	Patients, n	Follow-up, mo	Symptom Score Baseline	Post-TUNA[†]	Percent Change	Peak Flow Rate Baseline	Post-TUNA[†]	Percent Change
US/Pilot Study (Issa et al.)	12	6	25.5	9.8	-61	7.8	13.5	+73
US/Multicenter Study (Roehrborn et al.)	130	12	23.7	11.9	-50	7.8	14.6	+68
US/Multicenter Randomized Study (Bruskewitz et al.)	65	12	24.7	11.1	-55	6.7	15.0	+72
Brussels, Belgium (Schulman et al.)	36	12	21.5	7.8	-64	9.9	16.8	+69
	25	24	21.6	8.5	-61	9.9	15.5	+57
	17	36	21.6	7.6	-65	9.9	16.2	+64
Harlow, UK (Virdi et al.)	71	12	22.3	10.0	-55	7.0	13.8	+97
	71	24	22.3	9.4	-58	7.0	14.8	+111
	71	35	22.3	7.4	-67	7.0	14.2	+103
Milan, Italy (Campo et al.)	72	12	20.8	6.2	-70	8.2	15.9	+93
	42	18	20.8	5.7	-67	8.2	14.1	+71
European Multicenter (Ramon et al.)	68	12	22.0	7.5	-66	8.4	11.6	+33
Sheffield, UK (Chapple et al.)	58	12	22.0	10.0	-54	8.8	11.6	+30
Ioannina, Greece (Giennekopoulos et al.)	50	12	22.4	9.1	-59	7.6	16.8	+121
Johannesburg, South Africa (Steele et al.)	41	12	22.4	7.0	-68	5.6	10.2	+54
	38	24	22.4	9.5	-57	6.6	11.0	+66
Australia (Millard et al.)	20	12	19.0	8.2	-56	3.0	11.4	+280
Summary[‡] (world literature)	546	12	22.2	9.1	-58	7.8	13.8	+77
	176[‡]	24	21.8	8.5	-60	7.6	13.9	+82
	88	36	22.1	7.4	-66	7.5	14.5	+92

*For complete reference information, see Issa et al. [36].
[†]P = 0.01 to 0.0001.
[‡]First, second, and third rows summarize average improvement at first, second, and third years.
[§]Includes one series with 18-month follow-up.

FIGURE 4-48. Following the first series of 12 transurethral needle ablation procedures performed in the United States in 1994 [33], hundreds of patients have been treated worldwide under standardized protocols. The clinical results in terms of symptom score improvements and peak urinary flow rate improvements were recently reviewed by Issa et al. [35]. Overall, at 12 months, a decrease in symptom score from 22.2 to 9.1 (-60%) as well as at 3 years (-66%). Similarly, improvements in peak urinary flow rate from 7.8 to 13.8 mL/s at 1 year (+ 77%) were maintained at 2 years (+ 82%) and 3 years (+ 92%). However, the number of patients available for follow-up at 3 years as well as longer term follow-up is not available at this time. (*From* Issa *et al.* [35]; with permission.)

Detrusor Pressure Following Transurethral Needle Ablation of the Prostate

Study Group*	Patients, n	Follow-up, mo	Baseline	Post-TUNA	Percent Change	P Value
US/Pilot Study (Issa et al.)	12	6	91.8	70.9	-22.7	0.094
Milan, Italy (Campo et al.)	12[†]	6[†]	74.5[†]	56.3[†]	-24.4	0.046
	108	3	85.3	53.2	-37.6	<0.01
	86	6	85.3	61.3	-28.1	<0.01
	72	12	85.3	63.7	-25.3	<0.01
	42	24	85.3	67.8	-20.5	<0.01
Johannesburg, South Africa (Steele et al.)	41	1	92.4	77.0	-16.6	<0.05
	39	3	92.4	68.5	-25.8	<0.05
	34	6	92.4	54.8	-40.6	<0.05
	29	12	92.4	72.9	-21.1	<0.05
	12	24	92.4	56.9	-36.2	<0.05
Sheffield, UK (Chapple et al.)	39	3	97.0	79.0	-18.5	>0.05
	39	12	97.0	84.0	-13.4	>0.05
Australia (Millard et al.)	20	6	70.7	59.9	-15.8	0.90

Maximum Detrusor Pressure, cm H_2O

*For complete reference information, see Issa et al. [36].
[†]Indicates detrusor open pressure.

▶ **FIGURE 4-49.** Detrusor pressures following transurethral needle ablation of the prostate. Five investigators performed invasive pressure-flow urodynamic studies before and at various times after therapy. The percent reduction in the maximum detrusor pressure ranged from -13.4% to -14.6%. All but one investigator found a statistically significant decrease in the maximum detrusor pressure. (*From* Issa *et al.* [36]; with permission.)

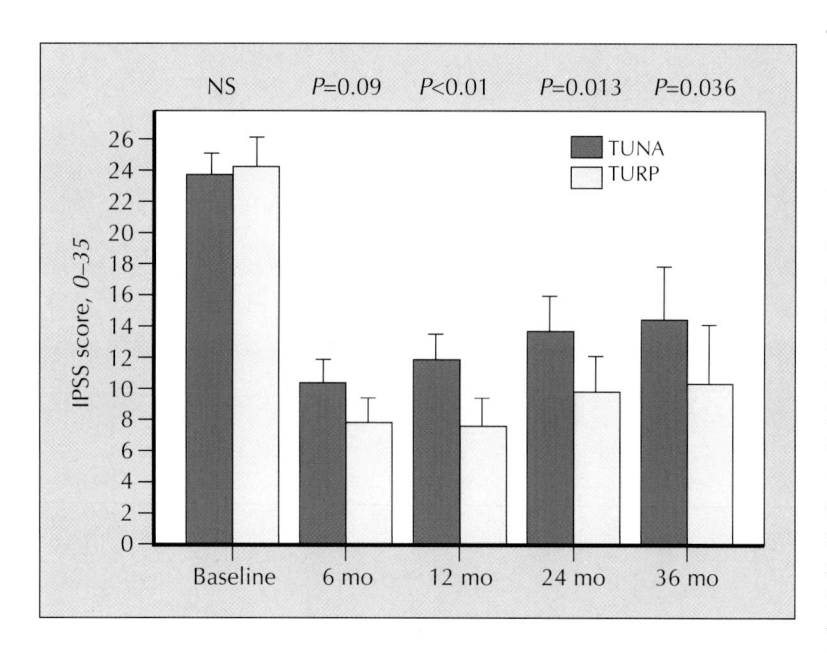

▶ **FIGURE 4-50.** Transurethral needle ablation (TUNA) versus transurethral resection (TURP) American Urological Association (AUA) symptom score. In the United States, a multicenter, randomized trial was initiated in which patients were randomly assigned to either TUNA or a standard TURP procedure. Entry criteria included men with lower urinary tract symptoms and benign prostatic hyperplasia over the age of 45 years, with an AUA symptom score of 13 or greater, a peak flow rate of 12 mL/s or less, a prostate volume between 25 and 75 mL by transurethral ultrasound (TRUS), and a prostate-specific antigen level of less than 10 ng/mL. Sixty-five patients were randomly assigned to TUNA and 56 to TURP. Both groups were well matched in terms of demographics and baseline parameters prior to treatment. The mean age was 66.1 (65.8) years, and mean AUA symptom score was 23.9 (24.1). Prostate volume was 36.2 mL (35.7 mL by TRUS). Three-year data are available that demonstrate a significant decrease in AUA symptom score from baseline at 6 months and all subsequent follow-ups. Although the initial decrease in AUA symptom score is almost identical between TUNA and TURP, a slight deterioration in symptom score is noted in the TUNA group for up to 2 years, after which no further change in symptom score occurs. IPSS—International Prostate Symptom Score; NS—not significant.

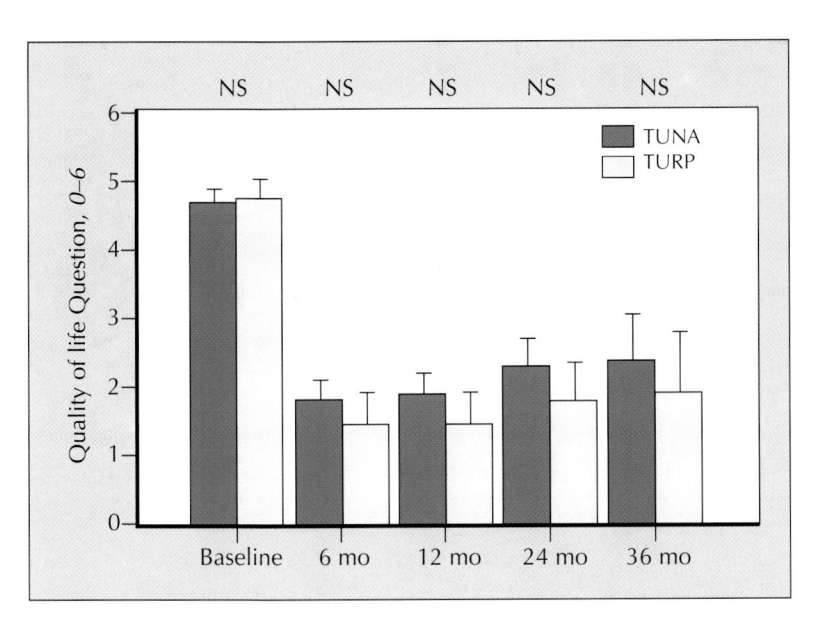

FIGURE 4-51. Quality of life score for transurethral needle ablation (TUNA) versus transurethral resection (TURP). Similar results are found for the quality of life score, which is equally improved in both TUNA and TURP groups with a slight deterioration in the TUNA group up to 2 years. (All differences from baseline in both groups are significant.) NS—not significant.

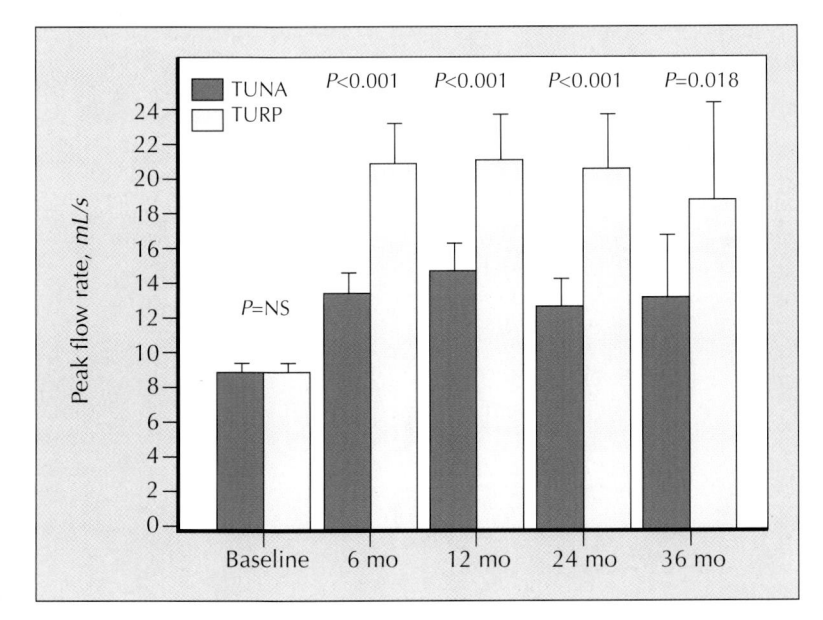

FIGURE 4-52. Transurethral needle ablation (TUNA) versus transurethral resection (TURP) peak flow rates. Although the TUNA-treated patients experience an improvement in peak urinary flow rate significantly different from baseline at all time points of follow-up, the TURP group achieved a statistically much larger improvement in flow rate that was maintained over the entire duration of follow-up.

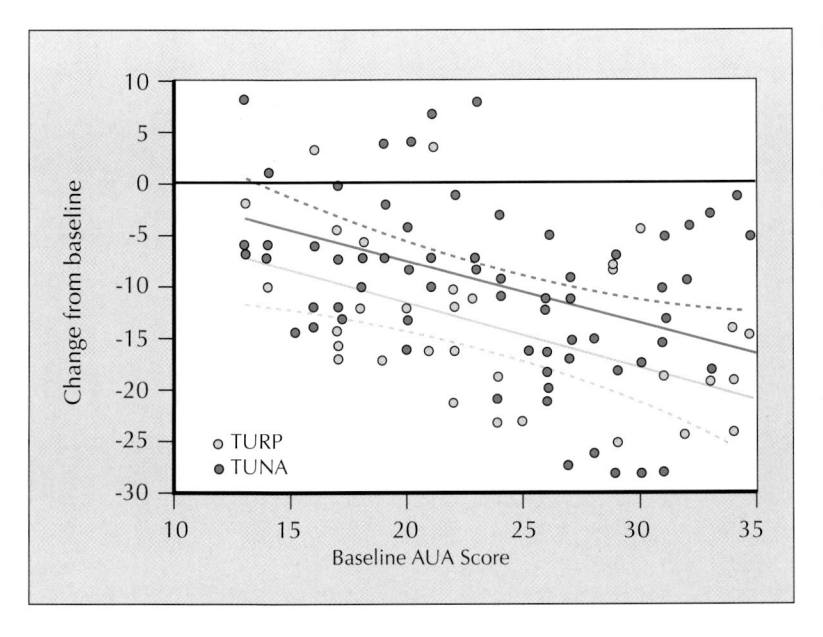

FIGURE 4-53. Transurethral needle ablation (TUNA) versus transurethral resection (TURP) baseline score versus change from baseline and linear regression. A convenient way to compare treatment efficacy in terms of symptom improvement is a plot depicting the baseline symptom severity score against the changes from baseline. It is evident that almost all patients with very few exceptions experienced a decrease from baseline (*ie*, below the 0 or no-change line). With more advanced symptom severity scores, more significant drops from baseline were observed. The regression lines for both TUNA- and TURP-treated patients indicate that across all symptom severity ranges, the TUNA-treated patients had almost the same symptomatic improvement as the TURP-treated patients. AUA—American Urological Association.

Baseline and 6-Month Data for TUNA and TURP

Parameter	TUNA Baseline	TUNA 6 mo	TURP Baseline	TURP 6 mo	P Value[†]
AUA SI	23.9	10.8	24.1	8.1	0.0288
	$P < 0.0001$*		$P < 0.0001$*		0.430
BII	7.1	2.3	8.1	1.8	0.170
	$P < 0.001$*		$P < 0.001$*		< 0.001
QOL	4.6	2.0	4.8	1.5	0.19
	$P < 0.001$*		$P < 0.0001$[†]		< 0.001
Qmax	8.8	13.5	75.8	54.9	
	$P < 0.0001$*		$P < 0.001$*		
P_{det} Qmax	78.7	64.5	58.3	10.9	
	$P < 0.036$*		$P < 0.001$*		
AG number	61.2	37.2			
	$P < 0.001$*				

*Comparison from baseline to 6 months within groups.
[†]Comparison at 6 months between groups.

FIGURE 4-54. Results of baseline and 6-month follow-up, pressure-flow urodynamic studies performed in the US randomized trial. The transurethral needle ablation–treated patients achieved a decrease in P_{det} (detrusor pressure) at Qmax from 78.7 to 64.5 cm H_2O ($P = 0.036$), whereas the transurethral resection–treated patients achieved a decrease from 75.8 to 54.9 cm H_2O ($P < 0.01$). The Abrams-Griffith (AG) number, calculated as P_{det} at Qmax minus two times Qmax, decreased significantly in both treatment groups. AUA SI—American Urological Association Symtom Index; BII—BPH Impact Index; QOL—Quality of Life Question.

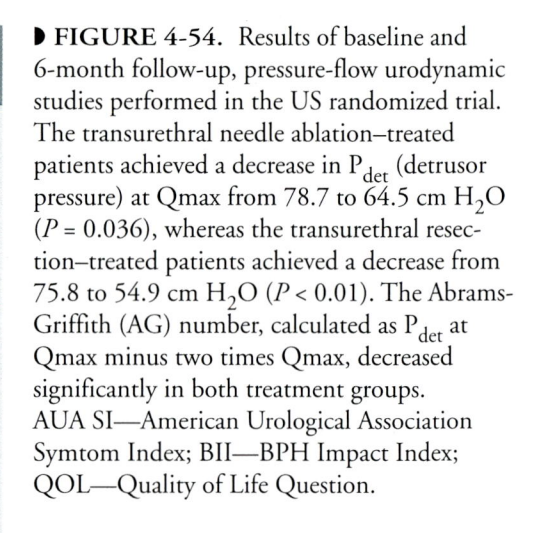

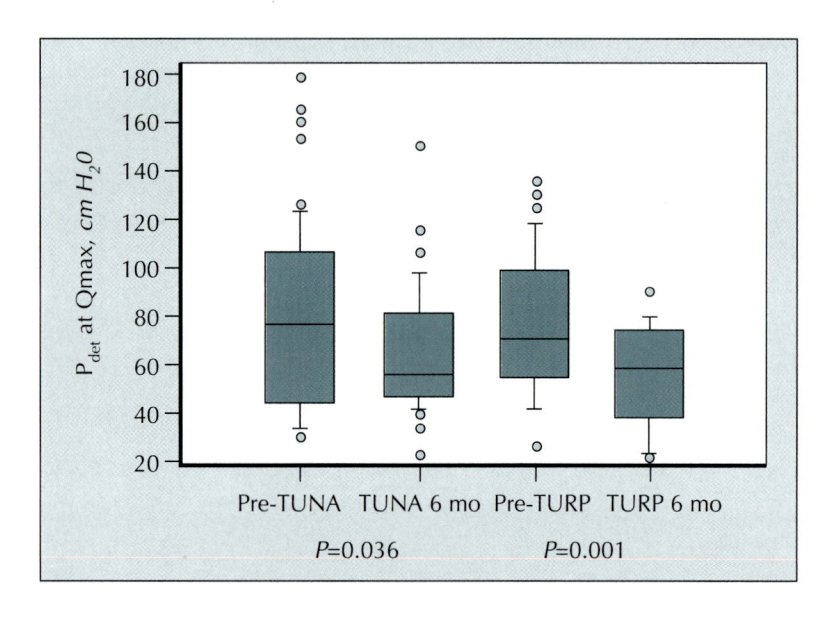

FIGURE 4-55. Baseline and 6-month data for transurethral needle ablation (TUNA) and transurethral resection (TURP). The P_{det} (detrusor pressure) at Qmax for both TUNA- and TURP-treated patients before and 6 months after therapy demonstrate the overall decrease of the P_{det} at Qmax in both treatment groups. There was no statistically significant difference at 6 months between the two groups ($P = 0.19$).

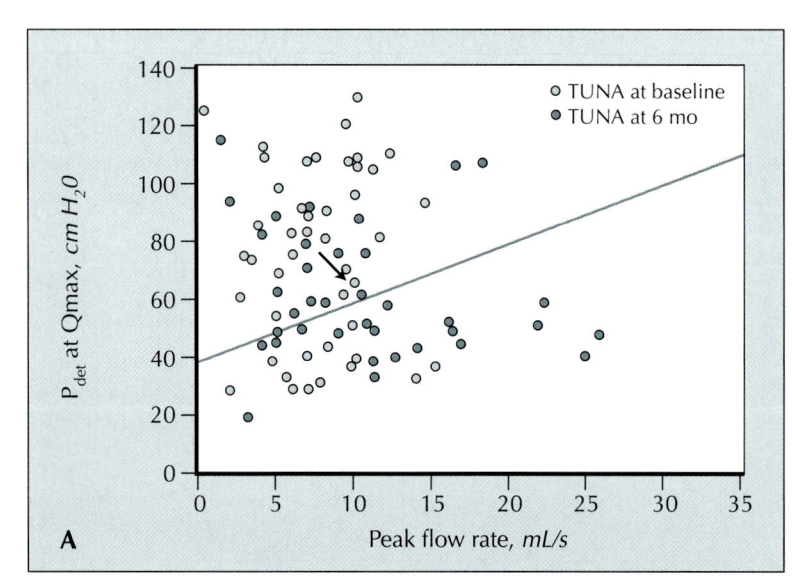

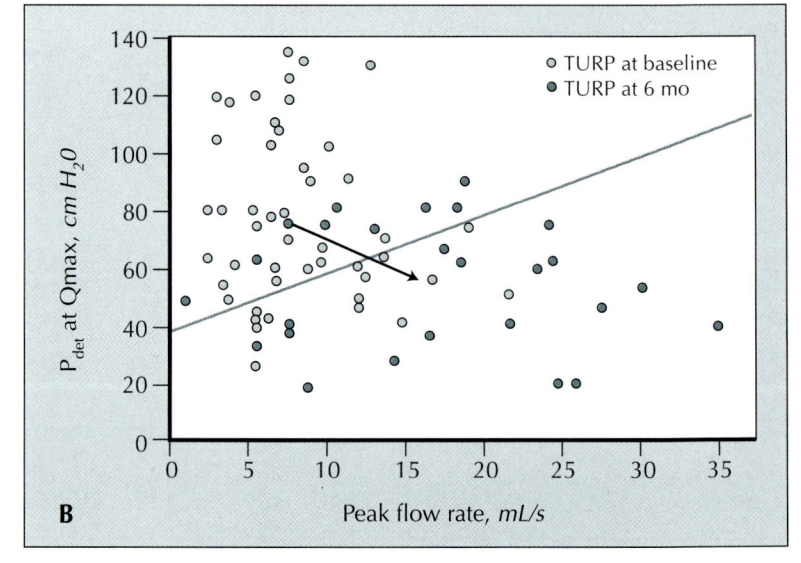

FIGURE 4-56. The P_{det} (detrusor pressure) Qmax versus Qmax for transurethral needle ablation (TUNA) (*panel A*) or transurethral resection (TURP) (*panel B*) treated patients at baseline and 6 months. When plotting P_{det} at Qmax versus Qmax in the traditional form of an Abrams-Griffith nomogram, it is apparent that overall the TURP-treated patients move from the obstructed to the equivocal and nonobstructed category (*arrow*), whereas the overall change in the TUNA-treated patients is less pronounced, and more patients remain in the obstructed category [36]. *Straight line* indicates equivocal.

TUNA Versus TURP Adverse Events

	TUNA, n (%)	TURP, n (%)
Bleeding	21 (32.3)	56 (100)
Retrograde ejaculation	0 (0)	21 (38.2)
Urinary tract infection	5 (7.7)	7 (12.7)
Urethral stricture	1 (1.5)	4 (7.3)
Erectile dysfunction	0 (0)	7 (12.7)
Incontinence	0 (0)	2 (3.6)
Dysuria	0 (0)	2 (3.6)

FIGURE 4-57. Transurethral needle ablation (TUNA) versus transurethral resection (TURP) adverse events. The TUNA procedure is remarkably free of adverse events. No cases of retrograde ejaculation, erectile dysfunction, or urinary incontinence were seen, and the most common adverse event noted was hematuria. Urinary retention has been reported between 13.3% and 41.6% [37]. The retention is transient and lasts usually less than 72 hours. Anesthetic requirements for the TUNA procedure vary from patient to patient and from physician to physician. Some investigators perform the TUNA procedure in an office setting with intraurethral lidocaine or intravenous solution only; others prefer an operating room setting with either monitored intravenous sedation or other forms of general anesthesia.

REFERENCES

1. Arrighi HM, Metter EJ, Guess HA, Fozzard JL: Natural history of benign prostatic hyperplasia and risk of prostatectomy. *Urology* 1991, 38:4–8.
2. Barry MJ: Epidemiology and natural history of benign prostatic hyperplasia. In *The Urologic Clinics of North America*. Edited by Lepor H, Walsh PC. Philadelphia: WB Saunders; 1990: 495–507.
3. Wasson JH, Reda DJ, Bruskewitz RC, et al.: A comparison of transurethral surgery with watchful waiting for moderate symptoms of benign prostatic hyperplasia: The Veterans Affairs Cooperative Study Group on Transurethral Resection of the Prostate. *N Engl J Med* 1995, 332:75–79.
4. McConnell JD, Barry MJ, Bruskewitz RC, et al.: *Benign Prostatic Hyperplasia: Diagnosis and Treatment. Clinical Practice Guideline, Number 8.* Edited by McConnell JD, Barry MJ, Bruskewitz RC, et al. Rockville, MD: Agency for Health Care Policy and Research, Public Health Service, US Department of Health and Human Services; 1994.
5. Harada T, Etori D, Kumazaki T, et al.: Microwave surgical treatment of disease of the prostate. *Urology* 1985, 26:572–576.
6. Astrahan MA, Sapozink MD, Cohen D, et al.: Microwave applicator for transurethral hyperthermia of benign prostatic hyperplasia. *Int J Hyperthermia* 1989, 5:283–296.
7. Abbou CC, Colombel M, Payan C, et al.: The efficacy of microwave induced hyperthermia in the treatment of BPH: The Paris Public Hospitals' experience. In *Benign Prostatic Hyperplasia: Recent Progress in Clinical Research and Practice*. Edited by Kurth KH, Newling DWW. New York: Wiley-Liss; 1994:449–454.
8. de la Rosette JJMCH, D'Ancona FCH, Debruyne FMJ: Current status of thermotherapy of the prostate. *J Urol* 1997, 157:430–438.
9. Madersbacher S, Kratzik C, Szabo N, et al.: Tissue ablation in benign prostatic hyperplasia with high-intensity focused ultrasound. *Eur Urol* 1993, 23 (suppl 1):39–43.
10. Ramon J, Goldwasser B, Shenfield O, et al.: Needle ablation using radio frequency current as a treatment for benign prostatic hyperplasia: experimental results in ex vivo human prostate. *Eur Urol* 1993, 24:406–410.
11. Schulman CC, Zlotta AR, Rasor JS, et al.: Transurethral needle ablation (TUNA): safety, feasibility, and tolerance of a new office procedure for treatment of benign prostatic hyperplasia. *Eur Urol* 1993, 24:415–423.
12. Rasor S, Zlotta AR, Edwards SD, Schulman CC: Transurethral needle ablation (TUNA): thermal gradient mapping and comparison of lesion size in a tissue model and in patients with benign prostatic hyperplasia. *Eur Urol* 1993, 24:411–414.
13. Schulman CC, Zlotta AR: Transurethral needle ablation of the prostate (TUNA): pathological, radiological and clinical study of a new office procedure for treatment of benign prostatic hyperplasia using low-level radiofrequency energy. *Sem Urol* 1994, 12:205–210.
14. Schulman CC, Zlotta AR: Transurethral needle ablation of the prostate for treatment of benign prostatic hyperplasia: early clinical experience. *Urology* 1995, 45:28–33.
15. Servadio C, Leib C: Hyperthermia in the treatment of prostate cancer. *Prostate* 1984, 5:205–211.
16. Roehrborn CG, Krongrad A, McConnell JD: Temperature mapping in the canine prostate during transurethrally-applied local microwave hyperthermia. *Prostate* 1992, 20:97–104.
17. Denis L, McConnell JD, Yoshida O, et al.: Recommendations of the International Scientific Committee: the evaluation and treatment of lower urinary tract symptoms (LUYS) suggestive of benign prostatic obstruction. In *4th International Consultation on Benign Prostatic Hyperplasia (BPH)*. Edited by Denis L, Griffiths K, Khoury S, et al. Plymouth PL67PY, UK: Health Publication; 1997: 669–684.
18. Bernier PA, Roehrborn CG: Thermal therapy in the treatment of benign prostatic hyperplasia. *Curr Opin Urol* 1997, 7:15–20.
19. Gibbons RP, Mebust W, Smith P, et al.: Interventional therapy. In *4th International Consultation on Benign Prostatic Hyperplasia (BPH)*. Edited by Denis L, Griffiths K, Khoury S, et al. Plymouth PL67Py, UK: Health Publication; 1997: 515–572.
20. de Wildt MJAM, D'Ancona FCH, Hubregtse M, et al.: Three-year followup of patients treated with low energy microwave thermotherapy. *J Urol* 1996, 156:1959–1996.
21. Dahlstrand C, Walden M, Geirsson G, Petterson S: Transurethral microwave thermotherapy versus transurethral resection for symptomatic benign prostatic obstruction: a prospective randomized study with a 2-year follow-up. *Br J Urol* 1995, 76:614–618.
22. de la Rosette JJMCH, de Wildt MJAM, Höfner K, et al.: High energy thermotherapy in the treatment of benign prostatic hyperplasia: results of the European Benign Prostatic Hyperplasia Study Group. *J Urol* 1996, 156:97–102.
23. Bosch JLHR: Urodynamic effects of various treatment modalities for benign prostatic hyperplasia. *J Urol* 1997, 158:2034–2044.
24. de la Rosette JJMCH, de Wildt JMAM, Höfner K, et al.: Pressure-flow study analyses in patients treated with high energy thermotherapy. *J Urol* 1996, 156:1428–1433.
25. de Wildt MJ, Tubaro A, Höfner K, et al.: Responders and nonresponders to transurethral microwave thermotherapy: a multicenter retrospective analysis [see comments]. *J Urol* 1995, 154:1775–1778.
26. Djavan B, Shariat S, Schafer B, Marberger M: Tolerability of high energy transurethral microwave thermotherapy with topical urethral anesthesia: results of a prospective, randomized, single-blinded clinical trial. *J Urol* 1998, 160:772–776.
27. Madersbacher S, Pedevilla M, Vingers L, et al.: Effect of high-intensity focused ultrasound on human prostate cancer in vivo. *Cancer Res* 1995, 55:3346–3351.
28. Foster RS, Bihrle R, Sanghvi N, et al.: Production of prostatic lesions in canines using transrectally administered high-intensity focused ultrasound. *Eur Urol* 1993, 23:330–336.
29. Foster RS, Bihrle R, Sanghvi NT, et al.: High-intensity focused ultrasound in the treatment of prostatic disease. *Eur Urol* 1993, 23 (suppl 1): 29–33.
30. Kirby RS, McConnell JD, Fitzpatrick JM, et al. (eds.): High intensity focused ultrasound. In *Textbook of Benign Prostate Hyperplasia*. Oxford, UK: Isis Medical Media; 1996:429–439.
31. Goldwasser B, Ramon J, Engelberg S: Transurethral needle ablation of the prostate using low-level radiofrequency energy: an animal experimental study. *Eur Urol* 1993;24:400–405.
32. Bihrle R, Foster RS, Sanghvi NT, et al.: High intensity focused ultrasound for the treatment of benign prostatic hyperplasia: early United States clinical experience. *J Urol* 1994, 151:1271–1275.
33. Madersbacher S, Kratzik C, Susani M, Marberger M: Tissue ablation in benign prostatic hyperplasia with high intensity focused ultrasound [see comments]. *J Urol* 1994, 152:1956–1960.

34. Ramon J, Goldwasser B, Shenfeld O, *et al.*: Needle ablation using radio frequency current as a treatment for benign prostatic hyperplasia: experimental results in ex vivo human prostate. *Eur Urol* 1993, 24:406–410.
35. Issa MM: Transurethral needle ablation of the prostate: report of initial US Clinical trial. *J Urol* 1996, 156:413–419.
36. Issa MM, Myrick SE, Symbas NP: The TUNA procedure for BPH: basic procedure and clinical results. *Infect Urol* 1998, Sept/Oct:148–154.
37. Burkhard FC, Roehrborn CG, Bruskewitz RC, *et al.*: The effects of transurethral needle ablation (TUNA) and transurethral resection (TURP) of the prostate on pressure flow urodynamic parameters. Analysis of the US randomized study. *J Urol* 1999, in press.

Laser Prostatectomy

Aaron P. Perlmutter & John N. Kabalin

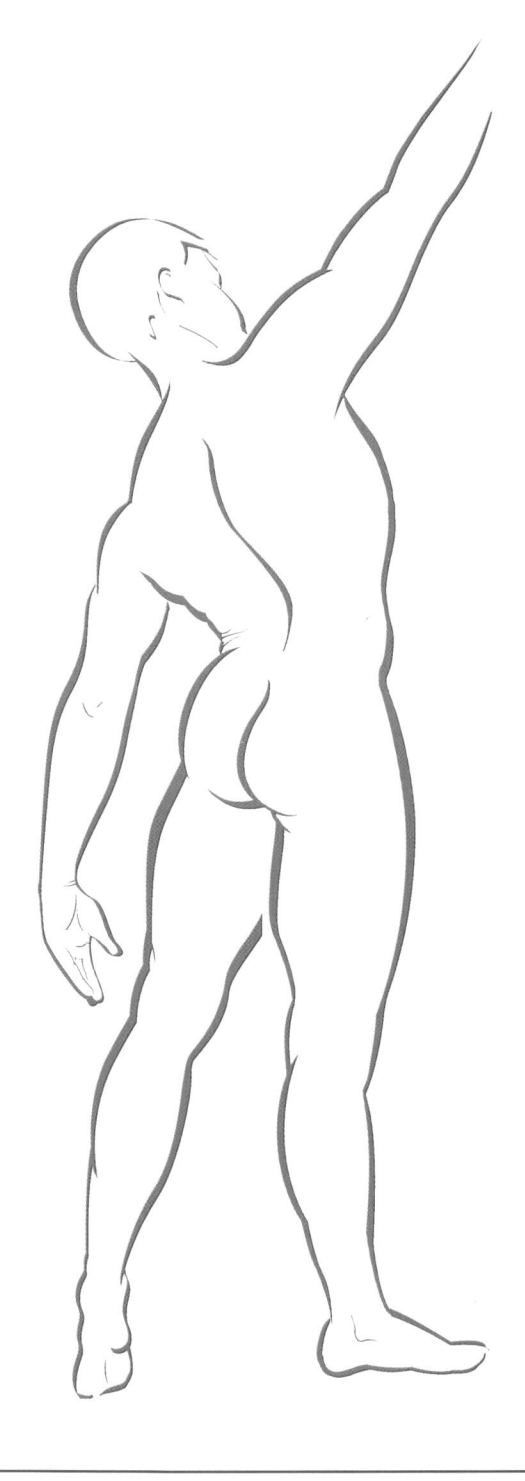

NONCANCEROUS DISEASE SECTION

Laser prostatectomy can remove obstructing benign prostatic hyperplasia (BPH) tissue without the hospitalization, bleeding, and perioperative and postoperative morbidity caused by transurethral resection of the prostate (TURP). Laser wavelengths suitable for urologic applications can be delivered through small semiflexible fibers that pass through standard endoscopes. The tissue effects of laser energy usually involve virtually instantaneous attainment of temperatures greater than 60°C to create coagulation or greater than 100°C to create vaporization. Laser energy can be delivered via a free-beam delivery system to create coagulation necrosis, vaporization, or tissue cutting. In addition, a diffusing laser fiber can be placed directly into the adenoma for interstitial treatment, to create coagulation necrosis.

Laser prostatectomy has undergone an amazingly rapid evolution since its introduction in the late 1980s. The free-beam coagulation technique is not commonly used, and has been replaced by the holmium resection technique when the immediate effect of TURP is desired, and by interstitial techniques when a delay in clinical improvement can be tolerated. Laser techniques in the prostate continue to evolve as urologists pursue the goal of removing the obstructing adenoma with minimal side effects and maximum clinical improvement.

Laser	Wavelength, nm	Treatment/Fiber	Primary Tissue Effect
Nd:YAG	1064	Free beam/low energy density	Coagulation necrosis
		Free beam/high energy density	Vaporization and coagulation
		Interstitial	Coagulation necrosis
Semiconductor diode	800–1000	Free beam/low energy density	Coagulation necrosis
		Interstitial	Coagulation necrosis
KTP	532	Free beam/high energy density	Vaporization
Holmium:YAG	2140	Free beam	Cutting with vaporization

Lasers and Their Tissue Effects

▶ **FIGURE 5-1.** Lasers and their tissue effects with delivery fibers commonly used for prostate treatment.

TRANSURETHRAL ULTRASOUND-GUIDED LASER-INDUCED PROSTATECTOMY

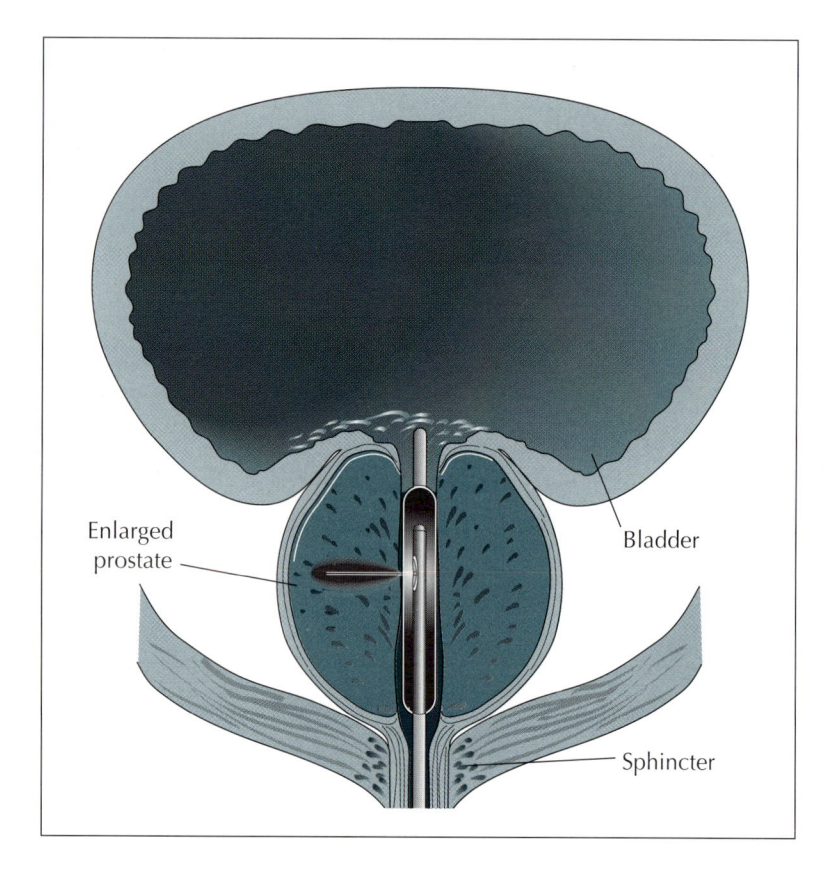

▶ **FIGURE 5-2.** The first delivery system purposely designed for the performance of free-beam laser prostatectomy was developed in the late 1980s [1]. The transurethral ultrasound-guided laser-induced prostatectomy (TULIP [Intrasonix Inc., Burlington, MA]) device was a uniquely engineered apparatus consisting of a 22-F rigid urethral probe containing an Nd:YAG (neodymium:yttrium-aluminum-garnet) delivery fiber with a deflecting prism mechanism. It was the first system developed to laterally deflect laser energy into the prostatic lateral lobes in order to produce coagulation necrosis. Clinical results demonstrated substantial efficacy [2], although less than that of transurethral resection of the prostate (TURP), but the device and ultrasound imaging proved cumbersome, and the procedure disappeared. However, the efforts of the TULIP investigators inspired much of the subsequent development of free-beam laser prostatectomy.

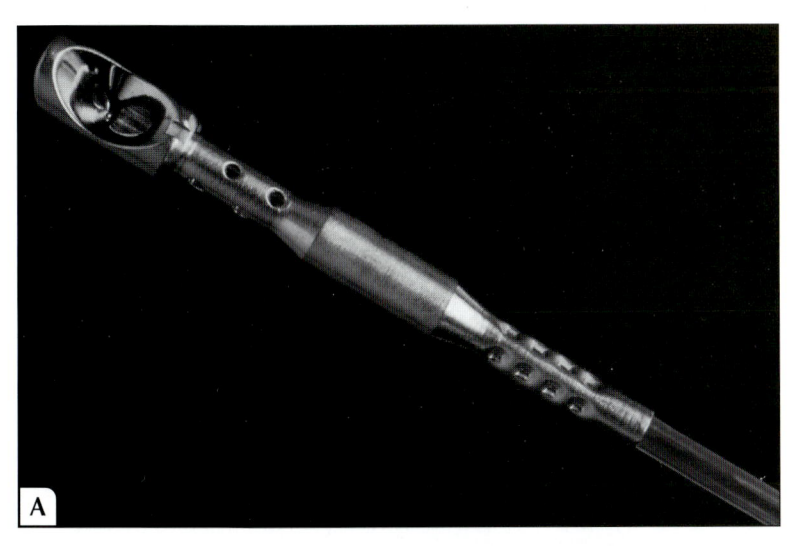

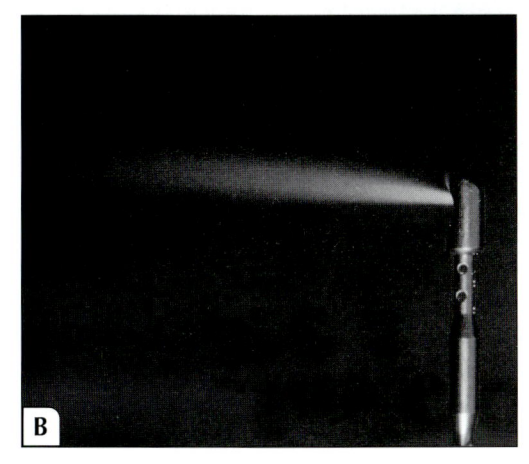

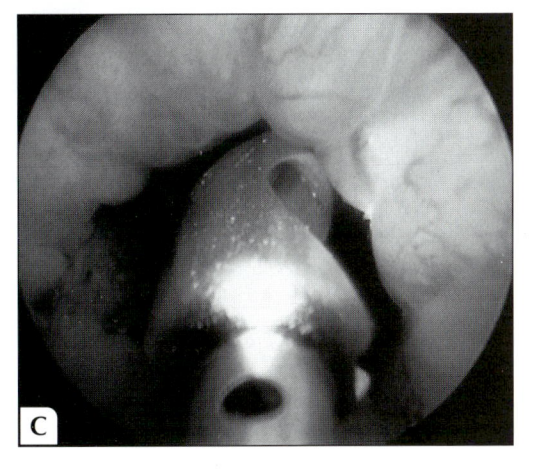

ND:YAG FREE-BEAM LASER PROSTATECTOMY

FIGURE 5-3. The Nd:YAG wavelength is well suited for transmission through flexible fibers, which are easily manipulated through standard urologic endoscopes and applied under direct vision [3]. This allows for visually guided prostatic irradiation. **A,** Distal reflecting mirror of the side-firing Nd:YAG laser delivery fiber for prostatic irradiation (Urolase, CR Bard and Trimedyne; Covington, GA). **B,** This fiber allows the laser beam to be aimed directly at the lateral or median lobe of the prostate under direct vision. **C,** Visual cystoscopic appearance of the laser fiber in use. The fiber is directed at obstructing tissue and held in place during the irradiation.

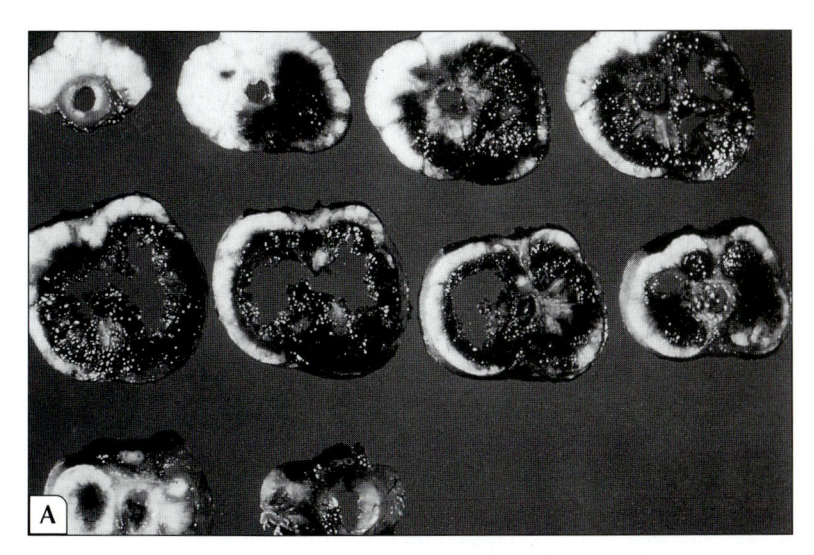

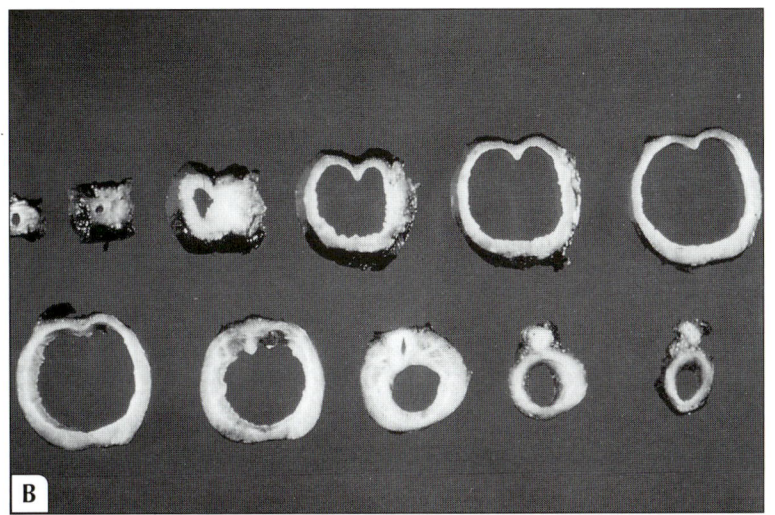

FIGURE 5-4. Because the Nd:YAG wavelength is relatively poorly absorbed by water, there is a slow energy transfer to tissue when it is used at lower energy density applications. Thus, tissue coagulation is favored over tissue vaporization. In canine feasibility studies, Johnson *et al.* [4] demonstrated that the Nd:YAG laser created a large volume of coagulation necrosis, and that resolution of this lesion resulted in enlargement of the prostatic fossa. This pioneering work led to clinical investigations of safety and efficacy in humans with benign prostatic hyperplasia. **A,** Serial transverse section of the canine prostate immediately after Nd:YAG irradiation demonstrating the area of coagulation necrosis (*dark tissue*). **B,** The cavity formed 7 weeks later. (*From* Johnson *et al.* [4]; with permission.)

Laser Prostatectomy

5.3

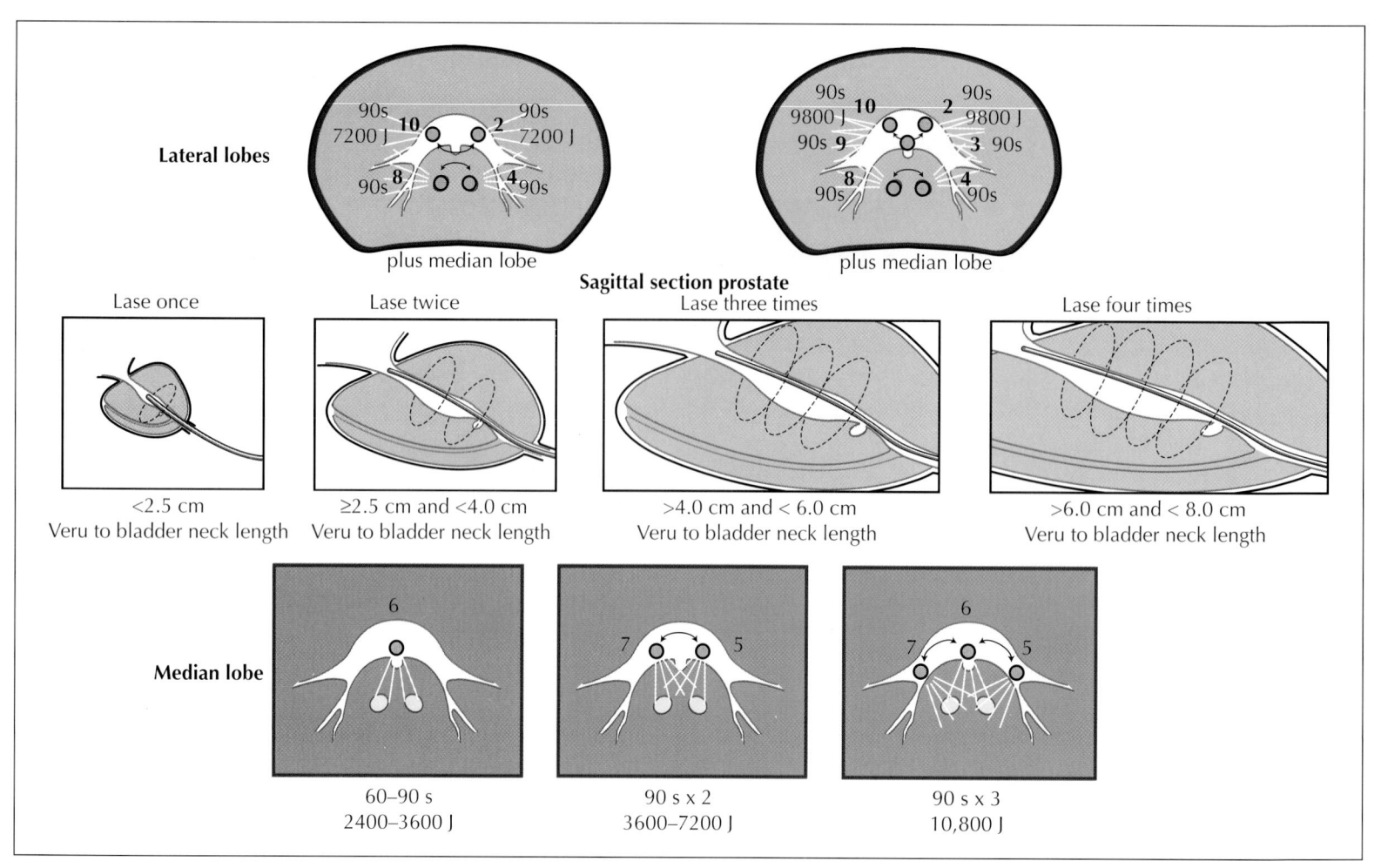

FIGURE 5-5. Prostatectomy using Nd:YAG laser typically is performed under regional or general anesthesia. A cystoscope of relatively small caliber (≤ 22 F) accommodates almost all side-firing laser fibers used for Nd:YAG laser prostatectomy. Because Nd:YAG laser coagulation seals blood vessels, preventing both bleeding and intraoperative fluid absorption (and, thus, transurethral resection syndrome), sterile water or saline irrigation commonly is used. Room temperature irrigation dissipates the heat more effectively, and thus is preferred over warm irrigation. In the spot coagulation technique described by Kabalin [5], the Nd:YAG laser fiber is held in close approximation, without touching the obstructing benign prostatic hyperplasia tissue. Laser energy is applied for a minimum of 60 to 90 seconds, and power settings between 40 W and 60 W are used, depending on the degree of divergence of the emitting laser fiber. If the laser is applied without causing tissue char, the depth of coagulation necrosis is approximately 1.5 cm. Areas of coagulation necrosis eventually slough per urethra during micturition.

The goal is to treat all lateral lobe tissue. The number of irradiations in the anterior-posterior direction depends on the size of the gland. The larger the anterior-posterior distance, the more irradiations are required to create lesions that coagulate the majority of the tissue. The number of irradiations in the sagittal plane also increases with increasing prostate size. Again, the goal is to place lesions no more than 1.5 cm apart to avoid leaving untreated areas of obstructing tissue. The middle lobe requires complete treatment.

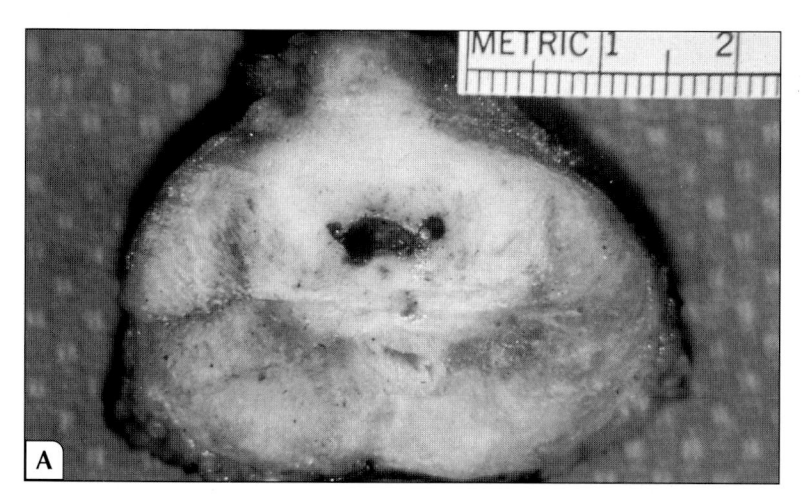

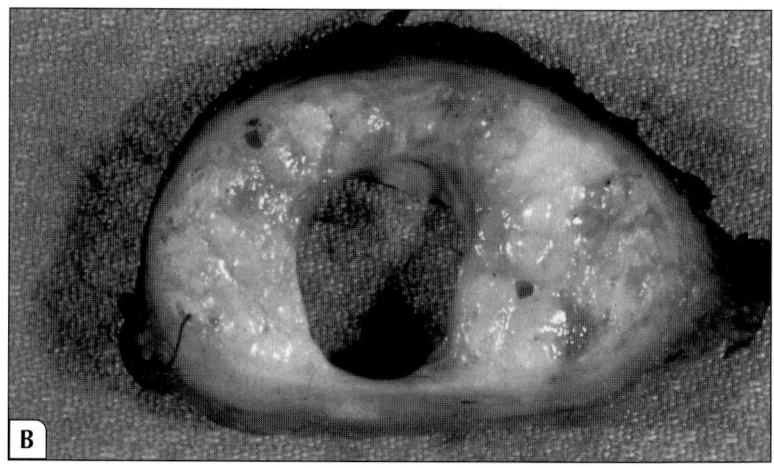

FIGURE 5-6. The acute and chronic tissue effects of Nd:YAG laser spot applications effects have been demonstrated *in vivo* by Kabalin *et al.* [6]. **A**, A transverse section through a human prostate removed immediately after Nd:YAG laser spot applications. The transition zone shows extensive coagulation necrosis. **B**, A transverse section through a human prostate removed 1 year after Nd:YAG laser spot applications. The transition zone slough is complete, leaving a large laser defect.

A. Complications of Nd:YAG Laser Prostatectomy in 230 Men With 1-year Minimum Postoperative Follow-up

	Incidence, n (%)
Acute complications	
Significant hemorrhage/transfusion	0 (—)
Transurethral resection syndrome	0 (—)
Prostatic perforation/extravasation	0 (—)
Postoperative prostatitis	6 (2.6)
Long-term complications	
Stress urinary incontinence	0 (—)
Urethral stricture	4 (1.7)
Bladder neck contracture	10 (4.3)
Reoperation for residual tissue	13 (5.7)

B. Voiding Outcomes of Nd:YAG Laser Prostatectomy from 20 Combined Series Reporting 3 to 12 Months' Postoperative Follow-up

	Preoperative (n)	Postoperative (n) 3 mo	6 mo	12 mo
Peak flow rate, mL/s	8.0 (1765)	16.2 (1306)	16.2 (1433)	17.2 (600)
Post-void residual, mL	189 (1295)	63 (1104)	61 (1044)	72 (576)
AUA symptom index	21.3 (1851)	8.4 (1308)	7.4 (1466)	7.0 (618)

C. Long-term Voiding Outcomes of Nd:YAG Lower Prostatectomy

	Preoperative (n)	Postoperative (n) 1 y	2 y	3 y
Peak flow rate, mL/s	7.7 (290)	16.9 (193)	17.1 (84)	19.7 (18)
Post-void residual, mL	334 (273)	120 (175)	117 (84)	111 (17)
AUA symptom index	19.9 (289)	7.8 (218)	8.8 (101)	5.7 (20)

FIGURE 5-7. Complications of Nd:YAG laser prostatectomy. A, In a detailed analysis of acute and long-term complications following Nd:YAG laser prostatectomy, a complication rate of 14.3% was found in 230 men with a minimum 12-month follow-up and median 35-month follow-up. No significant bleeding, transfusion requirement, transurethral resection syndrome, or prostatic perforation was observed. B, The voiding outcomes from 20 combined series reporting 3 to 12 months postoperative follow-up. C, Follow-up of up to 3 years from the series of Kabalin [7].

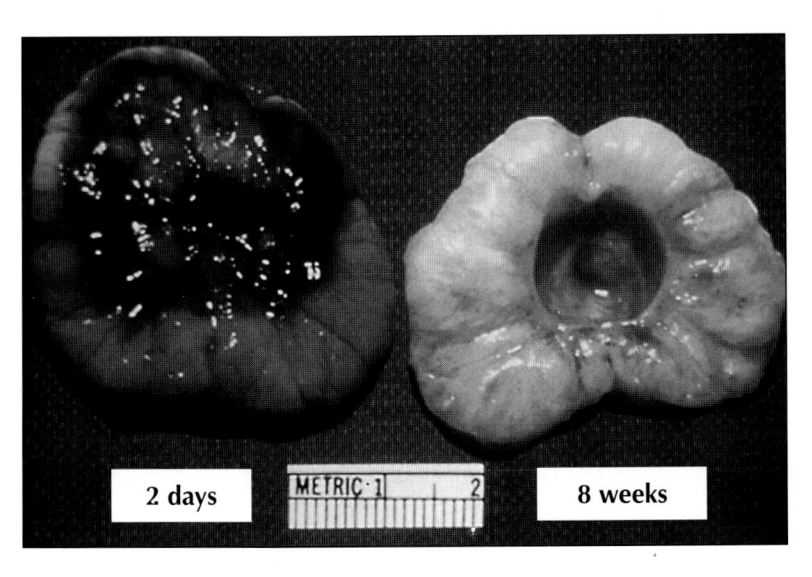

FIGURE 5-8. Result of Nd: YAG vaporization at 2 days and 8 weeks. The Nd:YAG laser prostatectomy is one of the most studied surgical therapies for benign prostatic hyperplasia (BPH). Efficacy is similar to that of transurethral resection of the prostate (TURP) in some series, but a great variation in response has been seen by different investigators. The major drawback is the prolonged postoperative catheterization requirement compared with TURP and the delayed onset of improvement. The occurrence of irritative postoperative voiding symptoms for some patients led to a decrease in its use by many urologists.

HO:YAG LASER RESECTION OF THE PROSTATE

A. Steps in the Resection of the Middle Lobe

1–2: Incise BN deeply at 5 and 7 o'clock
3–4: Connect incisions in front of veru
5: Undermine or excise median lobe
6: Consider division into smaller pieces

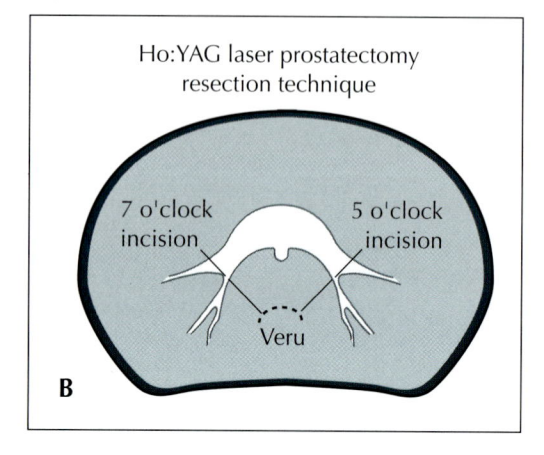

▶ **FIGURE 5-9.** Holmium:yttrium-aluminum-garnet (Ho:YAG) laser prostatectomy. The Ho:YAG laser wavelength (2140 nm) is highly absorbed by tissue water, causing rapid heating with vaporization or incision of irradiated tissues. Initial clinical trials by Kabalin [12] showed Ho:YAG vaporization to be safe, but also demonstrated the inefficiency of trying to vaporize large volumes of BPH with existing fiber delivery systems. This led to the development of a much more practical and efficient technique for Ho:YAG laser resection of the prostate (HoLRP) by Kabalin [13] in the United States and Gilling *et al.*[14] in New Zealand, who showed that this technique provides a more rapid and more consistent outcome than the Nd:YAG coagulation prostatectomy.

The procedure allows a true prostatic resection, which removes the obstructing tissue, to be performed. Because the Ho:YAG laser allows tissue cutting and vaporization with excellent hemostasis, postoperative catheterization and recovery is much quicker than with standard transurethral resection of the prostate (TURP).

The resection begins with removal of the middle lobe, and then the two lateral lobes are removed. The laser fiber is able to create a hemostatic plane between the adenoma and the surgical capsule, so the same landmarks for removal that are observed during open suprapubic prostatectomy are used for HoLRP. **A,** Steps in resection of the middle lobe. **B,** Beginning of the resection.

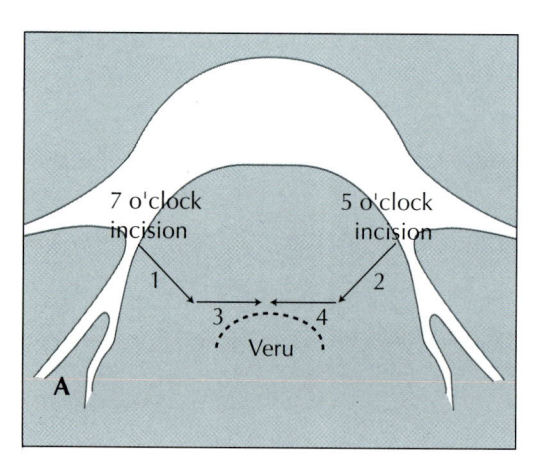

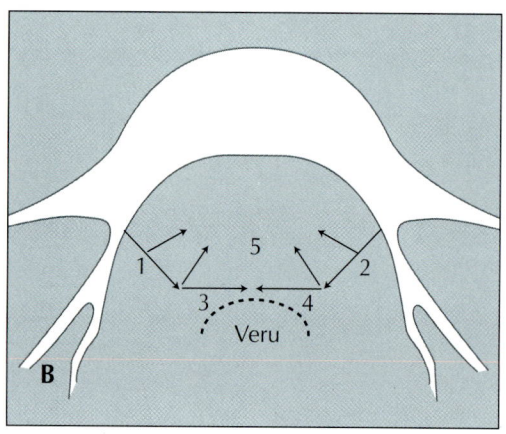

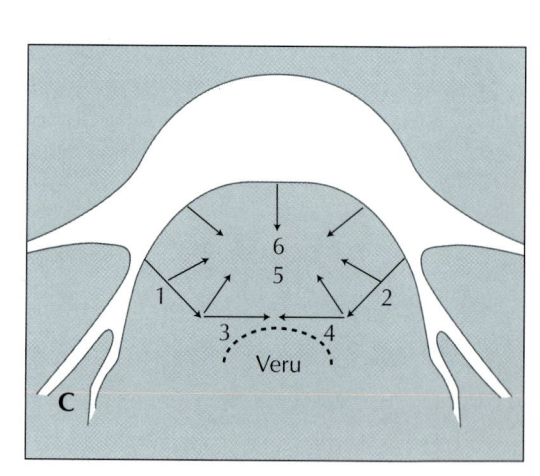

▶ **FIGURE 5-10.** Completion of middle lobe removal. **A,** Incisions joined in midline. **B,** Median lobe is detached. **C,** Lobe may be divided into smaller pieces.

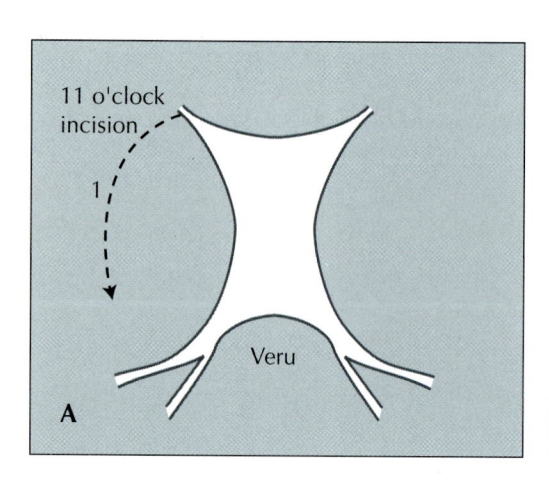

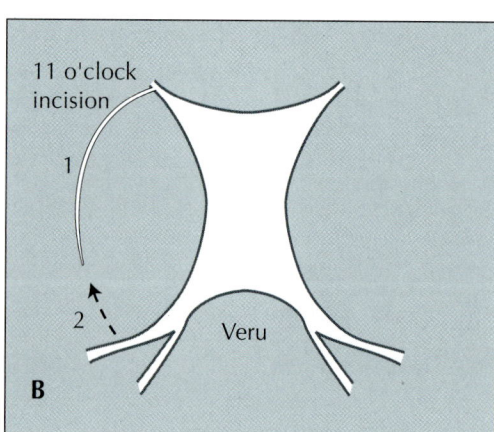

▶ **FIGURE 5-11.** Steps in the lateral lobe resection. The lateral lobe is resected in the same anatomic plane used for open prostatectomy. **A,** "Template" incisions are made to capsule bilaterally at 1 and 11 o'clock. **B,** The lateral lobes are undermined.

(*Continued on next page*)

II. The Prostate

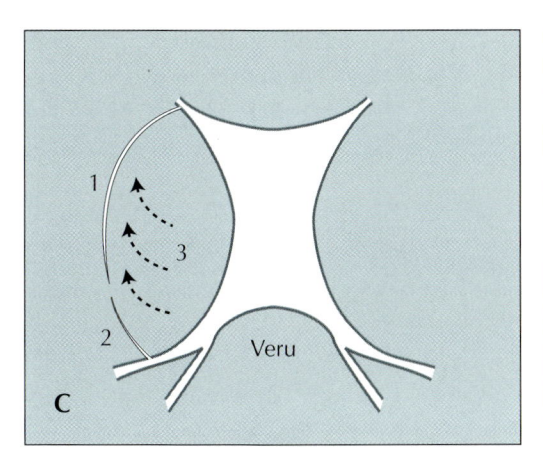

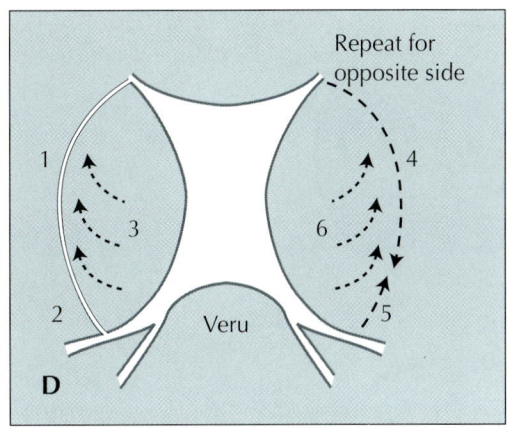

▶ **FIGURE 5-11.** *(Continued)* **C,** The lateral lobes are detached from capsule. **D,** Division into smaller pieces can be considered.

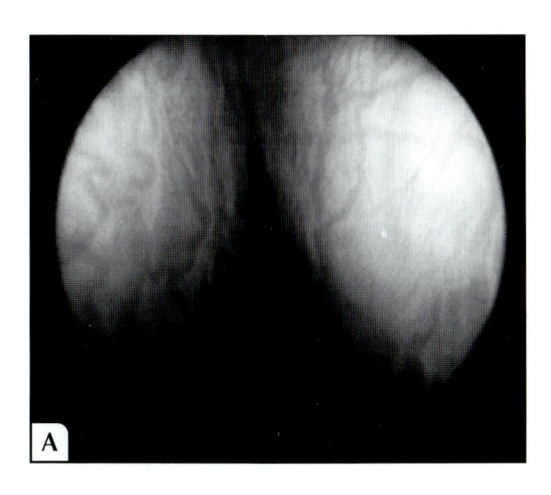

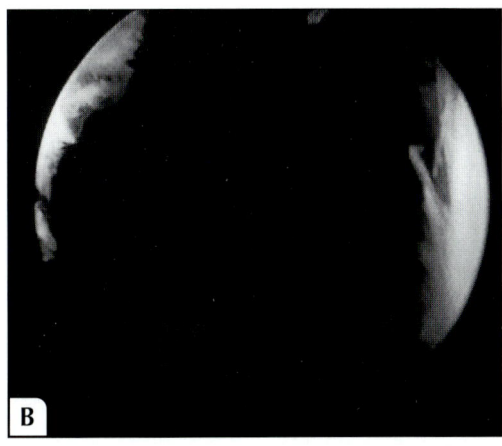

▶ **FIGURE 5-12.** Complete hemostatic removal of the obstructing adenoma. The procedure results in an immediate cavity. Pre- (*panel A*) and post- (*panel B*) Ho:YAG laser resection of the prostate (HoLRP) images. This feature makes this type of laser prostatectomy most like the standard transurethral resection of the prostate (TURP).

Results of Ho:YAG Laser Resection of the Prostate

	Preoperative	1 mo	3 mo	6 mo	12 mo
AUA symptom score	24 (14–33)	8 (0–16)	4 (0–12)	5 (1–6)	4 (0–9)
Peak flow rate, mL/s	8 (3–15)	21 (0–30)	20 (1–30)	21 (12–32)	22 (8–41)

▶ **FIGURE 5-13.** Results of Ho:YAG laser resection of the prostate (HoLRP) demonstrate the efficiency of the HoLRP and the similarity to the outcomes of electrosurgical transurethral resection of the prostate (TURP). (*Data from* Gilling *et al.* [14].)

INTERSTITIAL LASER PROSTATECTOMY

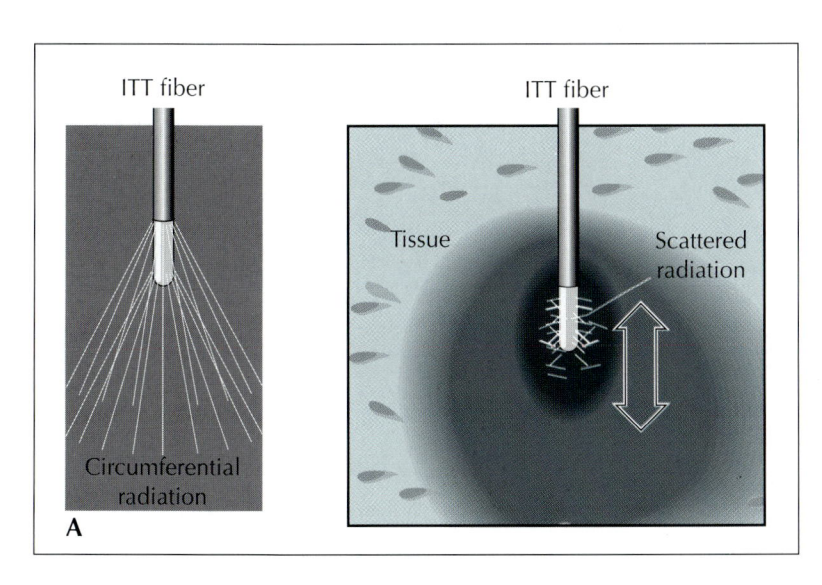

▶ **FIGURE 5-14.** Interstitial laser coagulation (ILC) is performed using laser delivery fibers placed directly into the obstructing hyperplastic prostatic adenoma. In contrast to the free-beam laser irradiation approach, the objective of ILC is to achieve coagulation necrosis inside the adenoma, rather than at its urethral surface. Interstitial coagulation is thought to result in secondary atrophy and regression of the prostatic lobes, thus relieving the obstruction [14]. **A,** A region of coagulation necrosis is created using a laser diffusing fiber. The volume of coagulation necrosis is produced by the diffusion of laser energy and the conduction of heat to adjacent tissue.

(Continued on next page)

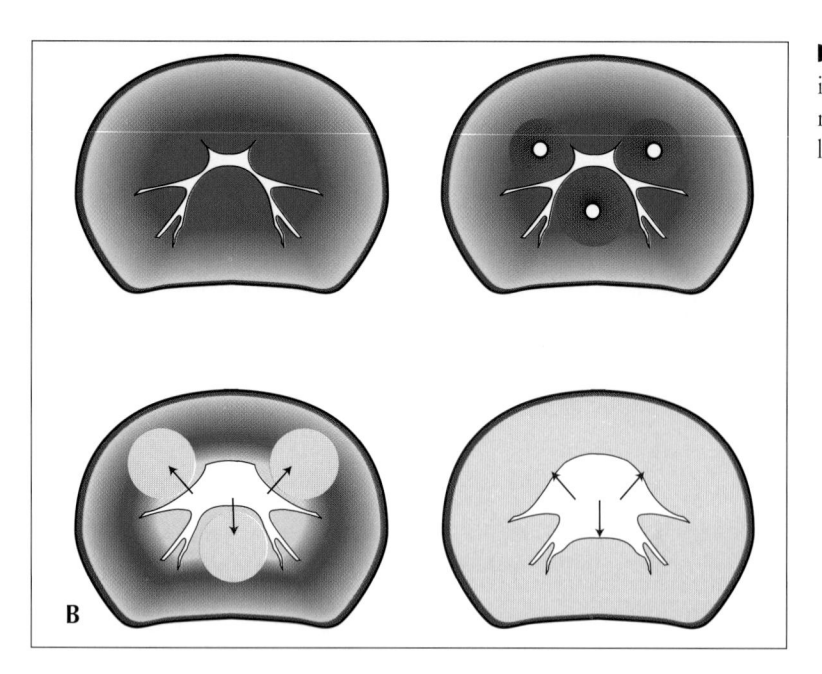

▶ **FIGURE 5-14.** *(Continued)* **B,** A hypothetical ILC prostate treatment is illustrated showing the areas of coagulation necrosis with eventual resolution and a reduction in prostatic tissue and opening of the urethral lumen. ITT— interstitial thermal therapy.

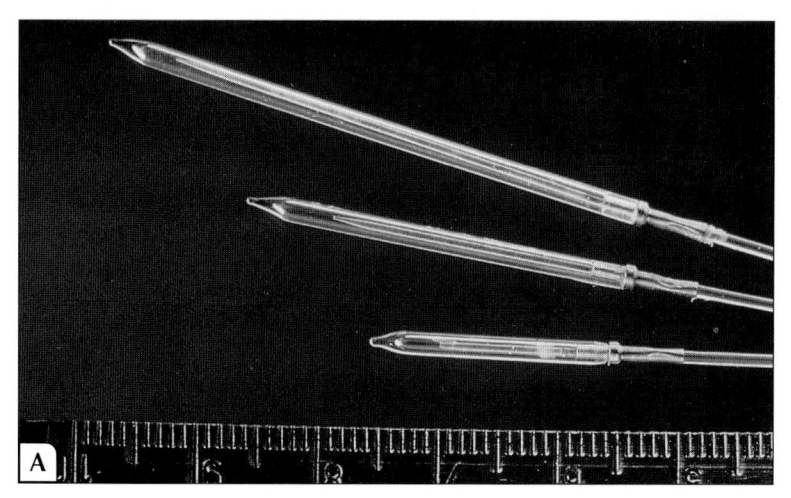

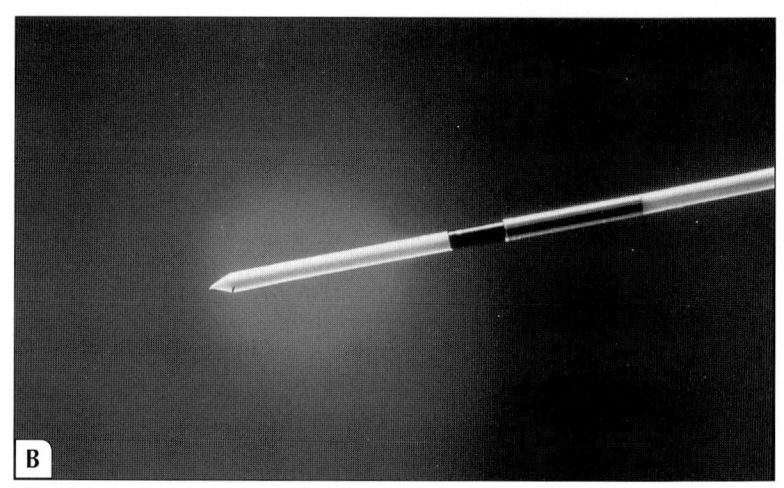

▶ **FIGURE 5-15.** *(See Color Plate)* The laser fibers used for interstitial laser coagulation (ILC). **A,** The sizes of glass-diffusing tip fibers produced by Dornier MedTech (Marietta, GA) for use with the Nd:YAG laser. The sharp point facilitates easy tissue puncture, and multiple sizes are available for treating different tissue volumes. These fibers originally were placed via the transperineal route using ultrasound guidance. Currently they are placed under vision via a standard cystoscope. **B,** The fiber designed by Indigo Medical (Cincinnati, OH) for the 830-nm semiconductor diode laser shown with laser energy emission. The *red area* demarcates the region around the fiber that is penetrated by the laser light.

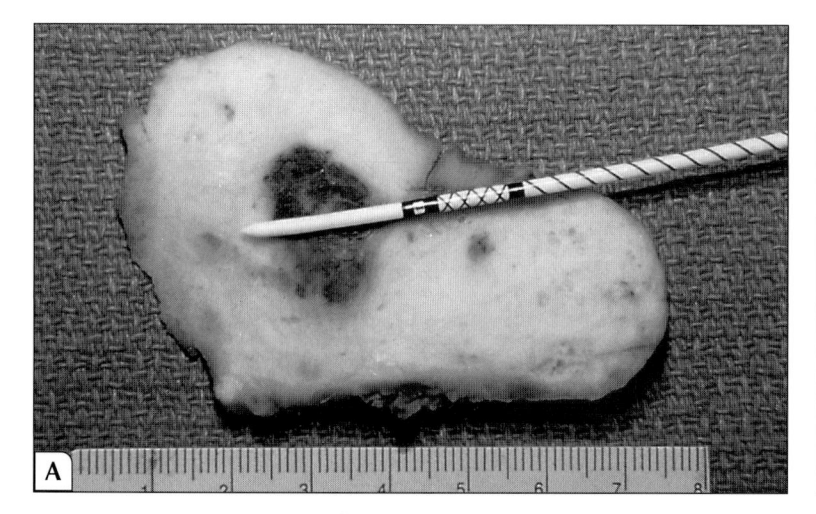

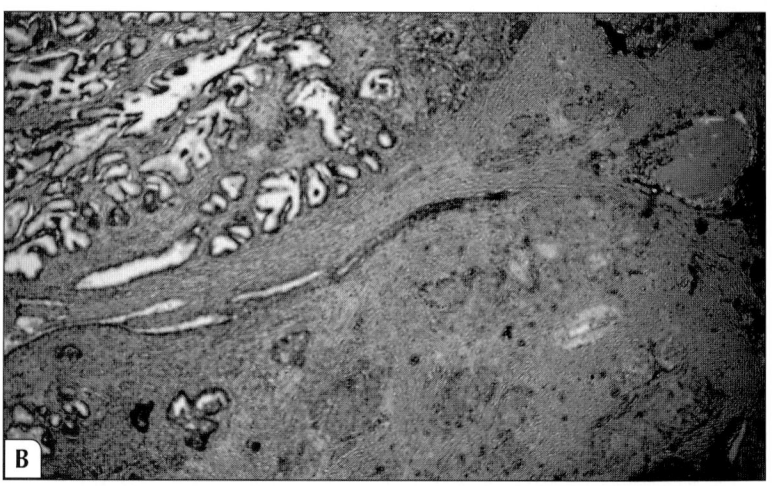

▶ **FIGURE 5-16.** Regions of coagulation necrosis in a prostatectomy specimen. **A,** An open prostatectomy specimen removed 5 days after interstitial laser coagulation with the laser fiber positioned to recreate treatment conditions. The *dark area* represents coagulation and hemorrhagic necrosis. The coagulation zone correlates with the predicted region of treatment based on the diffusing delivery fiber. **B,** A photomicrograph demonstrating the necrosis grossly identified in *panel A*. The lower half demonstrates necrosis. Note the sharp demarcation between the treated zone and the untreated benign prostatic hyperplasia (BPH) tissue.

II. The Prostate

Clinical Outcomes of Interstitial Laser Coagulation

Study	Patients, n	Follow-up, mo	AUA Score Preoperative	AUA Score Postoperative	Peak Flow, mL/s Preoperative	Peak Flow, mL/s Postoperative
Arai et al. [17]	70	6	18.9	7.7	6.7	10.0
De la Rosette et al. [18]	25	3	20.6	6.9	9.1	20.3
Henkel et al. [19]	35	12	21	8	5.3	10.0
Horninger et al. [20]	12	12	29	6	8.3	16.9
Martov and Kilchukov [21]	25	6	19.9	13.5	8.7	13.5
McNicholas and Alsudani [22]	36	12	22	7	9.4	14.6
Muschter and Hofstetter [23,24]	239	12	25.4	6.1	7.7	17.8
Muschter et al. [25]	48	12	31.0	2.3	9.4	19.7
Muschter et al. [26]	112	6	20.9	7.9	8.0	14.2
Muschter et al. [27]	42	3	22.1	4.2	8.2	24.9
Orovan and Whelan [28]	16	3	16.3	5.8	8.8	11.9
Roggan et al. [29]	27	2	14	5	8.0	13.0
Schettini et al. [30]	20	3	22.6	9.2	7.9	15.0
Zhenghua and Ciling [31]	78	3	22.5	8.5	9.8	16.5

▶ FIGURE 5-17. Clinical outcomes of interstitial laser coagulation (ILC).

Complications of Interstitial Laser Coagulation

	Muschter and Hofstetter (n=239)	Muschter et al. (n=112)	Muschter et al. (n=42)
Blood transfusion	0.5%	0	0
Transurethral resection syndrome	0	0	0
Clot retention	2%	0	0
Incontinence	0	0	0
Bladder neck stricture	1.7%	0	0
Urethral stricture	5.4%	0	0
Epididymitis	1.5%	0	0
Erectile dysfunction	0	0	0
Retrograde ejaculation	6.7%	3%	11.9%
Irritative symptoms	12.6%	11%	12.2%
Urinary tract infection	35%	27%	16.5%

▶ FIGURE 5-18. Complications of interstitial laser coagulation. (*Data from* Muschter and Hofstetter [23,24] and Muschter et al. [25,26].)

Retreatment Rate of Interstitial Laser Coagulation

Study	Patients, n	Retreatment, n (%)	Follow-up, mo
Arai et al. [17]	70	5 (7.1)	6
De La Rosette et al. [18]	25	0 (0)	3
Handke et al. [32]	13	2 (15.4)	2
Henkel et al. [19]	35	3 (8.6)	12
Horninger et al. [20]	12	0 (0)	12
Martov and Kilchukov [21]	25	0 (0)	6
McNicholas and Alsudani [22]	36	0 (0)	12
Meagher [33]	36	3 (8.3)	No data
Muschter and Hofstetter [23,24]	239	23 (9.6)	12
Muschter et al. [25]	48	4 (8.3)	12
Muschter et al. [26]	112	3 (2.7)	6
Muschter et al. [27]	42	5 (11.9)	3
Orovan and Whelan [28]	16	0 (0)	3
Roggan et al. [29]	27	1 (4)	6
Schettini et al. [30]	20	1 (5)	3
Zhenghua and Ciling [31]	78	0 (0)	3

FIGURE 5-19. Retreatment rate of interstitial laser coagulation (ILC).

REFERENCES

1. Roth RA, Aretz HT: Transurethral ultrasound guided laser induced prostatectomy (TULIP): a canine feasibility study. *J Urol* 1991, 146:1128–1135.

2. McCullough D, Roth RA, Babayan RK, *et al.*: Transurethral ultrasound guided laser induced prostatectomy: National Human Cooperative Study results. *J Urol* 1993, 150:1607–1611.

3. Johnson DE, Levinson AK, Greskovitch FJ, *et al.*: Transurethral laser prostatectomy using a right angle delivery system. *SPIE Proceedings* 1991, 1421:36–41.

4. Johnson DE, Price RE, Cromeens DM: Pathologic changes occurring in the prostate following transurethral laser prostatectomy. *Lasers Surg Med* 1992, 12:254–263.

5. Kabalin JN: Laser prostatectomy performed with a right angle firing Nd:YAG laser fiber at 40 watts power setting. *J Urol* 1993, 150:95–99.

6. Kabalin JN, Terris MK, Mancianti ML, *et al.*: Dosimetry studies utilizing the urolase right angle firing Nd:YAG laser fiber in the human prostate. *Lasers Surg Med* 1996, 18:72–80.

7. Kabalin J: Invasive therapies for benign prostatic hyperplasia: 1. *Menographs in Urology* 1997, 18:2.

8. Kabalin JN: Laboratory and clinical experience with Nd:YAG laser prostatectomy. *SPIE Proceedings* 1996, 2671:274–287.

9. Kabalin JN, Bite G, Doll S: Neodymium:YAG laser prostatectomy: 3 years of experience with 227 patients. *J Urol* 1996, 155:181–185.

10. Kabalin JN: *Monographs in Urology* 1997, 18:39–79.

11. Costello AJ, Lusaya DG, Crowe HR: Transurethral laser ablation of the prostate: long term results. *World J Urol* 1995, 13:119–122.

12. Kabalin JN: Clinical development of holmium:YAG laser prostatectomy. *SPIE Proceedings* 1996, 2671:292–299.

13. Kabalin JN: Holmium:YAG laser prostatectomy: results of US pilot study. *J Endourol* 1996, 10:453–457.

14. Gilling PJ, Cass CB, Creswell MD, Fraundorfer MR: Holmium laser resection of the prostate: preliminary results of a new method for the treatment of benign prostatic hyperplasia. *Urology* 1996, 47:48–51.

15. Muschter R: Interstitial laser therapy. *Curr Opinion Urol* 1996, 6:33.

16. Perlmutter AP: Interstitial laser prostatectomy. *Mayo Clin Proc* 1998, 73:903–907.

17. Arai Y, Ishitoya S, Odubo K, Suzuki Y: Transurethral interstitial laser coagulation for benign prostatic hyperplasia: treatment outcome and quality of life. *Br J Urol* 1996, 77:93.

18. De La Rosette JJMCH, Muschter R, Lopez MA: Interstitial laser coagulation in the treatment of BPH using a tissue adaptive laser system. *J Endourol* 1996, 10 (suppl l.1):S93.

19. Henkel TO, Greschner M, Luppold T, Alken P: Transurethral and transperineal interstitial laser therapy of BPH. In *Laser-Induced Interstitial Thermotherapy*. Edited by Muller G, Roggan A. Bellingham, WA: SPIE Press; 1995: 416–425.

20. Horninger W, Janesheck G, Pointner J, Watson G, Bartsch G: Are TULIP, interstitial laser and contact laser superior to TURP? *J Urol* 1995, 153:413A.

21. Martov AG, Kilchukov ZI: Interstitial laser induced coagulation of BPH: 6 months follow-up. *J Endourol* 1996, 10(suppl 1):S191.

22. McNicholas T, Alsuldani M: Interstitial laser coagulation therapy for benign prostatic hyperplasia. *SPIE Proceedings* 1996, 2671:300.

23. Muschter R, Hofstetter A: Interstitial laser therapy outcomes in benign prostatic hyperplasia. *J Endourol* 1995, 9:129–135.

24. Muschter R, Hofstetter A: Technique and results of interstitial laser coagulation. *World J Urol* 1995, 13:109–114.

25. Muschter R, De La Rosette JJMCH, Whitfield H, *et al.*: Initial human clinical experience with diode laser interstitial treatment of benign prostatic hyperplasia. *Urology* 1996, 48:223–228.

26. Muschter R, Ehasn A, Stepp HG, Hofstetter A: Clinical results of LITT in the treatment of benign prostatic hyperplasia. In *Laser-Induced Interstitial Thermotherapy*. Edited by Muller G, Rogagn A. Bellingham, WA: SPIE Press; 1995: 434–442.

27. Muschter R, Sroka R, Perlmutter AP, *et al.*: High power interstitial laser coagulation of benign prostatic hyperplasia. *J Endourol* 1996, 10 (suppl 1):S197.

28. Orovan WL, Whelan JP: Neodymium YAG laser treatment of BPH using interstitial thermotherapy: a transurethral approach. *J Urol* 1994, 151:230A.

29. Roggan A, Handke A, Miller K, Muller G: Laser induced interstitial thermotherapy of benign prostatic hyperplasia: basic investigations and first clinical results. *Minimal Invasive Medizin* 1994, 5:55.

30. Schettini M, Diana M, Fortunato P, *et al.*: Results of interstitial laser coagulation of the prostate. *J Endourol* 1996, 10 (suppl 1):S191.

31. Zhenchua G, Ciling C: ITT combined with vaporized incision for treatment of BPH. *J Endourol* 1996, 10 (suppl 1):S192.

32. Handke A, Roggan A, Andreesen R, Miller K: Laserinduzierte interstitielle thermotherapic (LITT) bei BPH. *Urologe A* 1994, 33(suppl): S81.

33. Meagher M: Interstitial laser prostatectomy (abstract). *J Endourol* 1996, 155(supp): 318.

Transurethral Resection of the Prostate, Transurethral Incision of the Prostate, and Open Prostatectomy for Benign Prostatic Hyperplasia

NONCANCEROUS DISEASE SECTION

Winston K. Mebust & Mark J. Noble

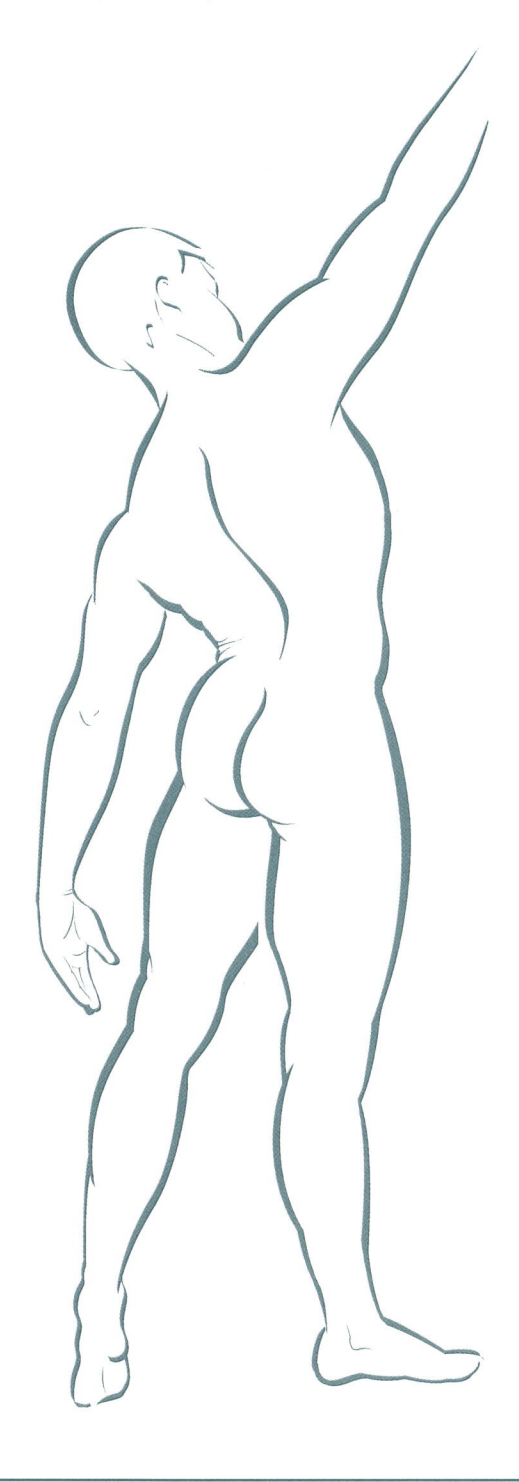

Transurethral prostatectomy (TURP) became possible with the introduction of the resectoscope in 1932. Development of the resectoscope depended on other scientific advances, such as the incandescent lamp, developed by Edison in 1879, which permitted direct visualization of the prostate. The vacuum tube developed by deForest in 1908 made possible the development of an electrosurgical unit for coagulation and cutting of tissue. Finally, Young (see Nesbit [1]) introduced the fenestrated tube. Since then, additional advances such as the Hopkins rod lens system and fiberoptic light source have improved visualization of the prostate. In most academic institutions today, transurethral resection is done by using a television camera and viewing the operation on a screen, which has vastly improved the ability to teach the operation.

The most common reason for intervening in patients with bladder outlet obstruction secondary to benign prostatic hyperplasia (BPH) is to alleviate the symptoms. In addition to the patient's symptoms, certain complications of benign prostatic hyperplasia are considered a definite requirement for intervention, preferably a transurethral resection of the prostate (TURP). These complications are acute refractory urinary retention, recurrent urinary tract infection, recurrent hematuria, bladder stones, and renal insufficiency secondary to obstructing BPH. Although TURP continues to be the operation most commonly done for benign disease of the prostate, the number of TURPs performed declined by 52% between 1989 and 1995 (Holtgrewe, AUA Health Policy Brief). This decline represents the impact of newer medical treatments as well as the availability of less invasive surgical treatments. The morbidity and mortality or TURP is quite low, but still exists. Many patients select a treatment modality that may not be as effective as TURP but is associated with less morbidity.

Indications for transurethral incision of the prostate (TUIP) are similar to those for TURP—primarily the patient's symptoms and the complications of bladder outlet obstruction, *ie*, acute refractory urinary retention. The procedure is best done in smaller glands with a minimal amount of lateral lobe tissue and a high posterior lip of the bladder, forming what has been called a primary bladder contracture configuration.

Indications for open prostatectomy are similar to those for TURP. The open procedure usually is reserved for patients with larger, benign glands (*ie*, > 70 g), however. The decision whether to do a TURP or open prostatectomy depends on the urologist's training and surgical skills in resecting larger glands. TURP in patients with very large glands (*ie*, 100 g or larger) can be associated with significant fluid absorption, intraoperative bleeding, and intraoperative and immediate postoperative complications.

American Urological Association Symptom Index for Benign Prostatic Hyperplasia

	Not at All	Less Than 1 Time in 5	Less Than Half the Time	About Half the Time	More Than Half the Time	Almost Always
1. Over the past month, how often have you had a sensation of not emptying your bladder completely after you finished urinating?	0	1	2	3	4	5
2. Over the past month, how often have you had to urinate again < 2 h after you finished urinating?	0	1	2	3	4	5
3. Over the past month, how often have you found you stopped and started again several times when you urinated?	0	1	2	3	4	5
4. Over the past month, how often have you found it difficult to postpone urination?	0	1	2	3	4	5
5. Over the past month, how often have you had a weak urinary stream?	0	1	2	3	4	5
6. Over the past month, how often have you had to push or strain to begin urination?	0	1	2	3	4	5
7. Over the past month, how many times did you most typically get up to urinate from the time you went to bed at night until the time you got up in the morning?	None	One time	Two times	Three times	Four times	≥ Five times

The American Urological Association Symptom Score equals the sum of questions A1 through A7.

▶ **FIGURE 6-1.** American Urological Association (AUA) Symptom Index. Although many symptom scores have been developed to provide a more objective assessment of patient symptoms (*eg*, Boyarsky and Madsen-Iversen), the AUA Symptom Index, developed by Barry *et al.* [2] of the AUA as part of the guideline on evaluation and management of BPH, has received the greatest worldwide acceptance. The AUA Symptom Index has been validated as to test-retest reliability, internal consistency, and overall validity. The AUA Symptom Index is not disease-specific but does give the physician a method for evaluating the severity or frequency of patient symptoms. The AUA Symptom Score equals the sum of questions A1 through A7.

---

1. Over the past month, how much physical discomfort did any urinary problems cause you?
   - [0] None   [1] Only a little   [2] Some   [3] A lot

2. Over the past month, how much did you worry about your health because of any urinary problems?
   - [0] None   [1] Only a little   [2] Some   [3] A lot

3. Overall, how bothersome has any trouble with urination been during the past month?
   - [0] Not at all bothersome   [1] Bothers me a little   [2] Bothers me some   [3] Bothers me a lot

4. Over the past month, how much of the time has any urinary problem kept you from doing the kinds of things you would usually do?
   - [0] None of the time
   - [1] A little of the time
   - [2] Some of the time
   - [3] Most of the time
   - [4] All of the time

▶ **FIGURE 6-2.** The benine prostatic hyperplasia (BPH) Impact Index. The American Urological Association (AUA) Symptom Index does not assess the degree of "bother" or impact of the obstructing BPH on the patient's quality of life. The International Prostate Symptom Score (I-PSS) is the same as the AUA Symptom Index, with one additional question that addresses the impact of BPH on the patient's quality of life. Barry *et al.* [2] also developed a four-question instrument that could be used to assess the "bother" caused by the patient's symptoms and their impact on his quality of life. This instrument was introduced in 1993. The BPH Impact Index equals the sum of questions B1 through B4.

Recommended, Not Recommended, and Optional Tests in the Evaluation of Patients With Lower Urinary Tract Symptoms

Highly recommended tests
  Medical history
  AUA Symptom Index or International Prostate
    Symptom Score plus Quality of Life Question
  Voiding diary (if nocturia is dominant symptom)
  Physical examination plus digital rectal examination
  Urinalysis
  Renal function (serum creatinine)
  Prostate-specific antigen (if life expectancy > 10 y)

Recommended tests
  Flow rate
  Residual urine
Optional tests
  Urine culture
  Intravenous urogram
  Ultrasonography
  Endoscopy
  Transrectal ultrasonography plus biopsy

Optional test for specific indications
  Pressure-flow studies
Not recommended tests
  Retrograde urethrography
  Urethral pressure profile
  Voiding cystourethrography
  Electromyography of external urinary sphincter

▶ **FIGURE 6-3.** Recommended, not recommended, and optional tests in the evaluation of lower urinary tract symptoms. Evaluation of patients with lower urinary tract symptoms is based on the Agency for Health Care Policy and Research (AHCPR) Guideline on benine prostatic hyperplasia (BPH), which was published in 1994. These guidelines were further refined at the 4th World Health Organization Consultation on BPH held in 1997 [4]. AUA—American Urological Association.

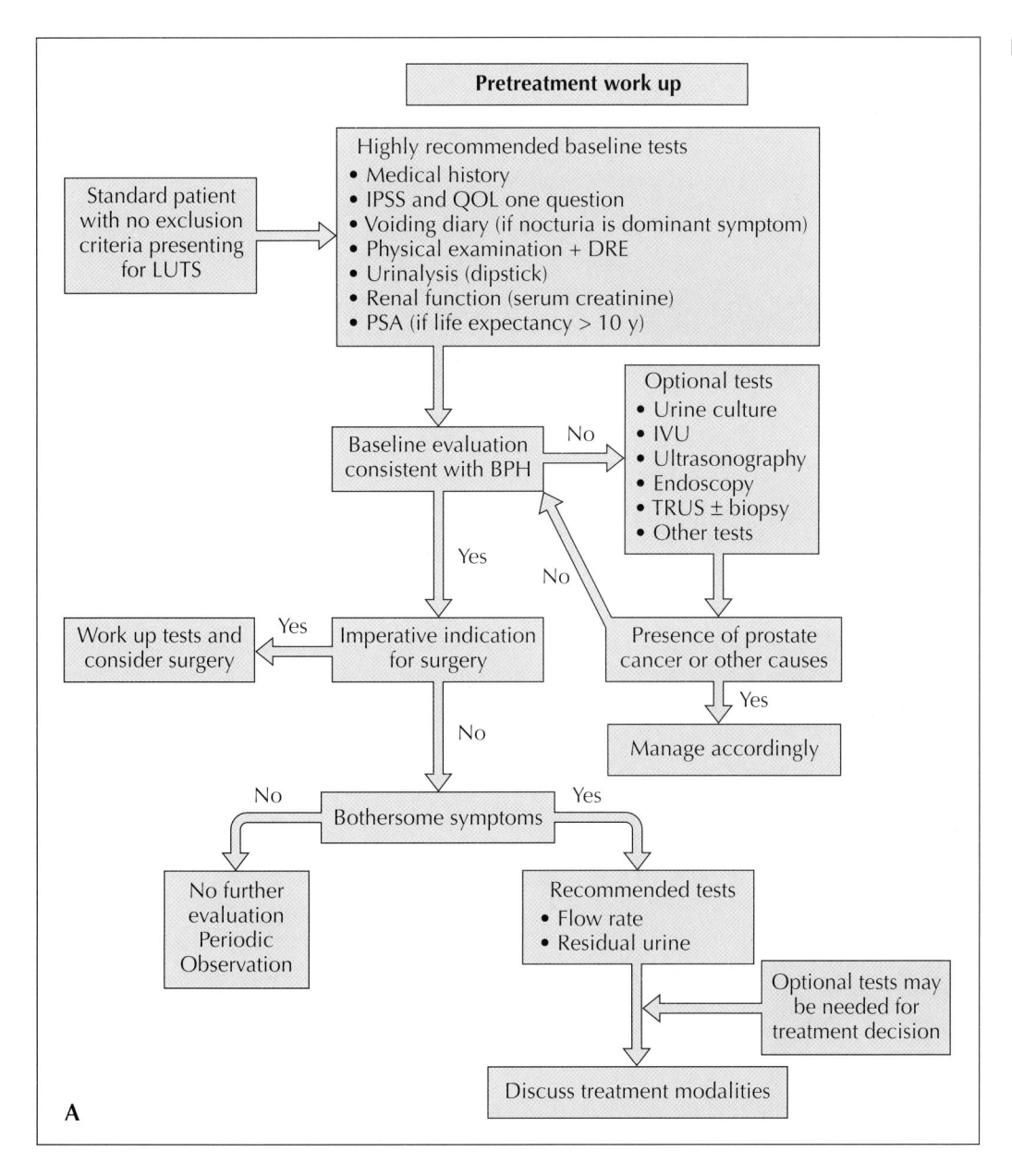

▶ **FIGURE 6-4.** Treatment algorithm (*panel A*)
(Continued on next page)

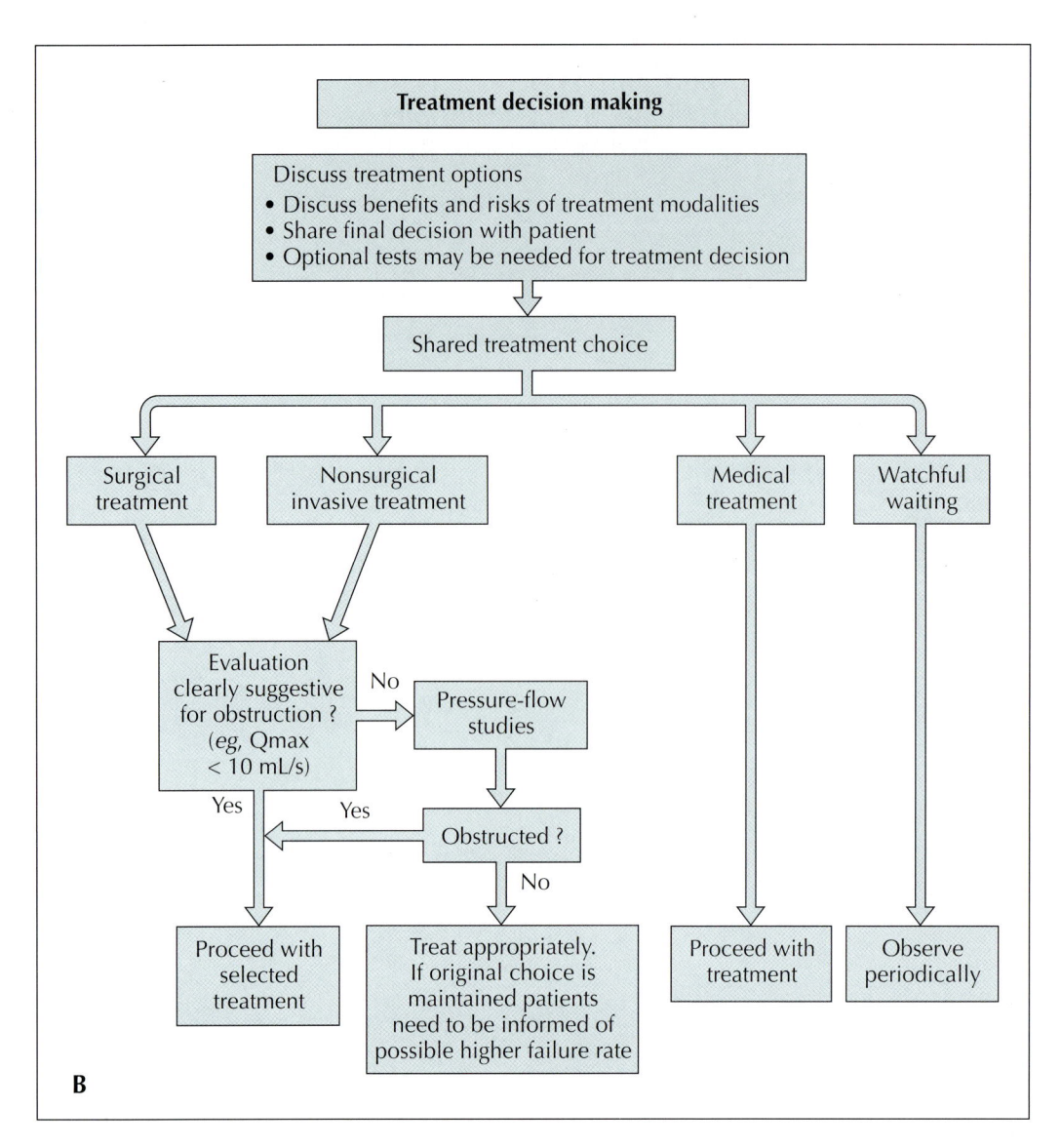

FIGURE 6-4. *(Continued)* and treatment decision (*panel B*) for benign prostatic hyperplasia (BPH). IPSS—International Prostate Symptom Score; LUTS—lower urinary tract symptoms; QOL—quality of life.

SURGICAL TECHNIQUES

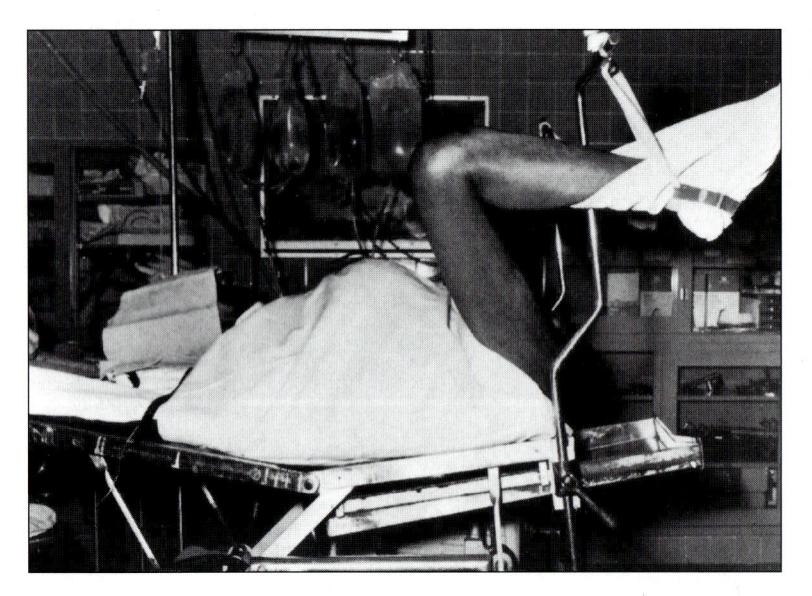

FIGURE 6-5. Patient positioning. The patient is positioned on the operating table in a somewhat exaggerated lithotomy position.

II. The Prostate

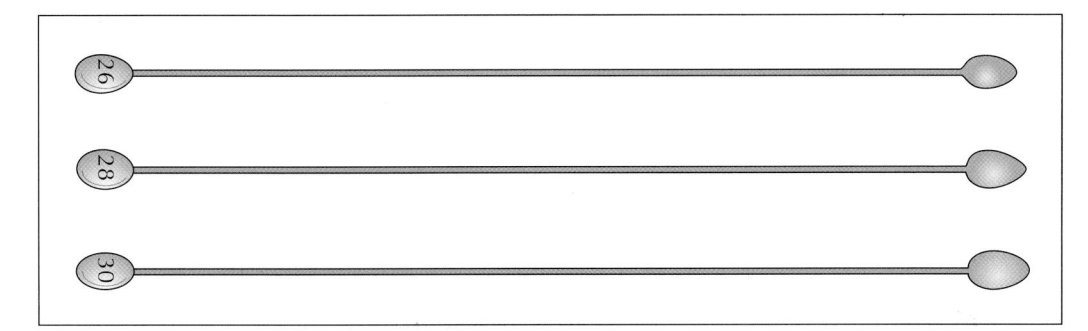

FIGURE 6-6. Examples of bougie-á-boules. The urethra should be calibrated with bougie-á-boules before the resectoscope is inserted. Emmett *et al.* [5] reported that 80% of men usually calibrate at 28 F or larger. More tissue can be resected in less time with a 28-F than a 24-F resectoscope. With today's excellent equipment, however, it is feasible to resect even glands larger than 75 g with a 24-F resectoscope, thereby avoiding the complication of instrument-induced urethral stricture.

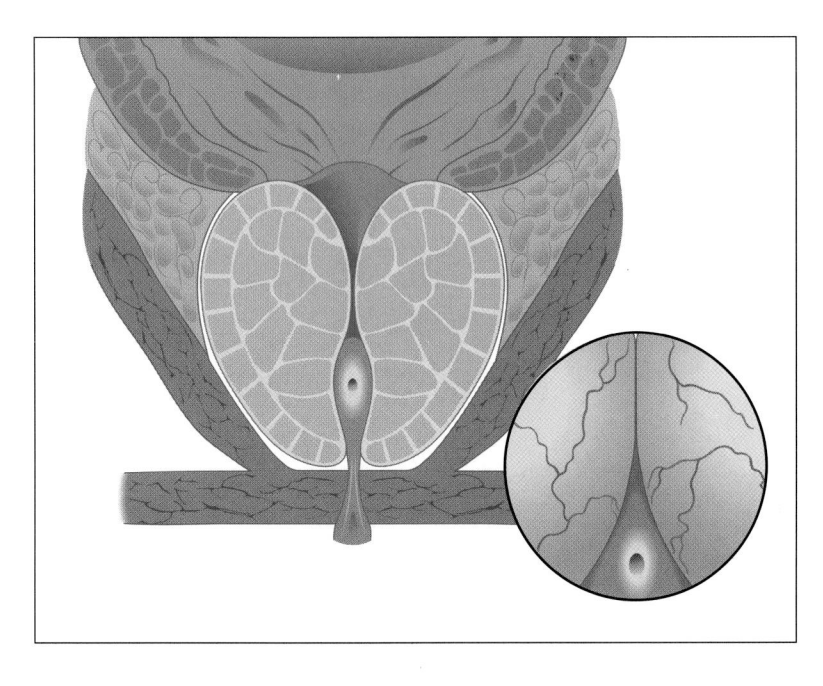

FIGURE 6-7. Benign prostatic hyperplasia. Frontal view showing the relationship of the prostate to the bladder and verumontanum.

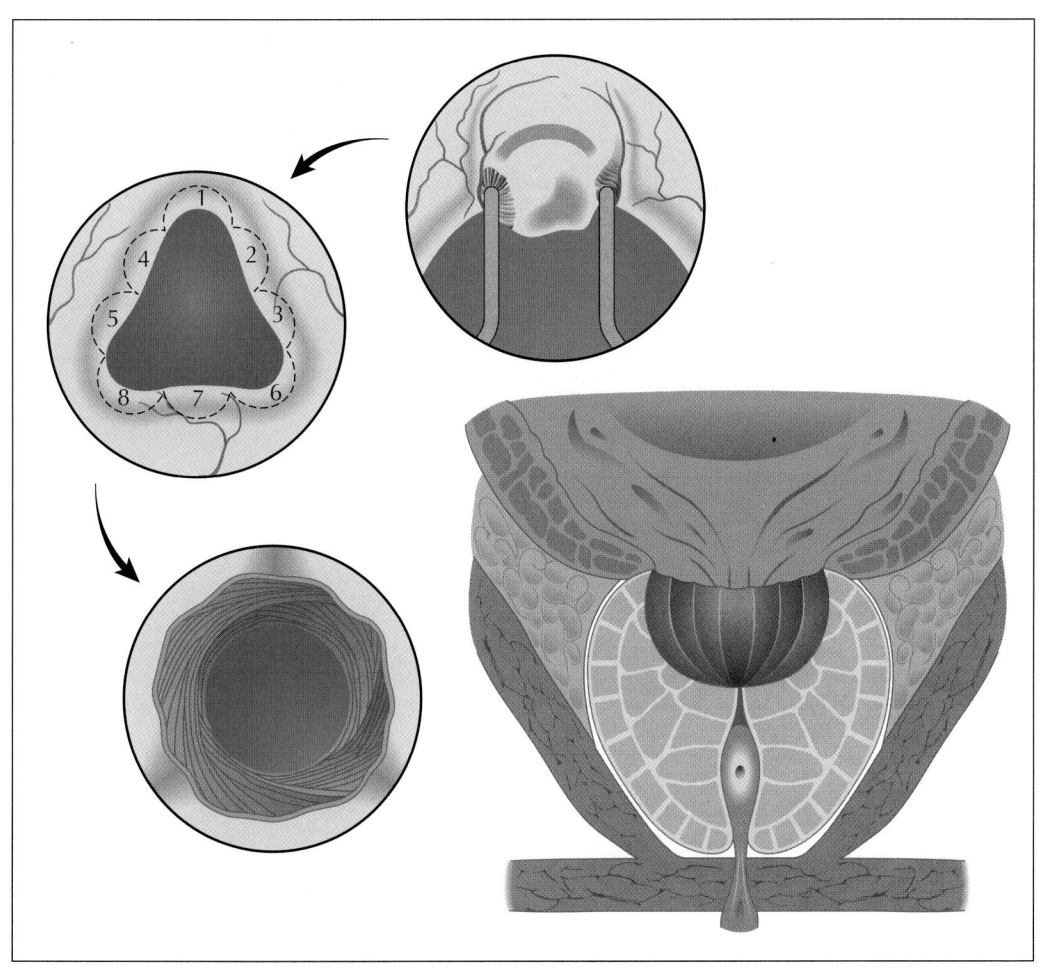

FIGURE 6-8. Resection of the prostate: stage 1. There are a number of ways of resecting the prostate, but all should be done in a step-by-step, orderly fashion to control the bleeding so that a precise anatomic dissection of the adenoma can be done. We use the Nesbit three-staged technique, which is illustrated here. The bladder is distended with approximately 100 mL of fluid to demarcate more clearly the prostate, the bladder neck, and the bladder wall. An initial cut is made anteriorly at 12 o'clock with the resectoscope loop. The incision is carried deeply until the seemingly circular fibers of the bladder neck are exposed. The resection is carried to approximately the 3 o'clock position, and bleeding points are carefully controlled. The resection is then continued counterclockwise from 12 to 9 o'clock, in a similar fashion. The resection is completed from the 3 to 9 o'clock position.

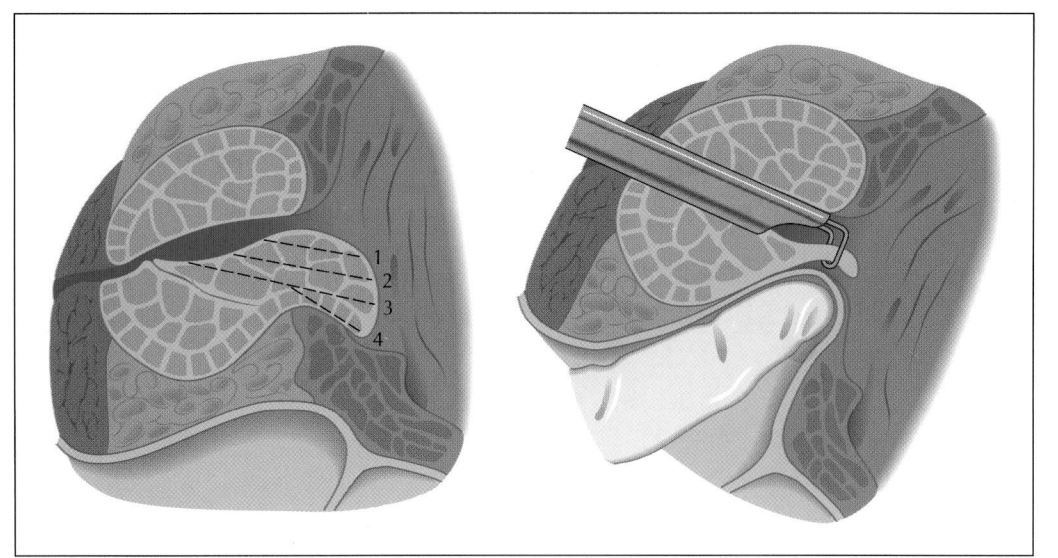

▶ **FIGURE 6-9.** Resecting the median lobe. The median lobe is resected by going back and forth (left to right then right to left) and resecting it level by level 1 to 4 (*left*). At this point, manipulation of the prostate floor and median lobe with the finger in an O'Connor rectal sheath (*right*) facilitates the resection. If the anatomy of the gland is that of a primary vesical neck contracture, or what has been called a "median bar," a 6 o'clock incision is made through the bladder neck at the end of the procedure if the neck is very prominent.

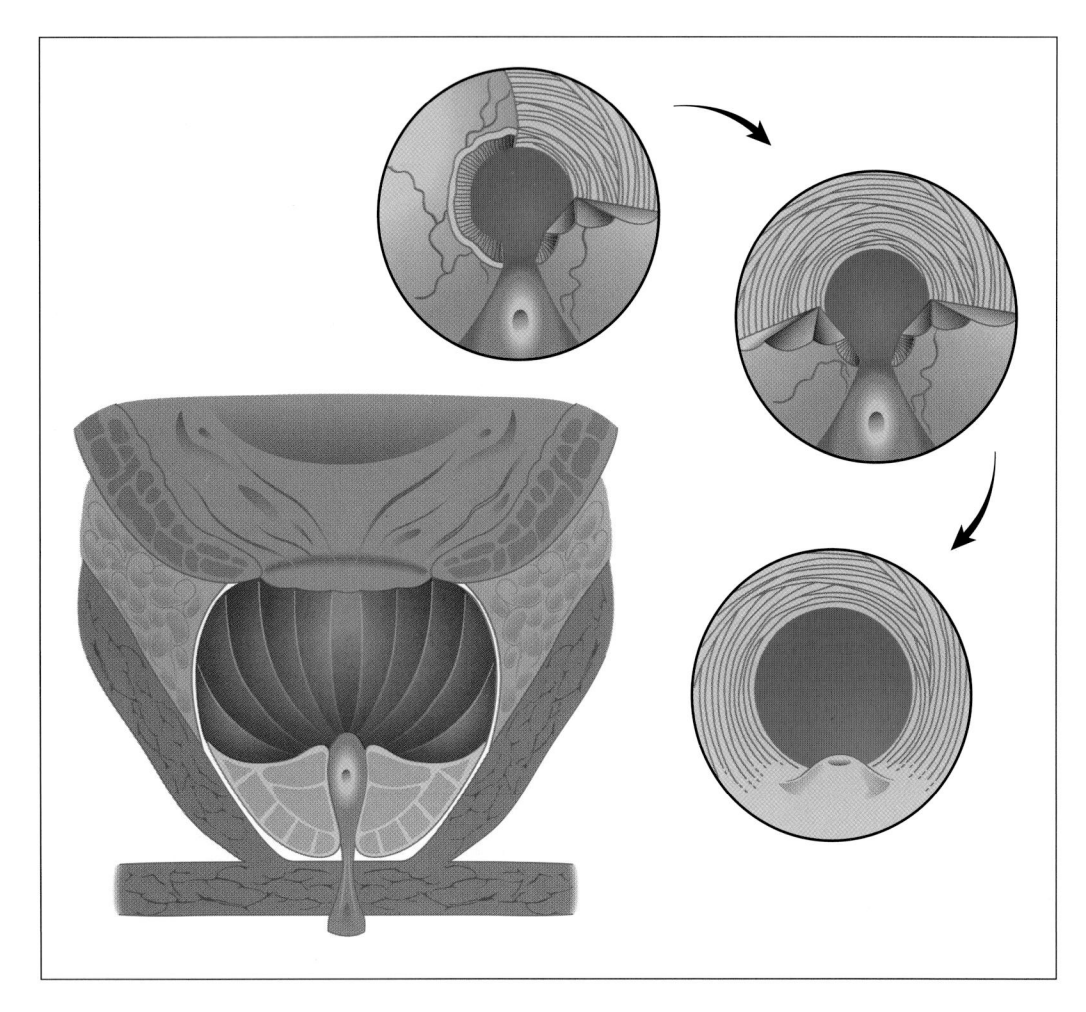

▶ **FIGURE 6-10.** Resection of the prostate: stage 2. Depending on the length of the prostatic fossa, the resectoscope is placed in front of the verumontanum and the resection is begun at the 12 o'clock position. Resection is done again by quadrants, first from 12 to 3 o'clock, with bleeding points controlled as necessary. Resection is carried down until the surgical capsule of the prostate is identified. The quadrant from 12 to 9 o'clock is resected. When resecting the two posterior quadrants, we usually take the resection down from the 9 o'clock to the 7 o'clock position, resecting most of the bulk of the lateral lobe. We then move to the other posterior quadrant and resect it similarly from 3 to 5 o'clock. We resect the floor last, manipulating the tissue with the finger in the O'Connor sheath. Fibers readily identified on the roof and sides of the prostate usually are not as apparent on the floor.

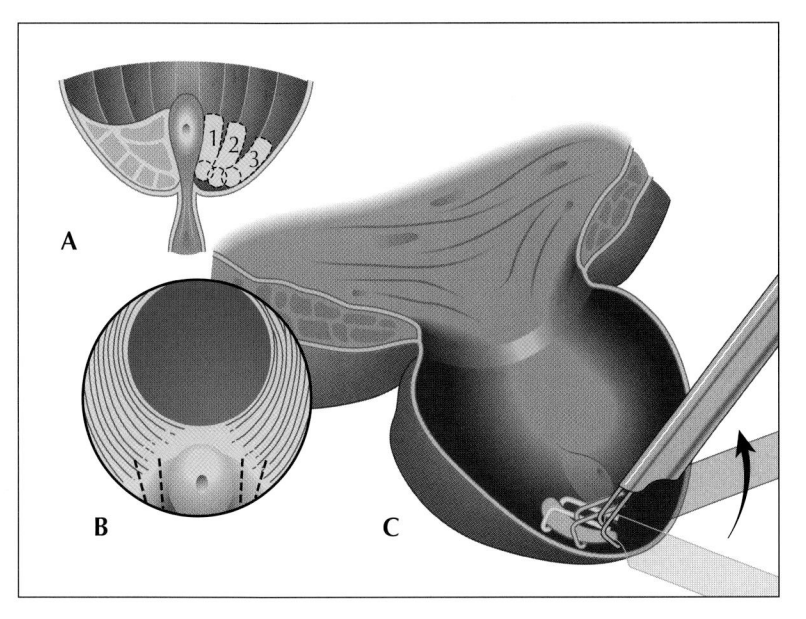

◗ **FIGURE 6-11.** Resection of the prostate: stage 3. The external sphincter and the verumontanum are identified. The tissue lying next to the verumontanum at the 5 and 7 o'clock positions is removed carefully with the resectoscope. The resection now is begun at the apex, proceeding from 7 to 12 o'clock. Use of a lateral-to-medial sweep of the resectoscope loop in response to the concavity of the gland can be helpful as adenomatous tissue is removed. Care must be taken not to advance the scope inward or, more significantly, not to retract the scope out during the resection, thereby inadvertently injuring the external sphincter. The resection is then carried out similarly from 5 to 12 o'clock. Bleeding is carefully controlled. In a very large gland, the lateral lobe tissue of the apex may project beyond the verumontanum into the sphincter area. In such cases, it is advisable to leave a thin rim of apical prostatic tissue rather than risk inadvertently resecting the sphincter.

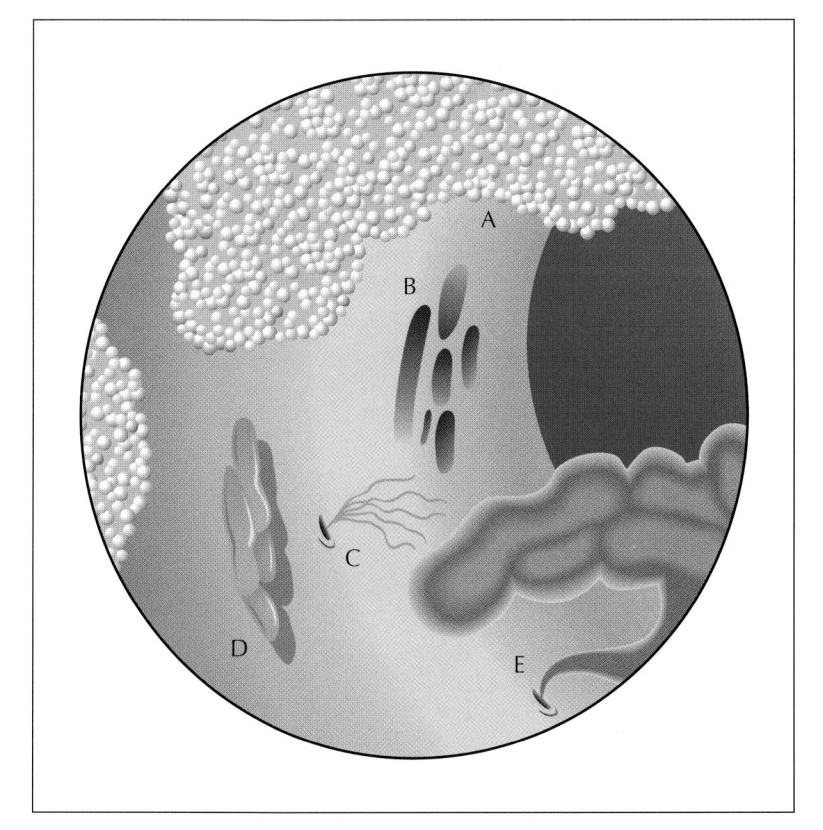

◗ **FIGURE 6-12.** Surgical landmarks for transurethral prostatectomy. **A**, The granular snowlike appearance of adenoma. **B**, Coarse striations of the surgical prostatic capsule. **C**, Arterial bleeding points. **D**, Venous sinuses exposed with globules of fat protruding. If there has been extensive resection of the prostatic capsule, it will be necessary to terminate the operation because of excessive absorption of fluid into the periprostatic tissue and venous complexes. **E**, Venous bleeding appears cloudlike when the water flow is reduced.

Benign Prostatic Hyperplasia Treatment Outcomes

	Surgical Options				Nonsurgical Options		
	Balloon Dilation	TUIP	Open Surgery	TURP	Watchful Waiting	α-Blockers	Finasteride
Chance for improvement of symptoms (90% CI)	37–76	78–83	94–99.8	75–96	31–55	59–86	54–78
Degree of symptom improvement (percent reduction in symptom score)	51	73	79	85	Unknown	51	31
Morbidity or complications associated with surgical or medical treatment (90% CI), ≈ 20% of all complications assumed to be significant	1.78–9.86	2.2–33.3	6.98–42.7	5.2–30.7	1–5 (complications from BPH progression)	2.9–43.3	13.6–18.8
Chance of dying within 30–90 d of treatment (90% CI)	0.72–9.78 (high risk/elderly patients)	0.2–1.5	0.99–4.56	0.53–3.31	0.8% chance of death ≤ 90 d for 67-year-old man		
Risk of total urinary incontinence (90% CI)	Unknown	0.06–1.1	0.34–0.74	0.68–1.4	Incontinence associated with aging		
Need for operative treatment for surgical complications in future (90% CI)	Unknown	1.34–2.65	0.6–14.1	0.65–10.1	0		
Risk of impotence (90% CI)	No long-term follow-up available	3.9–24.5	4.7–39.2	3.3–34.8	2% of men aged 67 become impotent per year; long-term data on α-blockers not available		2.5–5.3; also decreased volume of ejaculate
Risk of retrograde ejaculation (percent of patients)	Unknown	6–55	36–95	25–99	0	4–11	0
Loss of work time, d	4	7–21	21–21	7–21	1	3.5	1.5
Hospital stay, d	1	1–3	5–10	3–5	0	0	0

▶ **FIGURE 6-13.** Outcomes of treatment modalities for benign prostatic hyperplasia. TUIP—transuretheral incision of the prostate; TURP—transuretheral resection of the prostate. (*Data from* McConnell *et al.* [6].)

TRANSURETHRAL INCISION OF THE PROSTATE

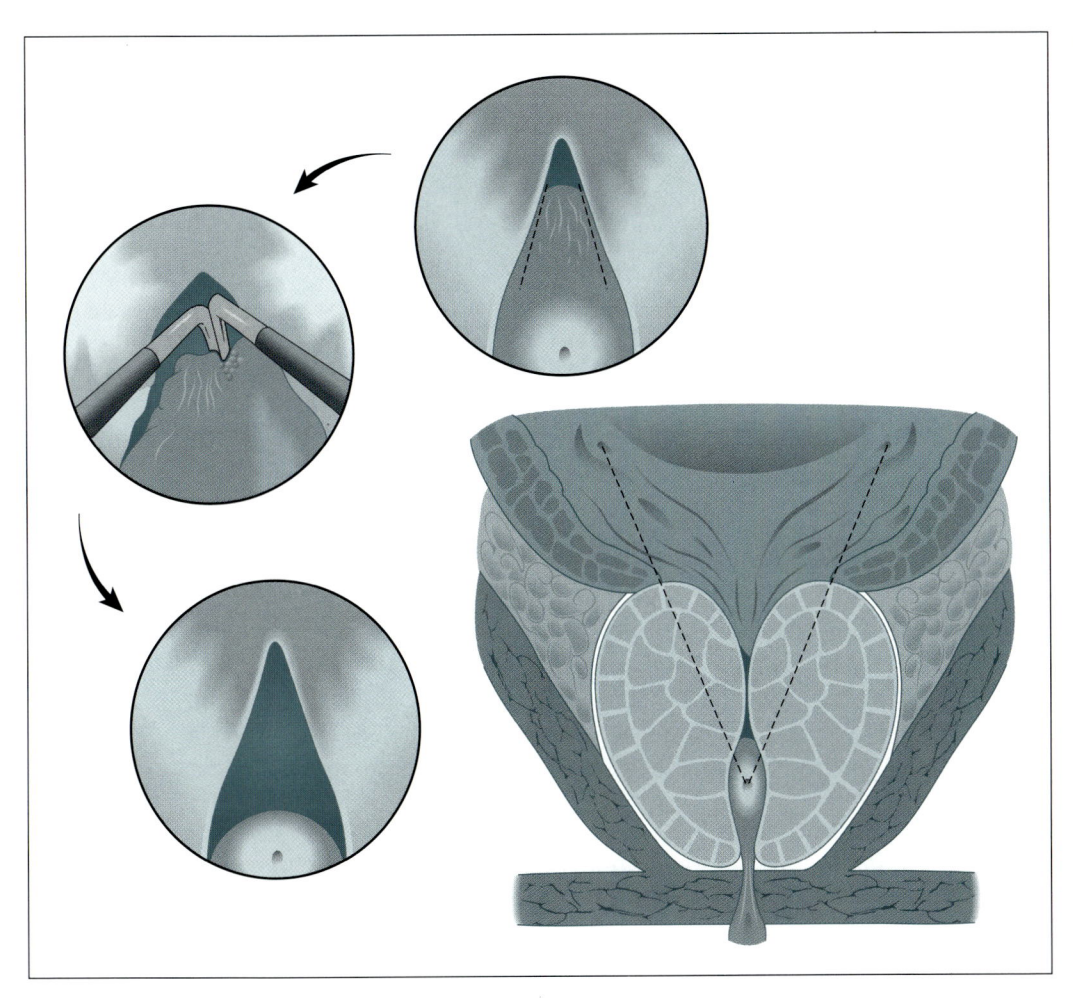

FIGURE 6-14. Incision for transurethral incision of the prostate. Resection is started at the right ureteral orifice and continued through the bladder neck. The depth through the bladder neck should expose the shiny, filmy fibers at the vesical–prostate junction. The incision is then carried through the floor of the prostate down to the capsule. The resection is carried out similarly from the left ureteral orifice to the verumontanum. Bleeding is carefully controlled and a catheter inserted.

POSTOPERATIVE CARE

Treatment Outcomes

	TUIP	TURP
Chance of symptom improvement	78–83 (80)	75–96 (88)
Degree of symptom improvement	73	85
Morbidity: 20% significant	2.2–33	5.2–30.7 (16)
Mortality: 30–90 d	0.2–1.5	0.53–3.31
Total incontinence	0.061–1.1	0.68–1.4
Operative treatment for surgical complications	1.34–2.65	0.68–10
Impotence	3.9–24.5	3.3–34.8
Retrograde ejaculation	6–55	25–99

FIGURE 6-15. Treatment outcomes. Harms and benefits of transurethral incision of the prostate (TUIP) as compared with transurethral resection of the prostate (TURP). (*Data from* McConnell *et al.* [6].)

OPEN PROSTATECTOMY

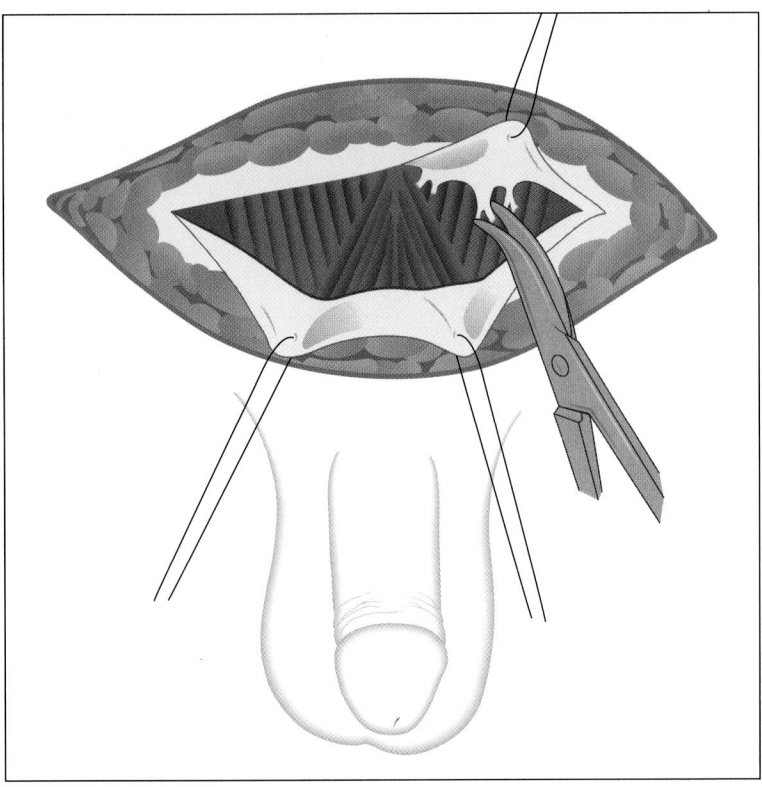

FIGURE 6-16. Skin incision. The incision is started approximately 2 cm above the pubic bone and curved upward toward the anterior iliac spine, staying within the skin lines to reduce postoperative skin scar. Elevation of the anterior rectus fascia exposes the rectus and pyramidalis muscle. The muscles are separated in the midline, exposing the retropubic space. If a wider exposure is needed, the tendinous insertion of the rectus on the pubis can be partially incised and reapproximated at the end of the procedure.

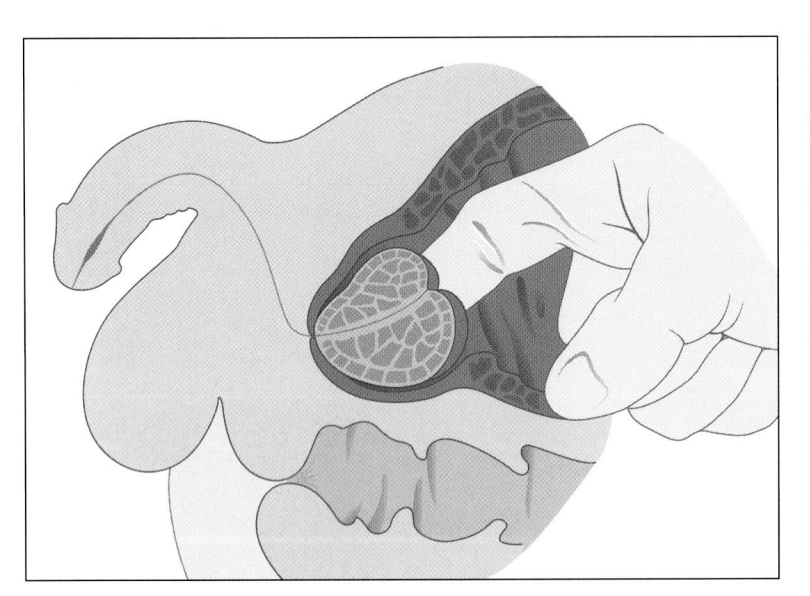

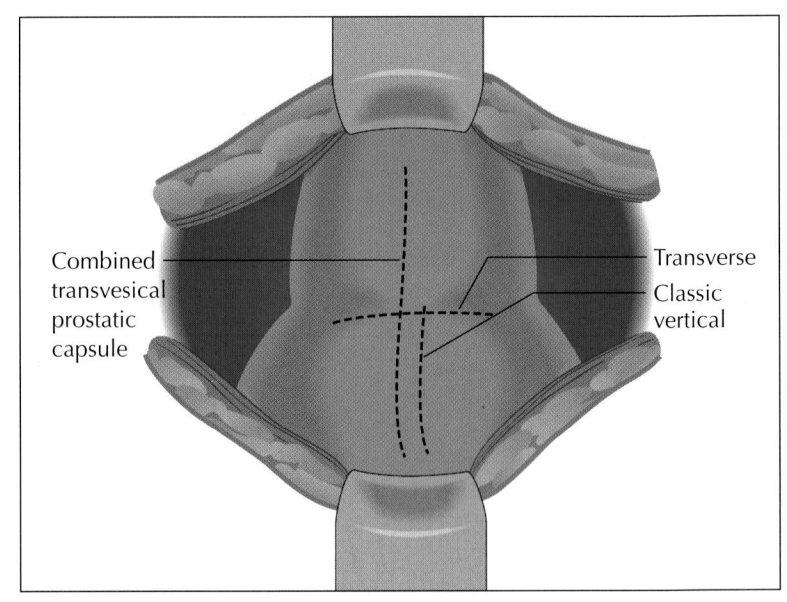

FIGURE 6-17. Bladder incision. Classically, a suprapubic or transvesical prostatectomy is performed through a midline bladder incision. The incision starts just cephalad to the bladder neck. Alternatively, a transverse incision approximately 1 cm above the bladder neck may be used. The combined incision is in the midline of the bladder and extends into the capsule of the prostate. With extension into the muscle of the prostate, it may be necessary to place a deep chromic stitch into the capsule of the prostate to control bleeding from the dorsal vein complex.

FIGURE 6-18. Blunt enucleation of the prostate. The bladder has been filled to 300 mL of fluid and entered through a standard vertical incision. Enucleation is begun by cutting through the anterior commissure of the prostate. The surgeon then finds the plane between the compressed prostatic capsule and the adenoma. Alternatively, the surgeon may incise the mucosa overlying the prostate at the vesical junction and bluntly or sharply find the plane between the adenoma and surgical capsule. The adenoma is then enucleated. The apex can then be pinched off as it meets the prostatic urethra. Care must be taken not to distract the apex cephalad and inadvertently damage the more distal portion of the external sphincter mechanism. If the vertical incision has been extended into the prostatic capsule, the urethra can be divided from the prostate more precisely with better exposure of the area.

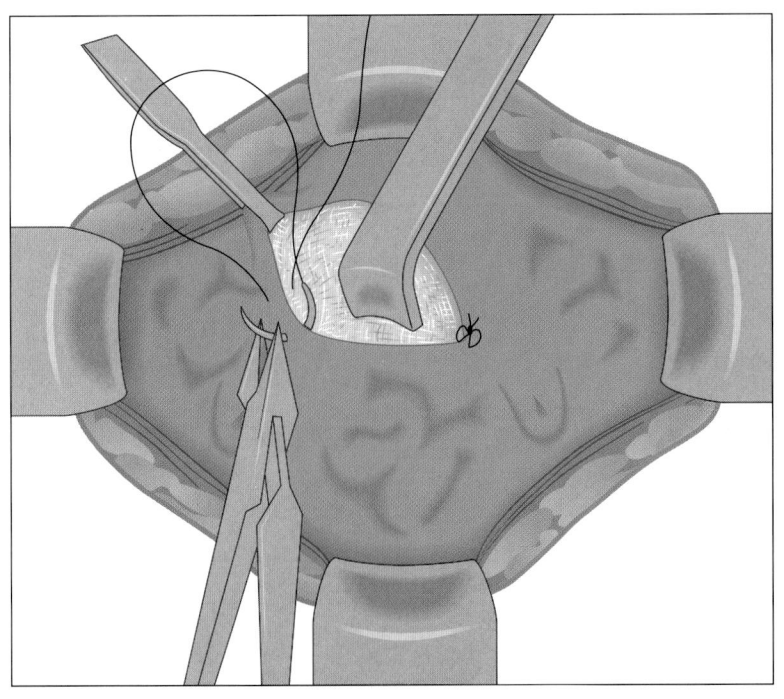

▶ **FIGURE 6-19.** Control of bleeding. A warm, moist gauze pack is placed firmly in the prostatic fossa to tamponade venous bleeding after a transvesical prostatectomy. Figure-of-eight 0 chromic catgut sutures are placed at 5 and 7 o'clock to control bleeding from major arterial branches to the prostate. Bleeding within the fossa is controlled via individual suture ligatures of 3-0 chromic, or, alternatively, bleeding points can be cauterized using the ball electrode.

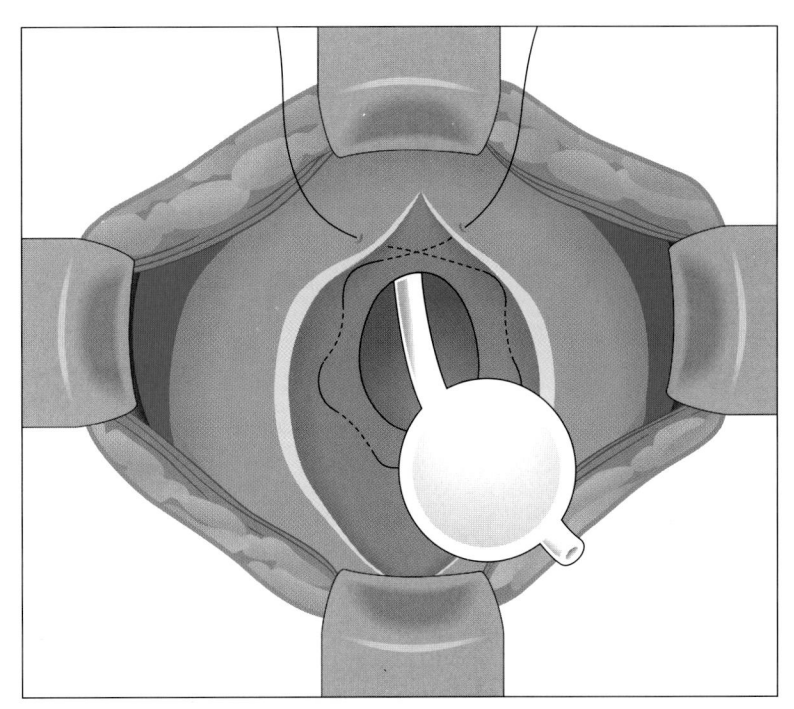

▶ **FIGURE 6-20.** Pursestring suture. Bleeding from the prostatic fossa may also be controlled by using a pull-out suture of heavy nonabsorbable suture to pursestring the bladder neck. With a pursestring pulled tight to approximate the bladder neck, a Foley catheter is snugged up to the bladder neck.

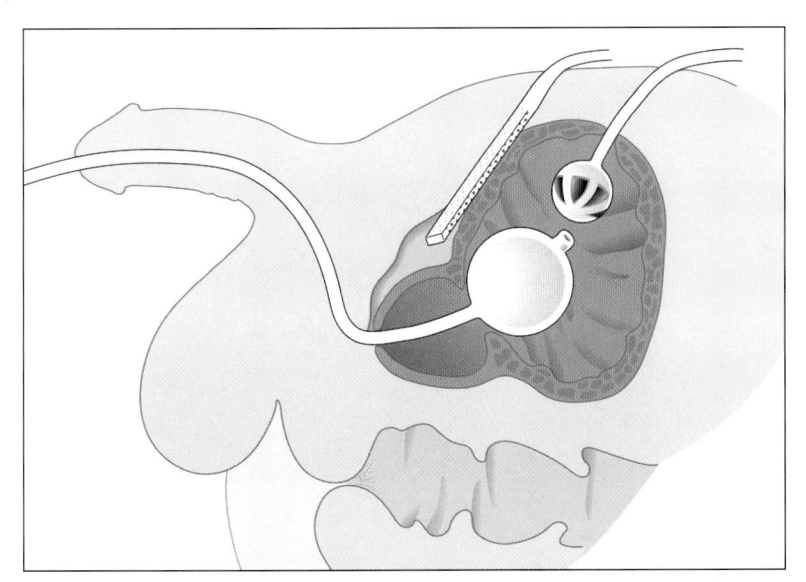

▶ **FIGURE 6-21.** Suprapubic prostatectomy drainage. A suprapubic tube (26-F Malecot) is placed through the dome of the bladder after the bleeding is controlled. An indwelling urethral catheter is left to permit through-and-through irrigation to wash out clots. A suction drain (*eg*, Jackson-Pratt) is left in the space of Retzius. The bladder is closed in two layers using 2-0 chromic catgut running suture on the mucosa and interrupted 0 chromic catgut suture on the serosa and muscular area.

RETROPUBIC PROSTATECTOMY

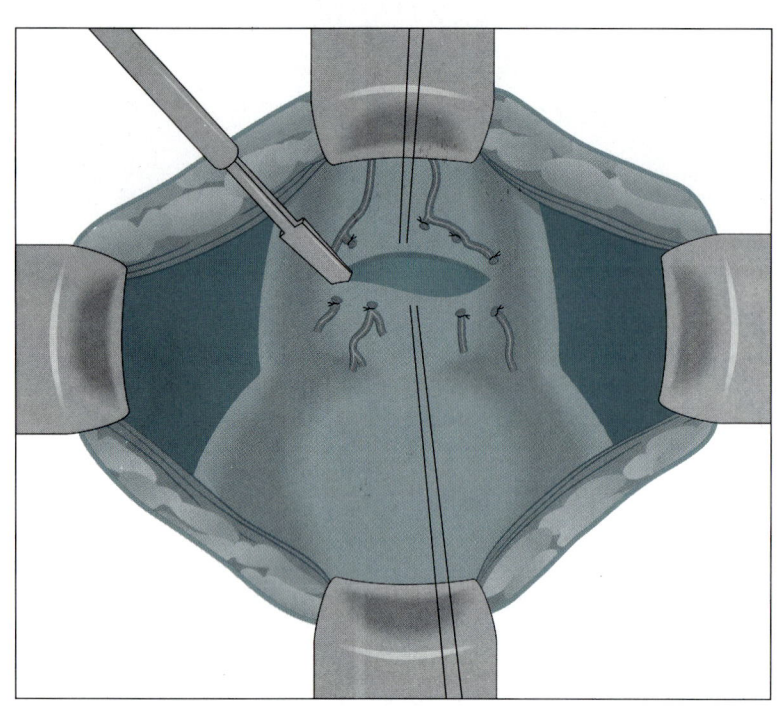

▶ **FIGURE 6-22.** Incision of the prostate capsule. A transverse capsular incision is made through the prostate midway between the apex of the prostate and bladder neck. Stay sutures are used to elevate the surgical capsule, exposing the adenoma. Venous capsular bleeders are suture ligated or cauterized as necessary.

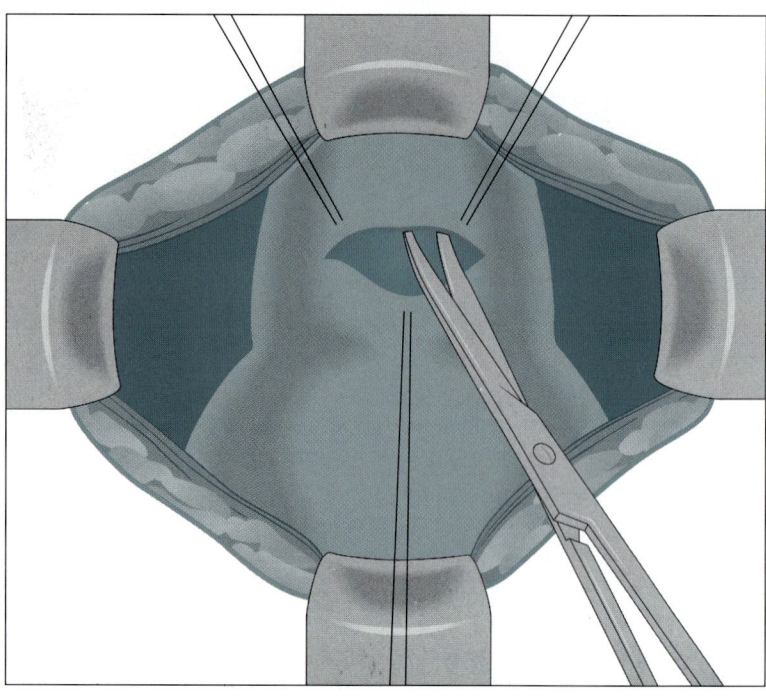

▶ **FIGURE 6-23.** Sharp dissection of the adenoma. A plane between the capsule and the adenoma is identified and, using curved scissors, the adenoma is sharply dissected away from the surgical capsule of the prostate. The urethral mucosa attachment can be transected with scissors and careful dissection of the lateral lobes of the prostate accomplished. The adenoma is then grasped with a tenaculum and dissection carried out sharply, removing the adenoma up to the bladder neck. At this point, the mucosa at the bladder neck is sharply incised and the adenoma removed.

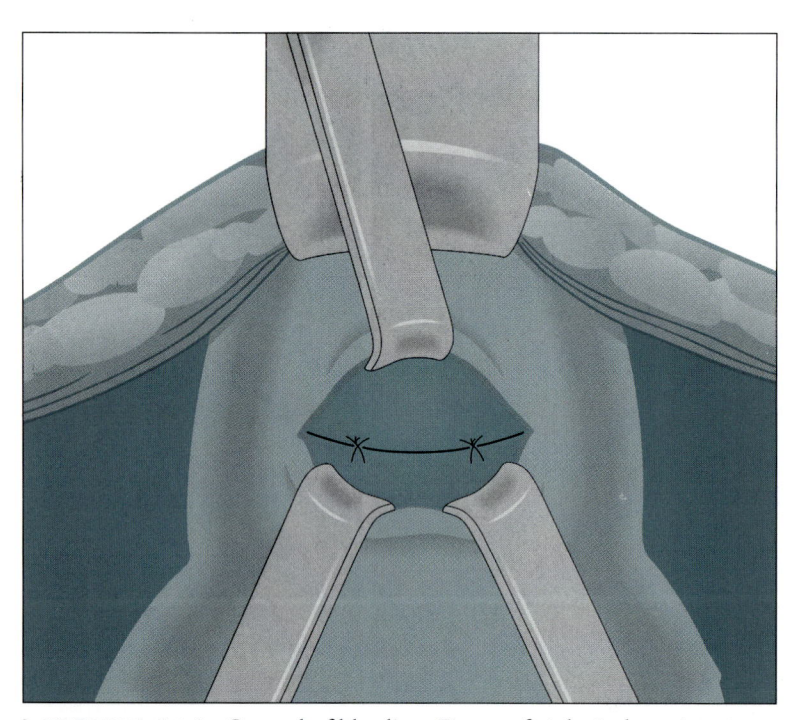

▶ **FIGURE 6-24.** Control of bleeding. Figure-of-eight 0 chromic sutures are placed at 5 and 7 o'clock in the bladder neck to control arterial bleeding.

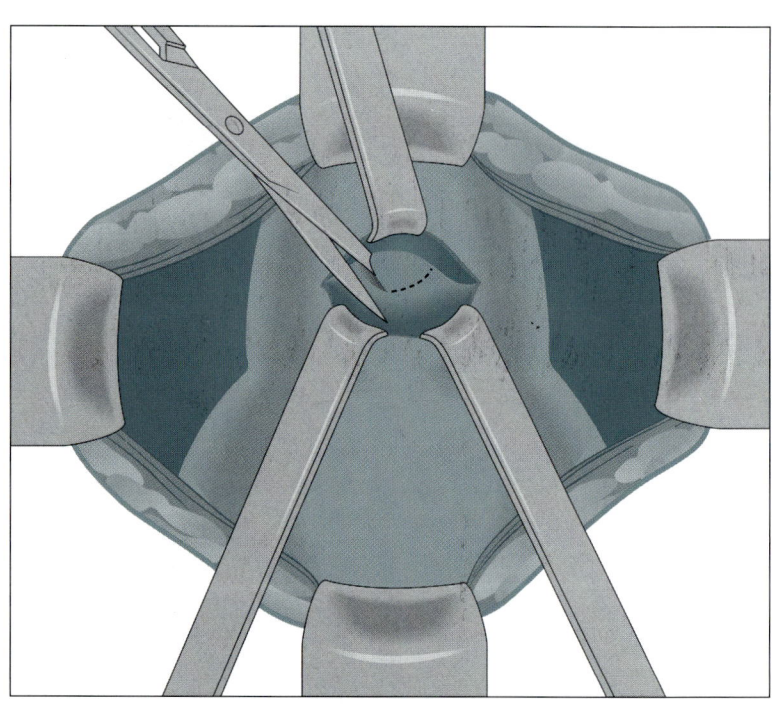

▶ **FIGURE 6-25.** Wedge resection of bladder neck. After retropubic prostatectomy, a V-shaped wedge of bladder neck may be removed if the bladder neck appears to be partially obstructed.

II. The Prostate

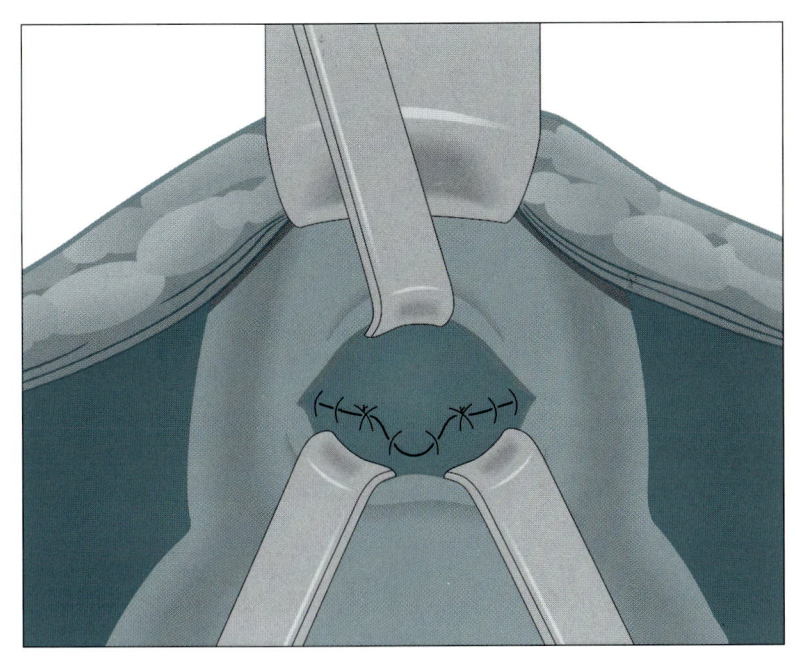

FIGURE 6-26. Closure of wedge resection of the bladder neck. After a wedge of bladder neck is removed, the bladder mucosa is advanced over the cut edge and secured to the prostatic fossa. This may prevent a secondary vesical neck contracture. Bleeding within the prostatic capsule has been controlled with suture ligatures and cautery as needed. If bleeding is insignificant at this point, a suprapubic tube may be unnecessary. A three-way catheter is inserted into the bladder for continuous irrigation with normal saline in the postoperative period. The capsule of the prostate is closed with interrupted 0 chromic catgut. A suction drain is placed into the retropubic space and brought out through a separate stab wound in the anterior abdominal wall. The abdominal fascia and skin are closed in the usual manner.

REFERENCES

1. Nesbit RM: *Transurethral Prostatectomy.* Springfield, IL: Charles C. Thomas; 1943.
2. Barry MJ, Fowler JR, O'Leary MP, *et al.*: The American Urological Association Symptom Index for benign prostatic hyperplasia. *J Urol* 1992, 148:1549–1557.
3. Barry MJ, Fowler FJ, O'Leary MP, *et al.*: Measuring disease-specific health status in men with benign prostatic hyperplasia. *Medical Care* 1995, 33:AS145–AS155.
4. Denis L, Yoshida O, Khoury S, *et al.* (eds): *The 4th International Consultation on BPH Proceedings.* UK: Plymbridge Distibutor; 1998: 669–684.
5. Emmett JL, Rous SN, Greene LF, *et al.*: Preliminary internal urethrotomy in 1036 cases to prevent urethral stricture following transurethral resection: caliber of normal adult male urethra. *J Urol* 1963, 89:829–835.
6. McConnell JD, Barry MJ, Bruskewitz RC, *et al.*: *Benign Prostatic Hyperplasia: Diagnosis and Treatment.* Clinical Practice Guideline Number 8. AHCPR Publication No. 94–0582. Rockville, MD: Agency for Health Care Policy and Research, Public Health Service, US Department of Health and Human Services, 1994.
7. Turner-Warwick R: A urodynamic review of bladder outlet obstruction in the male and its clinical implications. *Urol Clin North Am* 1979, 6:171–192.

Prostatitis: Definition and Clinical Approaches

NONCANCEROUS DISEASE SECTION

John N. Krieger

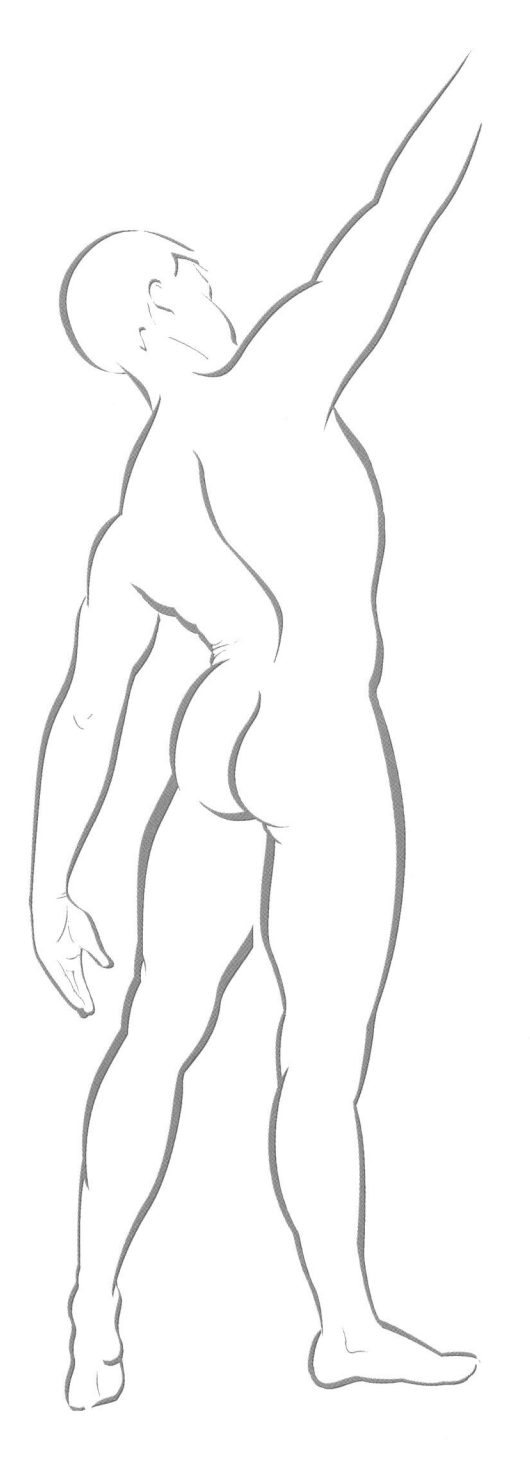

We tell our medical students that the prostate is easy. There are only three problems: 1) prostate cancer, which is a very common cause of death among adult men; 2) benign prostatic hypertrophy (BPH), which is also a common cause of morbidity among adult men and represents an indication for considerable medical and surgical therapy; and 3) prostatitis. Prostatitis also causes considerable morbidity and loss of productivity, and is a frequent cause of visits to physicians in the United States [1,2]. Of the three conditions, prostatitis is by far the least well understood. Perhaps the problem with prostatitis is that we do not have a good abbreviation!

There are several definitions of prostatitis. One of the real problems is that it matters very much which literature one is reviewing. The definition is remarkably different depending on how one approaches this problem. There are different definitions in the pathology literature, in the urology literature, in the infertility literature, and in clinical practice. The aim of this chapter is to examine many of these definitions and to propose a new classification of prostatitis.

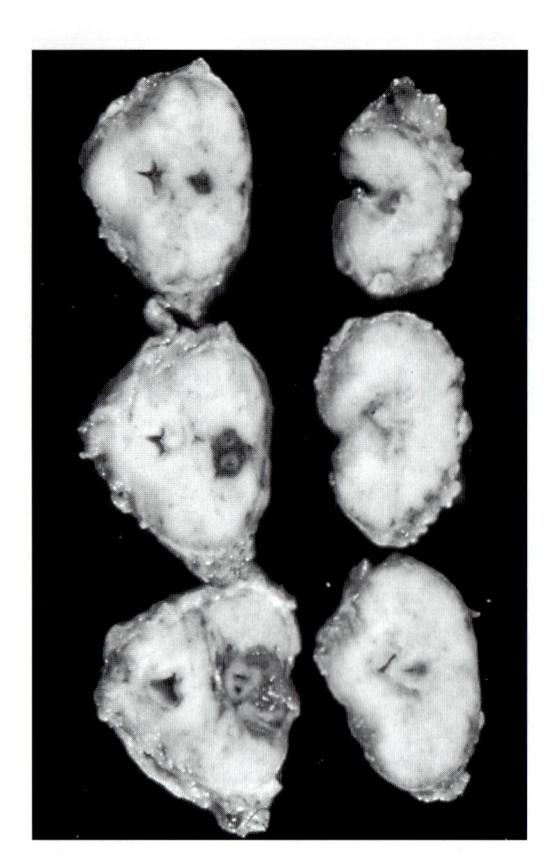

▶ **FIGURE 7-1.** Step-sections of a "normal prostate" from the bladder base through the urethra. Note that there is a focus of gross inflammation apparent in this specimen, illustrating that areas of pathologic prostatitis are commonly seen in autopsy material.

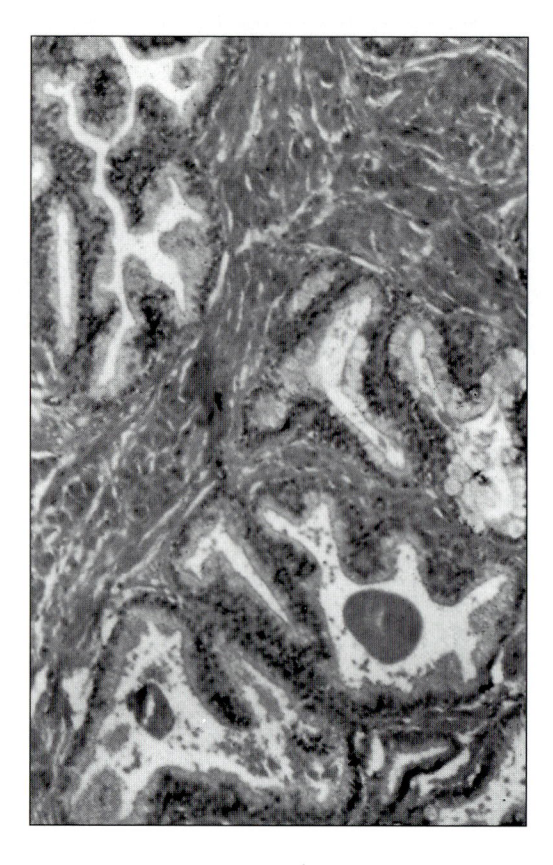

▶ **FIGURE 7-2.** Normal prostate showing the typical histologic appearance of benign-appearing glands and stroma. Note the corpora amylacea.

Histopathologic Criteria for Prostatitis Diagnosis

Examination of tissue
  Benign prostatic hypertrophy
  Definition and categorization of prostatitis
  Inflammatory infiltrates
    Presence
    Characteristics

▶ **FIGURE 7-3.** Criteria for prostatitis diagnosis. In pathology, diagnosis of prostatitis is based on the histologic picture. Pathologists seldom have access to clinical history or physical examination, or microbiologic findings. Thus, diagnosis of prostatitis by pathologists is based entirely on histopathologic criteria.

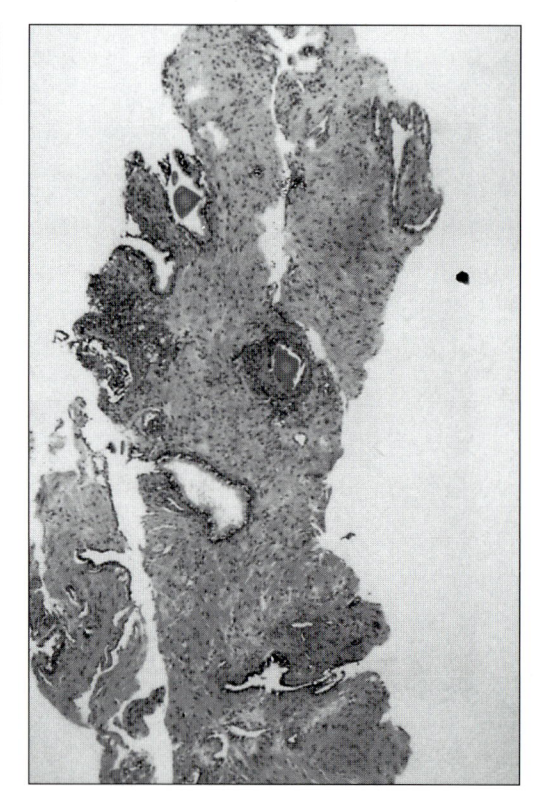

▶ **FIGURE 7-4.** Typical low-power view of a prostate chip from a transurethral resection specimen showing areas of obvious inflammation. This image represents a very unusual patient from the pathologic perspective—unusual because of the documented clinical history and microbiologic data. The patient is a 67-year-old man with acute urinary tract obstruction due to acute bacterial infection with *Escherichia coli* (>10^6 cfu/mL). Bladder drainage and antimicrobials resolved his infection. Unfortunately, he was unable to resume normal voiding. Several weeks later we did a transurethral resection of the prostate, which resolved his bladder outflow obstruction.

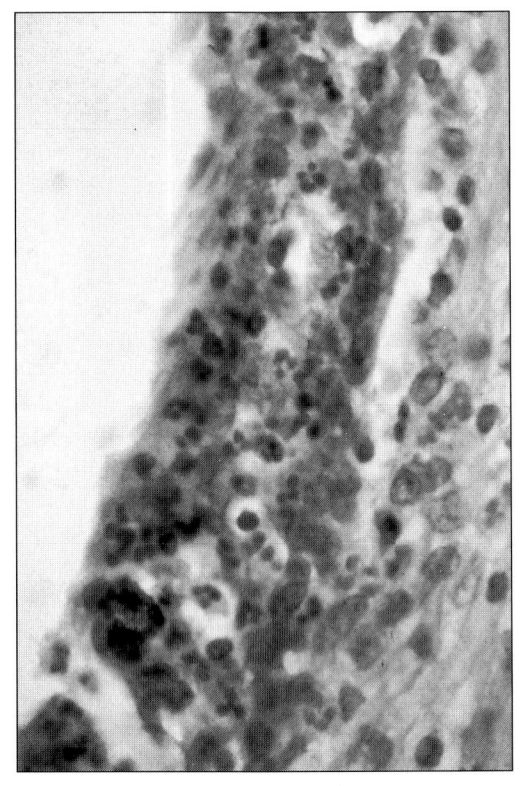

▶ **FIGURE 7-5.** High-power view showing an acute inflammatory infiltrate. The pathologic diagnosis was acute prostatitis.

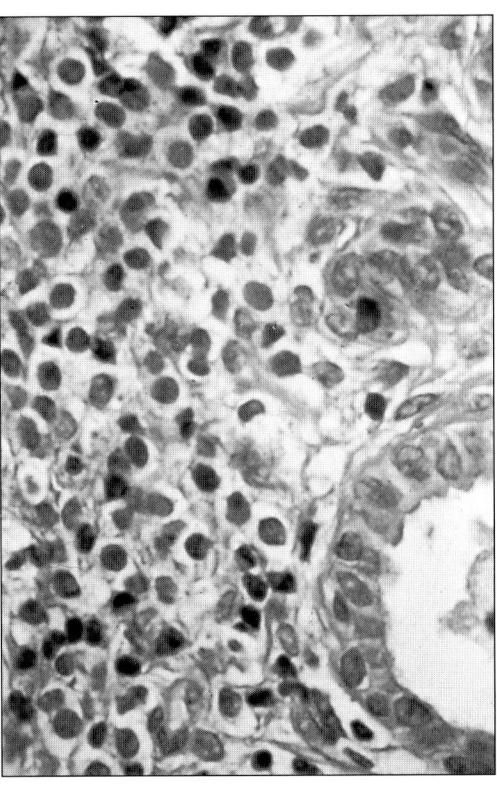

▶ **FIGURE 7-6.** Another case with a chronic inflammatory infiltrate. The pathologic diagnosis was chronic prostatitis.

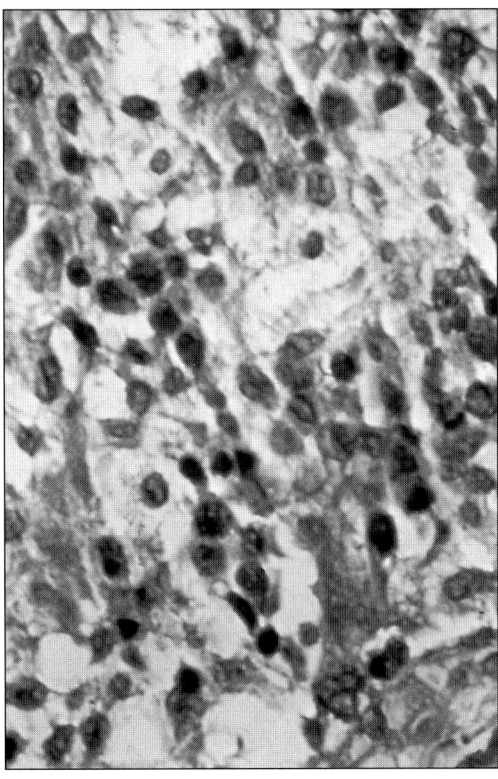

▶ **FIGURE 7-7.** A case of eosiniphilic prostatitis with characteristic red-staining eosinophils predominating in the inflammatory infiltrate. These cases are often associated with allergic reactions.

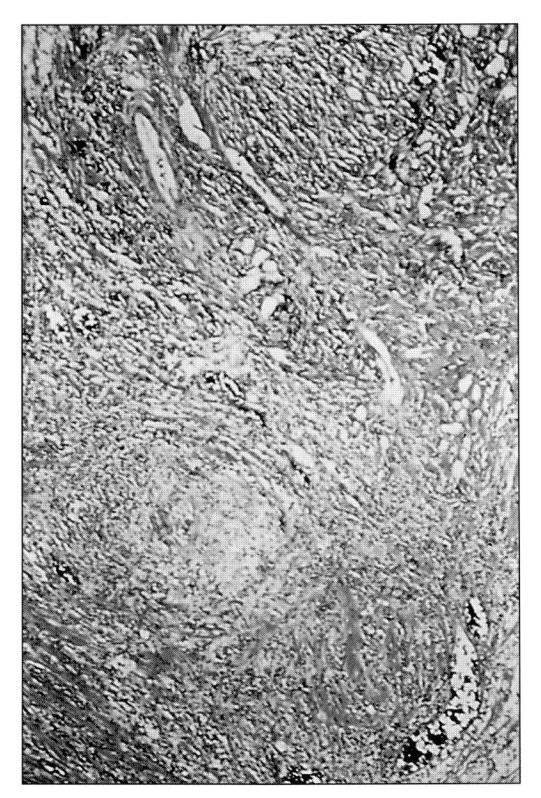

▶ **FIGURE 7-8.** Pathologic diagnosis of granulomanous prostatitis. Granulomanous prostatitis is the characteristic histologic reaction of the prostate to a variety of different causes. Many of these cases are idiopathic, including this case.

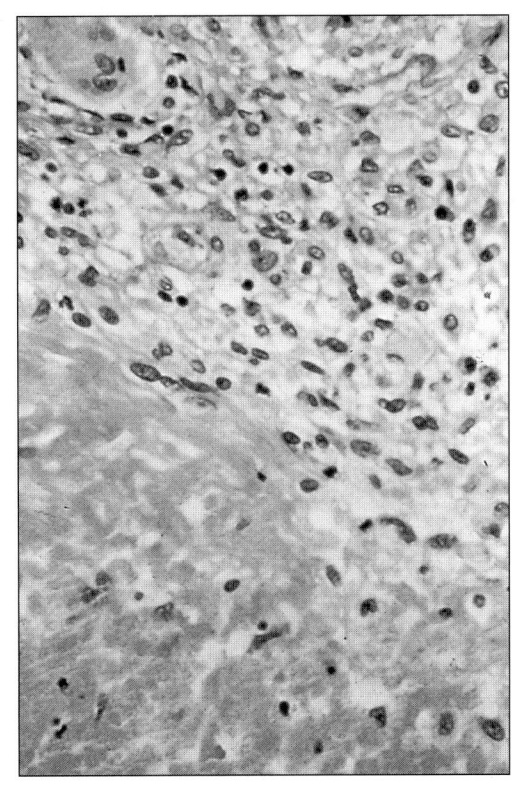

▶ **FIGURE 7-9.** Granulomanous prostatitis due to tuberculosis. Other cases of granulomanous prostatitis are related to urologic surgery or to specific infections, such as tuberculosis, bacille Calmette-Guérin therapy, or fungal infections. Note the caseous necrosis and Langhan's giant cells.

Problems With the Pathologic Definition and Classification of Prostatitis

Population
Inflammation or infection may be focal
Not well correlated with clinical findings
Many men with no history of prostatitis have histologic findings of prostatitis

▶ **FIGURE 7-10.** Problems with the pathologic definition and classification of prostatitis. First, the population studied is approximately 20 years older than the typical population of patients with symptoms of chronic prostatitis. The second problem is that step sections of prostates removed at autopsy show that inflammation and infection may be focal, affecting some areas of the prostate but not other areas. The pathologic diagnoses and findings have not been well correlated with clinical findings. In the older literature, pathology has rarely been found to be helpful in the clinical management of patients with prostatitis symptoms. Finally, in our practice many men with no history of prostatitis who undergo prostatectomy for benign or malignant disease have histologic findings of prostatitis.

The Traditional Definition of Prostatitis

Meares-Stamey (research definition)
  Lower urinary tract localization
    VB1, VB2, EPS, VB3 (cultures or microscopy)
  Four clinical syndromes
    Acute bacterial prostatitis
    Chronic bacterial prostatitis
    Nonbacterial prostatitis
    Prostatodynia

▶ **FIGURE 7-11.** The traditional definition of prostatitis. The traditional definition used in the urology literature has been based on the Meares-Stamey definition and classification [3–5]. This research definition is based on careful lower urinary tract localization studies. These studies include examination of the following: VB1 (voided bladder 1 or first-void urine), VB2 (voided bladder 2, or midstream urine), expressed prostatic secretions (EPS) and VB3 (voided bladder 3, or postmassage urine), using quantitative cultures and microscopy. The four clinical syndromes that have classically been described are listed in this figure.

Distinctions Among the Four Clinical Syndromes of Prostatitis

Syndrome	Symptoms	EPS leukocytes	Bacteriuria	Physical Examination
Acute bacterial	+	+	+	+
Chronic bacterial	+	+	+	
Nonbacterial	+	+		
Prostatodynia	+			

▶ **FIGURE 7-12.** Distinctions among the four clinical syndromes of prostatitis. Acute bacterial prostatitis is associated with characteristic symptoms of acute urinary tract infection. On occasion, the patient may be septic and present with a systemic illness. The physical examination is frequently impressive with local bladder tenderness, an exquisitely tender and tense prostate on rectal examination, and occasionally signs of systemic infection. The patient has bacteriuria defined as presence of uropathogens in the midstream urine. The expressed prostatic secretions have leukocytes and pathogenic bacteria.

Chronic prostatitis is characterized by recurrent symptoms of acute urinary tract infection. There are increased numbers of leukocytes in the prostatic secretions and uropathogens are present episodically in the midstream urine. The physical examination may or may not be impressive. The characteristic clinical feature of chronic bacterial prostatitis is recurrent urinary tract infections caused by the same bacterial species.

In contrast, nonbacterial prostatitis and prostatodynia are not associated with bacteriuria. These patients are symptomatic. The distinction between nonbacterial prostatitis and prostatodynia is based on the presence of increased numbers of expressed prostatic secretions (EPS) leukocytes in patients with nonbacterial prostatitis, but not in patients with prostatodynia.

Characteristics of Acute Bacterial Prostatitis

Systemic symptoms of tissue-invasive infection ("flu")
  Malaise, myalgias, fever
Urinary tract symptoms of bacteriuria
  Frequency, dysuria, and obstructive voiding
  Physical examination finds "tense," exquisitely tender prostate
Responds dramatically to antimicrobial therapy

▶ **FIGURE 7-13.** Characteristics of acute bacterial prostatitis. Acute bacterial prostatitis is associated with systemic symptoms of a tissue-invasive infection. The patient may present with a flulike syndrome characterized by malaise, myalgias, and fever. The patient will have urinary tract symptoms of bacteriuria characterized by increased urinary frequency, dysuria, and often obstructed voiding. On physical examination the prostate may be "tense" and exquisitely tender. Fortunately, these patients respond dramatically to appropriate antimicrobial therapy for recognized uropathogens. Many agents that do not get into the prostate under noninflamed conditions work very well in this syndrome. This is usually not a difficult or subtle diagnosis.

Characteristics and Treatment of Chronic Bacterial Prostatitis

Recurrent bacteriuria in adult men
Often asymptomatic between episodes of bacteriuria
Treatment strategies
    Antimicrobials that penetrate prostate
    Curative: long course, full dose
    Suppressive: continuous, low dose

FIGURE 7-14. Characteristics of chronic bacterial prostatitis. Chronic bacterial prostatitis is the most common cause of recurrent bacteriuria in adult men. It is noteworthy that these patients may be totally asymptomatic between acute episodes of bacteriuria.

There are a number of treatment strategies using antimicrobial agents that penetrate the prostatic parenchyma. One can use curative treatment strategies, meaning a long course (in my practice, 6 weeks to 3 months) of full-dose antimicrobial therapy, usually using a drug such as fluoroquinolone or trimethoprim-sulfamethoxazole. This regimen will cure 30% to 50% of patients. For patients who cannot be cured, one can use a strategy of suppression with continuous low-dose therapy using nightly or every-other-night dosing of a low-dose agent to suppress bladder bacteriuria. This is the United States Food and Drug Administration's definition of prostatitis, but it represents very few patients seen in clinical practice.

Diagnosis Localization Cultures in Some Cases of Chronic Bacterial Prostatitis

Organism	VB1	VB2	EPS	VB3
Escherichia coli	1200	1200	15,000	4400
Escherichia coli	0	0	4000	110
Escherichia coli	100	200	2700	110
Escherichia coli	240	140	2700	270
Escherichia coli	0	0	100	0
Pseudomonas aeruginosa	0	0	50,000	300
Enterobacter cloacae	0	0	1500	10

FIGURE 7-15. Diagnostic localization cultures in some cases of chronic bacterial prostatitis [6]. In each case the patient had recurrent episodes of bacteriuria caused by the same organism that we localized to the prostate using the four-glass test. Many of these patients required more than one study for definitive localization. Note that these organisms are all recognized uropathogens. These seven patients all had gram-negative rod infections. It is possible to have a gram-positive result, but it is important to document recurrent episodes of bacteriuria caused by that organism. The characteristic localization pattern is a tenfold increase when the VB3 sample is compared with the VB1 sample. If that criterion fails, one can compare the expressed prostatic secretion (EPS) sample with the VB1. VB1—voided bladder 1; VB2—voided bladder 2; VB3—voided bladder 3.

Problems With the Urologic Definition of Prostatitis

Represents < 10% of all bacterial prostatitis cases (acute or chronic)
    Studies concern a small subset of patients
    Only group of interest to US FDA for drug development
Localization seldom done in clinical practice
    Laboratory problems
    Subtleties in technique
    Usually negative or not helpful

FIGURE 7-16. Problems with the urologic definition of prostatitis. First and foremost, this definition represents less than 10% of bacterial prostatitis seen in clinical practice. Much of the literature concerns a very small subset of highly selected patients. Localization studies, although described very carefully and thoroughly in research settings, are seldom done in clinical practice. This is for a number of reasons, such as problems setting up the laboratory studies and subtleties in technique. However, most clinicians believe that these studies are usually negative and thus are not particularly helpful or cost-effective for most patients. US FDA—US Food and Drug Administration.

Assumptions Made by the Traditional Definition

Nonbacterial prostatitis indicates a physical problem
    Fastidious microorganisms
        (many classified as bacteria, eg, Chlamydia trachomatis)
    Inflammatory disorder (noninfectious)
    Allergy
    Stones
    Other organic pathology

FIGURE 7-17. Assumptions implicit in the traditional urologic definition of prostatitis. The first is that patients with nonbacterial prostatitis have a physical problem, such as the presence of fastidious microorganisms. Many of these potential organisms are classified as bacteria, such as *Chlamydia trachomatis* [7]. Thus, nonbacterial prostatitis is in fact a misnomer. Others have suggested that nonbacterial prostatitis is an inflammatory disorder that may be noninfectious (see Krieger [8]). Other theories in the literature are that nonbacterial prostatitis is related to allergy, prostate stones, or other organic pathology, such as voiding dysfunction or reflux of sterile urine into the prostatic ducts.

Causes of Prostatodynia
Neuromuscular: genitourinary diaphragm
"Pelvic floor tension myalgia"
Primary voiding disturbance
Bladder neck obstruction
External sphincter spasm
Treatment includes TURP, TUIP, cystoprostatectomy, hyperthermia, diazepam, α-blockers
Primary psychologic disturbances

▶ **FIGURE 7-18.** Prostatodynia. The syndrome of prostatodynia has been ascribed to a variety of causes, such as neuromuscular dysfunction of the genitourinary diaphragm. Some suggest that this is "pelvic floor tension myalgia" [8]. Others suggest that this is a primary voiding disturbance with abnormalities at the bladder neck or external sphincter spasm. Treatment recommendations include transurethral resection or incision of the prostate. Other procedures described in the recent literature include cystoprostatectomy, hyperthermia, and use of α-blockers. Such treatments may help some patients, although our clinic is full of patients in whom such therapies failed. Still other authors suggest that there is a primary psychologic disturbance in these patients, and that "psychiatric counseling should be seriously pursued, because these patients have serious personality disturbances and defects in sexual identification" [4]. TUIP—transurethral incision of the prostate; TURP—transurethral resection of the prostate.

Experiential Findings Regarding Prostatitis and Prostatodynia
Symptoms similar in nonbacterial prostatitis and prostatodynia
EPS findings variable
Fastidious organisms isolated from both populations
Both groups are often frustrated, depressed
Psychologic abnormalities common among patients with chronic diseases associated with pain
Gastric ulcer and *Helicobacter pylori*

▶ **FIGURE 7-19.** In our experience symptoms are often similar in patients with nonbacterial prostatitis and prostatodynia. Further, findings in the prostatic fluid of individual men may be variable [9]. We have isolated fastidious organisms from both populations. Both groups of men are often frustrated and depressed. However, psychologic abnormalities are very common among patients with chronic diseases associated with pain, and one must not forget that gastric ulcer, once ascribed to personality disorders, now is recognized as an infectious disease.

Another Definition of Prostatitis Based on the Fertility Literature
Seminal fluid analysis
Various terms in addition to prostatitis
Leukocytospermia
Pyosemia
Prostatoseminal vesiculitis
Epididymo-prostato-vesiculitis
Male accessory gland infection
Seminal inflammation (preferred)

▶ **FIGURE 7-20.** Still another definition of prostatitis used in the fertility literature. This definition is based on identification of inflammation in the seminal fluid. Various terms are used in this literature in addition to prostatitis [10].

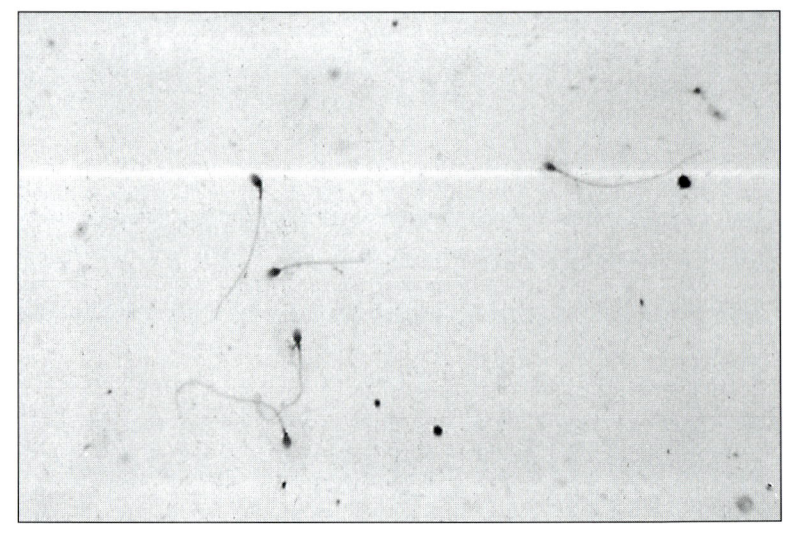

▶ **FIGURE 7-21.** A normal seminal fluid specimen that has been stained with Papanicolaou stain. Sperm and a few leukocytes are shown.

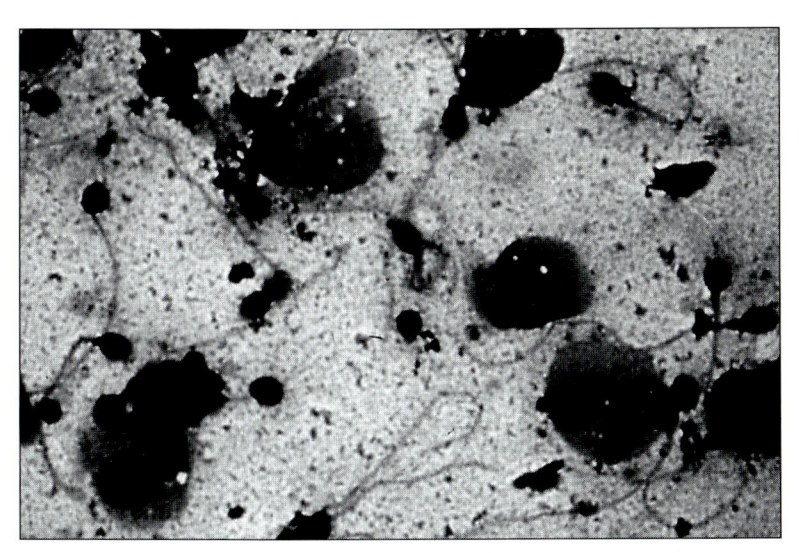

▶ **FIGURE 7-22.** A seminal fluid sample with increased numbers of polymorphonuclear leukocytes. Note that the slide is stained with Bryan-Leishman's stain to facilitate differentiation of leukocytes from sperm forms. Cells with pink cytoplasm are leukocytes, whereas cells with gray cytoplasm are germ cells.

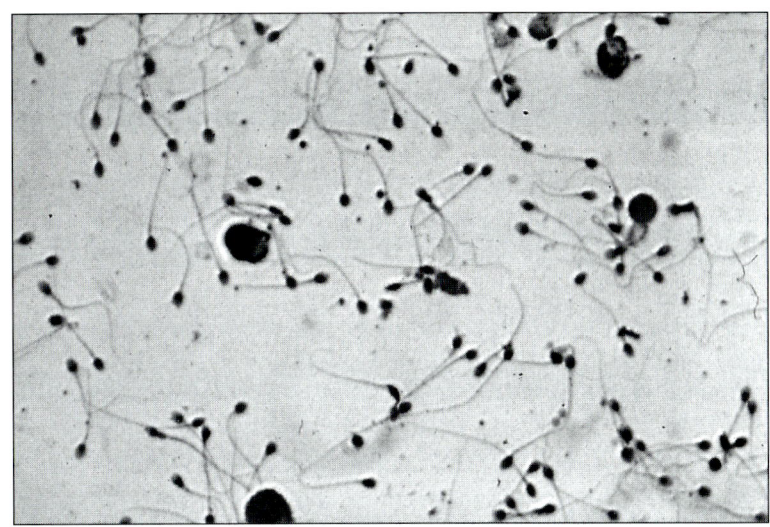

▶ **FIGURE 7-23.** A monoclonal antibody–stained preparation (HLe1), illustrating that the inflammatory cells are indeed leukocytes.

Problems with the Andrology Definition of Prostatitis

Population studied
Methods
   Staining: distinguish leukocytes from sperm
   Definition of inflammation
      > 10^6 leukocytes per milliliter of semen
      > 6 leukocytes per 100 sperm
Possible relationship of leukocytospermia to:
   Infection
   Infertility

▶ **FIGURE 7-24.** Problems with the andrology definition of prostatitis. The first problem is the populations studied, which are predominantly patients with infertility as their chief complaint, not prostatitis. A second problem concerns the methods. Many studies used "round cell" counts in unstained specimens. Staining is necessary to distinguish leukocytes from sperm. Third, there have been varying definitions of inflammation (numbers or concentrations of leukocytes) used in this literature. Fourth, the question of the relationship between leukocytospermia and either infection or infertility is incompletely defined.

Other problems include the fact that leukocytes in semen can come from multiple sites besides the prostate. Most studies in this literature, however, seldom evaluate other sites, such as the urethra or expressed prostatic secretions, for presence of inflammation. Many studies lack data on patients' symptoms or physical findings. Finally, limited data correlate seminal fluid analysis findings with either findings in the prostatic secretions or with histology of the prostate.

Standard Clinical Definition of Prostatitis

Based on symptoms
Limited laboratory evaluation
Repeated courses of empirical therapy

▶ **FIGURE 7-25.** The clinical definition of prostatitis. Stamey [4] describes this definition as "a wastebasket of clinical ignorance used to describe any condition associated with prostatic inflammation or prostatic symptoms . . . most commonly diagnosed in patients who have no history of bladder infection despite the presence of perineal aching, low back pain, or urinary discomfort."

The standard clinical definition of prostatitis is based entirely on symptoms. Most patients undergo limited laboratory evaluation. In contrast, they have repeated courses of empirical therapy using a variety of agents. This does have one overriding advantage: the clinical definition does address what patients actually suffer from.

Genitourinary Symptoms of Chronic Prostatitis

General agreement in literature
   Certain pain symptoms common, *ie*, perineal, back, and genital
Marked disagreement regarding:
   Voiding complaints
   Sexual dysfunction

▶ **FIGURE 7-26.** The genitourinary symptoms of chronic prostatitis. Careful review of the literature found general agreement on the presence of certain pain symptoms, such as perineal, back, and genital pain [11]. However, there was marked disagreement on the prevalence of voiding complaints and sexual dysfunction.

Problems With the Clinical Definition of Prostatitis

Characteristic symptoms poorly defined
No diagnostic physical finding or laboratory test
Therapy is entirely empirical and often unsatisfactory

FIGURE 7-27. Problems with the clinical definition of prostatitis. The model used for benign prostatic hypertrophy (BPH) may prove valuable. In the new BPH model, the American Urological Association symptom score proved critical for developing new therapies, although we still do not completely understand the cause of BPH.

Genitourinary Symptoms of Prostatitis

Stress and psychologic abnormalities common
Patients present to urologists with somatic symptoms
Concentrated on the urogenital complaints
  Pain complaints
  Voiding complaints
  Sexual dysfunction

FIGURE 7-28. Genitourinary symptoms of prostatitis. What we do know about the genitourinary symptoms of prostatitis is that stress and psychologic abnormalities are very common. Many of these patients present to urologists with somatic symptoms; therefore, we and others have concentrated on developing instruments that evaluate the genitourinary complaints of these patients. We found that most complaints can be classified as either pain complaints, voiding complaints, or sexual dysfunction complaints [11].

To summarize, prostatitis causes considerable morbidity. It is neglected in terms of research and new clinical initiatives compared with the other prostate diseases. Although there are at least four definitions, none of them work well for the great majority of patients.

A. Aspects of the Working Definition of "Chronic Prostatitis"

Symptoms: pain complaints are primary component
Closer to patient presentation and clinical practice
New synonym for chronic prostatitis: CPPS

B. Automatic Exclusion Criteria for Chronic Prostatitis

Duration < 3 mo
Genitourinary cancer (*eg*, TCC, CIS, prostate cancer)
Active stone disease
Active infection
  Bacteriuria, herpes, genitourinary tuberculosis
Gastrointestinal disorders
  Inflammatory bowel disease
  Perirectal disease (*eg*, fissure, fistula)
Radiation/chemical cystitis
Acute urethritis
Acute epididymitis
Acute orchitis
Urethral stricture
Neurologic disease affecting bladder

FIGURE 7-29. Consensus working definition of "chronic prostatitis." As a first step in addressing these problems, a new working definition for chronic prostatitis was developed by an expert panel convened by the National Institute of Diabetes and Digestive and Kidney Diseases (NIDDK). **A,** This new definition, which has yet to be validated, concentrated on patients' symptoms using pain complaints as a primary component. In this respect it is much closer to patient presentation and clinical practice. In addition there is a new synonym for chronic prostatitis: chronic pelvic pain syndrome (CPPS).

B, Exclusion criteria. These criteria include duration less than 3 months, presence of genitourinary cancers such as transitional cell carcinoma (TCC), carcinoma *in situ* (CIS), or carcinoma of the prostate. Other exclusions include presence of active stone disease, because a distal ureteral stone or crystaluria can cause lower tract symptoms. Presence of active infection, such as bacteriuria, herpes or genitourinary tuberculosis, presence of genitourinary disease, such as inflammatory bowel disease or perirectal disease such as fissure or fistula, also exclude patients from the NIDDK definition. Other automatic exclusions are also listed in this figure.

A. Symptomatic Prostatitis Syndromes

Bacterial prostatitis
  Acute and chronic
Chronic prostatitis
  CPPS or "abacterial" prostatitis

B. Aspects of Acute and Chronic Prostatitis

Acute
  Bacteriuria
    Uropathogens
  Possible systemic illness
Chronic
  Recurrent episodes of bacteriuria
  Organism "localizes" to prostate

C. Chronic Prostatitis or Chronic Pelvic Pain Syndrome

Inflammatory
  Leukocytes in EPS, semen, VB3
Noninflammatory
  No leukocytes

FIGURE 7-30. Prostatitis syndromes. The National Institute of Diabetes and Digestive and Kidney Diseases consensus classification of prostatitis considers prostatitis syndromes as either symptomatic or asymptomatic. A, The symptomatic prostatitis syndromes include bacterial prostatitis, either acute or chronic, and chronic prostatitis or chronic pelvic pain syndrome (CPPS), also known as "abacterial" prostatitis. B, Aspects of acute and chronic bacterial prostatitis. Acute bacterial prostatitis is characterized by presence of bacteriuria caused by recognized uropathogens. Some patients may have a systemic illness. The hallmark of chronic bacterial prostatitis is recurrent episodes of bacteriuria caused by the same organism that localizes to the prostate on segmented cultures. C, The third syndrome is chronic prostatitis or chronic pelvic pain syndrome, which has an inflammatory subtype, characterized by presence of leukocytes in prostatic secretions, semen, or postmassage urine, and a noninflammatory subtype, characterized by absence of leukocytes. EPS—expressed prostatic secretions; VB3—voided bladder 3.

Characteristics of Asymptomatic Inflammatory Prostatitis

Increased PSA level
Histology indicates prostatitis
Infertility is only symptom

FIGURE 7-31. Finally, there is a category termed "asymptomatic inflammatory prostatitis." For example, an asymptomatic patient presents with an increased prostate-specific antigen (PSA) and this leads to a biopsy. The most common noncancer diagnosis is prostatitis. There are also patients with infertility, but who have no symptoms other than their infertility, and have prostatitis based on seminal fluid findings. Such patients are characterized as having asymptomatic inflammatory prostatitis.

The New Consensus Classification of Prostatitis Syndromes

Acute bacterial prostatitis
Chronic bacterial prostatitis
Chronic prostatitis or CPPS
  Inflammatory
  Noninflammatory
Asymptomatic inflammatory prostatitis

FIGURE 7-32. Summary of the new classification of prostatitis. CPPS—chronic pelvic pain syndrome.

REFERENCES

1. Krieger J: How common is prostatitis? [editorial comment] *J Urol* 1998, in press.
2. Collins EA: How common is prostatitis? *J Urol* 1998, in press.
3. Meares E, Jr., Stamey T: Bacteriologic localization patterns in bacterial prostatitis and urethritis. *Invest Urol* 1968, 5:492.
4. Stamey T: Urinary infections in males. In *Pathogenesis and Treatment of Urinary Tract Infections*. Baltimore: Williams & Wilkins; 1980: 342.
5. Krieger J, McGonagle L: Diagnostic considerations and interpretation of microbiologic findings for evaluation of chronic prostatitis. *J Clin Microbiol* 1989, 27:240.
6. Krieger J, Egan K: Comprehensive evaluation and treatment of 75 men referred to chronic prostatitis clinic. *Urology* 1991, 38:11–19.
7. Krieger J, Riley D: Prokaryotic DNA sequences in patients with chronic idiopathic prostatitis. *J Clin Microbiol* 1996, 34:3120.
8. Krieger J: Prostatitis syndromes. In *Sexually Transmitted Diseases*. Edited by Holmes K, Sparling P, Mardh P-A. New York: McGraw-Hill; 1998.
9. Wright ET, Chmiel J, Grayhack J, Schaeffer R: Prostatic fluid inflammation in prostatitis. *J Urol* 1994, 152:2300.
10. Krieger J, Berger R, Ross S, *et al.*: Seminal fluid findings in men with nonbacterial prostatitis and prostatodynia. *J Androl* 1996, 17:310.
11. Krieger J, Egan K, Ross S, *et al.*: Chronic pelvic pains represent the most prominent urogenital symptoms of "chronic prostatitis." *Urology* 1996, 48:715.

Section II — Cancerous Disease

Peter T. Scardino

Cancer of the prostate is the most common cancer in men throughout the Western world and is the second leading cause of cancer deaths among men in the United States. In 1999, it is anticipated that 179,000 men in the United States will be newly diagnosed with prostate cancer and 39,000 men will die from this disease. Prostate cancer accounts for about 3% of all deaths among men over 50 years of age. It has been estimated that nearly one million men now alive and over age 50 will eventually die of prostate cancer.

This disease perplexes physicians and epidemiologists because of the enormous disparity between the high prevalence of histologically recognizable malignant cells in the prostate and much lower clinical evidence of the disease or of death from prostate cancer. Cancer can be found in the prostates of over half of all men over 50 years of age. However, only 20% to 25% of these cancers will be clinically manifest during the patient's lifetime and only 6% to 8% will prove fatal.

Today, systematic, periodic testing with prostate-specific antigen (PSA) and the digital rectal examination (DRE) can detect almost all cancers before they metastasize. The difficult challenge is distinguishing the indolent from the potentially lethal cancers and assigning treatment that is appropriate to the threat that each cancer poses to the individual patient.

In this section, we provide an overview of the early detection and treatment of prostate cancer as it is currently practiced. We have emphasized those practical, clinical aspects of diagnosis and local and systemic therapy that are widely accepted and have withstood the test of time. The consensus indicates that the appropriate methods for screening and early detection include regular, annual use of PSA and DRE. If either of these tests are abnormal, the patient should be referred for ultrasound-guided systematic needle biopsies of the prostate.

In contrast, considerable controversy surrounds the optimal treatment, especially for clinically localized cancers. Surgeons debate the merits of perineal versus retropubic prostatectomy, focusing on the need for pelvic lymph node dissection, differences in expected blood loss, and the rate of positive surgical margins, as well as the frequency of recovery of erections after the operation. Radiation oncologists debate the value of external-beam radiotherapy versus brachytherapy, alone or in combination, focusing on costs, convenience, local tumor control, and long-term gastrointestinal and erectile dysfunction. Cryoablation has been advocated as a means to control the local tumor with greater efficacy than irradiation therapy and fewer complications than surgery, but its position in the therapeutic armamentarium today is far from secure. Hormonal therapy—androgen ablation—revolutionized the treatment of prostate cancer in 1941 when Hudgins and Hodges first described immediate regression of metastatic prostate cancer after medical or surgical castration. We are now on the threshold of an era of effective nonhormonal systemic agents—chemotherapy, vaccines, and, possibly, gene or cellular therapy.

In this section, internationally respected scholars present each of these aspects of prostate cancer clearly and succinctly. We hope these chapters help clarify an often confusing and contentious field and will lead to better care of the patient with prostate cancer.

Clinical Aspects of Prostate Cancer

8
CANCEROUS DISEASE SECTION

H. Ballentine Carter & Alan W. Partin

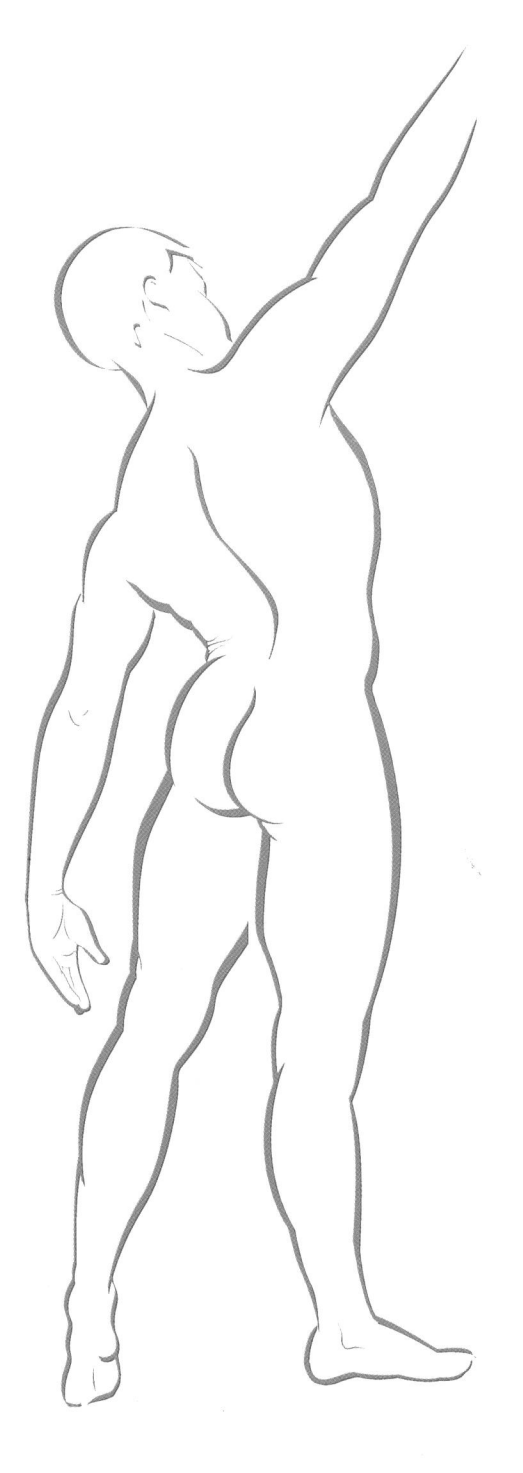

An understanding of the gross anatomic relationship of the prostate to other structures within the male pelvis is of great medical importance. Because benign prostatic hyperplasia and adenocarcinoma of the prostate are common conditions of aging men, a clear understanding of the anatomic relationships among the prostate, seminal vesicles, and bladder is important for developing the concepts necessary to understand the clinical aspects of prostate cancer.

▶ **FIGURE 8-1.** Digital rectal palpation of the prostate. The prostate is the largest of the male sex accessory glands. It consists of glandular and fibromuscular elements. Normally, the prostate is the size of a horse chestnut or a walnut ($\approx$ 20 g). It is found low in the male pelvis, above the rectum and below the pubis, situated between the bladder superiorly and the urethra inferiorly. It surrounds a major portion of the urethra. The prostate is enclosed by a dense sheaf of fascia known as the endopelvic fascia of the prostate. On its anterior surface, the prostate is enveloped in a vast network of venous channels (the prostatic venous plexus), which are responsible for the majority of blood loss during radical removal of the prostate. Blood supply to the prostate emanates primarily from the internal pudendal, the inferior vesicle, and the middle rectal arteries. The lymphatic drainage of the prostate terminates primarily in the internal iliac and sacral lymph nodes. Nerve supply to the prostate emanates from the inferior hypogastric plexus and travels in close approximation with the neurovascular bundle that contains the nerves essential for erectile function. The seminal vesicles, situated at the base of the bladder and anterior to the rectum, are attached to the base of the prostate at the site of entry of the ejaculatory duct. During radical removal of the prostate for prostate cancer, these structures are removed intact with the prostate. This figure demonstrates how the prostate can be palpated rectally. The anterior wall of the rectum and the rectovesicle septum separate the examiner's finger from the posterior surface of the prostate. In some instances, the seminal vesicles can be palpated per the rectum. (*Adapted from* Laurenson [1]; with permission.)

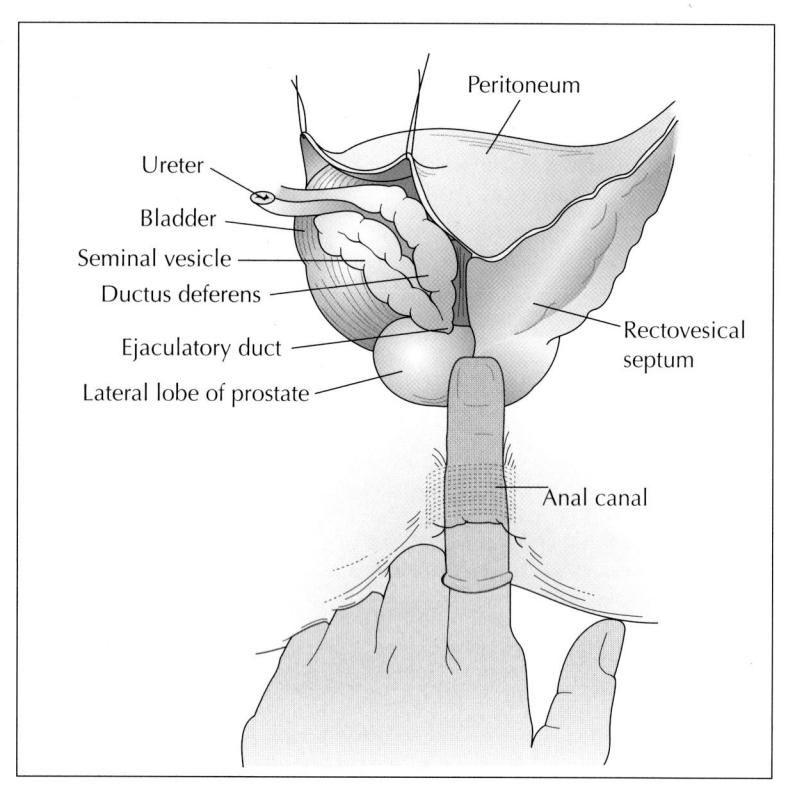

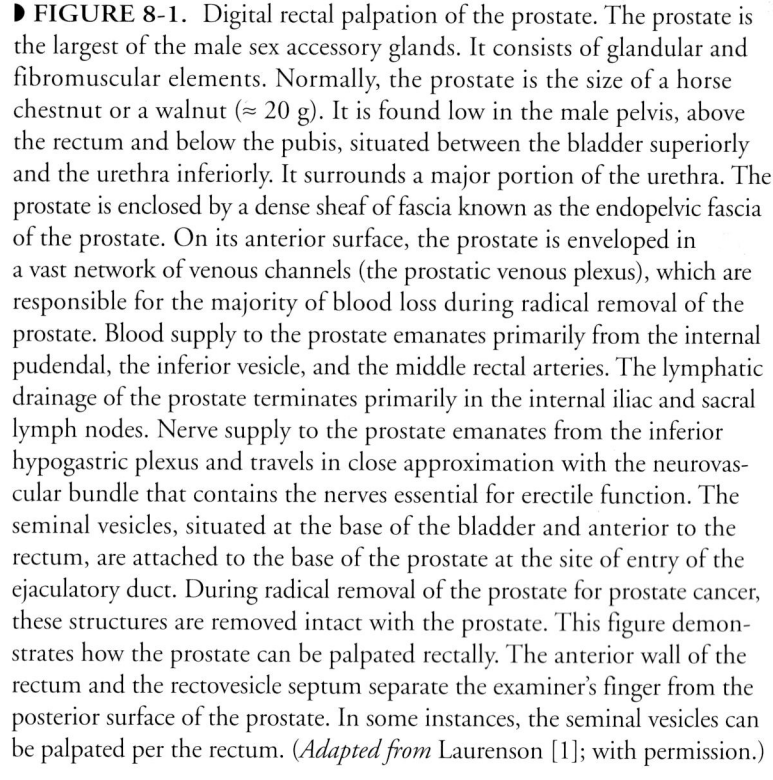

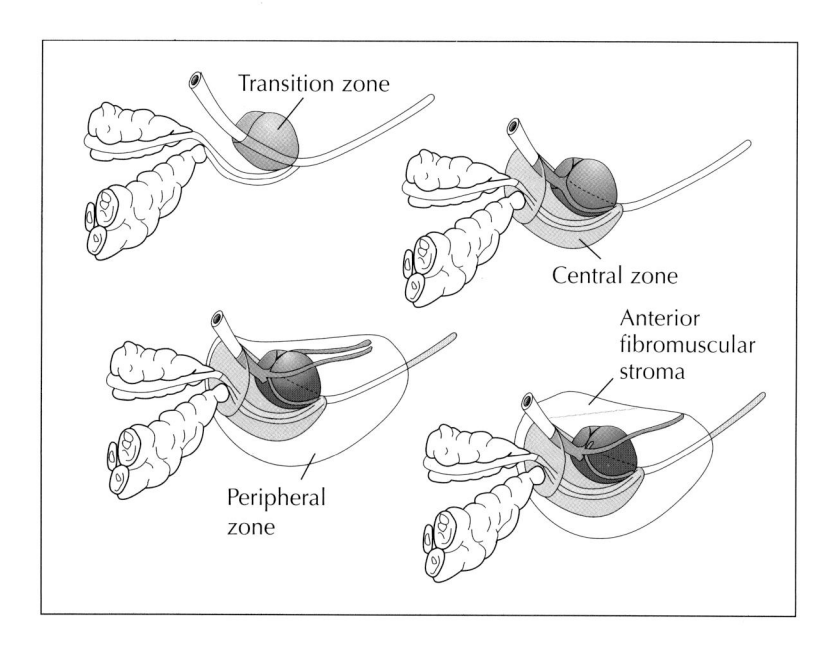

▶ **FIGURE 8-2.** Surgical anatomy. The glandular structure of the prostate can be divided into three zones. The peripheral zone (PZ) includes 70% of the glandular elements, primarily at the apical, posterior, and lateral region; the central zone surrounds the ejaculatory ducts (20% of glandular elements); and the transition zone (TZ), or site of development of benign prostatic hyperplasia, surrounds the proximal urethra (10% of glandular elements). The anterior fibromuscular stroma, a zone with few glandular elements, extends from the bladder neck (base of the prostate) to the striated urethral sphincter (apex of the prostate). Prostate cancer most often is a multifocal, bilateral, PZ disease. Most of the tumor mass in palpable (stage T2) and nonpalpable (stage T1c) prostate cancers is detected by prostate biopsy specimens taken from within the PZ. The PZ location of most prostate cancers is important clinically because 1) cancer arising away from the urethra rarely causes symptoms until it has reached an advanced stage; 2) proximity to the rectal surface allows detection of some early cancers by palpation; and 3) removal of centrally located transition zone tissue for benign prostatic enlargement does not remove the area at highest risk for development of prostate cancer. The TZ is the predominant location of the tumor in less than 20% of cases. TZ cancers are more likely than are PZ cancers of similar size to be confined because of natural barriers to extension (*eg*, urethra, anterior fibromuscular stroma, and fibrous plane between transition and peripheral zone), and, perhaps, a lower biologic potential. Common sites of extraprostatic extension for TZ cancers are the anterolateral gland and bladder neck. (*Adapted from* Greene *et al.* [2]; with permission.)

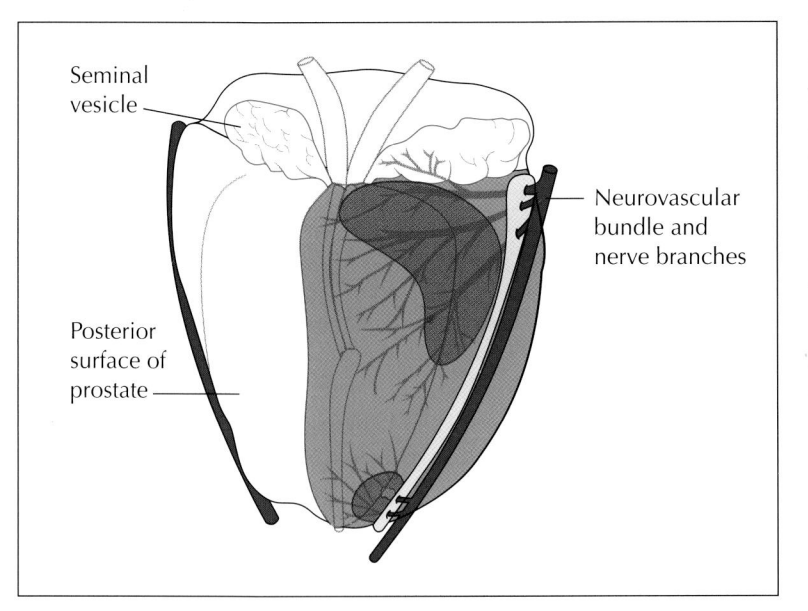

FIGURE 8-3. Posterolateral surface of the prostate gland. Branches of the neurovascular bundles (NVB) enter the prostate on the posterolateral surface. Local extension of peripheral zone (PZ) cancers most commonly occurs posteriorly and posterolaterally via invasion of the perineural space where branches of the neurovascular bundle enter the prostate. More extensive local extraprostatic extension may involve the seminal vesicles (SV) at the base of the prostate. Metastatic spread of prostate cancer most commonly affects the pelvic lymph nodes surrounding the iliac vein and within the obturator fossa, as well as the bony pelvis and lower spine. Other sites of metastatic spread, such as lung, are uncommon without the presence of lymph node and bone metastases. (*Adapted from* Stamey and McNeal [3]; with permission.)

EARLY DETECTION OF PROSTATE CANCER

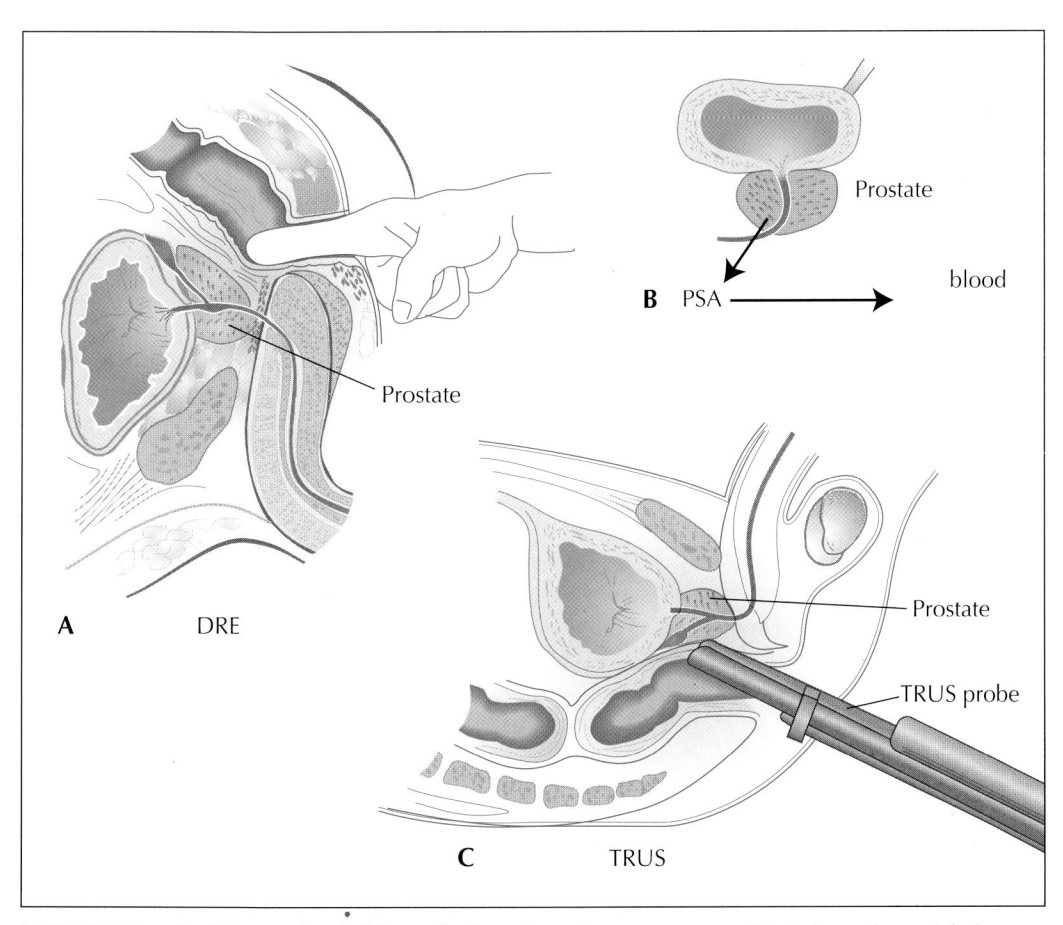

FIGURE 8-4. Diagnostic triad for early detection of prostate cancer. Digital rectal examination (DRE), measurement of the protein prostate-specific antigen (PSA) in sera, and transrectal ultrasound (TRUS)–directed prostatic biopsy comprise a diagnostic triad for early detection of prostate cancer. **A,** DRE usually is performed with the patient bent at the waist 90° over the examining table, feet spread about 2 feet apart, and knees slightly bent. The normal prostate should have the consistency of the thenar eminence of the thumb when the thumb is apposed to the little finger. Prostate cancer should be suspected when the consistency is firmer than normal, or distinct nodules are present. **B,** PSA can be detected in sera by immunoassay and most commonly is elevated in the presence of prostate disease that occurs with age. **C,** TRUS is performed, with the patient on his side, by gently inserting an ultrasound probe into the rectum. Prostate biopsies can be visually directed using a biopsy gun loaded onto the TRUS probe.

Although controversy exists regarding the benefits of early diagnosis, it has been demonstrated that an early diagnosis of prostate cancer is best achieved using a combination of DRE and PSA as first-line tests to assess the risk of prostate cancer being present. When DRE and PSA are used to detect prostate cancer, detection rates are higher with PSA alone than with DRE alone, and highest with a combination of the two tests. Because DRE and PSA do not always detect the same cancers, the tests are complementary. TRUS is not recommended as a first-line screening test because of its low predictive value for early prostate cancer and the high cost of the examination. TRUS-guided, systematic needle biopsy currently is the most reliable method to ensure accurate sampling of prostatic tissue in those men at high risk for harboring prostatic cancer based on DRE abnormalities or PSA elevations. (*Adapted from* Resnick and Older [4] and Tanagho [5]; with permission.)

Chance of Cancer on Biopsy

	PSA< 4.0 ng/mL, %	PSA> 4.0 ng/mL, %
+DRE findings	6–9	12–32
–DRE findings	10–21	42–72

▶ **FIGURE 8-5.** Chance of cancer as a function of serum prostate-specific antigen (PSA) level and findings on digital rectal examination (DRE). Men with abnormalities on DRE, or PSA elevations—regardless of DRE findings— should undergo transrectal ultrasound–guided prostatic biopsy because of the higher risk of prostate cancer. With the advent of PSA testing, the majority of prostate cancers (>60%) are detected in men with PSA elevations but no suspicion of prostate cancer on DRE. Among men with PSA elevations and nonsuspicious rectal examinations, the chance of cancer is 20% to 30% when PSA levels are below 10.0 ng/mL. Thus, most men with PSA elevations do not have cancer (*ie*, the PSA test is not specific among men without prostate cancer). This high false-positive rate among men without cancer has led to a number of approaches to decrease false-positive tests, including PSA density, PSA velocity, age-specific PSA, and percent free PSA. (*Adapted from* Carter and Partin [6].)

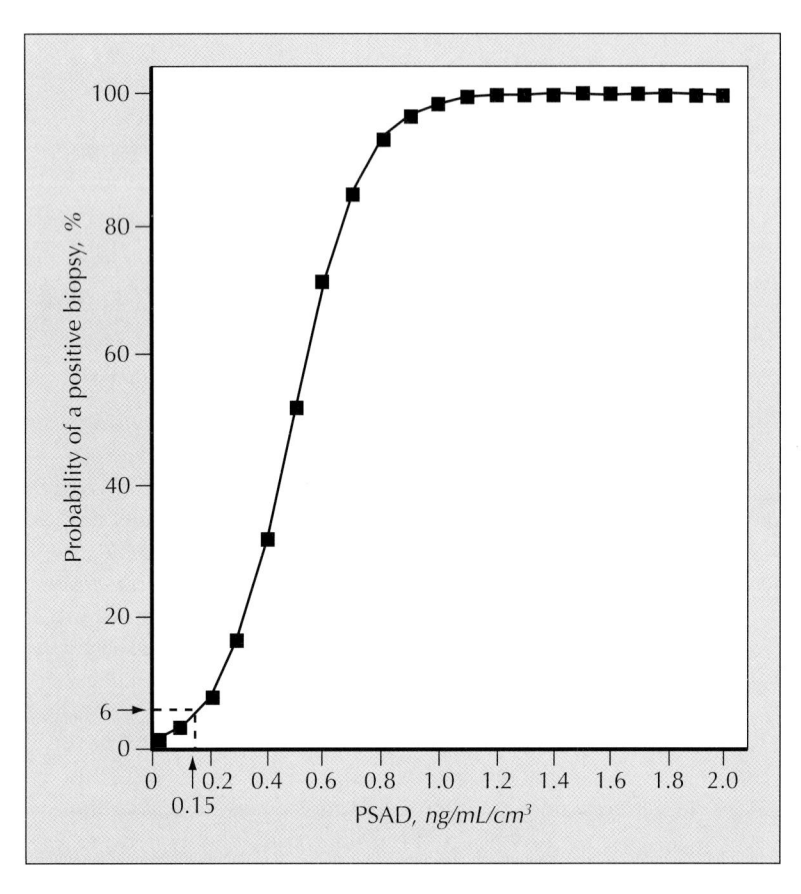

▶ **FIGURE 8-6.** Probability of a positive prostate biopsy (percent) as a function of prostate-specific antigen (PSA) density (PSAD) among men with PSA levels between 4.0 and 10.0 ng/mL.

More than 80% of men with PSA elevations have levels in the range of 4.0 to 10.0 ng/mL. The most likely reason for the elevation of PSA in these men is prostate enlargement rather than prostate cancer. Adjusting the PSA according to the ultrasound-determined prostate size by calculating the quotient of PSA and prostate volume (PSAD) is one method of distinguishing between men with PSA elevations caused by prostatic enlargement and those caused by prostate cancer. There is a direct relationship between PSAD and the chance of cancer: a PSAD of 0.15 or greater has been proposed as the threshold for recommending prostate biopsy in men with PSA levels between 4.0 and 10.0 ng/mL and no suspicion of cancer on DRE or TRUS. The major determinant of serum PSA in men without prostate cancer is the transition zone epithelium (zone of origin of benign prostatic hyperplasia [BPH]). Because BPH represents an enlargement of the transition zone, and serum PSA levels are primarily a reflection of transition zone histology in men with BPH, adjusting PSA for transition zone volume may help distinguish between BPH and prostate cancer. Although PSAD is an imperfect predictor of cancer, it is an additional method of risk assessment that is potentially useful for counseling men with intermediate PSA levels (4.0 to 10.0 ng/mL) regarding their need for prostate biopsy. (*Adapted from* Beduschi and Oesterling [7].)

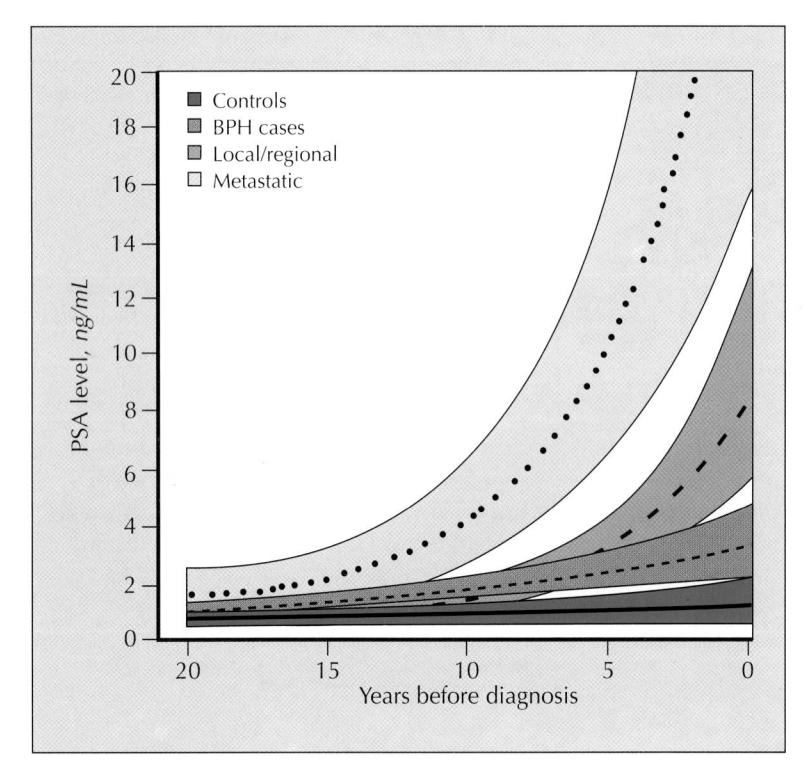

▶ **FIGURE 8-7.** Average prostate-specific antigen (PSA) levels (95% CI) for men with and without prostate cancer. The rate of rise in PSA (PSA velocity) is greater in men with prostate cancer than men without prostate cancer. Substantial changes or variability in serum PSA (10% to 20%) can occur between measurements in the presence or absence of prostate cancer. The short-term changes in PSA between repeated measurements are primarily caused by physiologic variation. Changes in serum PSA between measurements can be adjusted (corrected) for the elapsed time between the measurements, a concept known as PSA velocity or rate of change in PSA. In one study, when three PSA measurements were used to calculate PSA velocity over a 2-year period, 5% of men without prostate cancer had a rate of change in PSA of more than 0.75 ng/mL per year, whereas 70% of men with cancer had a rate of change in PSA more than 0.75 ng/mL per year. In a large prospective screening study, the cancer detection rate was 47% among men with a PSA velocity more than 0.75 ng/mL per year, compared with 11% among men with a PSA velocity less than 0.75 ng/mL per year. Separate studies have calculated the minimal length of follow-up time over which changes in PSA should be adjusted for PSA velocity to be useful in cancer detection to be approximately 18 months. Evaluation of three repeated PSA measurements to determine an average rate of change in PSA optimizes the accuracy of PSA velocity for cancer detection. (*From* Carter *et al.* [8]; with permission.)

	Based on 95% Specificity*		Based on 95% Sensitivity†	
Age Decade	White [9]	Black [10]	White [10]	Black [10]
40	0–2.5	0–2.4	0–2.5	0–2.0
50	0–3.5	0–6.5	0–3.5	0–4.0
60	0–4.5	0–11.3	0–3.5	0–4.5
70	0–6.5	0–12.5	0–3.5	0–5.5

"Normal" PSA Ranges (ng/mL) Among White and Black Men in the United States

*Upper limit of normal PSA determined from 95% percentile of PSA among men without prostate cancer.
†Upper limit of normal PSA required to maintain 95% sensitivity for cancer detection.

▶ **FIGURE 8-8.** Age- and race-specific prostate-specific antigen (PSA) levels. The 95th percentile of PSA levels seen in men without prostate cancer (95% specificity) and the PSA range required to maintain the detection of 95% of prostate cancers (95% sensitivity) have been used to establish "normal" age-specific reference ranges among black and white men. PSA increases with age, primarily because of increases in prostate size, and age-adjustment of PSA are ways of accounting for this size increase with age. It has been suggested that use of an age-adjusted PSA rather than a single PSA cutoff for all ages may lead to increased cancer detection in younger men more likely to benefit from treatment and minimize unnecessary evaluations in older men who are less likely to benefit from treatment. It has been shown that PSA levels are higher in black men without prostate cancer than in white men without prostate cancer of the same age. It has not definitely been shown, however, that use of age- or race-specific reference ranges has an advantage in detecting curable cancer over the use of a single cut-point of 4.0 ng/mL. Currently, the data suggest that a cut-point of 4.0 ng/mL—using the Tandem assay (Hybritech, San Diego, CA)—is an effective threshold for maximizing prostate cancer detection and minimizing unnecessary biopsies in men between the ages of 50 and 70 years. The optimal PSA threshold, *ie*, the cutoff that will result in detection of clinically significant cancers in those men who are most likely to benefit from treatment, is not known. For younger men, a greater index of suspicion is warranted at PSA levels below 4.0 ng/mL because the relative risk of cancer is increased even at PSA levels between 2.0 and 4.0 ng/mL: these men have the most to gain from early diagnosis and treatment of prostate cancer. A greater suspicion of prostate cancer at lower PSA levels is especially important in the setting of known risk factors of family history and black race. The use of higher PSA thresholds among older men, who are less likely to benefit from prostate cancer treatment, should take into consideration the overall health and life expectancy of the individual.

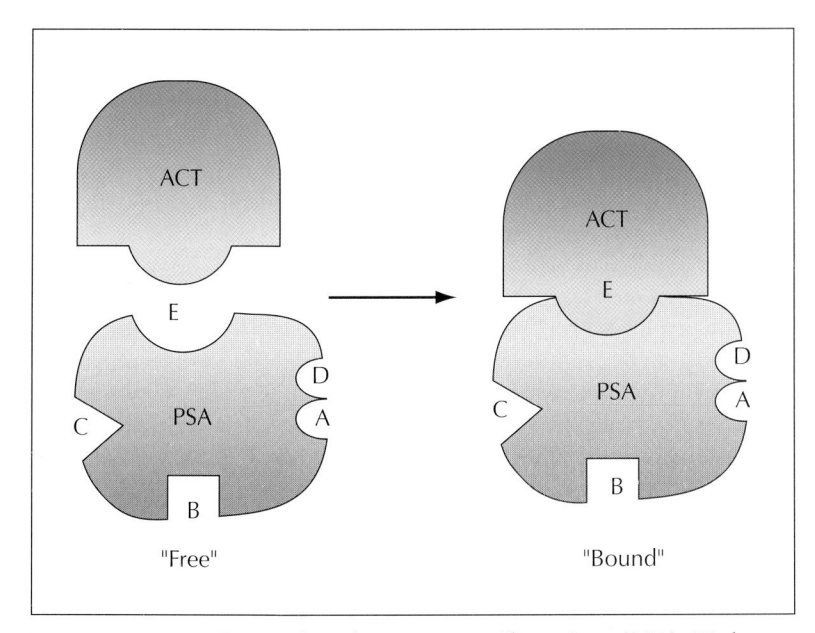

▶ **FIGURE 8-9.** Free and total prostate-specific antigen (PSA). Little controversy exists regarding the clinical utility of serum PSA measurements for detection, staging, and monitoring of men with prostate cancer. However, total serum PSA levels between 4.0 and 10.0 ng/mL (the diagnostic "gray zone") have led physicians to perform biopsies of nearly all their patients with prostate cancer in an attempt to identify the 25% who ultimately will harbor malignancy and potentially require therapy. The goal of any modification to the total PSA test is to maintain its sensitivity for cancer detection as close to 100% as possible while improving specificity. The recently introduced modification to the standard total PSA test, percent *free* PSA, may provide the best means of distinguishing prostate cancer from benign prostatic conditions within this diagnostic gray zone. The free form of PSA represents an enzymatically inactive nonprotein-bound form of PSA that ranges anywhere from 5% to 50% of total measured PSA. The complexed form of PSA, PSA-α_1-antichymotrypsin (ACT), represents an enzymatically inactive form of PSA that is irreversibly bound to an endogenous protease inhibitor. PSA-ACT can be found in concentrations ranging from 50% to 90% of total measured PSA. Several investigations have demonstrated that percent-free PSA best distinguishes prostate cancer from other benign prostatic conditions in men who have serum PSA levels between 4.0 and 10.0 ng/mL. Data from a multi-institutional prospective trial have demonstrated that using the Hybritech percent-free PSA assay and a cut-off of 25% free PSA, 95% of prostate cancers are still detected and 20% of unnecessary biopsies are avoided. Considering this, it is important to note that the new assays designed by various manufacturers have been demonstrated to perform differently. When using this new test, investigators should discuss with their reference laboratories the recommended criteria for sample collection, storage conditions, and shipping, as well as the recommended cut-offs of and the clinical trials supporting the data for the assay being used. Percent-free PSA may improve our diagnostic armamentarium for decision-making in men who have normal digital rectal examination findings but elevated serum total PSA. The best use of this assay at present is in determining the need for repeat biopsies among men who fit these criteria and have had at least one previous negative biopsy. (*Modified from* Partin [11]; with permission.)

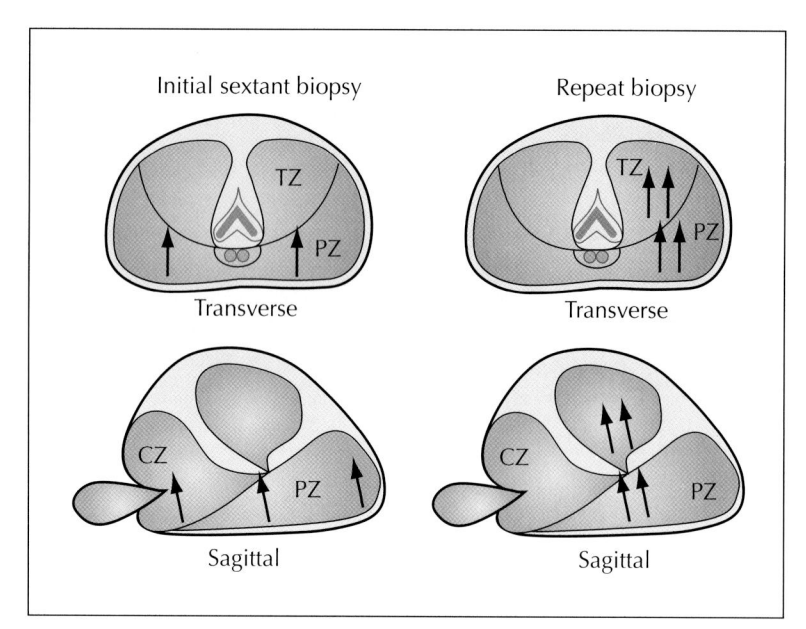

FIGURE 8-10. Use of transrectal ultrasound for diagnosis of prostate cancer. The diagnosis of prostate cancer is made solely through histologic examination of prostate tissue. Isolation and identification of adenocarcinoma from histologic tissue is possible only through biopsy techniques. Recently, advances in the knowledge of prostate-specific antigen and ultrasound technology have made it easier to identify men who have prostate cancer. The history of prostate biopsy dates back to the early 1930s, when transperineal, digitally guided biopsies first were performed. Between the 1960s and 1980s, aspiration techniques with very fine needles were popularized in Europe; these never gained popularity in the United States, however. In the early 1980s, advances in ultrasound technology and the development of a transrectal ultrasound probe made imaging and biopsy access to the prostate from a transrectal approach possible. Sextant, or systematic, biopsies were first introduced in the late 1980s and have become the gold standard method for obtaining prostate tissue for diagnostic purposes. Stamey *et al.* from Stanford University were the first to carefully describe the methodology and rationale behind the use of sextant biopsies for diagnosis of prostate cancer. To perform transrectal ultrasound-guided biopsies of the prostate, it is essential to understand the zonal anatomy of the prostate (transition and peripheral zones). Performance of ultrasound-guided biopsy should proceed according to an established routine to maximize the likelihood of identifying any malignancy that may be present. A preliminary diagnostic scan should be performed to allow calculation of prostate size and indicate the presence of ultrasound abnormalities that may guide directed biopsies following the sextant biopsy procedure. Biopsy specimens of all palpable lesions and specific lesions suspicious on ultrasound should be obtained as well as the collection of guided sextant biopsy material. Transition zone biopsies are not performed routinely, but they often are recommended when a patient has had a previous histologically negative biopsy but has a persistent elevation of PSA (4.0 to 10.0 ng/mL). Biopsy of the transition zone has been associated with increased pain; additionally the diagnostic yield of transition zone biopsies does not support the routine use of this technique on initial biopsy of the prostate. (*Adapted from* Terris *et al.* [12]; with permission.)

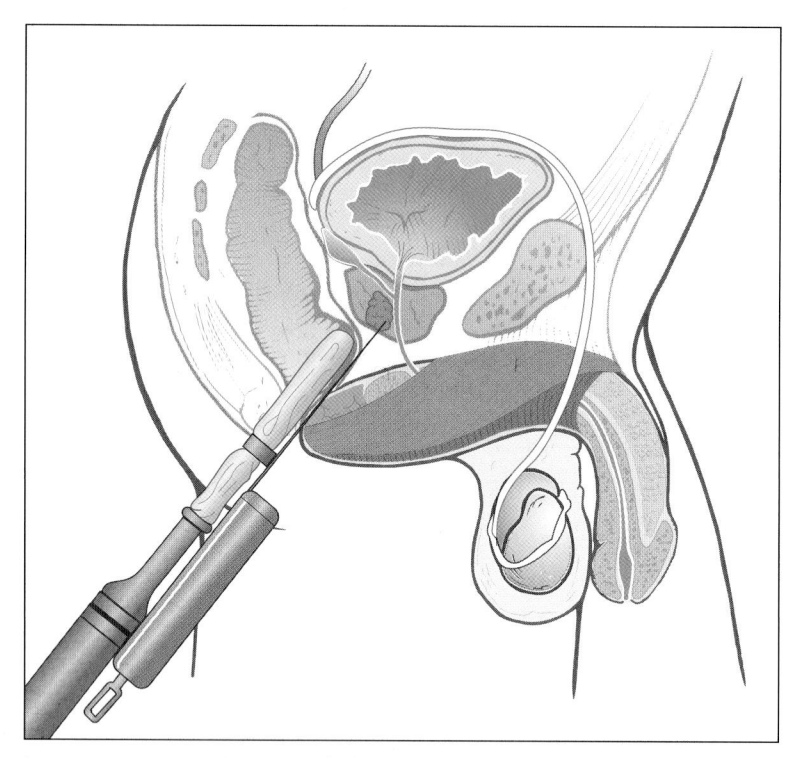

FIGURE 8-11. Transrectal ultrasound for early detection. When prostate cancer is suspected because of an elevated prostate-specific antigen (PSA) level or an abnormal digital rectal examination, histologic confirmation of adenocarcinoma of the prostate is essential before treatment decisions are made. The volume, location, and grade of tumor are the most critical issues involved in the decision to undergo definitive therapy, the choice of type of definitive therapy, and the urgency with which therapy should be delivered. Since transrectal ultrasound-guided biopsy was introduced, a number of different biopsy techniques have been used. The currently recommended method for biopsy of the prostate from the transrectal approach is to perform a sextant biopsy of palpable lesions. Various parameters can be determined from the transrectal ultrasound imaging: 1) the volume of the prostate (essential in calculating PSA density); 2) the degree of differentiation between the peripheral and central zones of the prostate; 3) the presence of abnormalities along the posterior border of the prostatic capsule and the lateral edges of the prostate suggestive of extensive capsular penetration; 4) asymmetry in the size and shape of the prostate gland; and 5) echo texture patterns within the prostatic tissue itself. Many prostate cancers demonstrate a hypoechoic feature when analyzed with TRUS. Unfortunately, because nearly 75% of prostate cancers originate within the peripheral zone of the prostate, which itself is hypoechoic in nature, use of this technique for location by hypoechoic nature is significantly limited. The use of color Doppler transrectal ultrasound coupled with enhancing agents for identifying vascular structures has increased the ability to characterize inflammatory, normal, and cancerous tissue within the prostate. Assessment of the volume of cancer, location of tumor, and histologic grade are necessary before treatment planning begins. Transrectal ultrasound plays a major role in this assessment. (*Adapted from* Kirby *et al.* [13]; with permission.)

II. The Prostate

STAGING OF PROSTATE CANCER

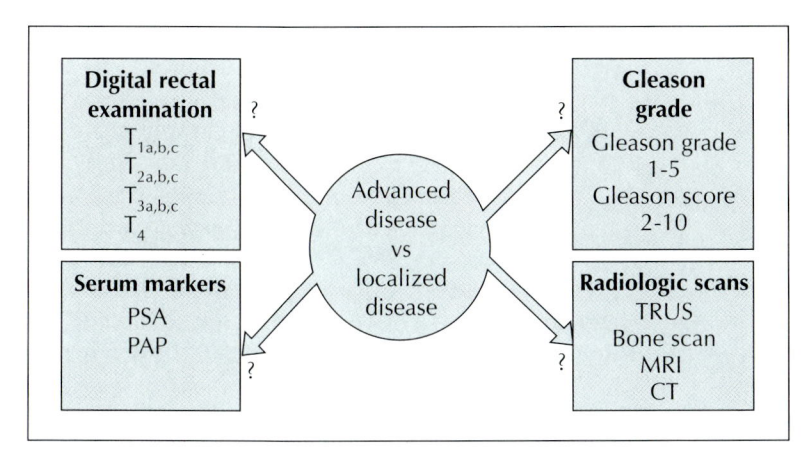

FIGURE 8-12. General concepts in the staging of prostate cancer. Decisions regarding the appropriate treatment modality for patients diagnosed with apparently clinically localized (curable) prostatic adenocarcinoma often are highly individualized. These decisions are based on the experience and opinions of the physician as well as the knowledge and the concerns of the patient. Educated decisions regarding the management of clinically localized prostate cancer also should be based on accurate and interpretable prognostic information. The most common modalities currently used by clinicians as prognostic markers for prostate cancer are digital rectal examination (DRE), histologic tumor grade (Gleason score), serum markers such as prostate-specific antigen (PSA) and prostatic acid phosphatase (PAP), and other radiologic studies such as transrectal ultrasound (TRUS), bone scan, magnetic resonance imaging (MRI), and computed tomography (CT). Although most of these clinical staging modalities are widely used, no single modality is either sufficiently sensitive or sufficiently specific to stand alone as the "ideal" prognostic marker for prostate cancer. (*Adapted from* Partin [14]; with permission.)

Prostate Cancer Clinical Staging Systems

TNM Stage	Description	Whitmore-Jewett Stage	Description
T1a	Nonpalpable, with ≤ 5% of resected tissue with cancer, not high grade	A1	Same as TNM
T1b	Nonpalpable, with > 5% of resected tissue with cancer and/or high grade	A2	Same as TNM
T2a	Palpable, half of a lobe or less	B1N	Palpable, < one lobe surrounded by normal tissue
		B1	Palpable, < one lobe
T2b	Palpable, > half of one lobe but not both lobes	B1	Palpable, < one lobe
		B2	Palpable, one entire lobe or more
T2c	Palpable, involves both lobes	B2	Palpable, one entire lobe or more
T3a	Palpable, unilateral capsular penetration	C1	Palpable, outside capsule, not into seminal vesicles
T3b	Bilateral capsular penetration	C1	Same as TNM
T3c	Tumor invades seminal vesicles	C2	Same as TNM
T4	Tumor invades other structures (eg, bladder neck, levator muscle, or sphincter)	C2	Same as TNM

FIGURE 8-13. Prostate cancer clinical staging systems. Clinical staging for prostate cancer requires making an accurate assessment of the extent of disease spread, which can be determined through digital rectal examination (DRE), serum tumor markers, histologic grade, and various imaging modalities. The determination of the local extent of disease (T stage) is performed primarily through digital rectal examination. This table presents a description of the digital rectal findings for various T stages, and also characterizes clinical staging of prostate cancer in an older, ABCD (Whitmore-Jewett) classification system. Pathologic stage, a more accurate representation of the extent of disease, can be described only following histologic examination of the surgical material removed at the time of radical prostatectomy. Although pathologic stage is more useful than is clinical staging in the prediction of prognosis, it cannot be determined with presurgical information. Thus, this currently accepted TNM clinical staging system for prostate cancer has been used to subcategorize patients based on their likelihood of disease spread prior to definitive therapy. (*Adapted from* Carter and Partin [6].)

Clinical Aspects of Prostate Cancer

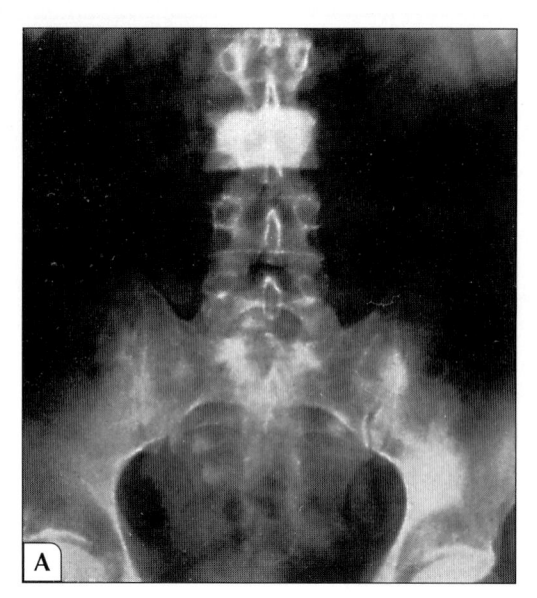

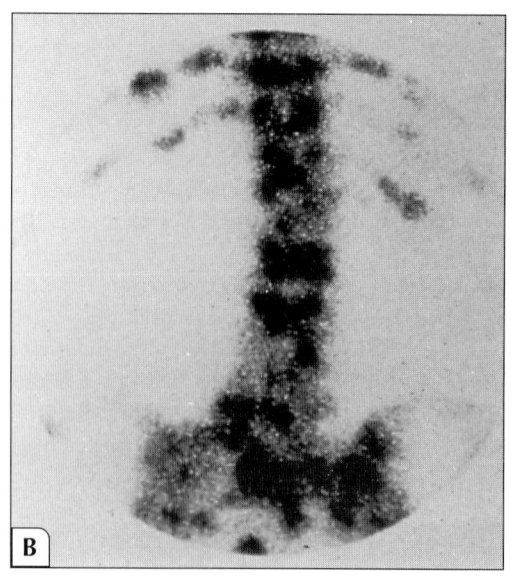

FIGURE 8-14. Bone scan for staging of prostate cancer. **A,** Plain film. **B,** Bone scan. Accurate prediction of extraprostatic disease spread before therapeutic decision making is fundamental to prediction of prognosis and staging. Accurate radiographic information that supports the presence or absence of extraprostatic disease provides the basis for making major decisions regarding therapeutic options. The radionuclide bone scan is widely used for detecting distant bony metastases in men with newly diagnosed prostate cancer before therapy. However, opinions regarding its application vary widely. Recent studies suggest that bone scans can be omitted in patients with serum prostate-specific antigen (PSA) levels less than 10 ng/mL. Other authorities continue to recommend bone scans, even in patients with low to normal PSA values because these data provide a baseline should the patient require further bone scan studies following a treatment failure. It must be recognized, however, that although the sensitivity of a bone scan is high, the specificity is extremely poor. In addition, data using PSA as part of the staging evaluation for men with newly diagnosed prostate cancer suggest that the radionuclide bone scan may not be cost-effective. (*Adapted from* ICI Pharmaceutical [15]; with permission.)

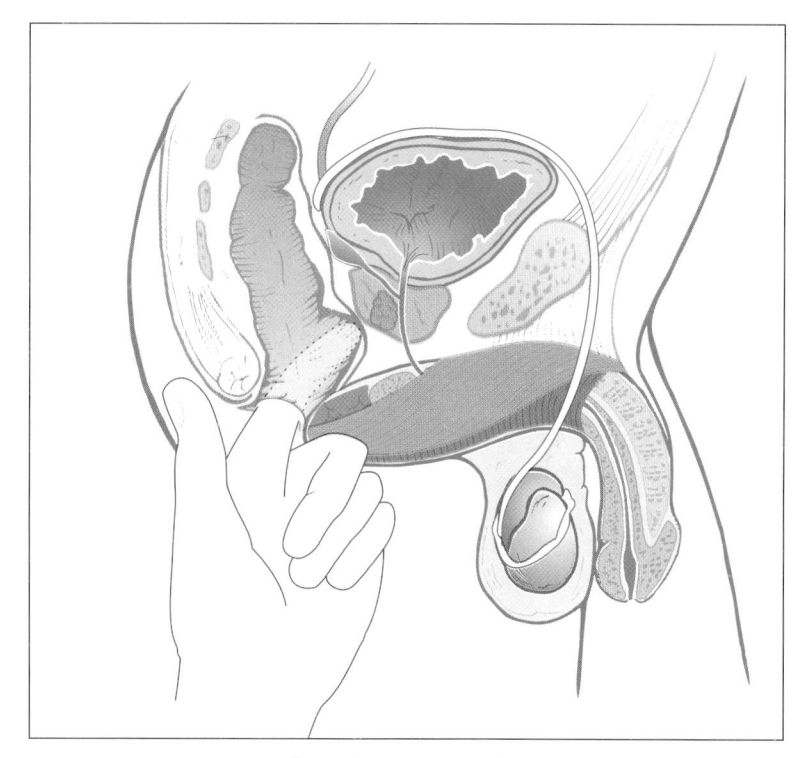

FIGURE 8-15. Digital rectal examination (DRE). DRE was the "gold standard" for detection and determination of prognosis of prostate cancer long before the development of modern urologic practice. Performing a DRE as part of a routine physical examination has become a common practice among general practitioners in recent years, partly as a result of increased public awareness of prostatic disease. Although DRE is cost-effective and generally is accepted by the public as a standard of care for routine prostate examination, the palpability of a prostate cancer depends on its location and the volume of the tumor. Tumors infiltrating centrally or basally located tumors are difficult to palpate, whereas larger peripheral or apical tumors are relatively easy to palpate. Thus, even when DRE is performed by a highly experienced physician, the positive biopsy rate per suspicious DRE is poor, reaching only 40% in large screening studies. However, DRE is currently strongly recommended for the initial detection of prostate cancer and is likely to remain so. Large tumor volume and the presence of palpable disease outside the prostate are poor prognostic signs. Jewett [16] was the first to subclassify prostate cancers according to the local extent of the tumor as determined by the DRE. Because of the subjective nature of the DRE, both understaging and overstaging have been demonstrated when the pathologic extent of the disease following prostatectomy has been correlated with the DRE findings. Within one large series of 565 men in whom DRE suggested organ-confined disease (clinical stage T2), only 52% actually demonstrated organ-confined disease, whereas 31% demonstrated capsular penetration, and the remaining 17% had either invasion of the seminal vesicles or pelvic lymph node involvement. Within that same series, of 36 men in whom extraprostatic disease was suspected on DRE (clinical stage T3a), seven (19%) in fact had organ-confined disease on final pathologic analysis. This represents a sensitivity of 52% and a specificity of 81% for prediction of organ-confined status by DRE alone. (*Adapted from* Kirby *et al.* [13].)

Serum Markers as Predictors of Prognosis

Prostate-specific, *not* prostate cancer–specific
Produced by prostate epithelial cells (luminal)
Increased serum PSA indicates prostatic disease
Interpretation of PSA elevation limited
Not normally accurate for staging or prognosis prediction

FIGURE 8-16. Serum prostate-specific antigen (PSA) for clinical staging of prostate cancer. PSA is a serine protease made exclusively by prostatic luminal epithelial cells, both normal and cancerous. The major role of PSA is to liquefy the seminal coagulum. In certain prostatic disease states, PSA can "leak" into the intravascular spaces and its presence can be detected in the serum. The use of PSA as a prognostic marker has been limited secondary to the fact that it is produced in higher-than-normal amounts by the prostates of men with benign prostatic hyperplasic (BPH) as well as by men with prostatic adenocarcinoma. Serum PSA levels in men with prostate cancer ultimately depend on prostate volume, tumor volume, and the degree of tumor differentiation. Tumors of higher grade often are associated with levels of PSA production lower than expected. In general, a pretreatment PSA level greater than 100 ng/mL represents advanced disease and is associated with a poor prognosis. By contrast, serum PSA levels lower than normal (< 4.0 ng/mL) are often associated with less aggressive tumors. Most men with prostate cancer (> 75%) present with serum PSA levels between these two extreme values. Within this range, the serum PSA level alone, although directly correlating with disease extent, is by no means an accurate method for staging prostate cancer.

The contribution of BPH to overall serum PSA has been estimated to be from 0.15 to 0.3 ng/mL per gram of BPH tissue. An accurate assessment of the BPH contribution to overall serum PSA level currently is not possible for an individual patient because 1) the epithelial component of BPH is the major source of PSA; 2) BPH tissue contains variable amounts of epithelium and stroma; and 3) no minimally or noninvasive methods currently are available to distinguish between epithelium and stroma within BPH tissue. Another confounding factor demonstrated by Partin suggests that men with prostate cancer presenting at a more advanced stage and higher grade have higher volume tumors, which produce less PSA per gram of epithelial cells. (*Adapted from* Partin [14]; with permission.)

Prediction of Pathologic Stage by Imaging Techniques

Technique	Sensitivity, %	Specificity, %
Extracapsular penetration		
TRUS	(50–89)	(50–94)
CT	(35–75)	(60–73)
MRI	(35–77)	(57–88)
Seminal vesicle involvement		
TRUS	(20–100)	(85–100)
CT	(33–36)	(60–96)
MRI	(50–83)	(88–97)
Pelvic lymph nodal involvement		
CT	(0–100)	(86–96)
MRI	(44–69)	(95–100)

FIGURE 8-17. Prediction of pathologic stage by imaging techniques. Imaging techniques, including transrectal ultrasound (TRUS), CT, and magnetic resonance imaging (MRI), both body and endorectal, have proved to be disappointing as pretherapy predictors of pathologic stage. TRUS and MRI are useful mainly in determining the local extent of prostate cancer. Pelvic imaging with either CT or MRI for the detection of lymph node metastasis has not been routinely useful secondary to low sensitivity. (*Adapted from* Gishman and deVere White [17]; with permission.)

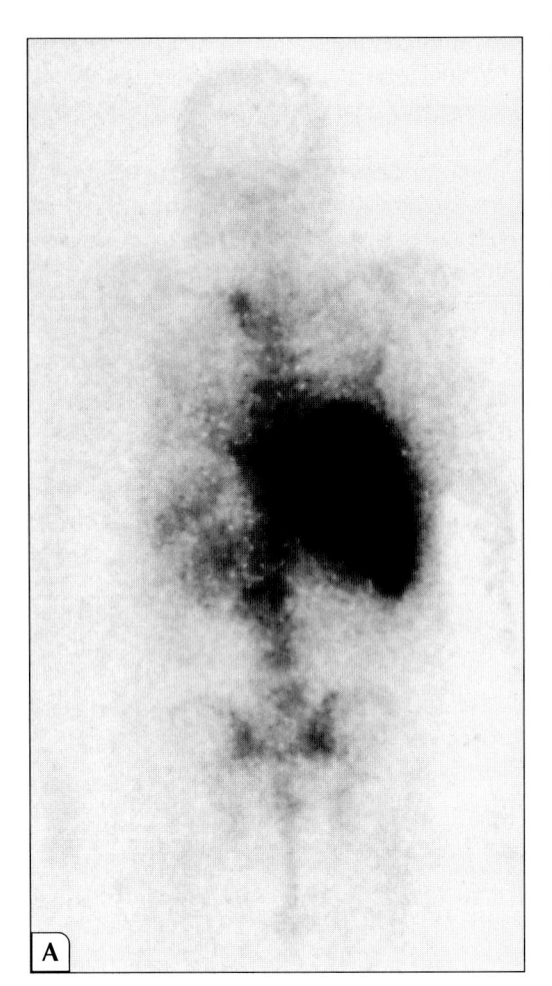

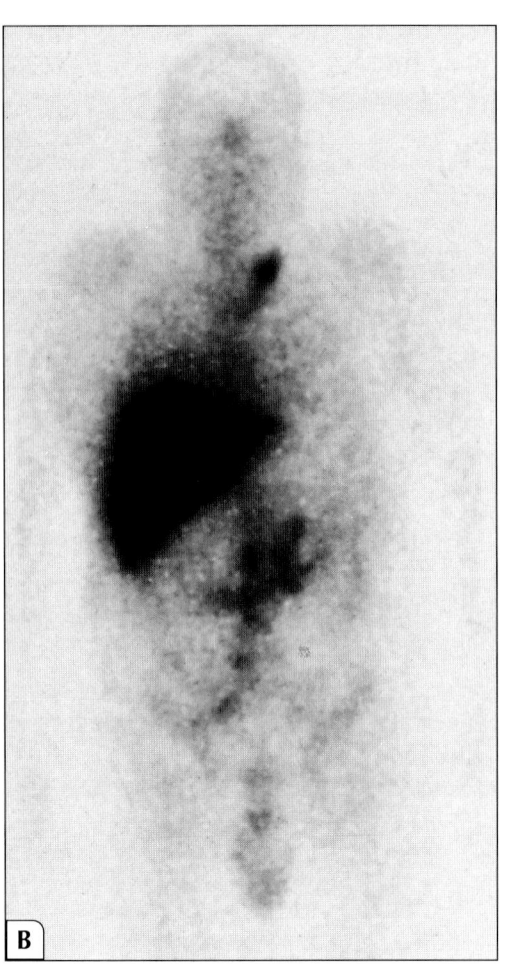

▶ **FIGURE 8-18.** Immunoscintigraphy (ProstaScint; Cytogen Corp., Princeton, NJ). **A,** Immediate posterior day-1 scan. **B,** Delayed anterior day-4 scan. These ProctaScint images demonstrate abdominal soft tissue prostate cancer metastasis. ProctaScint recently was approved as a diagnostic imaging agent for patients with newly diagnosed, clinically localized prostate cancer who are at high risk for pelvic and abdominal lymph node metastases. This radiolabeled monoclonal antibody targets a membrane-associated antigen on prostate cells (prostate-specific membrane antigen [PSMA]). PSMA is more highly expressed in malignant than in nonmalignant prostate cells. PSMA also appears to be more highly expressed in metastatic soft tissue lesions than in primary prostate cancers. Preliminary data suggest that immunoscintigraphy with ProctaScint might be used to identify possible sites of disease metastases both before therapy in patients with relatively high risk for nodal involvement and in patients with biochemical evidence (detectable PSA levels) of recurrent or residual disease following prostatectomy. Preliminary data presented to the Food and Drug Administration demonstrated that ProctaScint provided a sensitivity of 62% and a specificity of 72%. In the same group of patients, CT was less accurate in detecting soft tissue metastases. The ProctaScint scan has been useful in documenting the presence of soft tissue metastases beyond the pelvis that are not amenable to adjuvant pelvic radiation therapy. Recent data also have demonstrated that modifications to radiation fields in the presence of pelvic recurrence based on the findings of the ProctaScint scan has provided some improved benefit. Preliminary data have demonstrated that use of clinical, pathologic, and ProctaScint imaging information can improve the prediction of local recurrence versus distant metastases and help in rational decision making with respect to adjuvant therapy for recurrent or occult metastatic prostate cancer. (Courtesy of M. Haseman, MD.)

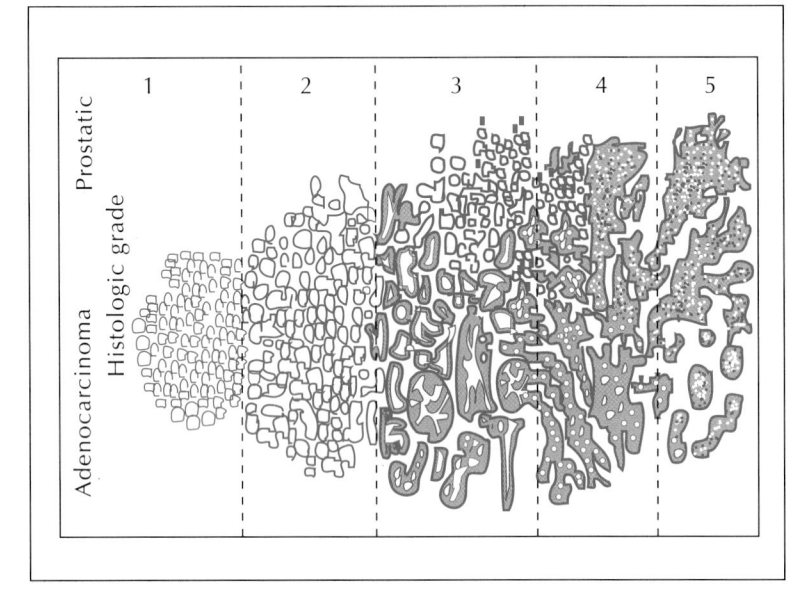

▶ **FIGURE 8-19.** Gleason grading system. In the 1960s, as part of a pathologic analysis of prostate cancer specimens collected during the Veterans Administration Cooperative Urologic Research Group studies, Gleason introduced a prostate cancer grading system based on low-magnification microscopic assessment of glandular patterns of prostate tissue. A Gleason grade from 1 to 5 is assigned to the primary tumor pattern and also to the secondary tumor pattern based on the degree of disorder of the tissue. A Gleason score is obtained by combining these numbers. Thus, a patient with a diagnosis of prostate cancer may have a Gleason score of between 2 and 10. For example, a patient with a large amount of grade 2 tumor and a small amount of grade 3 tumor will have a Gleason score of 2 + 3 = 5, whereas a patient with a large amount of grade 4 tumor and a small amount of grade 3 tumor will have a Gleason score of 4 + 3 = 7. When only one tumor pattern is evident, the grade is doubled to give the score. Based on current practice, the correlation between Gleason score and prognosis is accurate for specific populations. Men with Gleason scores on the outer edges of the range (*ie*, 2 to 4 or 8 to 10), who constitute only 20% of the total population, demonstrate a marked correlation between Gleason score and prognosis. Unfortunately, most men (> 75%) demonstrate Gleason scores of 5 to 7. For this group of men, the correlation between grade and prognosis is very poor. We conclude that Gleason score alone has prognostic value; however, for men with Gleason scores of 5 to 7, it has provided little or poor prognostic information. Improvements in our methods for histologic grading system are desperately needed. (*Adapted from* Gleason [18]; with permission.)

II. The Prostate

Nomogram for Prediction of Final Pathologic Stage

	PSA 0.0–4.0 ng/mL Clinical Stage							PSA 4.1–10.0 ng/mL Clinical Stage						
Gleason Score	T1a	T1b	T1c	T2a	T2b	T2c	T3a	T1a	T1b	T1c	T2a	T2b	T2c	T3a
Organ-Confined Disease														
2–4	90	80	89	81	72	77	—	84	70	83	71	61	66	43
5	82	66	81	68	57	62	40	72	53	71	55	43	49	27
6	78	61	78	64	52	57	35	67	47	67	51	38	43	23
7	—	43	63	47	34	38	19	49	29	49	33	22	25	11
8–10	—	31	52	36	24	27	—	35	18	37	23	14	15	6
Established Capsular Penetration														
2–4	9	19	10	18	25	21	—	14	27	15	26	35	29	44
5	17	32	18	30	40	34	51	25	42	27	41	50	43	57
6	19	35	21	34	43	37	53	27	44	30	44	52	46	57
7	—	44	31	45	51	45	52	36	48	40	52	54	48	48
8–10	—	43	34	47	48	42	—	34	42	40	49	46	40	34
Seminal Vesicle Involvement														
2–4	0	1	1	1	2	2	—	1	2	1	2	4	5	10
5	1	2	1	2	3	3	7	2	3	2	3	5	6	12
6	1	2	1	2	3	4	7	2	3	2	3	5	6	11
7	—	6	4	6	10	12	19	6	9	8	10	15	18	26
8–10	—	11	9	12	17	21	—	10	15	15	19	24	28	35
Lymph Node Involvement														
2–4	0	0	0	0	0	0	—	0	1	0	0	1	1	1
5	0	1	0	0	1	1	2	1	2	0	1	2	2	3
6	1	2	0	1	2	2	5	3	5	1	2	4	4	9
7	—	6	1	2	5	5	9	8	12	3	4	9	9	15
8–10	—	14	4	5	10	10	—	18	23	8	9	16	17	24

(Table continued on next page)

▶ **FIGURE 8-20.** Nomograms to predict pathologic stage. The prognostic value of any clinical marker used to predict pathologic stage is limited for the individual patient with prostate cancer when used alone. Staging accuracy for prostate cancer can be significantly enhanced through combinations of these markers. Partin *et al.* [19], in a multi-institutional study combining more than 4000 patients from The Johns Hopkins Medical Institutions, the Baylor College of Medicine, and the University of Michigan combined clinical staging (TNM stage), serum prostate-specific antigen (PSA) level, and Gleason histologic score from prostate biopsy specimens to develop nomograms to allow patients and their treating physicians to assess the probability of pathologic stage from preclinical variables. The numbers within the nomograms represent the percent probability of having a given pathologic stage based on logistic regression analyses for all three variables combined (95% CIs were provided within the original publication). This information has been very useful in counseling men with newly diagnosed prostate cancer about treatment alternatives and the probability of complete eradication of tumor. For example, a man with a serum PSA level of 3.0 ng/mL who has a clinical stage T2a cancer with a Gleason score of 5 has a 68% chance of having organ-confined disease, whereas a man with a serum PSA of 15 ng/mL with a clinical stage T2a cancer and a Gleason score of 8 has only a 14% chance of having organ-confined disease. This type of nomogram may help patients and physicians make more informed decisions based on the probability of a pathologic stage. An individual's risk tolerance and the values placed on various potential outcomes will then be used to guide treatment decisions. Use of these nomograms may aid in rational selection of patients to undergo definitive therapy for clinically localized prostate cancer with the hope of improving the percentage of cancers found to be organ-confined and, potentially, cured with definitive therapy alone. (*Adapted from* Partin *et al.* [19] and TAP Pharmaceuticals [20]; with permission.)

(Continued on next page)

Nomogram for Prediction of Final Pathologic Stage (Continued)

	PSA 10.1–20.0 ng/mL Clinical Stage							PSA >20.0 ng/mL Clinical Stage						
Gleason Score	T1a	T1b	T1c	T2a	T2b	T2c	T3a	T1a	T1b	T1c	T2a	T2b	T2c	T3a
Organ-Confined Disease														
2–4	76	58	75	60	48	53	—	—	38	58	41	29	—	—
5	61	40	60	43	32	36	18	—	23	40	26	17	19	8
6	—	33	55	38	26	31	14	—	17	35	22	13	15	6
7	33	17	35	22	13	15	6	—	—	18	10	5	6	2
8–10	—	9	23	14	7	8	3	—	3	10	5	3	3	1
Established Capsular Penetration														
2–4	20	36	22	35	43	37	—	—	47	34	48	52	—	—
5	33	50	35	50	57	51	59	—	57	48	60	61	55	54
6	—	49	38	52	57	50	54	—	51	49	60	57	51	46
7	38	46	45	55	51	45	40	—	—	46	51	43	37	2
8–10	—	33	40	46	38	33	26	—	24	34	37	28	23	17
Seminal Vesicle Involvement														
2–4	2	4	2	4	7	8	—	—	9	7	10	14	—	—
5	3	5	3	5	8	9	15	—	10	9	11	15	19	26
6	—	4	4	5	7	9	14	—	8	8	10	13	17	21
7	8	11	12	14	18	22	28	—	—	22	24	27	32	36
8–10	—	15	20	22	25	30	34	—	20	31	33	33	38	40
Lymph Node Involvement														
2–4	0	2	0	1	1	1	—	—	4	1	1	3	—	—
5	3	5	1	2	4	4	7	—	10	3	3	7	7	11
6	—	13	3	4	10	10	18	—	23	7	8	16	17	26
7	18	24	8	9	17	18	26	—	—	14	14	25	25	32
8–10	—	40	16	17	29	29	37	—	51	24	24	36	35	42

▶ **FIGURE 8-20. *continued*** Nomograms to predict pathologic stage.

PATHOLOGIC CONSIDERATIONS

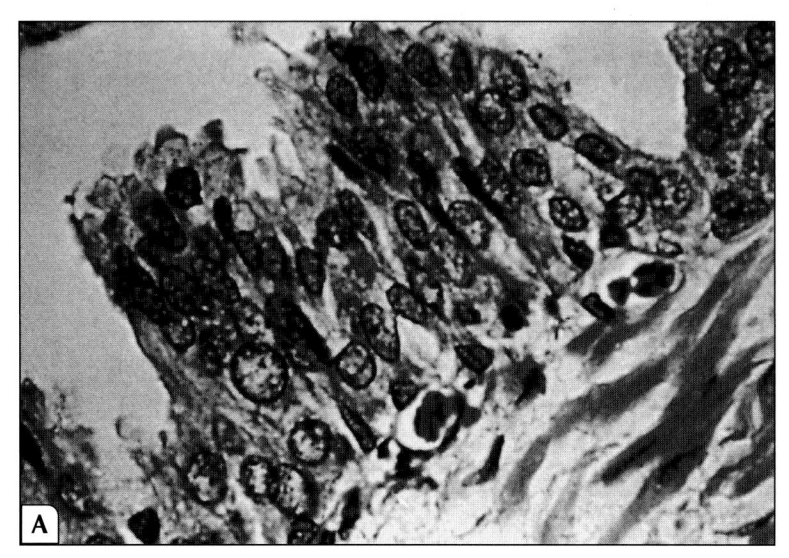

▶ **FIGURE 8-21.** Prostatic intraepithelial neoplasia. Several pathologic criteria are of great clinical importance in the early detection and staging of prostate cancer. The invention of the minimally invasive "skinny" needle biopsy guided with transrectal ultrasound (TRUS) increased public awareness, and increases in screening using serum prostate-specific antigen (PSA) have brought about a dramatic increase in the number of needle biopsies performed with the intention of diagnosing adenocarcinoma of the prostate. The precursor lesion to invasive carcinoma of the

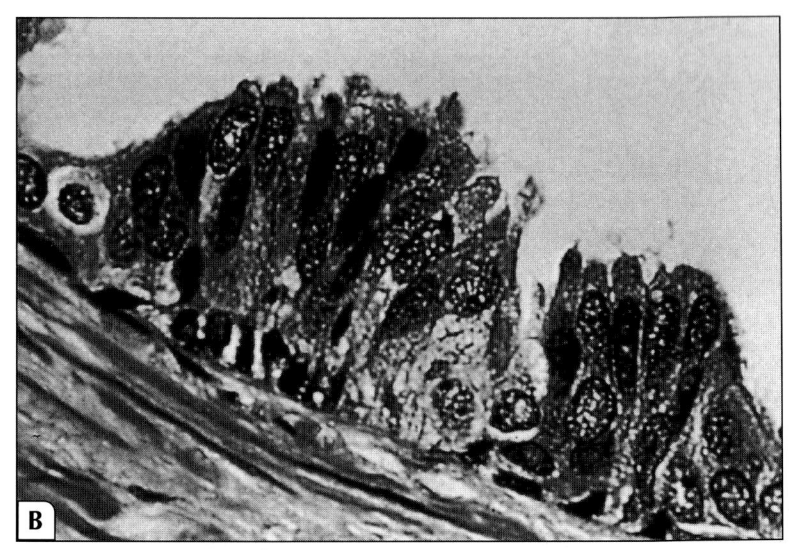

(Continued on next page)

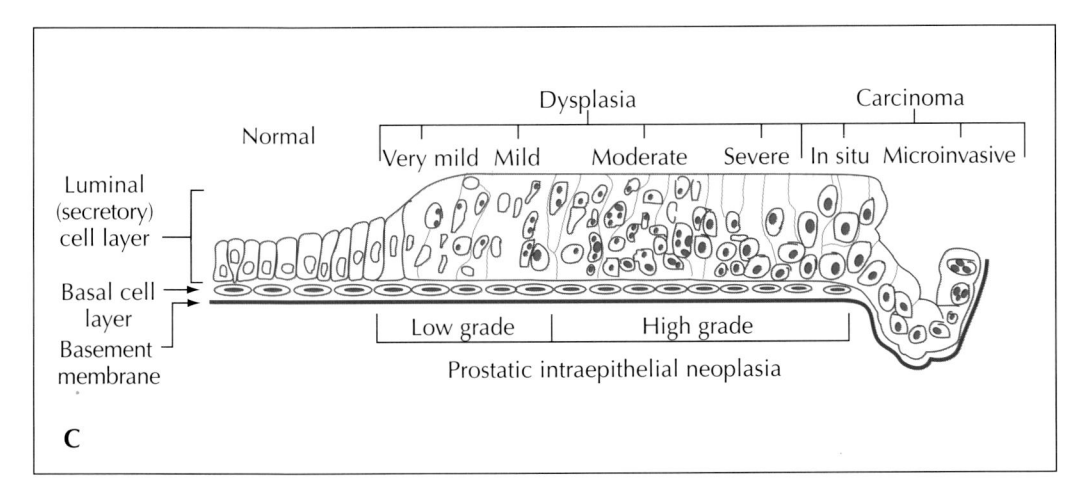

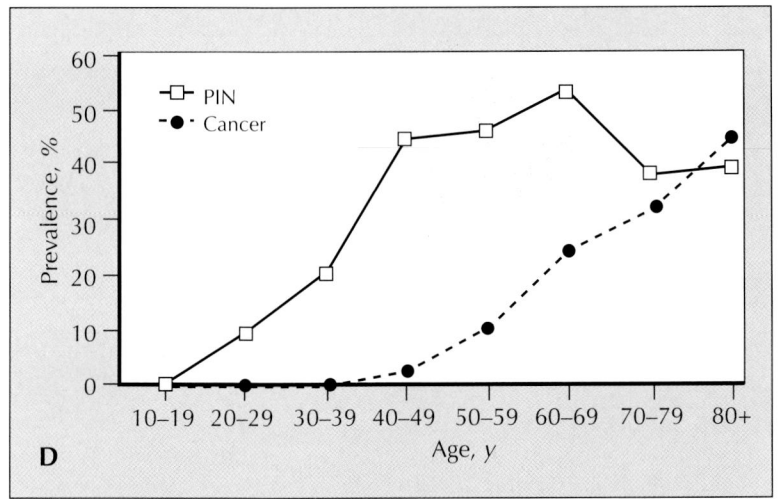

FIGURE 8-21. *(Continued)* prostate, prostatic intraepithelial neoplasia (PIN), and the Gleason grading system are practical pathologic points that are essential for urologists to understand when treating patients with newly diagnosed adenocarcinoma of the prostate.

Prostatic intraepithelial neoplasia is an architecturally benign prostate gland lined with cytologically atypical cells. This pathologic entity, first described by Bostwick and Brawer in 1987, replaced previously described pathologic lesions of the prostate such as atypical and intraductal dysplasia. Originally, PIN was divided into three categories: PIN-1, mild dysplasia (*panel A*); PIN-2, moderate dysplasia; and PIN-3, severe dysplasia (*panel B*). Currently, the only pathologic entity of clinical significance is believed to be PIN-3 or high-grade PIN. Pathologic studies have demonstrated that the reproducibility of low-grade PIN as a diagnosis is limited. In addition, when low-grade PIN (PIN-1 or -2) is diagnosed via needle biopsy, men were found to be at no greater risk of having prostatic carcinoma on repeat biopsies.

Panels A and *B* demonstrate the histologic difference between low-grade PIN and high-grade PIN. *Panel C* shows the histologic continuum proposed by Bostwick and Brawer in which normal columnar prostatic epithelium can differentiate into the various forms of prostatic intraepithelial neoplasia and on into carcinoma in situ and invasive cancer. High-grade PIN shares several histologic characteristics with invasive prostate cancer: 1) marked variation in nuclear size and shape; 2) increased heterogeneity in chromatin texture patterns; 3) increased number and variability of nucleoli; and 4) a decrease in the architectural order with which cells are arranged on the basement membrane. In addition, several phenotypic similarities have been noted between high-grade PIN and carcinoma of the prostate. Immunohistochemical studies have demonstrated a decrease in PSA, prostatic acid phosphatase (PAP), and other markers of prostatic neoplasia, as well as progressive increases in various tissue factors such as type IV collagenase, acidic mucin and other markers of invasive prostate cancer. Finally, *panel D* demonstrates the parallel increase in histologic diagnosis of PIN and prostate cancer from autopsy series. Current clinical recommendations dictate repeat prostatic biopsies when a diagnosis of high-grade PIN has been made. When high-grade PIN is found on needle biopsy, there is a 30% to 50% risk of finding carcinoma on subsequent biopsies. PIN by itself does not, however, give rise to elevated serum PSA levels. When PIN has been diagnosed, repeat biopsies should include wide sampling of the prostate in addition to the area in which PIN was found. (*Panel C modified from* Bostwick [21]; with permission.)

Clinical Aspects of Prostate Cancer

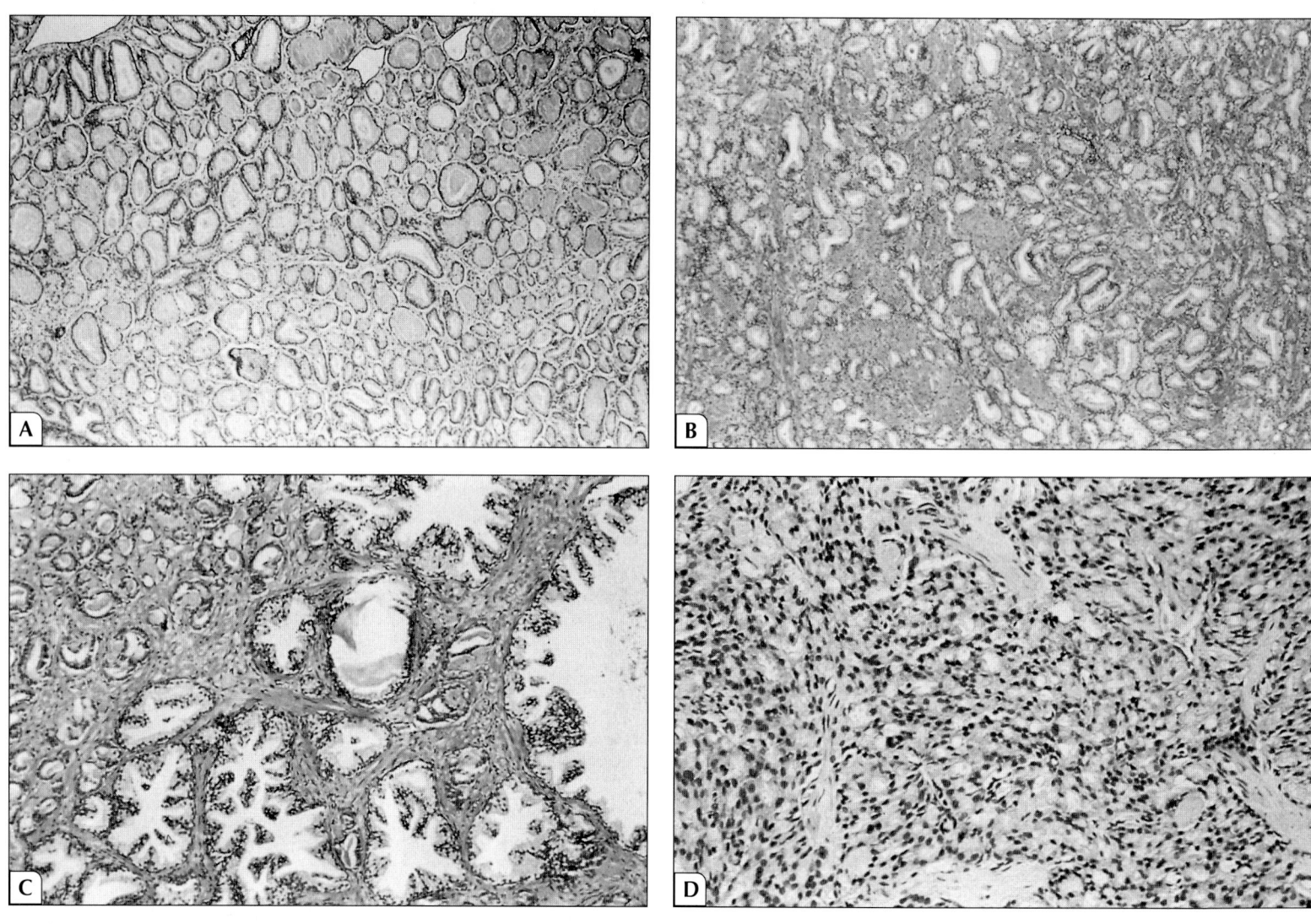

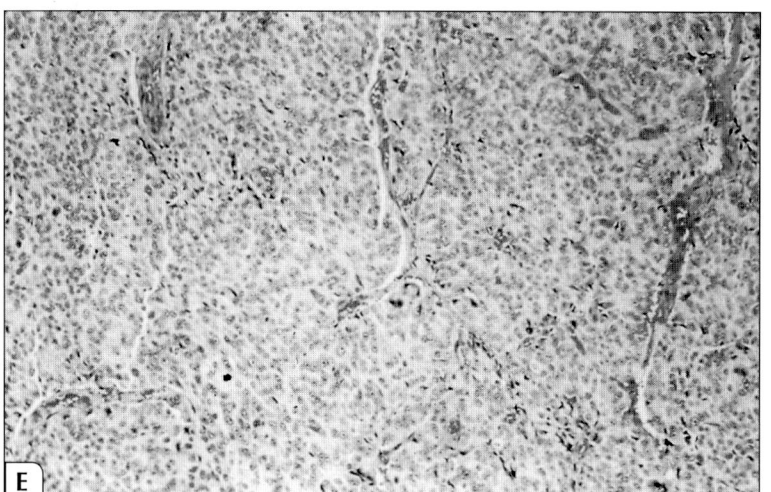

FIGURE 8-22. Histologic representation of Gleason grades 1 through 5. Various histologic grading systems for prostate cancer have been recommended over the years. One grading system, the Gleason grading system, has gained wide acceptance. This grading system is based primarily on the low-power glandular pattern of the tumor. Nuclear and cytologic features are not considered. The Gleason grading system assigns a grade from 1 to 5 for the primary (predominant) and the secondary (second most prevalent) architectural patterns identified within the tumor. A score of 1 represents prostate cells whose differentiation is most like normal prostate cells (*panel A*), whereas a grade of 5 represents the least differentiated prostate tissue (*panel E*). Panels A through E demonstrate the histologic patterns identified by each of the Gleason grades. When the Gleason grading system has been compared with long-term survival rates in both radical prostatectomy and radiation therapy series, the correlation between this grading system and survival generally has been good. Several previous grading systems have attempted to group the Gleason scores into three distinct categories (*eg*, grade I [Gleason score 2–4], grade II [Gleason score 5 to 7], and grade III [Gleason score 8 to 10]). It recently has become evident that a Gleason score of 7 has a significantly worse prognosis than a Gleason score of 5 or 6. Gleason score 7 tumors, however, are not believed to be as aggressive as Gleason score 8 to 10 cancers. Recognition of Gleason pattern 4 (*panel D*) in a tumor carries a significantly worse prognosis than does a biopsy with pure Gleason pattern 3 (*panel C*). In the past the Gleason grading system has been criticized for poor interobserver and intraobserver reproducibility, but recent studies have documented improvements in interobserver and intraobserver reproducibility (agreement within 1 Gleason sum). At this time, the Gleason scoring system represents the best prognostic marker available for clinically localized adenocarcinoma of the prostate. Careful understanding and recognition of the histologic patterns of this grading system are critical for urologists studying the clinical aspects of prostate cancer.

CONCLUSIONS

Characteristics of Nonpalpable Prostate Cancer in the Prostate-specific Antigen Era

		Patients, n (%)*	
Study	Population	Potentially Unimportant[†]	Potentially Significant[‡]
Humphrey et al. [22]	Screened (n=78)	18 (23)	60 (77)
Epstein et al. [23]	Referral (n=157)	41 (26)	116 (74)

*Men with nonpalpable prostate cancer and PSA elevations.
[†]Tumor < 0.5 cm^3 with no poorly differentiated components.
[‡]Tumor < 0.5 cm^3, or tumor with poorly differentiated components.

FIGURE 8-23. Characteristics of nonpalpable prostate cancer in the prostate-specific antigen (PSA) era. Most prostate cancers detected (>70%) are nonpalpable and are detected by prostate needle biopsy of the peripheral zone in men suspected of prostate cancer based on PSA elevations. The widespread use of PSA testing has led to earlier detection of prostate cancers before they can be felt on digital rectal examination (DRE), and this has resulted in virtual elimination of metastatic disease in serially screened populations. However, about 25% of nonpalpable cancers detected with PSA testing are potentially unimportant (< 0.5 cm^3 with no poorly differentiated elements), and it may not be necessary to treat them aggressively, especially in older men. Identification of those men with significant tumors (> 0.5 cm^3 or with poorly differentiated elements) that need aggressive treatment is an important challenge in the PSA era.

Criteria for Prediction of a Significant Tumor

Criteria	Observations Predictive of a Significant Tumor
PSA density	≥ 0.1
Pathology of needle biopsy	
Grade	Gleason score ≥ 7
Cores with cancer, n	≥ 2 involved
Percentage of core with cancer	≥ 50% involved

FIGURE 8-24. Prostate cancer detectable by prostate-specific antigen (PSA). The pretreatment criteria based on PSA density and needle biopsy findings are predictive of a significant cancer in men who have a PSA-detected nonpalpable prostate cancer. If the PSA density (PSA divided by ultrasound-determined prostate size) is 0.1 or greater, or if there is unfavorable pathology on needle biopsy (Gleason score 7 or higher, or more than two cores involved, or involvement of 50% or more), then 86% of the men will have a tumor larger than 0.5 cm^3 (significant cancer). If none of the above observations predictive of a significant cancer are present, 79% of men will have a tumor smaller than 0.5 cm^3 with no poorly differentiated elements (potentially insignificant cancer). For those men thought to have potentially insignificant cancers, expectant management or watchful waiting may be a reasonable option. (*Adapted from* Epstein *et al.* [23].)

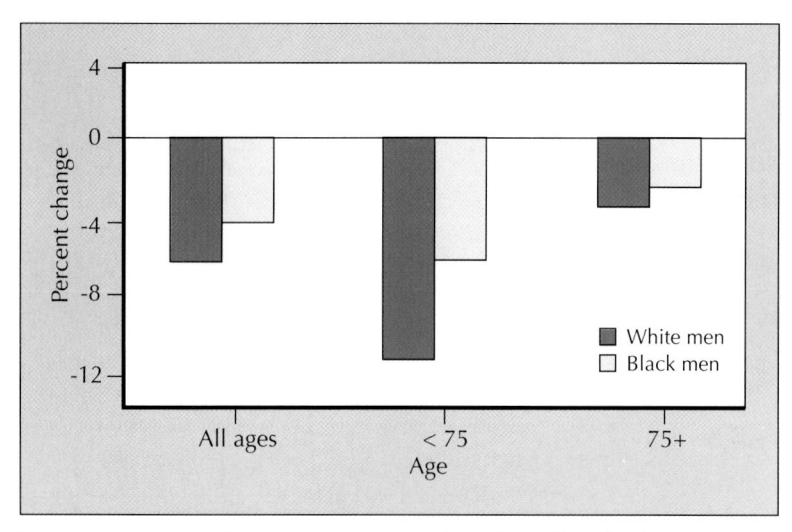

FIGURE 8-25. Prostate cancer mortality after a decade of prostate-specific antigen (PSA) testing and American Cancer Society Prostate Cancer Screening Guidelines. The American Cancer Society recently convened a multidisciplinary conference to evaluate the guidelines for screening for prostate cancer. The following statement summarizes the American Cancer Society's position in 1997 [24] regarding screening for prostate cancer:

"Both prostate-specific antigen (PSA) and digital rectal examination (DRE) should be offered annually, beginning at age 50 years, to men who have at least a 10-year life expectancy, and to younger men who are at risk. Information should be provided to patients regarding potential risks and benefits of intervention."

These recommendations highlight the interaction between physicians and patients regarding the need for prostate cancer screening. A full understanding of the potential risks, benefits, and further laboratory and diagnostic testing that will follow should these screening tests be abnormal must be discussed. It is also important to note that the American Cancer Society now recommends screening only for men who have a life expectancy of at least 10 years. High-risk groups also are now identified (*eg*, familial history, African-American descent), and earlier screening is recommended for these high-risk groups. The American Cancer Society also has pointed out that screening for prostate cancer in asymptomatic men has led to a decrease in the detection rate of advanced stage cancers. There has also been a reduction in mortality from prostate cancer in the United States; this, however, cannot be directly related to prostate cancer screening. The American Cancer Society currently recognizes an abnormal PSA value (> 4.0 ng/mL) and an abnormal digital rectal examination as abnormal results requiring further diagnostic evaluation.

Prostate cancer mortality has decreased for the first time 10 years after the introduction of a test (PSA) that has greatly decreased the presence of metastatic disease in a serially tested population. In the next decade, population data may reveal more substantial decreases in mortality among those more intensively screened (*eg*, white vs African-American men), similar to the data that now support routine cervical cancer screening. (*Figure adapted from* National Center for Health Statistics [25]; with permission.)

REFERENCES

1. Laurenson RD: *An Introduction to Clinical Anatomy by Dissection of the Human Body.* Philadelphia: WB Sauders; 1968.
2. Greene DR, Shabsigh R, Scardino PT: Urologic ultrasonography. In *Campbell's Urology*, edn 6. Edited by Walsh PC, Retik AB, Stamey TA, Vaughan ED, Jr. Philadelphia: WB Saunders; 1992:344–393.
3. Stamey TA, McNeal JE: Adenocarcinoma of the prostate. In *Campbell's Urology*, edn 6. Edited by Walsh PC, Retik AB, Stamey TA, Vaughan ED, Jr. Philadelphia: WB Saunders; 1992:1181.
4. Resnick MI, Older RA: *Diagnosis of Genitourinary Disease*, edn 2. New York: Thieme; 1997.
5. Tanagho EA: Physical examination of the genitourinary tract. *Smith's General Urology*, edn 12. Edited by Tanagho EA, McAninch JW. Norwalk: Appleton and Lange; 1988:40–47.
6. Carter HB, Partin AW: Diagnosis and staging of prostate cancer. In *Campbell's Urology*, edn 7. Edited by Walsh PC, Retik AB, Wein AJ, Vaughan ED, Jr. Philadelphia: WB Saunders; 1998:2522.
7. Beduschi MC, Oesterling JE: Prostate-specific antigen density. *Urol Clin North Am* 1997, 24:323–332.
8. Carter HB, Pearson JD, Metter JE, *et al.*: Longitudinal evaluation of prostate-specific antigen levels in men with and without prostate disease. *JAMA* 1992, 267:2215–2220.
9. Oesterling JE, Jacobson SJ, Chute CG, *et al.*: Serum prostate-specific antigen in a community-based population of healthy men: establishment of age-specific reference ranges. *JAMA* 1993, 270:860–864.
10. Morgan TO, Jacobson SJ, McCarthy WF, *et al.*: Age-specific reference ranges for serum prostate-specific antigen in black men. *N Engl J Med* 1996, 335:304–310.
11. Partin AW: The clinical utility of prostate-specific antigen: critical issues for 1997. *Advances in Prostate Cancer* 1997:2–4.
12. Terris MK, McNeal JE, Stamey TA, *et al.*: Detection of clinically significant prostate cancer by transrectal ultrasound-guided systematic biopsies. *J Urol* 1992, 148:829–832.
13. Kirby RS, Christmas TJ, Brawer MJ: *Prostate Cancer.* Wilmington, DE: Zeneca Press; 1996:82.
14. Partin AW: *Issues in the Diagnosis and Prognosis of Prostate Cancer: A Slide Lecture Series.* Oklahoma City: Cytodiagnostics (UROCOR); 1995.
15. *Prostate Cancer: Management of Advanced Disease.* Wilmington, DE: ICI Pharmaceutical; 1995.
16. Jewett HJ: The present status of radical prostatectomy for stages A and B prostatic cancer. *Urol Clin North Am* 1975, 2:105–124.
17. Gishman JR, de Vere White RW: Prostate cancer: screening, diagnosis, and staging. In *Clinical Urology.* Edited by Krane RJ, Siroky MB, Fitzpatrick JM. Philadelphia: JB Lippincott; 1994:947–948.
18. Gleason D: *Urologic Pathology: The Prostate.* Edited by Tannenbaum M. Philadelphia: Lea & Febiger; 1997:171–198.
19. Partin AW, Kattan MW, Subong ENP, *et al.*: Combination of prostate-specific antigen, clinical stage and Gleason score to predict pathological stage of localized prostate cancer: a multi-institutional update. *JAMA* 1997; 277:1445–1451.
20. *Using the Updated Partin Nomogram.* Deerfield, IL: TAP Pharmaceuticals; 1997.
21. Bostwick DG: *Issues in the Diagnosis and Prognosis of Prostate Cancer.* Oklahoma City: Cytodiagnostics (UROCOR) Speaker Support Program; 1995.
22. Humphrey PA, Keetch DW, Smith DS, *et al.*: Prospective characterization of pathological features of prostatic carcinomas detected via serum prostate-specific antigen based screening. *J Urol* 1996, 155:816–820.
23. Epstein JI, Walsh PC, Carmichael M, Brendler CB: Pathologic and clinical findings to predict tumor extent of non-palpable (stage T1c) prostate cancer. *JAMA* 1994, 271:368–374.
24. von Eschenbach A, Ho R, Murphy GP, *et al.*: American Cancer Society Guidelines for the early detection of prostate cancer. *Cancer* 1997, 80:1805–1807.
25. National Center for Health Statistics, 1998: http//www.cdc.gov/nchswwwdefault.htm

The Patient's Choice of Surgery for Clinically Localized Prostate Cancer

9
CANCEROUS DISEASE SECTION

Michael W. Kattan & Brian J. Miles

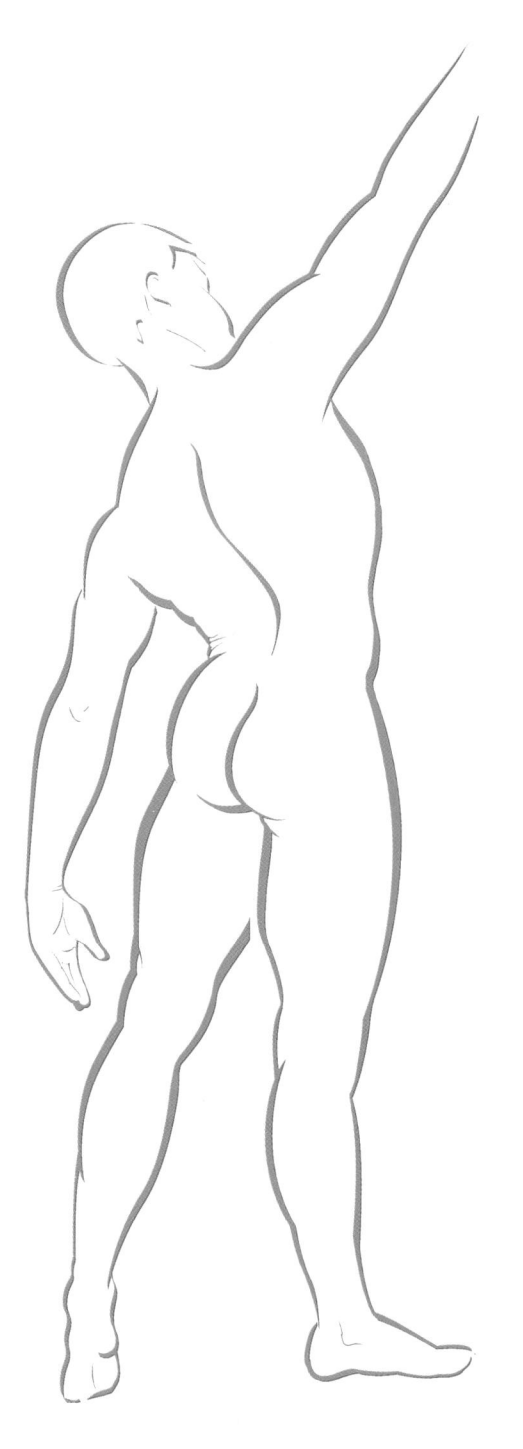

Treatment decision-making for patients with clinically localized prostate cancer can be difficult. Because of the age of men at diagnosis, survival benefits associated with aggressive therapies such as surgery typically are estimated to be small, and patient preferences are very influential in determining the preferred treatment. This chapter reviews two different methods for assisting patients in choosing the treatment that is best for them. First, we consider the decision analytic approach, which directly incorporates patient preferences and survival estimates in suggesting the appropriate treatment. Because this approach is difficult to perform at the bedside, we also discuss a second method, nomograms, which are mathematical models that predict outcomes for the individual patient.

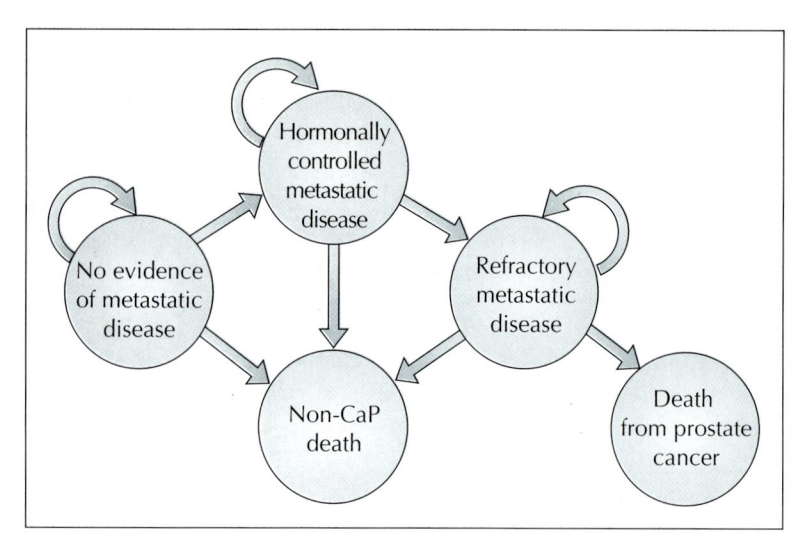

▶ **FIGURE 9-1.** Most decision analyses use computerized Markov models to represent treatment decisions. These models move patients through various health states (*eg*, healthy, sick, and dead). This figure represents a Markov model for clinically localized prostate cancer [1]. In this example, a theoretical cohort of patients begins in the health state ("no evidence of metastatic disease") (*left*). Every 6 months, a fraction of the cohort is allowed to progress in the direction of the arrows. The probabilities of progression are taken from the literature. *Circular arrows* indicate that it is possible for the patient to remain in that health state at the end of a 6-month period. The two death states are absorbing; they cannot be exited. Computerized Markov models such as this one allow survival estimation for various treatment strategies. If we assume that the patient will not prefer all health states equally, we may then be able to estimate quality-adjusted life expectancy by assigning different weights to the different health states. The quality-of-life adjustments, called *utilities*, can be estimated using several established techniques. (*From* Kattan *et al.* [1]; with permission.)

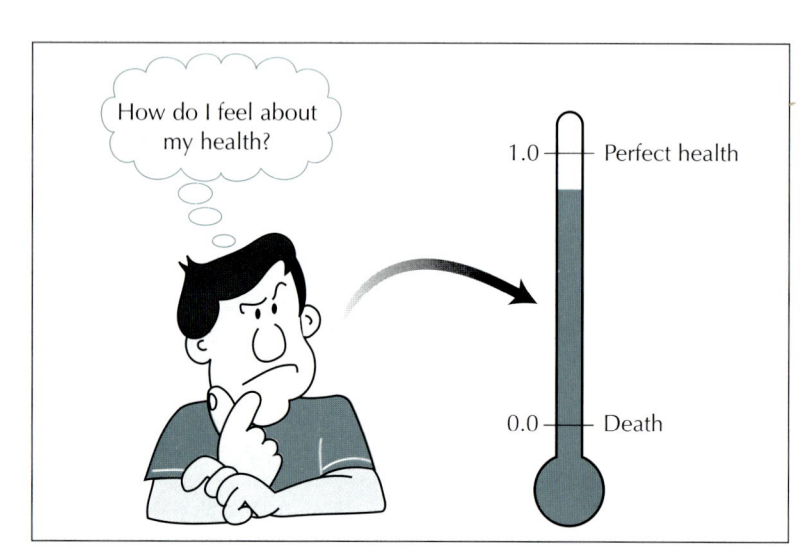

▶ **FIGURE 9-2.** Quality of life. There are numerous definitions of quality of life, from the psychologic to the social; in general, it can be understood as a patient's ability to function in a manner commensurate with his needs, desires, and abilities. Although all traditional definitions help us approach a sense of "quality of life," none can globally capture what it is for all people. Quality of life can be defined only by each individual. Therefore, measuring quality of life has been viewed as an inexact science fraught with misinterpretation, overinterpretation, biased questioning, or inadequate questioning. However, the science of quality-of-life evaluation has progressed to such an extent that dependable and reproducible results that allow investigators to estimate a patient's quality of life are achievable. For the purposes of decision algorithms and models, quality of life measurement must be reported numerically, on a scale from 0 to 1, in which 0 represents "death" and 1 represents "perfect health." The value of a utility is that all health states can be placed in this common scale.

Measuring Quality of Life

Self-report measures
Utility instruments
  Time tradeoffs
  Health-rating scales
  Standard gamble
  Consensus panel

▶ **FIGURE 9-3.** Measuring quality of life. In the decision analytic process, measuring quality of life is important in reflecting the impact that a disease (*eg*, prostate cancer) or its treatment has on the normal functioning of a patient's life.

We can measure quality of life in several ways. Patients can either present self-report measures of how they are doing, or, more commonly, utility instruments can be issued that evaluate how much a patient values one health state versus another health state. The four most common ways that utilities are measured are time tradeoff, health-rating scales, standard gamble, and a consensus panel. In time tradeoffs, a patient is given the option of living a longer life in the compromised state (*eg*, incontinence) as opposed to a shorter period of life in perfect health. The length of time in the health states is varied and presented to the patient for his selection of preference. The point at which the patient becomes indifferent to the two states is the time he is willing to trade off to live a perfectly normal life. Health-rating scales are a more global method of measurement, in which a patient indicates how he feels about his current state of health versus a perfect state of health. A standard gamble is a method of measuring what patients are willing to gamble to live a normal healthy life as opposed to one in an altered health state. Finally, there is the consensus panel, which to date is the most common way of evaluating quality-of-life issues. However, this method has the weakest methodology because a consensus panel of physicians defining how their patients feel in a particular health state does not reflect what patients themselves feel—a fact that has been demonstrated in a number of studies.

▶ **FIGURE 9-4.** The time tradeoff technique. One way of measuring utilities (*ie*, health state preferences) is to use the time tradeoff technique. This is one of the most common utility assessment techniques. With this method, the patient chooses between his current health/life expectancy and a guaranteed period of perfect health followed by immediate death. The duration of guaranteed perfect health is varied until indifference is reached, and utility is calculated as number of perfect health years divided by life expectancy. For example, patients might estimate the utility for impotence to be 0.8 and the utility for incontinence to be 0.7. This means that on average, patients would be willing to give up 10% of their life expectancy (0.8 − 0.7 = 0.1) to live with impotence rather than incontinence. Furthermore, a patient in this example would be willing to give up 20% of his life expectancy (1.0 − 0.8) to avoid impotence and remain in perfect health. As an example, the time tradeoff works as follows for evaluating the utility for a person's current state of health. First, find the minimum amount of life in perfect health that the patient is willing to trade for his current life expectancy. Then divide the number of perfect health years by the life expectancy to obtain the utility for his current health state.

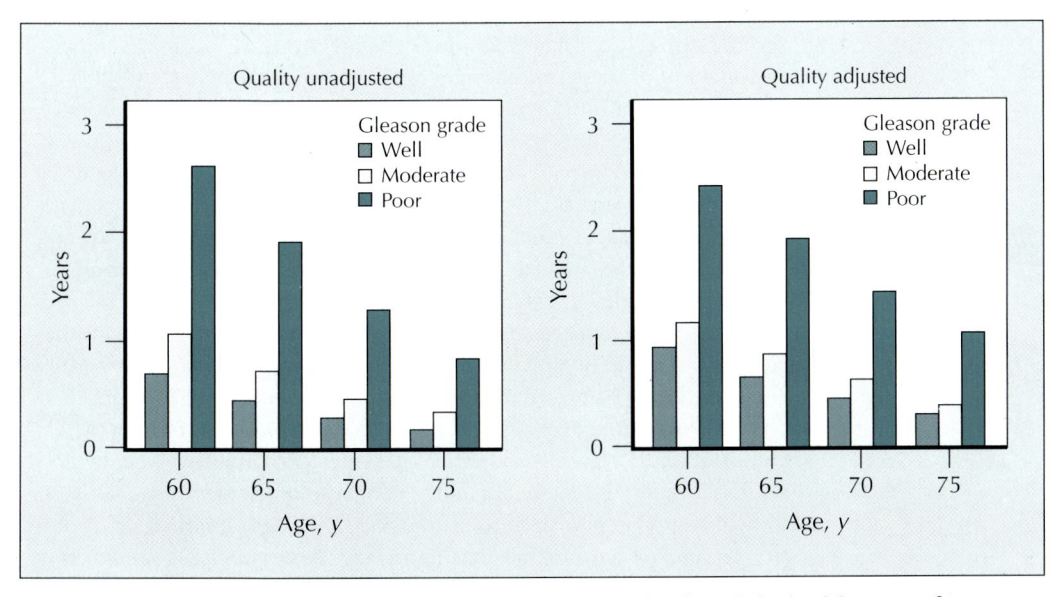

▶ **FIGURE 9-5.** Quality-adjusted survival. Once we have developed the health states of interest in a Markov model and reviewed the literature to obtain the probabilities of moving from one health state to another, and the utilities of the health states, we can estimate survival and survival adjusted for quality of life under different treatment strategies. Quality-adjusted survival is survival probability multiplied by quality of life (utility). This figure compares quality-adjusted survival with unadjusted survival. The values on the bars indicate how many years longer a radical prostatectomy patient is expected to live than is a watchful-waiting patient. For example, a 60-year-old man with poorly differentiated disease who chooses radical prostatectomy is expected to live 2.58 years longer than had he chosen watchful waiting. After adjusting for quality of life impact, that same man is expected to live an excess of 2.43 quality-adjusted years. Note that these estimates assume the patient has no comorbidity, and they do not specifically consider a particular patient's utilities. Instead, these estimates use group mean utilities. This is an important limitation because individuals of a group do not necessarily share the same utilities. (*From* Kattan *et al.* [5].)

The Patient's Choice of Therapy for Clinically Localized Prostate Cancer

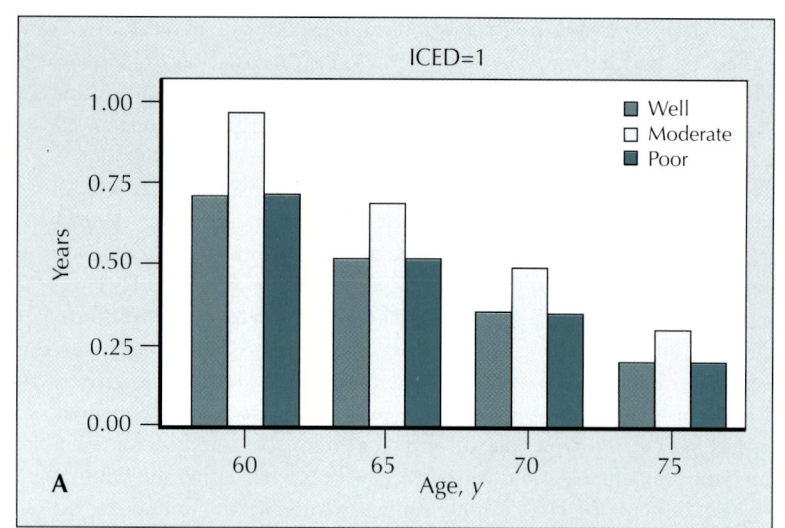

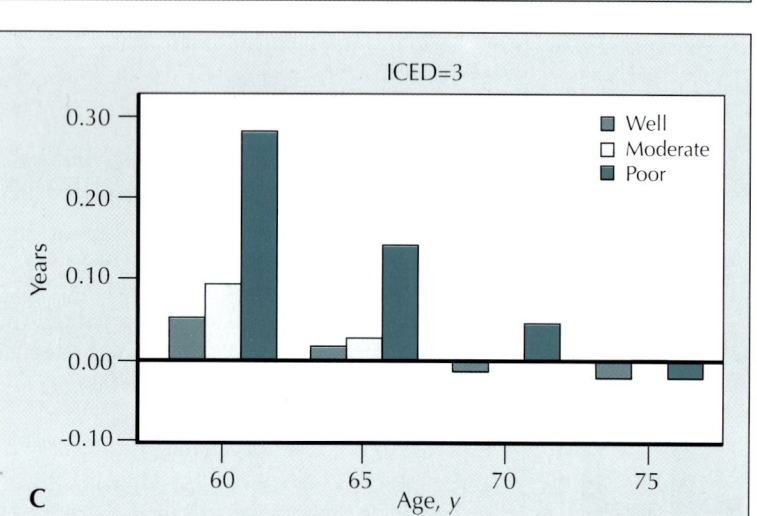

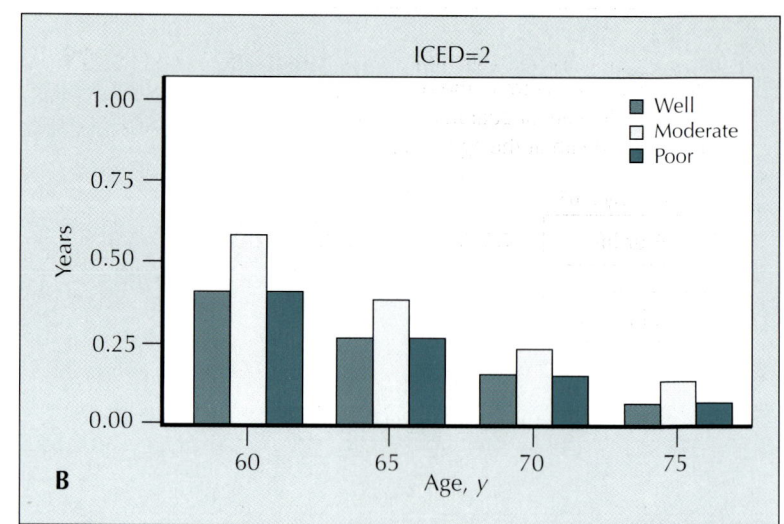

▶ **FIGURE 9-6.** Evaluating therapeutic options. It is necessary and important to consider the overall health of an individual when evaluating therapeutic options. In a very unhealthy patient (*eg*, with concomitant severe heart disease, diabetes, and Alzheimer's disease), aggressive surgical treatment of prostate cancer might be more immediately harmful than watchful waiting. This figure reflects the impact of comorbid conditions. As in Figure 9-5, the *vertical bars* indicate the additional quality-adjusted years of life that the patient is expected to derive from radical prostatectomy relative to watchful waiting.

The results of our model change when comorbidity is allowed to vary. The index of coexistent disease (ICED) is a measure from 0 (no comorbidity) to 3 (highest comorbidity). *Panels A–C* show the results for ICED levels 1, 2, and 3, respectively. The vertical axis in these plots represents the additional years of life (quality-adjusted) that a radical prostatectomy patient is expected to live beyond the life expectancy of a watchful-waiting patient. Notice the decreasing benefit of radical prostatectomy as the comorbidity increases. Also, notice that when comorbidity is very high, watchful waiting is preferred in older men with low-grade disease. Still, individual preferences need to be measured. Measuring individual utilities on each patient is time consuming and expensive, however. For this reason, we are developing a website that assesses utilities, and allows the physician to enter clinical information and then compute the quality-adjusted survival estimates for that patient in a customized fashion. The website should be available soon.

II. The Prostate

A. Nomogram for Prediction of Final Pathologic Stage

	PSA Level, 0.0–4.0 ng/mL						PSA Level, 4.1–10 ng/mL						PSA Level, 10.1–20 ng/mL						PSA Level, >20 ng/mL					
	Clinical Stage						Clinical Stage						Clinical Stage						Clinical Stage					
Score	T1a	T1b	T2a	T2b	T2c	T3a	T1a	T1b	T2a	T2b	T2c	T3a	T1a	T1b	T2a	T2b	T2c	T3a	T1a	T1b	T2a	T2b	T2c	T3a
Prediction of Organ-confined Disease																								
2–4	100	85	88	76	82	—	100	78	83	67	71	—	100	—	61	52	—	—	—	—	20	7	—	—
5	100	78	81	67	73	—	100	70	73	56	64	43	100	49	58	43	37	26	—	—	32	—	3	—
6	100	68	72	54	60	42	100	53	62	44	48	33	—	36	44	28	37	19	—	—	14	11	4	5
7	—	54	61	41	46	—	100	39	51	32	37	26	—	24	36	19	24	14	—	—	18	4	5	3
8–10	—	—	48	31	—	—	—	32	39	22	25	12	—	11	29	14	15	9	—	—	3	1	2	2
Prediction of Established Capsular Penetration																								
2–4	0	15	14	26	17	—	0	22	19	34	27	—	0	—	40	49	—	—	—	—	80	94	—	—
5	0	22	20	34	26	—	0	29	28	45	34	58	0	49	43	58	61	75	—	—	68	—	97	—
6	0	30	29	46	38	59	0	45	38	56	49	68	—	62	56	73	59	82	—	—	86	90	96	95
7	—	43	39	59	50	—	0	58	49	68	59	75	—	73	64	81	73	86	—	—	80	96	95	98
8–10	—	—	50	68	—	—	—	64	59	77	71	87	—	87	70	86	82	92	—	—	97	99	97	98

Numbers represent probability (%). Dash indicates lack of sufficient data to calculate probability.

B. Nomogram for Prediction of Final Pathologic Stage

	PSA Level, 0.0–4.0 ng/mL						PSA Level, 4.1–10 ng/mL						PSA Level, 10.1–20 ng/mL						PSA Level, > 20 ng/mL					
	Clinical Stage						Clinical Stage						Clinical Stage						Clinical Stage					
Score	T1a	T1b	T2a	T2b	T2c	T3a	T1a	T1b	T2a	T2b	T2c	T3a	T1a	T1b	T2a	T2b	T2c	T3a	T1a	T1b	T2a	T2b	T2c	T3a
Prediction of Seminal Vesicle Involvement																								
2–4	0	1	1	2	2	—	0	2	1	3	3	—	0	—	3	4	—	—	—	—	12	30	—	—
5	0	3	2	4	4	—	0	4	3	6	6	5	0	7	5	8	12	11	—	—	11	—	29	—
6	0	6	5	9	9	8	0	9	6	11	12	11	—	15	11	19	17	18	—	—	35	40	53	31
7	—	12	9	17	17	—	0	18	12	22	23	18	—	28	19	33	33	31	—	—	31	73	62	55
8–10	—	—	17	29	—	—	—	29	22	38	40	40	—	55	29	50	53	49	—	—	81	93	73	65
Prediction of Lymph Nodal Involvement																								
2–4	0	2	1	2	4	—	0	2	1	2	5	—	0	—	1	3	—	—	—	—	2	7	—	—
5	0	4	2	4	8	—	0	4	2	5	10	8	0	5	2	6	13	11	—	—	3	—	29	—
6	0	8	3	9	17	15	0	9	4	11	19	16	—	11	5	13	22	20	—	—	9	18	53	31
7	—	15	7	18	31	—	0	18	8	20	34	28	—	21	9	24	39	35	—	—	11	44	62	55
8–10	—	—	13	32	—	—	—	30	15	35	53	50	—	41	17	40	59	54	—	—	35	76	73	65

Numbers represent probability (%). Dash indicates lack of sufficient data to calculate probability.

▶ **FIGURE 9-7.** Nomograms. Markov's modeling is difficult to perform on individual patients [2]. Furthermore, Markov models are designed for use in population and cohort studies. Because of this difficulty of use, many physicians prefer to use nomograms. These are mathematical devices (usually tables or charts) that predict the probability of an outcome for an individual patient. The main attraction of a nomogram is that it precisely predicts probabilities, which is something that humans have difficulty doing. Numerous studies have shown that nomograms predict more accurately than do human experts under most conditions [3].

This figure shows the most popular nomogram for clinically localized prostate cancer: the original Partin nomogram. These tables indicate the predicted probability that a man has either organ-confined, capsular penetration (*panel A*), seminal vesicle invasion, or lymph node–positive disease (*panel B*). To make this final pathologic prediction, the nomogram requires the measurement of a man's preoperative prostate-specific antigen level, clinical stage, and Gleason sum of the biopsy. The nomograms are based on logistic regression analyses of several hundred men treated at Johns Hopkins University.

Although this nomogram predicted accurately on the sample of men at Johns Hopkins, one wonders how well it might do on future patients, especially those at another institution. The nomogram is of limited use if the patients are different such that the predictions are no longer accurate. In addition, it is not apparent how certain the probability estimates are. A measure of the confidence in the estimates is needed. (*Adapted from* Partin *et al.* [4]; with permission.)

Performance of the Partin Nomogram

Stage Predicted by Nomogram	When the Partin Nomogram Predicted This Probability of Pathologic Stage, %	Percentage of Men Actually Having the Corresponding Pathologic Stage
Organ confined (low)	20	25
Organ confined (high)	80	83
Extraprostatic extension (low)	20	15
Extraprostatic extension (high)	80	70
Seminal vesicle invasion (low)	20	25
Seminal vesicle invasion (high)	80	50
Positive lymph nodes (low)	20	15
Positive lymph nodes (high)	60	20

▶ **FIGURE 9-8.** Performance of the Partin nomogram. To investigate the accuracy of the widely popular Partin nomogram, Kattan *et al.* [5] conducted a validation study of its performance. They retrospectively ran information from more than 700 men through the nomogram using preoperative data and obtained the nomogram's predictions from final pathologic stage. They then compared these predictions with the actual pathologic stage of these men. The table shows some examples of the nomogram's predictions and what stage the men actually had. For example, of the men who had a 30% chance of having organ-confined disease based on the Partin nomogram, 25% actually had organ-confined disease. This table shows performance accuracy of the Partin nomogram at low and high extremes of each pathologic stage. The nomogram does not often predict probability of 0 or 1, so 20% and 80% were used except for the positive lymph nodes, where 80% of predictions were not found. Note that the nomogram predicted organ disease accurately but was not accurate when it predicted high probabilities of advanced disease. (*From* Kattan *et al.* [5]; with permission.)

Pathologic Stage Probabilities and 95% CIs

Clinical Stage	PSA	Gleason Sum	OC	ECE	SVI	LN
T1c	6	6	67(64–33)	30 (27–33)	2 (2–3)	1 (1–2)
T2c	15	7	15 (11–19)	45 (39–52)	22 (16–29)	18 (12–25)

▶ **FIGURE 9-9.** Updated version of the Partin nomogram. Issues regarding the lack of validation of the Partin nomogram motivated Partin and Kattan to produce an updated version [6], which featured improved methodology and 95% CIs to illustrate uncertainty. The uncertainty displayed in this updated version is important to convey to clinicians because no nomogram is perfect, and the user needs to know how accurate the nomogram is. This update was based on over 4000 men from three institutions. Internal validation was performed to ensure reliability in the predictions. This table illustrates two examples of predictions by the nomogram. PSA—prostate-specific antigen.

Predictive Value of Pathologic Stage

Pathologic Stage Grouping	Probability of PSA Recurrence at 5 Years, %
Organ confined	10
Non–organ confined	50
Negative lymph nodes	20
Positive lymph nodes	88

▶ **FIGURE 9-10.** Predictive value of pathologic stage. Although the updated Partin-Kattan nomogram corrects several deficiencies of the previous Partin nomogram, an important limitation remains. In the Partin validation paper, Kattan *et al.* pointed out that final pathologic stage often is not a suitable proxy for the efficacy of radical prostatectomy. Although having organ-confined disease is a good prognostic factor, not all patients are cured. Although nonconfined disease is a bad prognostic factor, the disease of many patients still does not recur. Providing patients with their probabilities of pathologic stage and the corresponding recurrence probabilities requires the patient to do a complex calculation to obtain his overall probability of recurrence. This process results in crude estimates because they are conditioned on pathologic stage.

FIGURE 9-11. Preoperative nomogram for recurrence of prostate cancer. Because prognosis, not final pathology, is important for treatment decision making, Kattan *et al.* developed a nomogram for recurrence at 5 years. Using prostate-specific antigen (PSA), clinical stage, and biopsy Gleason grade, the nomogram produces the probability of PSA recurrence within 5 years of radical prostatectomy. Validation of the nomogram suggested that it is accurate to within 10% of the true probability. Although the nomogram was derived from patients of a single surgeon, it performed at least as accurately on patients from five other surgeons. See Kattan *et al.* [7] for instructions to physician and patient. (*From* Kattan *et al.* [7]; with permission.)

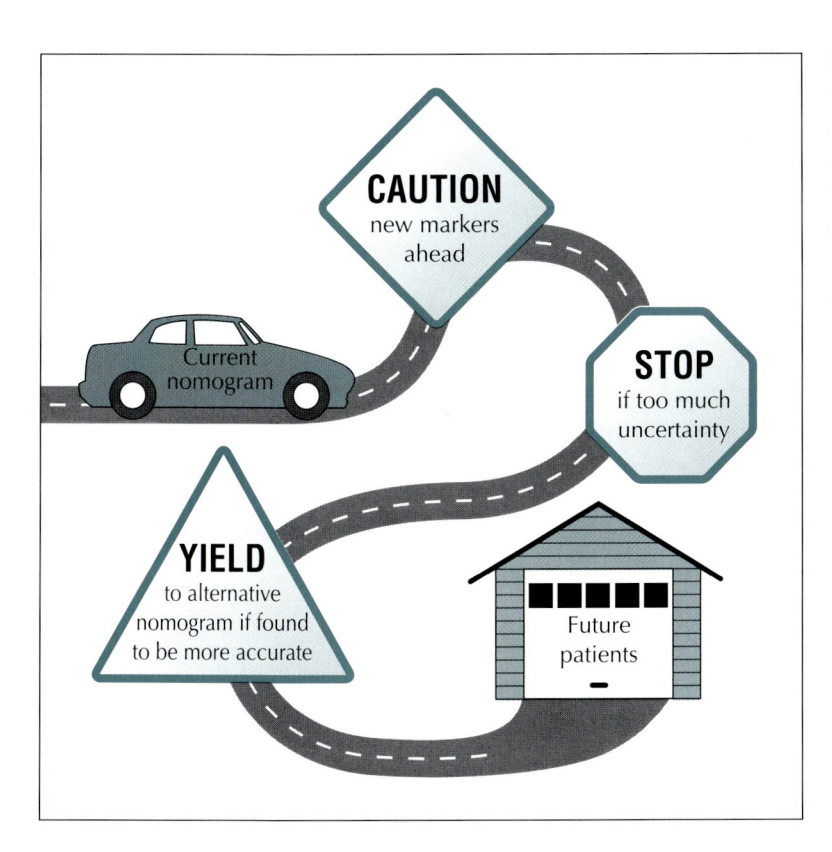

FIGURE 9-12. Nomograms are not without limitations. Keeping them current is difficult, given the rapid introduction and new markers for disease. Although it is difficult to say whether any markers for prostate cancer beside prostate-specific antigen, biopsy Gleason grade, and clinical stage have been shown to predict recurrence in large studies, other markers probably will emerge in the near future. Another issue to consider is the uncertainty inherent in the predictions of nomograms. No nomogram is perfect, and the clinician must be presented with an indicator of the error, such as a CI. Before use, nomograms must be validated with patients not previously used to construct the nomogram.

REFERENCES

1. Kattan MW, Cowen ME, Miles BJ: A decision analysis for treatment of clinically localized prostate cancer. *J Gen Intern Med* 1997, 12:299–305.
2. Cowen ME, Miles BJ, Cahill DF, *et al.*: The danger of applying group-level decision analyses for the treatment of localized prostate cancer to the individual. *Medical Decision Making* 1998, 18:376–380.
3. Kattan MW, Adams DA, Parko MS: A comparison of machine learning with human judgement. *J Manage Inf Surg* 1993, 9:37–57.
4. Partin AW, Yoo J, Carter HB, *et al.*: The use of prostate specific antigen, clinical stage and Gleason score to predict pathological stage in men with localized prostate cancer. *J Urol* 1993, 150:110–114.
5. Kattan MW, Stapleton AMF, Wheeler TM, Scardino PT: Evaluation of a nomogram for predicting pathological stage of men with clinically localized prostate cancer. *Cancer* 1997, 79:528–537.
6. Partin AW, Kattan MW, Subong ENP, *et al.*: Combination of PSA, clinical stage and Gleason score to predict pathological stage in men with localized prostate cancer: a multi-institutional update. *JAMA* 1997, 277:1445–1451.
7. Kattan MW, Eastham JA, Stapleton AMF, *et al.*: A preoperative nomogram for disease recurrence following radical prostatectomy for prostate cancer. *J Natl Cancer Inst* 1998, 90:766–771.

Radical Perineal Prostatectomy

CANCEROUS DISEASE SECTION

Lorne D. Sullivan

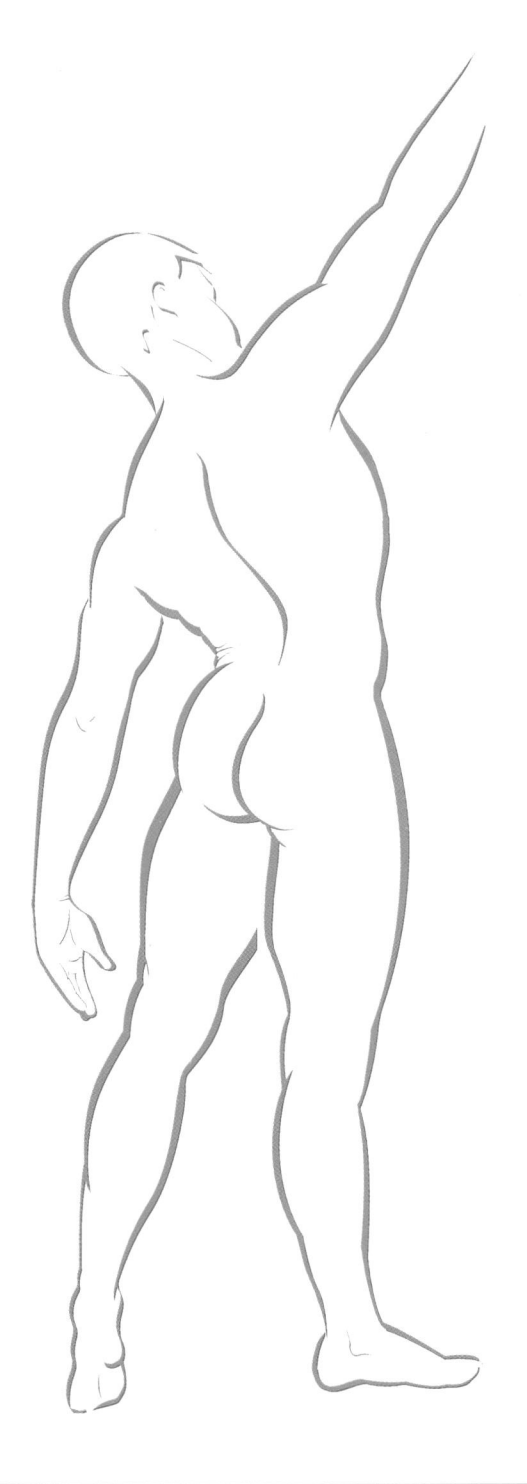

Radical perineal prostatectomy has been widely practiced to cure selected cases of localized prostate cancer for many decades [1,2]. The long-term survival data and disease-free survival have been excellent [3–5]. The indications for radical perineal prostatectomy initially were confined to the lesion described as B1, less than 1 cm in size, and usually well differentiated.

In the 1970s it became apparent with staging pelvic lymph node dissection before treatment of localized prostate cancer by brachytherapy that significant numbers of patients had positive lymph nodes [6]. Similar results were found with pelvic lymph node dissection before radical prostatectomy in patients with localized prostate cancer who did not conform to the classic B1 lesion, leading to the inclusion of pelvic lymph node dissection before radical prostatectomy as a staging criterion at many centers. Because the lower abdomen was opened for the pelvic node dissection, it was logical to proceed directly to retropubic prostatectomy; many centers moved away from the perineal approach.

With the introduction of the prostate-specific antigen (PSA) test and an increased public awareness of treatment options for localized prostate cancer during the past decade, we have seen a major change in staging patients presenting as possible candidates for radical prostatectomy [7].

Several authors recently identified groups of patients presenting with localized prostate cancer who are at extremely low risk for positive lymph nodes [8–10]. Nerve-sparing techniques by the perineal route with reasonable preservation of potency have been described by several authors [11].

These developments and the perceived advantages of radical perineal prostatectomy (*ie*, less invasive exposure, minimal use of analgesics, early return to ambulation and oral intake, excellent hemostasis and minimal requirement for blood transfusions, early discharge from hospital) have prompted renewed interest in the radical perineal prostatectomy. This chapter presents the surgical procedure for the perineal approach as described by Sullivan *et al.* [12].

Indications for Radical Perineal Prostatectomy

Usual indications
  Clinically localized prostate carcinoma on
    Digital examination
    Sextant rectal ultrasound (TRUS)–guided biopsies
  Ten-year life expectancy (<70 years of age)
  Minimal comorbidity
  Gleason scores < 8 (4+4)
  PSA level < 10 ng/mL
Unusual indications
  Gross obesity
  Previous multiple abdominal procedures
  Previous abdominal perineal surgery
  Previous arterial bypass grafts in the pelvis
  Previous extensive transurethral prostatic resection
  Salvage prostatectomy with delayed recurrence after radiotherapy

FIGURE 10-1. Indications for radical perineal prostatectomy. All of the usual indications must be present before radical perineal prostatectomy is considered. In cases in which the prostate-specific antigen (PSA) level is greater than 10 and the Gleason score is 5 or above on any single biopsy specimen, a radical perineal prostatectomy may be offered only after negative results have been obtained on an ileo-obturator node dissection and on a bone scan. Patients undergoing a node dissection often opt for concurrent radical retropubic node dissection under the same anesthetic.

Nerve sparing is offered to carefully selected patients who have normal preoperative sexual function and do not have a positive apical biopsy on the same side as the nerve to be spared, who have fewer than two positive biopsy results on the same side without evidence of capsular extension, and who have no Gleason 5 involvement on the ipsilateral side on biopsy analysis. Patients who normally would be considered candidates for retropubic prostatectomy sometimes are referred for the perineal approach because of unusual circumstances that make it more appropriate than the retropubic approach.

Preoperative Considerations

Preoperative work-up
  Medical evaluation: history, physical examination, and assessment
    of life expectancy
  Standard blood work
  Electrocardiogram
  PSA
  DRE
  Six zonal transrectal ultrasound–guided biopsies
  Ileo-obturator node dissection (recommended for selected cases;
    see Fig. 10-1)
  Blood type and screen (no cross-match)
Preoperative preparation of patient
  Bowel preparation (usually PEG) given at home the day before surgery
  Preoperative intravenous antibiotics, including cefazolin sodium;
    gentamicin, 1 mg/kg; and metronidazole, 500 mg. These are given
    on arrival in the preanesthetic area.

FIGURE 10-2. Preoperative considerations. The preoperative work-up involves blood work, biopsies, and a node dissection, if necessary. Because blood transfusions rarely are needed, only a type screen is done so that matched blood can be available within 20 minutes, if needed. If patients prefer autologous blood collection, two units can be stored. In a study comparing radical perineal prostatectomy with retropubic prostatectomy at our center, only one of 79 perineal patients required blood transfusion, and that patient was found to have von Willebrand's disease. (Sullivan *et al.*, Unpublished data.)

Preoperative preparation is done at home the night before the surgery, because the patient can be admitted on the day of surgery and already will have been seen at a preoperative assessment clinic. Minimal preanesthetic preparation is required. Blood loss usually averages 400 mL or less (Sullivan *et al.*, Unpublished data.), and extensive monitoring lines (*eg*, CVPs, arterial line) are not necessary, obviating the need for invasive anesthesia. DRE—digital rectal examination; PSA—prostate-specific antigen; PEG—polyethylene glycol.

Postoperative Care

Ambulation on arrival to the ward
Analgesia as required (usually minimal, oral)
Oral fluids on first postoperative day; full fluids to soft diet on second
  postoperative day
Removal of Penrose drain on first or second postoperative day
Discharge on second or third postoperative day
Removal of Foley catheter 3 weeks postoperative
Follow-up assessment, including prostate-specific antigen (PSA) levels,
  at 1, 3, 6, and 12 mo postoperation and once a year thereafter

FIGURE 10-3. Postoperative considerations. The postoperative care of the radical perineal prostatectomy patient is very straightforward. Patients should be encouraged to ambulate and start oral fluids the same day as the operation. Intravenous fluids are given until the patient is drinking adequate amounts. Minimal analgesia usually is required, although many patients may need one intramuscular injection of narcotic analgesia in the recovery room. Early discharge is possible as soon as the patient is taking a full diet and is stable.

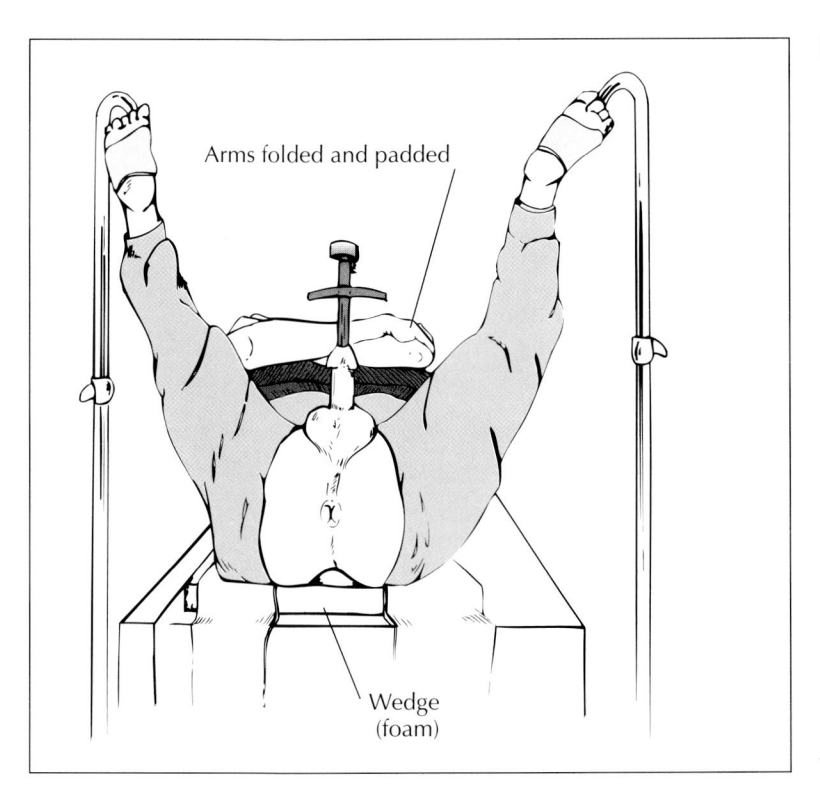

▶ **FIGURE 10-4.** Patient positioning. The patient is positioned in an exaggerated lithotomy position, using a standard operating table, shoulder support, and leg stirrups. The arms are folded over the chest and padded to avoid brachial plexus traction. (*From* Sullivan *et al.* [12]; with permission.)

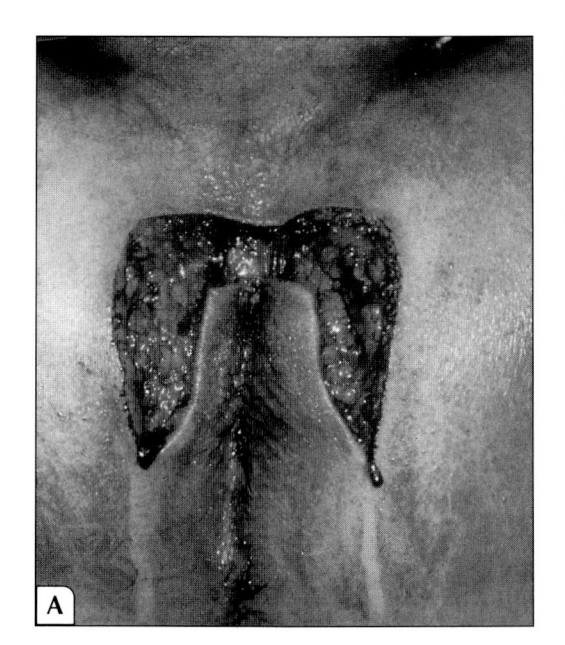

▶ **FIGURE 10-5.** **A** and **B**, Insertion of curved Lowsley retractor. A curved Lowsley retractor is inserted and the blades are opened. An inverted "U" incision should be made between the ischial spines exactly 2 cm anterior to the anal verge. The incision site can be confirmed by retraction of the skin bilaterally over the ischial spines. This method tents the skin over the subcutaneous anal sphincter, forming a defined line for the incision. The incision is carried 4 to 5 cm posteriorly on either side. (*Panel B adapted from* Paulson and Thrasher [13]; with permission.)

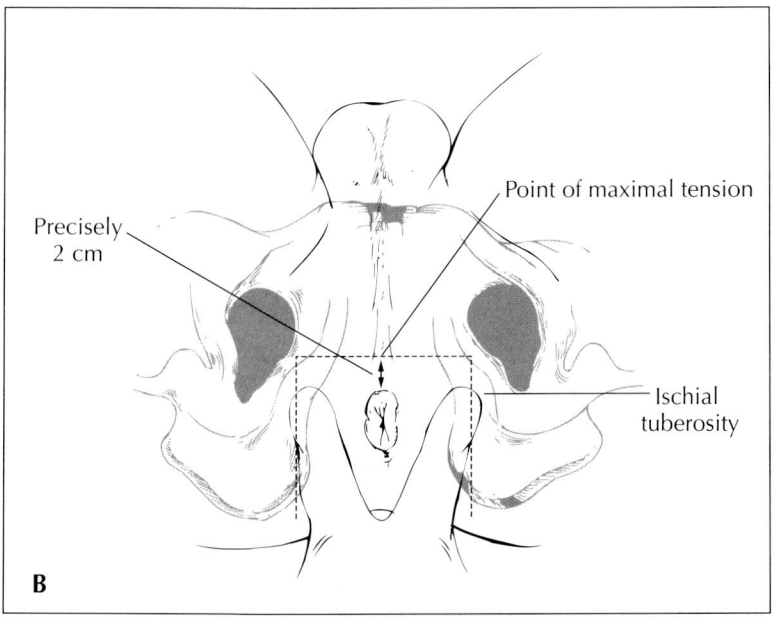

Radical Perineal Prostatectomy

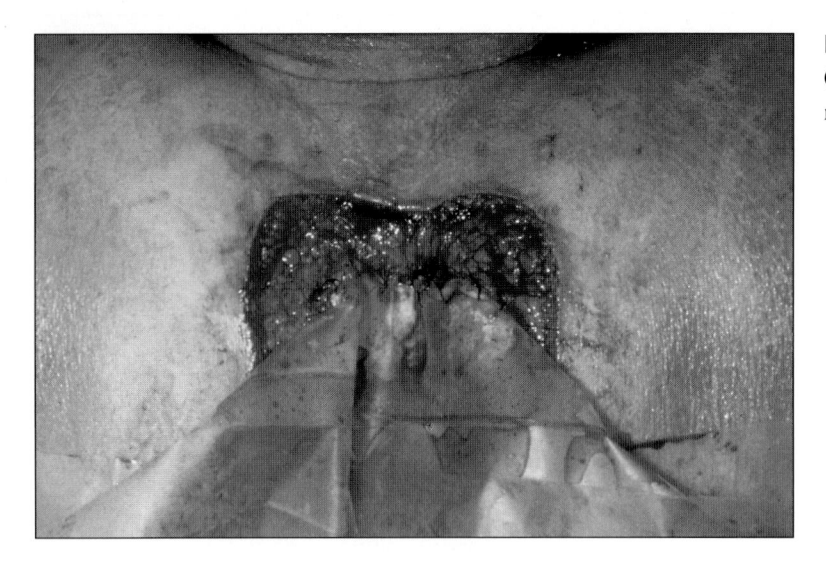

▶ **FIGURE 10-6.** Placement of sterile O'Connor drape. A lubricated O'Connor shield is sutured to the lower wound edge, providing sterile rectal access and allowing intraoperative assessment of the dissection.

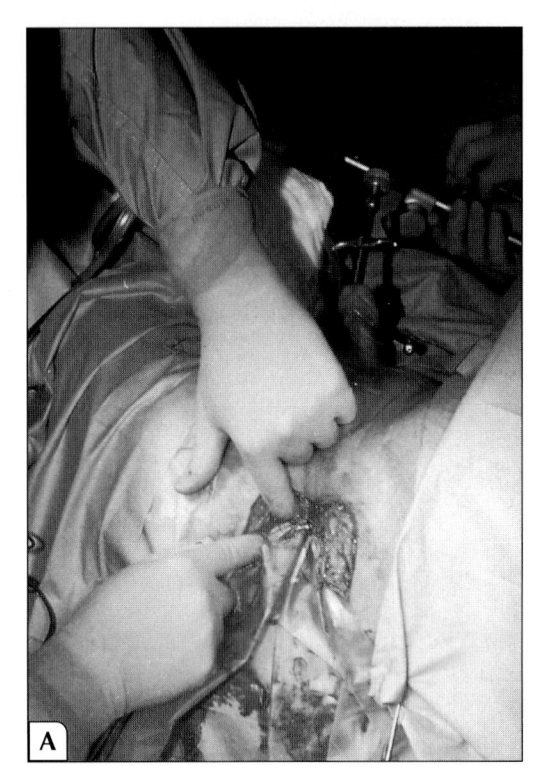

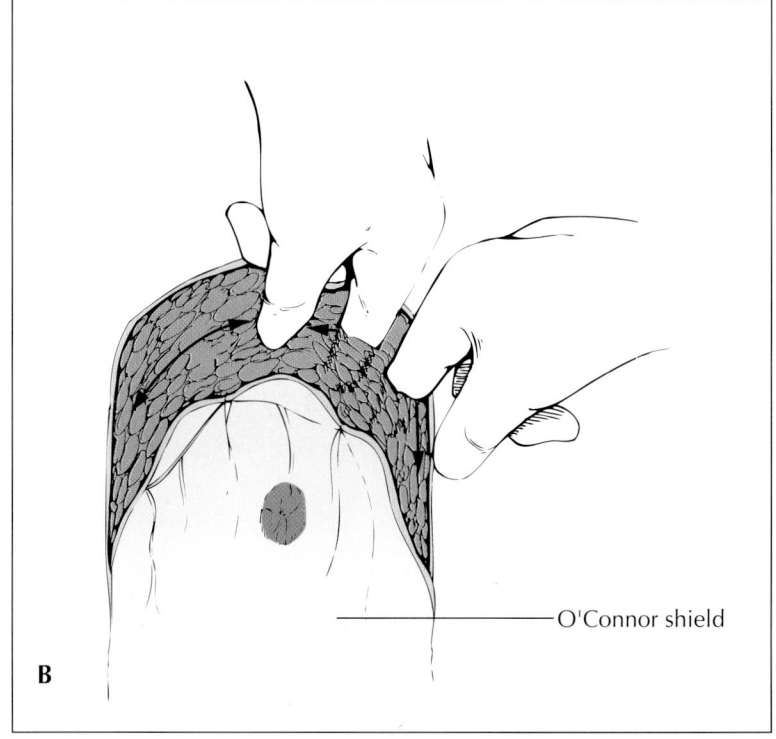

▶ **FIGURE 10-7.** A and B, Incision and blunt dissection of ischiorectal fat. Sharp dissection is used to develop the ischiorectal fossae on either side of the anus. The superficial fasciae is then incised at a 35° angle from the midline, causing the fat of the ischiorectal fossae to "bulge out." Blunt dissection of the remainder of the fossa can be performed by placing both index fingers into the fossa and dissecting superiorly and inferiorly until enough space is provided. Traction on the pudendal nerves and vessels in the apex of the fossa should be avoided. (*Panel B from* Sullivan *et al.* [12]; with permission.)

II. The Prostate

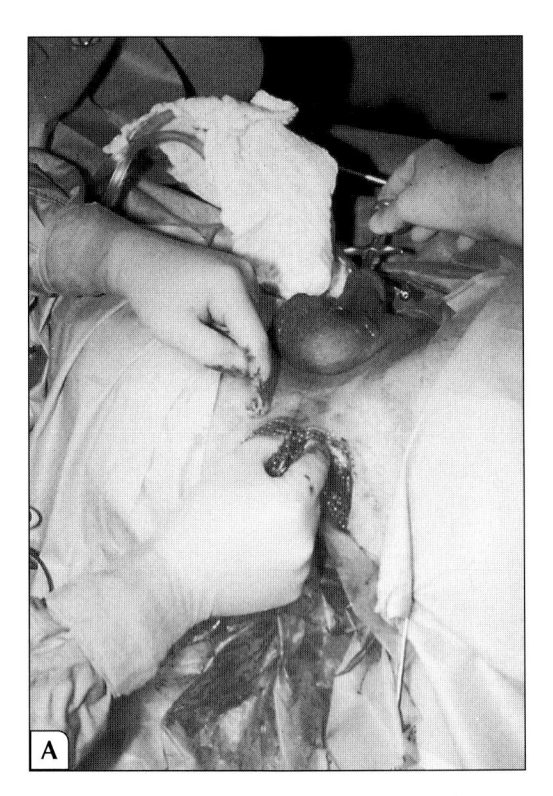

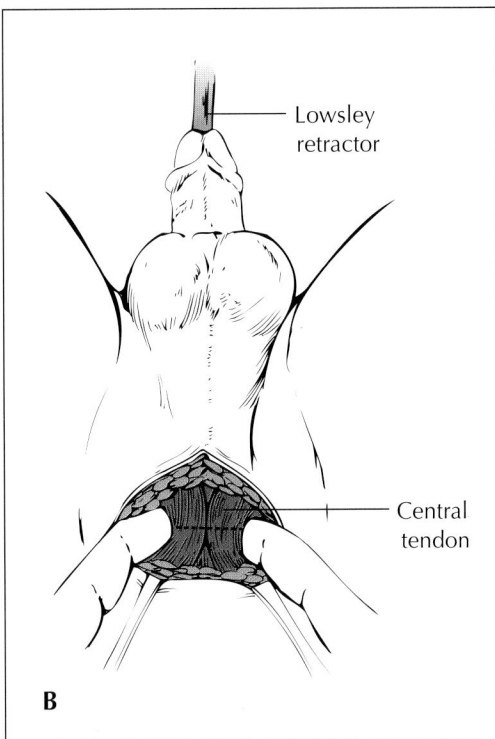

▶ **FIGURE 10-8.** Incision of the central tendon. **A,** The index finger and thumb are used to pinch the tissue in front of the anus and behind the central tendon of the perineum. This creates a safe space behind the tendon. **B,** The tendon can then be incised using cautery (*dotted line*). (*Panel B from* Paulson and Thrasher [13]; with permission.)

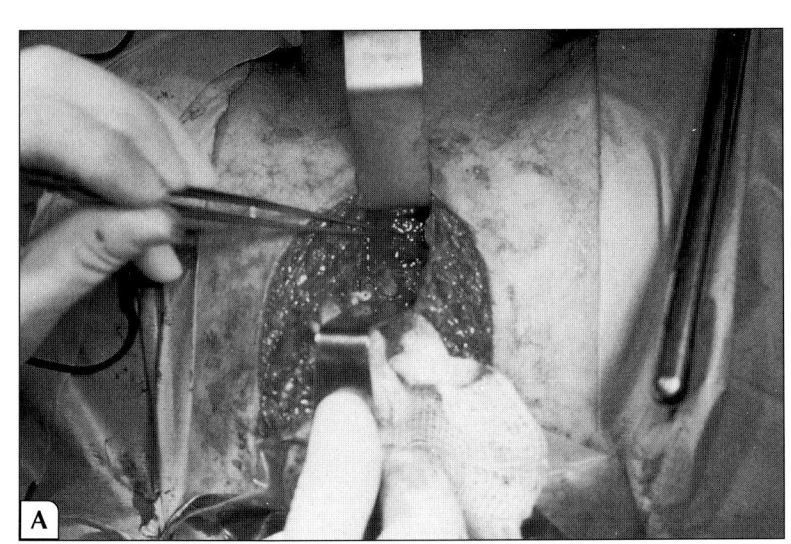

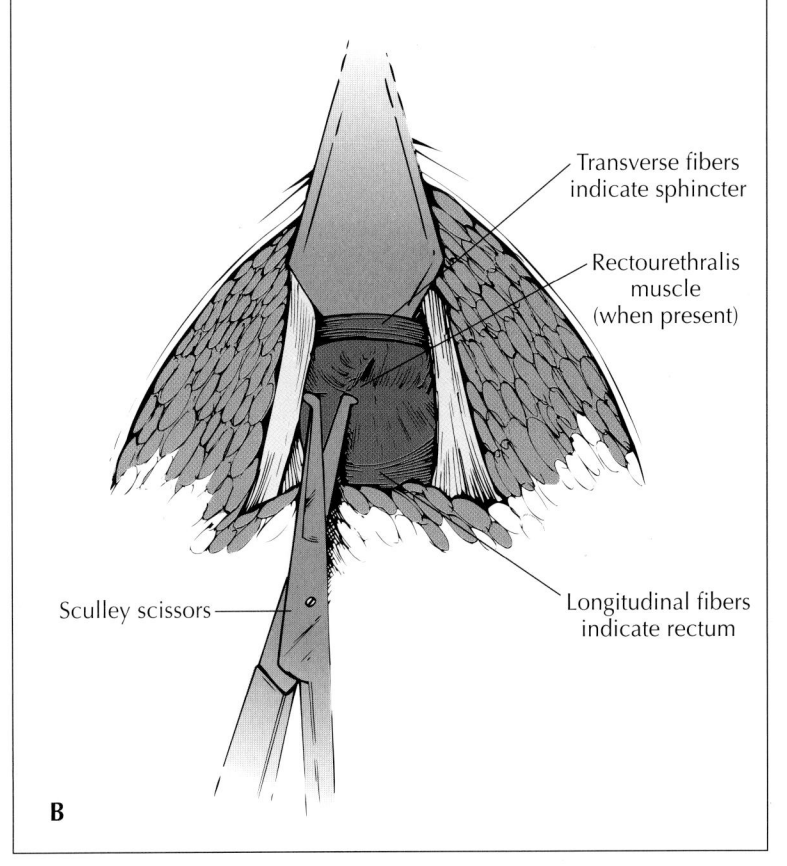

▶ **FIGURE 10-9.** **A** and **B,** Sharp dissection along longitudinal rectal fibers to horizontal fibers of striated sphincter. Horizontal fibers of the external anal sphincter run above the longitudinal rectal fibers and can be readily identified. This junction identifies the transsphincteric approach. Sculley scissors are used to perform a precise dissection along the rectal plane (longitudinal fibers). A retractor is used anteriorly to expose the striated urinary sphincter. The horizontal striated muscle fibers of the urethral sphincter complex are precisely elevated from the longitudinal rectal fibers to expose the apex of the prostate. The prostate can be rotated side to side with the curved Lowsley retractor to bring the prostate closer to the perineum, thus aiding visualization. Sharp and blunt dissection are used to dissect the posterior prostate from the rectum. If the perineal exposure allows, the surgeon has the advantage of taking a wide margin in selected cases, including, if necessary, the anterior rectal fascia, the neurovascular bundles, and even some levator fibers can be left covering the prostate. (*Panel B from* Sullivan *et al.* [12]; with permission.)

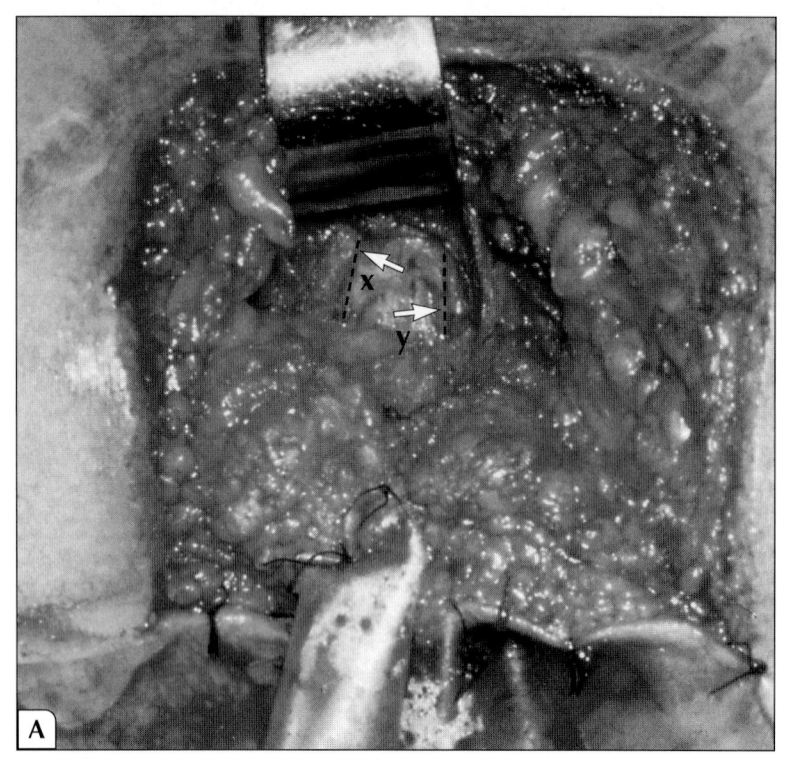

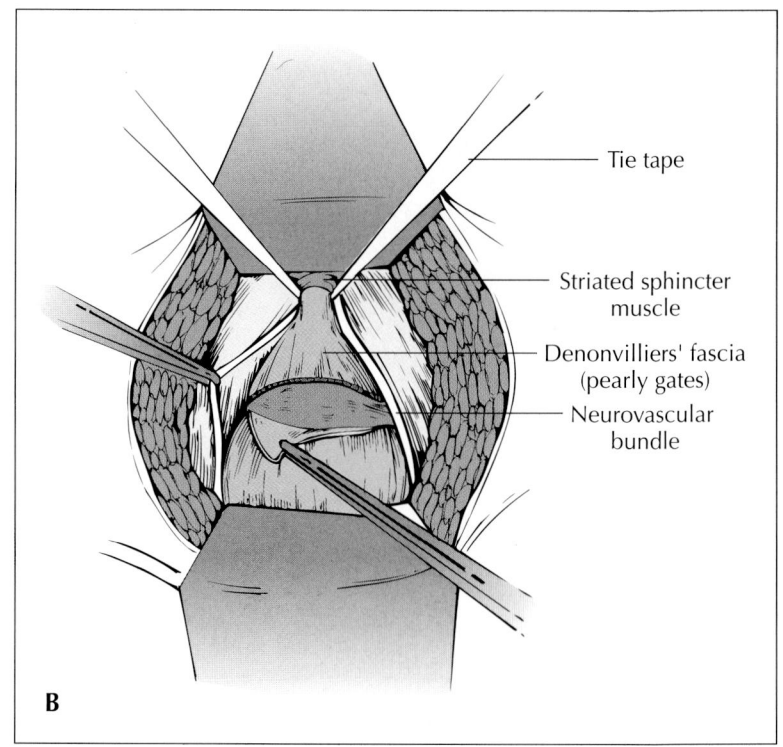

◗ **FIGURE 10-10.** Excision or preservation of neurovascular bundles and incision of posterior urethra. **A,** A Penfield dissector is used to dissect the neurovascular bundles from the posterior prostate (*x* and *y*). These can be resected widely with the prostate or conserved (see Figs 10-24B and 10-24C). Isolation of the neurovascular bundles may be difficult in some cases. During the perineal approach to radical prostatectomy, care should be taken to prevent neuropraxia. Neurovascular bundles may be difficult to isolate or identify in some cases, particularly after transurethral resection of the prostate or irradiation. (*Panel B adapted from* Weldon and Tavel [11].)

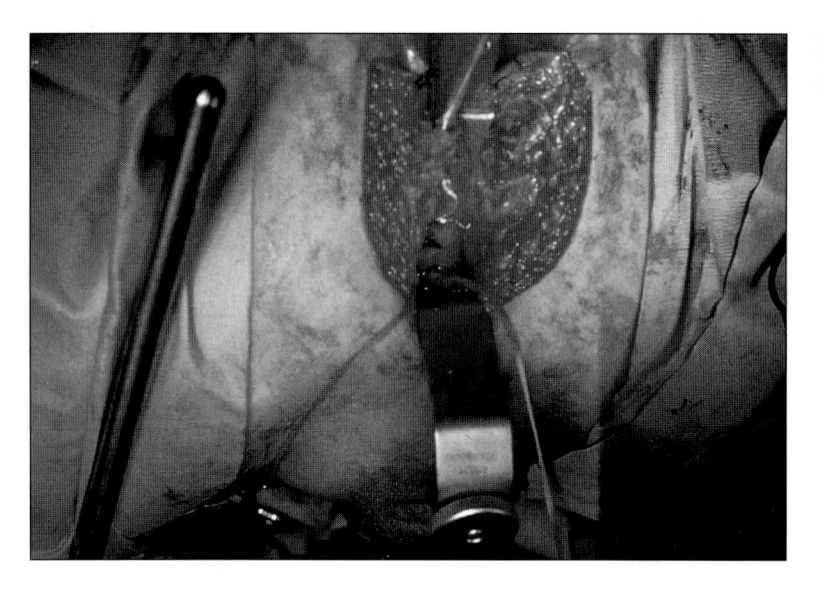

◗ **FIGURE 10-11.** Continuation of procedure. A Lauer forceps is passed around the urethra, and an umbilical tape is placed.

II. The Prostate

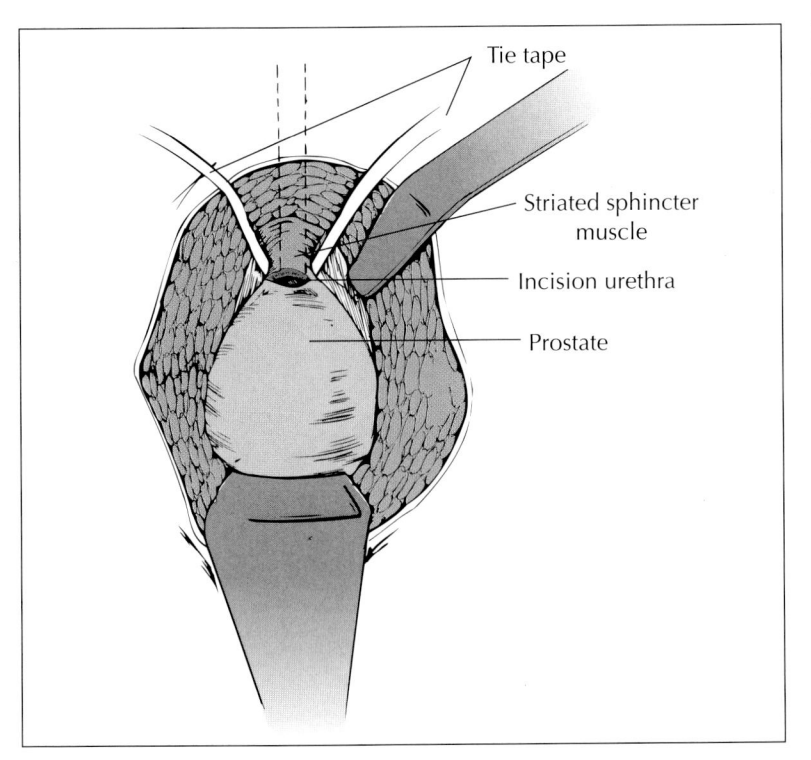

FIGURE 10-12. Division of urethra. The anterior (ventral) urethra is divided precisely at the junction with the prostate. Rush sections of the prostate apex are taken to confirm negative margins. The straight Lowsley retractor is placed into the urethra and the blades opened inside the bladder. The posterior (dorsal) urethra is precisely divided, preserving urethral length and the entire urethral sphincter mechanism. Gentle traction is applied to depress the prostate into the incision. (*Adapted from* Hudson [14]; with permission.)

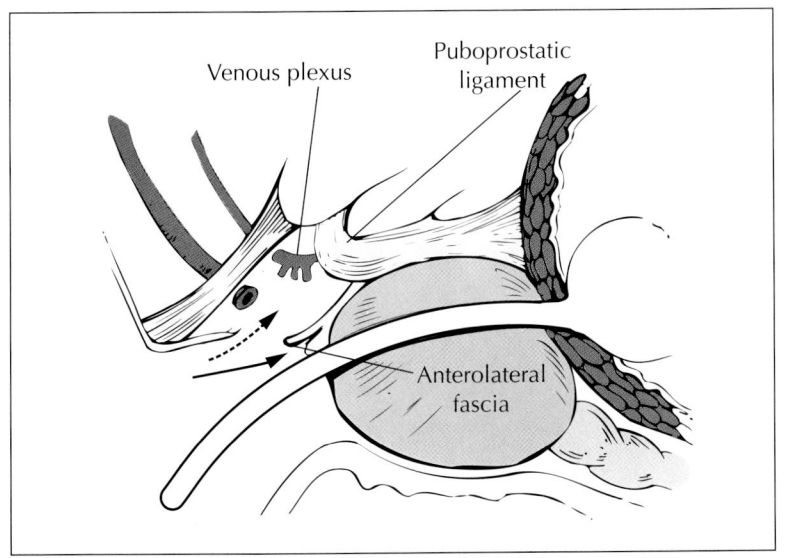

FIGURE 10-13. Retropubic dissection. Proper plane of dissection (*solid arrow*) beneath the anterolateral fascia and beneath the venous plexus. Dissection above this fascia (*dotted arrow*) may disrupt the venous sinus and cause significant bleeding [13]. Blunt dissection of the anterior prostate away from the puboprostatic ligaments is performed. In patients with transitional zone carcinoma, where wide margins are required, sharp dissection is used. (*Adapted from* Paulson and Thrasher [13].)

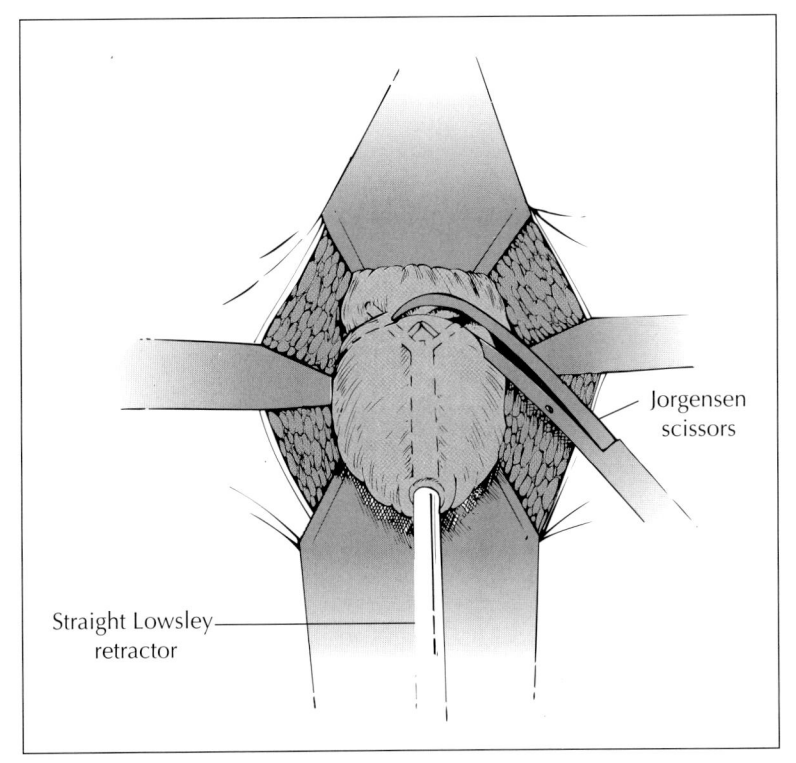

FIGURE 10-14. Lauer forceps are used to take the lateral pedicle of the prostate, including the prostatic arterial supply. These maneuvers facilitate homeostasis and retraction of the prostate into the incision. The blades of the Lowsley retractor become palpable at the bladder neck, and Jorgensen scissors are used to precisely incise the bladder neck. In patients with transition zone cancer, a cuff of anterior bladder neck may be taken with frozen sections to ensure a negative margin. (*Adapted from* Sullivan *et al.* [12]; with permission.)

Radical Perineal Prostatectomy

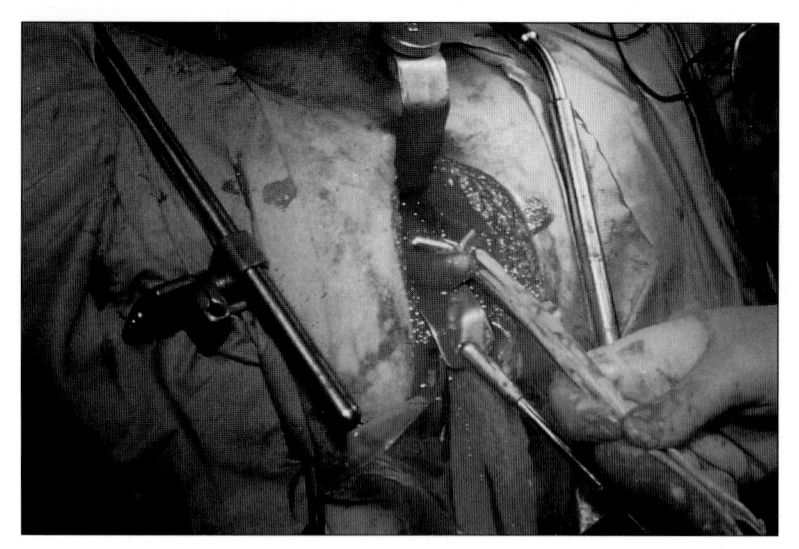

● **FIGURE 10-15.** Continuation of procedure. The Lowsley blades are then repositioned anterior to the bladder neck, exposing the trigone.

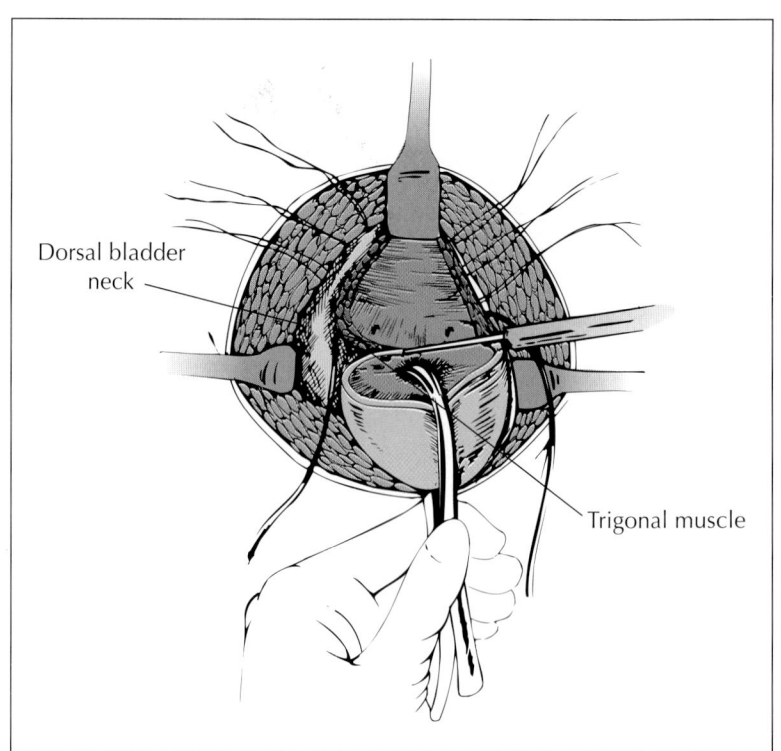

● **FIGURE 10-16.** Incision of the trigone. The trigone and the posterior bladder neck are incised under direct vision. Care must be taken to avoid the ureteric orifices. One ampule of indigo carmine is given intravenously before incision of the trigone. If indigo carmine is unavailable or the ureteric orifices are difficult to see, 4- or 5-F urethral catheters can be inserted. (*Adapted from* Hudson [14]; with permission.)

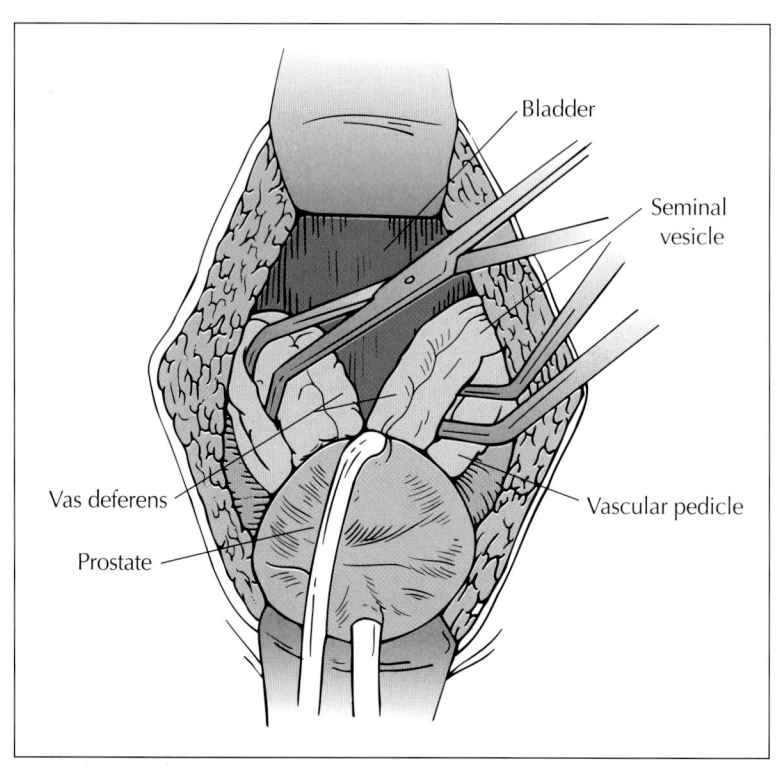

● **FIGURE 10-17.** Completion of dissection of pedicles, ejaculatory ducts, and seminal vesicles. Dissection is carried posteriorly, and seminal vesicles and ampullae of the vas deferens are dissected, clipped, and excised. Adequate retraction is essential. Parker or Deaver retractors may be needed to facilitate exposure and complete removal of the vesicles. Care is taken to avoid rectal or trigonal injury or traction on the neurovascular bundles if nerve sparing is a priority. (*Adapted from* Paulson and Thrasher [13]; with permission.)

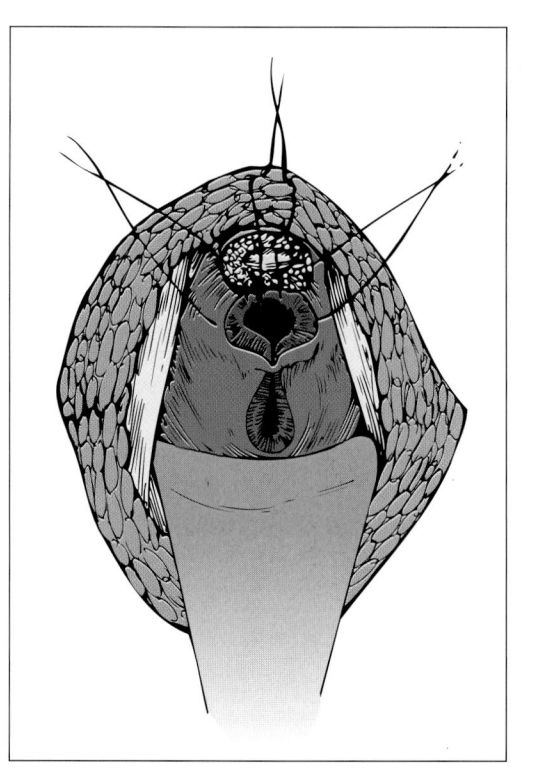

● **FIGURE 10-18.** Bladder neck reconstruction. The posterior bladder neck is closed with interrupted 2-0 chromic sutures, and the mucosa is everted over the bladder neck muscle and then closed with 4-0 chromic sutures to cover the bladder neck. (*Adapted from* Hinman [15]; with permission.)

II. The Prostate

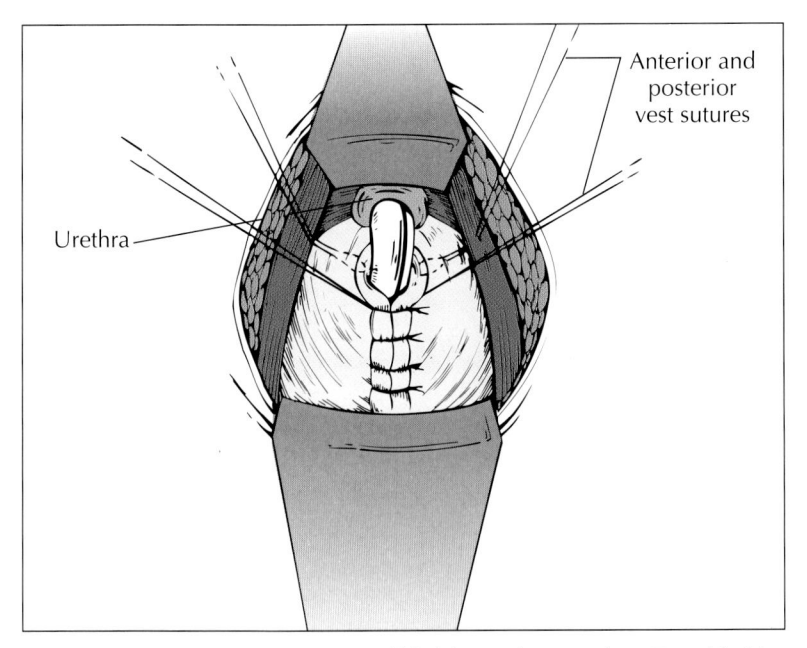

▶ **FIGURE 10-19.** Anastomosis of bladder neck to urethra. Four bladder neck sutures are left long for vest sutures. Urethrovesical anastomosis is performed using 2-0 chromic sutures anteriorly, and a 20-F Foley catheter is passed into the bladder. Posterior sutures are then tied, allowing direct visualization of the anastomosis. Vest sutures are passed through the superficial perineal muscles and lightly tied as stay sutures. (*Adapted from* Sullivan *et al.* [12]; with permission.)

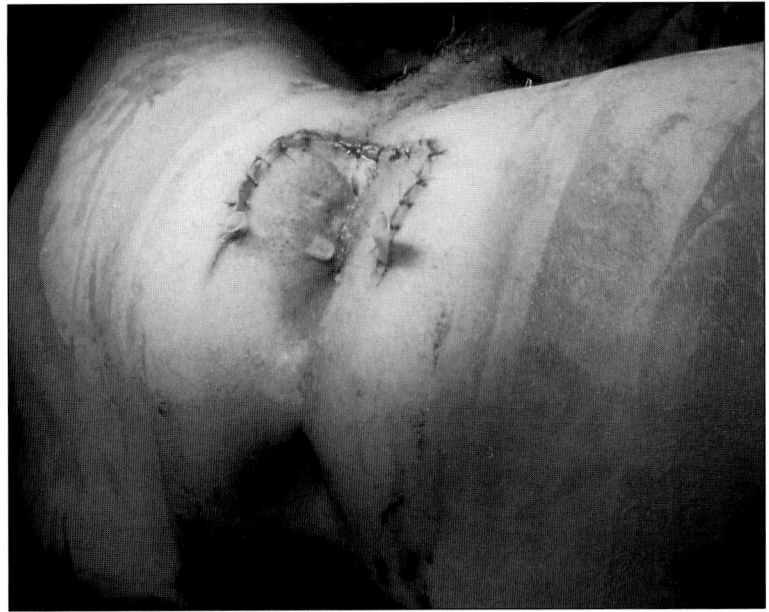

▶ **FIGURE 10-20.** Closure of central tendon and skin. The central tendon is closed with 2-0 chromic interrupted sutures. Two one-quarter inch Penrose drains are placed into the ischiorectal fossae, and the skin is then closed with 3-0 chromic sutures. Bupivacaine 1% is injected into the posterior aspect of the wound, and a single 50-mg diclofenac sodium suppository is placed in the rectum. The wound is appropriately dressed.

Incidence of Complications

	Sullivan et al.*†	Frazier et al. [16]	Harris and Thompson [17]	Mokulis and Thompson [18]
Fistula	1 (1.3)	1 (1)	1 (1)	2 (1.7)
Rectal injury	2 (2.5)	NA	NA	12 (10)
Urethral stricture	15 (19)	8 (7)	5 (5)	NA
Wound infection	1 (1.3)	1 (.8)	3 (3)	1 (.8)
Blood transfusions	1 (1.3)	NA	16 (16.7)	6 (5)

*Numbers in columns express number of patients and percentage (in parentheses).
†Unpublished data.

▶ **FIGURE 10-21.** Incidence of complications. The perineal approach results in few local complications. Urethral strictures occur in between 5% and 15% of patients and are easily managed with dilation performed in an outpatient or clinic setting. Rectal injury in the University of British Columbia (UBC) series occurred in only two patients: one following previous transurethral resection of the prostate, and one in a patient who underwent salvage prostatectomy [13]. The incidence of wound infection and fistulas is low. Additional complications occurring in the UBC series at a low incidence rate included perineal hematoma (1.3%), thrombosed external hemorrhoids (1.3%), ileus lasting 7 days (1.3%), and transient hydronephrosis caused by a small ureteral calculus requiring a temporary percutaneous nephrostomy tube. In most series the rate of blood transfusions is low. NA—not applicable.

Rate of Incontinence

Continent: 89% (*n* = 70/79)
Safety pads or stress incontinence: 9% (*n* = 7/79)
Severe incontinence (continuous pads): 3% (*n* = 2/79)

▶ **FIGURE 10-22.** Rate of incontinence. In the series by Sullivan *et al.* (Unpublished data) patients were assessed for continence 1 year postoperatively as part of a quality-of-life questionnaire (UCLA/RAND Prostate Cancer Index), which was independently reviewed. Thirty-six of 47 patients who were 1 year postoperative responded. The results were compared with the cohort of retropubic prostatectomy patients who were studied at the same time. There was no significant difference in overall scores between groups ($P = 0.79$).

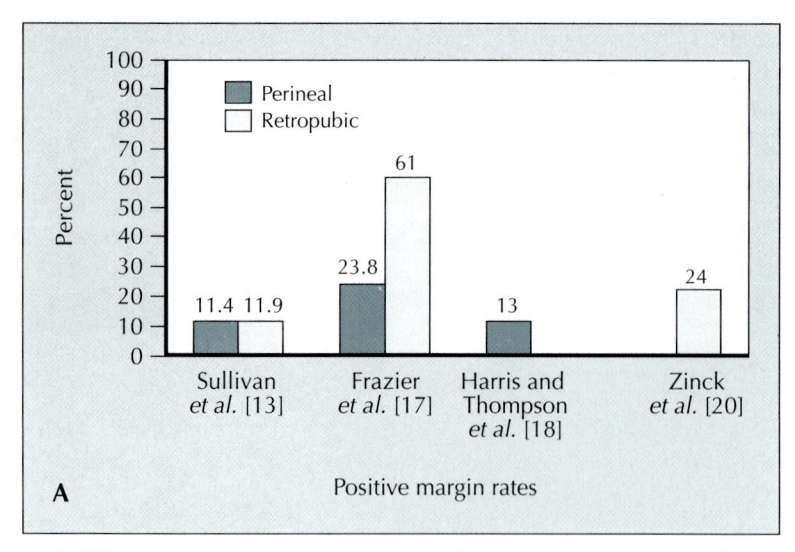

FIGURE 10-23. Cancer control rates. Positive margin rates (*panel A*) and prostate-specific antigen (PSA) detectability (>0.2 ng/mL) (*panel B*) are shown for Sullivan *et al.* (Unpublished data) and other series [16–20]. At the University of British Columbia (UBC) (Sullivan *et al.*, Unpublished data) there was no statistically significant difference in positive margin rates (chi-squared test, P=0.9) or PSA detectability (Kaplan-Meier log-rank test, P=0.44) between radical perineal and radical retropubic prostatectomy patients. Note that 77.2% of the perineal patients and 71.1% of the retropubic patients in the UBC series were treated with neoadjuvant hormones according to various protocols, which may explain the lower positive margin rates compared with that of other series. No clinical recurrence has been seen in this series of patients.

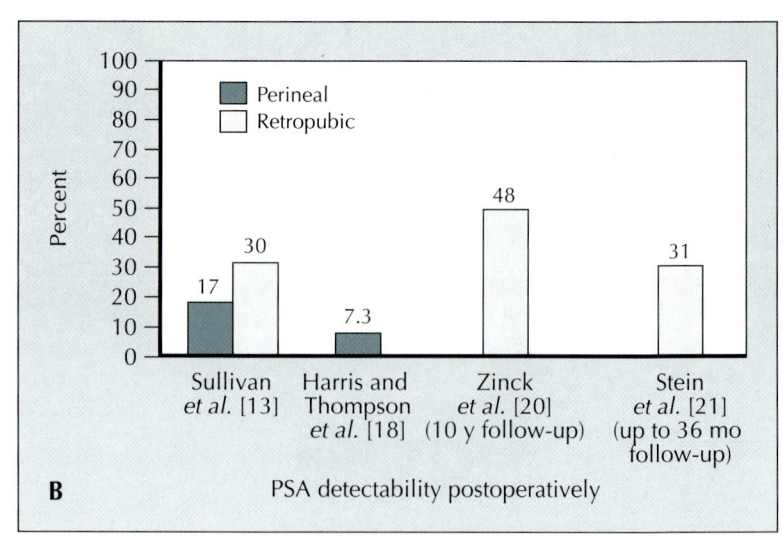

A. Recent Modifications to the Perineal Approach

Precise location of skin incision
Wide excision of the layer of tissue around the prostate in selected cases
Unilateral or bilateral nerve sparing

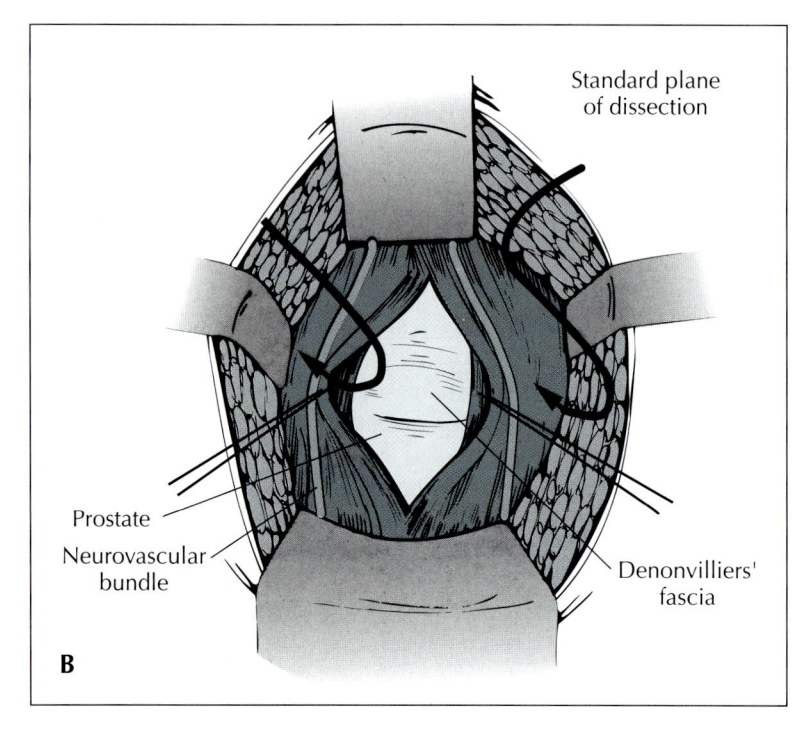

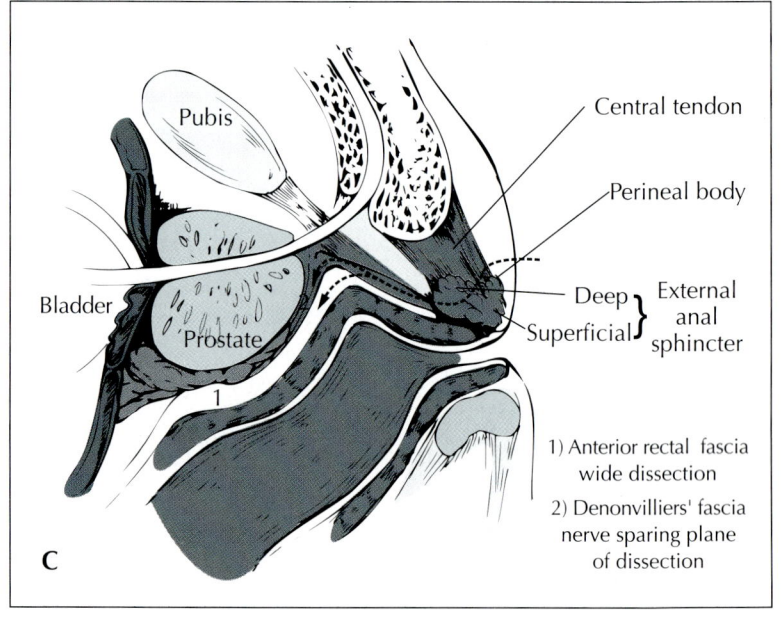

FIGURE 10-24. Recent modifications to the perineal approach. Modifications have been made to the perineal approach to radical prostatectomy since the mid-1990s (*panel A*). Attempts have been made to ensure a more precise location of the skin incision to position the surgeon reliably in the space between the superficial external sphincter and the longitudinal muscle fibers of the ureter (*panel B*; see Fig. 10-5).

In addition, attempts have been made to perform a wide excision of the layers of tissue around the prostate in selected cases in which positive margins are a potential concern. This allows the surgeon to remove the Denonvilliers' fascia completely, as well as, in selected cases, a layer of the rectal fascia, one or both of the neurovascular bundles, and some levator tissue en bloc, providing a wide surgical margin (*panel C*).

A third modification includes unilateral or bilateral nerve sparing, which can be performed as described by Weldon and Tavel [11]. Avoidance of traction on these nerves is essential. (*Panel C from* Sullivan *et al.* [12]; with permission.)

Management Options for Recurrent Disease

Watchful waiting
Adjuvant hormonal therapy
Radiotherapy

FIGURE 10-25. Management of recurrent disease. Patients should be followed carefully with postoperative prostate-specific antigen (PSA) tests at 3, 6, and 12 months, and then yearly thereafter. Digital rectal examinations should be performed once a year. Patients with a positive prostate-specific antigen test (>0.2 ng/mL) are offered watchful waiting or adjuvant hormonal therapy for a minimum of 6 months. If the PSA level rises again after 6 months of hormonal therapy, patients are offered intermittent hormone therapy [22]. Radiotherapy may be offered if there is positive, biopsy-proven local disease, but only after careful discussion with the patient about the risks related to continence and potency [23].

Preoperative Neoadjuvant Androgen Withdrawal Therapy: Effects on Prostate-specific Antigen Level

PSA reduction	84% reduction after 1 mo preoperative therapy; further 52% reduction after 3 to 8 mo of therapy
Time to reach nadir (<0.1 ng/mL):	
3 mo	22% of all patients
5 mo	42% of all patients
8 mo	84% of all patients
Positive margin rates	Overall, 4%

FIGURE 10-26. The effects of 8 months of preoperative neoadjuvant androgen withdrawal therapy before radical prostatectomy [24]. It has been shown that 8 months of neoadjuvant therapy results in low nadir prostate-specific antigen (PSA) levels preoperatively in the majority of patients, as well as low positive margin rates. The effect on survival remains unknown. It has also been shown, however, that patients with a PSA level of less than 4.0 ng/mL are likely to have organ-confined disease and are unlikely to benefit from preoperative neoadjuvant therapy [25].

REFERENCES

1. Young HH: The early diagnosis and radical cure of carcinoma of the prostate: being a study of 40 cases and presentation of a radical operation which was carried out in four cases. *Johns Hopkins Hosp Bull* 1905, 16:315–321.
2. Belt E, Ebert CE, Scurber AC, Jr: New anatomic approach to perineal prostatectomy. *J Urol* 1939, 41:482–497.
3. Jewett HJ: Radical perineal prostatectomy for palpable, clinically localized, non-obstructive cancer: experience at the Johns Hopkins Hospital 1909–1963. *J Urol* 1980, 124:492–494.
4. Gibbons RP, Correa RJ, Jr, Bannen GE, Weissman RM: Total prostatectomy for clinically localized prostatic cancer: long-term results. *J Urol* 1989, 141:564–566.
5. Paulson DF, Moul JW, Malther PJ: Radical prostatectomy for clinical stage T1-2N0M0 prostatic adenocarcinoma: long-term results. *J Urol* 1990, 144:1180–1184.
6. Sogani PC, Whitmore WF, Jr, Jilaris BS, Batata MA: Experience with interstitial implantation of iodine 125 in the treatment of prostatic carcinoma. *Scand J Urol Nephrol* 1980, 55 (suppl):205–211.
7. Denella JF, deKernion JB, Smith RB, Steckel J: Contemporary incidence of lymph node metastases in prostate cancer. *J Urol* 1993, 149:1488–1491.
8. Sullivan LD, Rabbani F: Should we reconsider the indications for ileo-obturator node dissection with localized prostate cancer? *Br J Urol* 1995, 75:3337.
9. Bluestein DL, Bostwick DG, Bergstralh EJ, Oesterling JE: Eliminating the need for bilateral pelvic lymphadenectomy in select patients with prostate cancer. *J Urol* 1994, 151:1315–1320.
10. Narayan P, Fournier G, Gajendran V, et al.: Utility of preoperative serum prostate-specific antigen concentration and biopsy Gleason score in predicting risk of pelvic lymph node metastases in prostate cancer. *Urology* 1994, 44:519–524.
11. Weldon VE, Tavel FR: Potency sparing radical perineal prostatectomy. *J Urol* 1988, 140:559–562.
12. Sullivan LD, Kinahan JF, Leone E: Radical perineal prostatectomy: a simplified approach. *Can J Urol* 1997, 4:386–391.
13. Paulson DF, Thrasher JB: Reappraisal of radical perineal prostatectomy. *Eur Urol* 1992, 22:1–8.
14. Hudson PB: Perineal prostatectomy. In *Campbell's Urology*, edn 5, vol 3. Edited by Walsh PC, Gittes RF, Perlmutter AD, Stamey TA. Philadelphia: WB Saunders; 1986:2776–2814.
15. Hinman F, Jr: Simple perineal prostatectomy. In *Atlas of Urologic Surgery*. Philadelphia: WB Saunders; 1989: 333–337.
16. Frazier HA, Robertson JE, Paulson DF: Radical prostatectomy: the pros and cons of the perineal versus retropubic approach. *J Urol* 1992, 147:888–890.
17. Harris JH, Thompson IM, Jr: The anatomic radical perineal prostatectomy: a contemporary and anatomic approach. *Urology* 1996, 48:762–768.
18. Mokulis J, Thompson I: Radical prostatectomy: is the perineal approach more difficult to learn? *J Urol* 1997, 157:230–232.
19. Zinck H, Oesterling JE, Blute ML, et al.: Long-term (15 years) results after radical prostatectomy for clinically localized (stage T2C or lower) prostate cancer. *J Urol* 1994, 152:1850–1857.
20. Stein A, deKernion JB, Dorey F: Prostatic specific antigen related to clinical status 1 to 14 years after radical retropubic prostatectomy. *Br J Urol* 1991, 67:626–631.
21. Paulson DF: Perineal surgery for prostatic carcinoma. In *The Perineum in Genitourinary Surgery*.
22. Akakura K, Bruchovsky N, Goldenberg SL, et al.: Effects of intermittent androgen suppression on androgen-dependent tumors: apoptosis and serum prostate-specific antigen. *Cancer* 1993, 71:278–290.
23. Syndikus I, Pickles T, Kostashuck E, Sullivan LD: Postoperative radiotherapy for stage pT3 carcinoma of the prostate: improved local control. *J Urol* 1996, 155:1983–1986.
24. Gleave ME, Goldenberg SL, Jones EC, et al.: Biochemical and pathological effects of 8 months of neoadjuvant androgen withdrawal therapy before radical prostatectomy in patients with clinically confined prostate cancer. *J Urol* 1996, 155:213–219.
25. Rabbani F, Sullivan LD, Goldenberg SL, Stothers L: Neoadjuvant androgen deprivation therapy before radical prostatectomy: who is unlikely to benefit? *Br J Urol* 1997, 79:221–225.

Nerve-sparing Radical Retropubic Prostatectomy

CANCEROUS DISEASE SECTION

Alan M.F. Stapleton & Peter T. Scardino

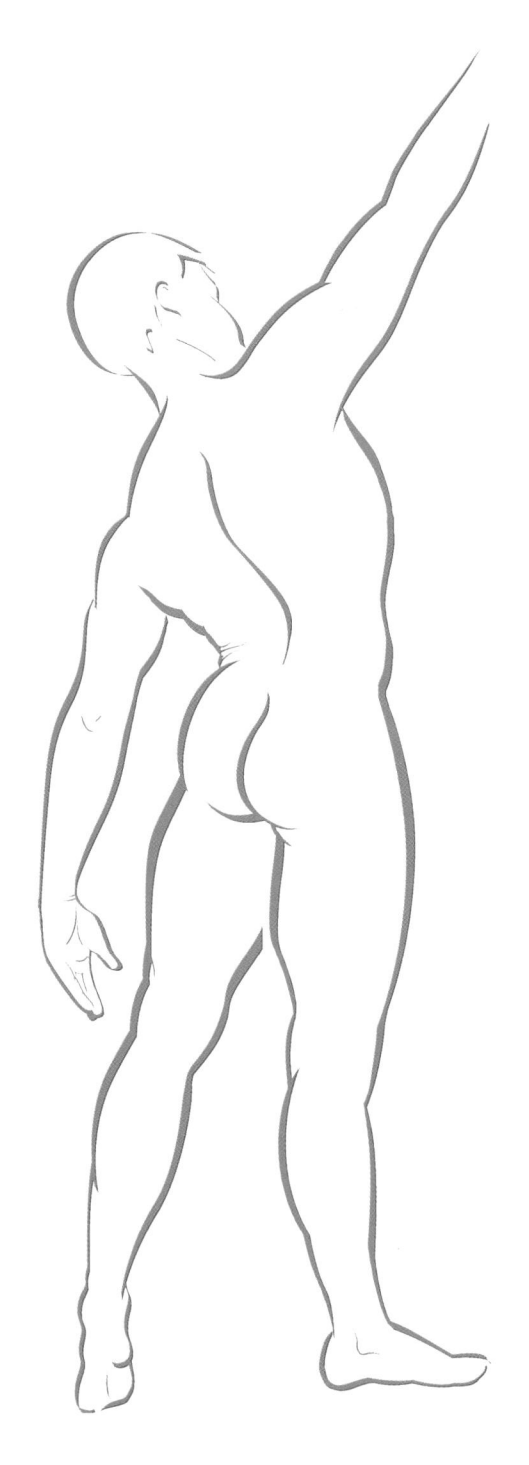

Prostate cancer is the leading internal malignancy diagnosed, and the second most common cause of cancer death in men in the United States [1]. Radical retropubic prostatectomy (RRP) can readily cure men with prostate cancer that is confined to the gland or immediate periprostatic tissue. Some controversy surrounds the selection of men who might benefit from this procedure given that there is considerable discordance between those with histologic evidence of prostate cancer (30% to 40% in men over age 50) [2,3] and those who develop clinically significant disease (10% to 20%) [4,5]. A detailed discussion of this point can be found in other sources [6–9].

The vast majority of prostate cancers detected by current diagnostic tests are clinically significant [10–12] and curative therapy in the form of RRP is a very effective treatment option for men with localized disease and a life expectancy of 10 or more years. An individual's comorbid features represent more important criteria for exclusion from surgical management than a definite age restriction. The average life expectancy of a 70-year-old American man today is 13 years [13], and the trend of improved life expectancy is predicted to continue. In contrast, the average man aged 65, 70, or 75 years with clinically localized prostate cancer of moderate grade treated conservatively can expect to lose 4.5, 4, and 3.3 years of life, respectively [8].

It is common practice to measure the efficacy of surgery not on patient survival (because of additional unrelated therapeutic options [*eg*, hormonal manipulation]), but on the presence and persistent rise of the serum prostate specific antigen (PSA) level postoperatively. The PSA level should remain in the undetectable range if all prostatic elements have been resected. Our analysis of 672 patients with clinically localized prostate cancer (T1 to 2, NXM0) treated by Scardino with intent to treat by RRP between 1983 and 1997 has revealed that the actuarial 5- and 10-year PSA-based nonprogression rates are 81% and 79%, respectively [14]. These data and those of others [15–19] strengthen the case for operative management of localized prostate cancer.

In this chapter we illustrate in detail our surgical technique for RRP in a patient with a high-grade palpable tumor on the right side of the prostate adjacent to the neurovascular bundle; hence, the left nerve is spared and the neurovascular bundle on the right is completely resected.

PREOPERATIVE CONSIDERATIONS

Preoperative Considerations Regarding RRP

Long-term complications	Microscopic hematuria	Pelvic lymph node dissection	Coexistent urologic disease	Anesthesia
Autologous blood banking	Thromboembolic disease	Antibiotic prophylaxis	Intestinal preparation	

▶ **FIGURE 11-1.** Long-term complications of RRP include urinary incontinence and erectile dysfunction. Patients incontinent before the operation will almost all remain incontinent afterward. Although the overall rate of severe incontinence is only 1% and stress incontinence 4% [25], the rate of incontinence varies with patient age, resection of the neurovascular bundles, and development of an anastomotic stricture. Similarly, many patients will recover erectile function after the operation, but risk factors for persistent erectile dysfunction include increasing patient age, status of erections before the operation, and degree of resection of the neurovascular bundles. The risks associated with these conditions need to be discussed with the patient preoperatively.

Intraoperative blood loss during RRP has been substantially reduced, largely because of the improved understanding of dorsal vein anatomy [20] and subsequent refinements of operative technique [21]. Intraoperative blood loss is on average less than 1 L [18,22]. In our series, only 11% of patients who did not donate preoperatively required allogeneic blood, whereas 30% of those who banked autologous blood were transfused [23]. A recent cost-benefit analysis indicates that advice in favor of autologous blood donation cannot be supported; however, an individual's request should be accommodated. Aspirin and nonsteroidal anti-inflammatory medications ought to be withheld for 10 days prior to surgery to improve the functional characteristics of platelets. Such medication can be safely restarted in the early postoperative period.

Microscopic hematuria, sometimes associated with prostate cancer, should be evaluated with cystoscopy and intravenous pyelogram preoperatively. The use of antibiotic prophylaxis is recommended for RRP, a "clean-contaminated" procedure. The initial dose of a broad-spectrum antibiotic with activity against common skin and uropathogens should be given intravenously at induction of anesthesia to achieve a satisfactory serum level at the time of the incision.

The use of prophylaxis against deep vein thrombosis and pulmonary embolism associated with RRP remains controversial [26]. Dorsiflexion exercises of the lower limb and early ambulation are to be encouraged; however, the use of compression devices to the lower limbs intraoperatively has not demonstrably lowered the risk of thromboembolic events [27].

Radical retropubic prostatectomy does offer several advantages over the perineal approach, including the opportunity to perform a pelvic lymph node dissection through the same incision. We no longer routinely perform frozen sections unless the nodes are grossly enlarged and highly suspicious for cancer, since the risk of positive nodes is only 2% to 3% today. We advocate the use of gross examination rather than frozen sections when the clinical stage is T2b, the PSA is less than 10 ng/mL and no high-grade cancer is present in the biopsy specimen, since the risk of detecting nodal disease in this group is less than 0.5% [28]. If the metastatic prostate cancer is diagnosed, the prostatectomy is abandoned. While lymph node metastases are not curable, patients with microscopic positive nodes survive for a median of more than 10 years and receive substantial palliative benefit for removal of the primary tumor. Other advantages of the retropubic approach include the more familiar anatomy, more consistent success with preservation of the neurovascular bundles, and greater flexibility to adapt the operation to the extent of each individual's cancer, minimizing risks of positive surgical margins.

The presence of synchronous urologic disease needs careful preoperative evaluation. A history of prior transurethral prostatic surgery is associated with diminished post-RRP urinary control, as are symptoms of bladder dysfunction such as urge incontinence [25]. The risks associated with these conditions need to be discussed with the patient preoperatively.

The use of antibiotic prophylaxis for major surgery is widespread and is recommended for RRP. The initial dose of a broad-spectrum antibiotic with good activity against common skin and uropathogens should be given to achieve a satisfactory serum level at the time of the incision (orally with anesthetic premedication, or more reliably by the intravenous route at induction of anesthesia). A second dose may not be advantageous, especially if the half-life of the antibiotic suggests more than 12 hours of adequate serum levels.

A liquid diet is recommended for the 24 hours prior to surgery and we routinely prepare the lower bowel with a phosphate enema on the morning of surgery. We recommend the routine use of stool-softening medication postoperatively.

General anesthesia with muscle relaxation allows for adequate pelvic exposure. The preoperative placement of an epidural catheter for supplementary anesthesia allows intraoperative controlled hypotension that can reduce blood loss, and also allows highly effective postoperative pain management. The catheter is typically withdrawn on or before postoperative day 2.

OPERATIVE TECHNIQUE

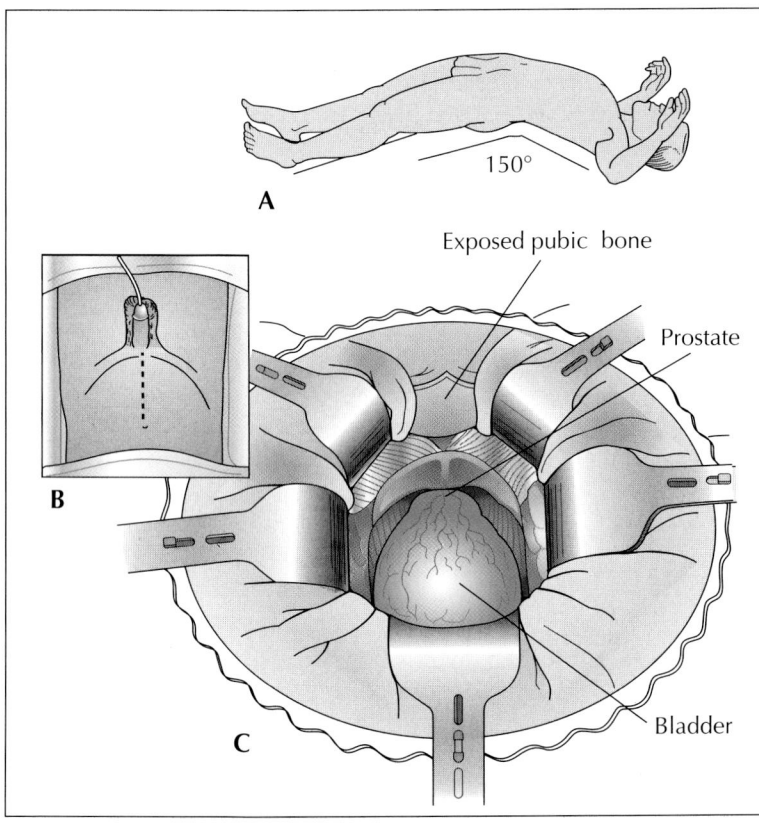

▶ **FIGURE 11-2.** Patient positioning. The patient is positioned supine with the table maximally flexed (~150°) and in mild Trendelenburg (**A**). The arms are abducted and externally rotated 90° with the elbows flexed at 90°, and the wrists fixed to a frame that is positioned across the head of the patient. A midline infraumbilical incision (**B**) and ring retractor provide adequate exposure of the pelvis (**C**).

Through a suprapubic midline incision that reaches toward the umbilicus, the transversalis fascia is incised sharply and the retropubic space entered. Care is taken not to sweep perivesical lymph nodes cephalad as the lateral pelvic walls are exposed back to the level of the obliterated umbilical arteries. A Turner Warwick self-retaining retractor (as shown) is a satisfactory device to provide adequate pelvic exposure. In those men with a narrow pelvis, additional exposure can be gained by releasing the medial attachments of the rectus abdominus tendons to the pubis. Occasionally, a bony spur protruding from behind the symphysis pubis will compromise the view of the prostatic apex; this can easily be removed using an osteotome and mallet.

Bilateral pelvic lymph node dissection is performed. Fatty tissue posterolateral to the prostate is also included with the nodal tissue and then the cleared endopelvic fascia is inspected. In an attempt to reduce intraoperative blood loss, bulldog clamps are placed across the hypogastric arteries just distal to the obliterated umbilical artery (see Fig. 11-3). Such application has not been consistently shown to reduce intraoperative bleeding [29,30], but because placement is generally easily and safely executed, we continue to recommend this maneuver.

The loose fatty tissue behind the symphysis pubis is gently teased out using nontoothed forceps to expose the superficial dorsal venous plexus. The prostate is mobilized by dividing the endopelvic fascia laterally, initially by puncturing with closed scissors into the deep natural groove between the prostate and the pelvic side wall (see Fig. 11-4), then by sharp dissection under vision distally and by blunt finger dissection posteriorly (see Fig. 11-5).

▶ **FIGURE 11-3.** The anatomic structures relevant to the pelvic lymph node dissection (**A**) and the position of a bulldog clamp on the distal right hypogastric artery (**B**). Bilateral pelvic lymph node dissection is performed. Fatty tissue posterolateral to the prostate is also included with the nodal tissue and then the cleared endopelvic fascia is inspected. To reduce intraoperative blood loss, bulldog clamps are placed across the hypogastric arteries just distal to the obliterated umbilical artery. Such application may reduce intraoperative bleeding [29,30], and placement is generally safe and easy. If the clamps are placed too far proximally, the abundant collateral circulation may lessen the effect.

Nerve-sparing Radical Retropubic Prostatectomy

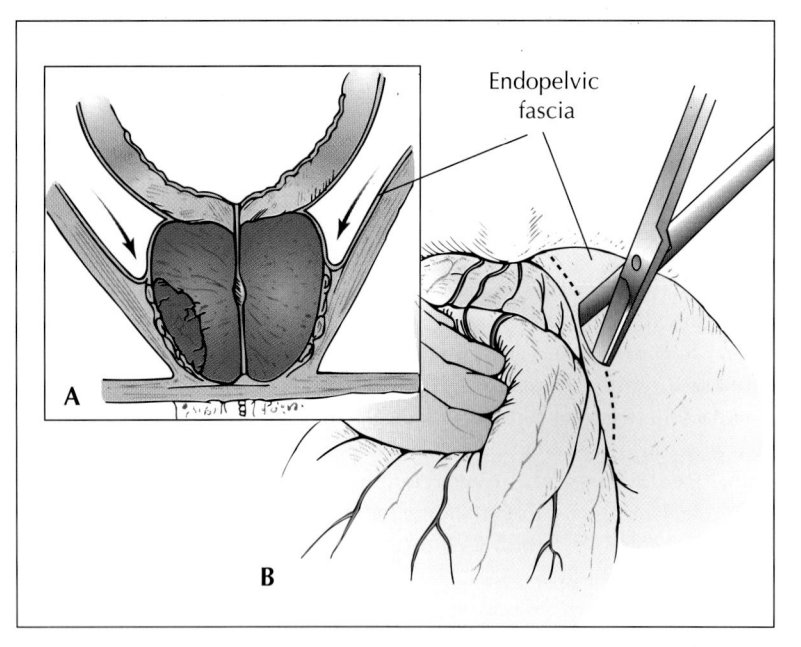

▶ **FIGURE 11-4.** Penetration of the endopelvic fascia with closed scissors deep in its caudal groove, adjacent to the midprostate. The loose fatty tissue behind the symphysis pubis is gently teased out using nontoothed forceps to expose the superficial dorsal venous plexus (**A**). The prostate is mobilized by dividing the endopelvic fascia laterally, initially by puncturing with closed scissors into the deep natural groove between the prostate and the pelvic side wall, then by sharp dissection under vision distally and by blunt finger dissection posteriorly (**B**) (see Fig. 11-5).

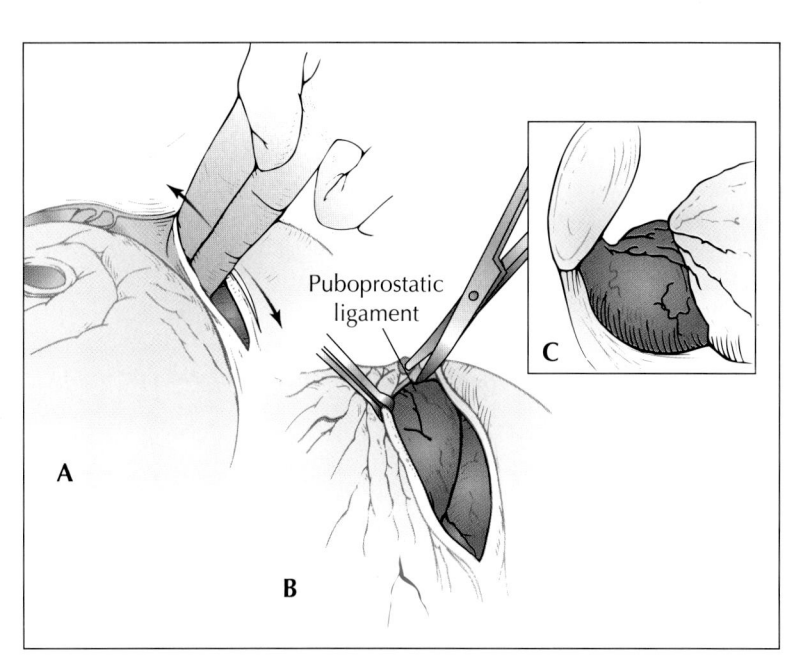

▶ **FIGURE 11-5.** Division of the endopelvic fascia in an anterior and posterior direction using both blunt finger (**A**) and sharp (**B**) dissection. Careful dissection with a Kitner (peanut) dissector (**C**) near the apex of the prostate can help delineate small branching vessels from the levator muscles that can be controlled with clips prior to the complete division of the puboprostatic ligaments. These ligaments are then divided sharply as close to the pubic bone as possible.

The puboprostatic ligaments are divided with scissors close to their bony origins. Venous channels can often be seen passing laterally from the tissue that surrounds the apex of the prostate and these can often be plied away from the prostate toward the levator ani muscle with gentle use of the peanut dissector, or alternatively, isolated and divided between small clips. The prostate is then carefully palpated for induration. This information, combined with preoperative information regarding the location of the cancer, will determine the feasibility and safety of a nerve-sparing procedure.

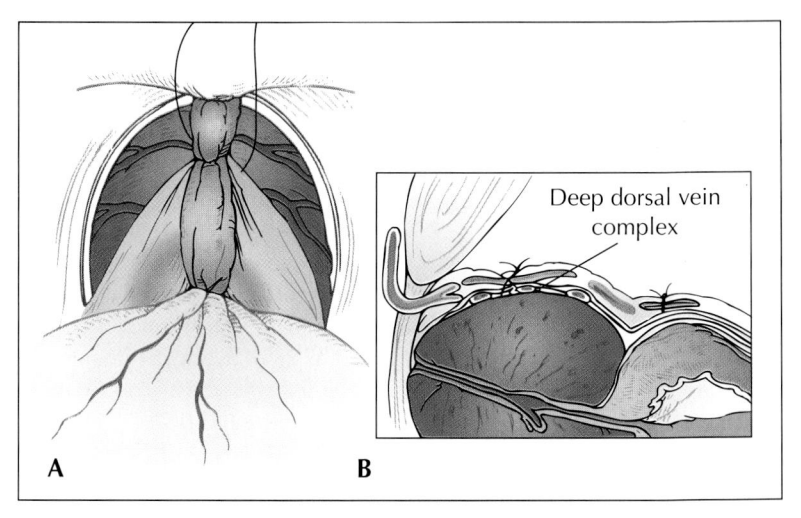

▶ **FIGURE 11-6.** Suture placement. The superficial dorsal venous complex is controlled with a suture approximately 1 cm cephalad to the bladder neck, which is determined by its relationship to the catheter balloon. This stitch serves to limit back bleeding and also marks the anterior limit of the proximal dissection at the bladder neck during the final stages of the removal of the prostate (**A**). The incised endopelvic fascia and deep dorsal vein complex are gathered in a figure-of-eight suture placed anteriorly over the apical half of the prostate (**B**). This suture is tagged with a hemostat and used as countertraction to aid finger dissection of the dorsal venous complex from the urethra distal to the apex of the prostate (see Fig. 11-7).

II. The Prostate

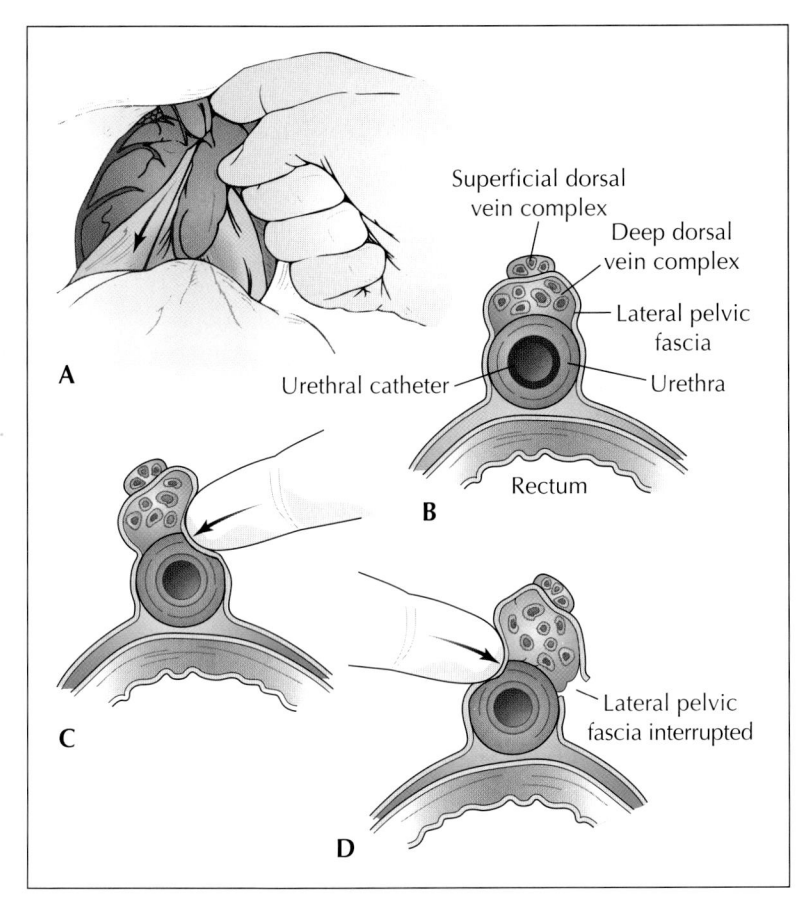

▶ **FIGURE 11-7.** Countertraction. Countertraction placed on the hemostatic figure-of-eight suture facilitates blunt finger dissection of the lateral pelvic fascia in the plane between the dorsal venous complex and the urethra (**A**). The lateral pelvic fascia (**B**) is broken with finger dissection applied from both sides (**C** and **D**).

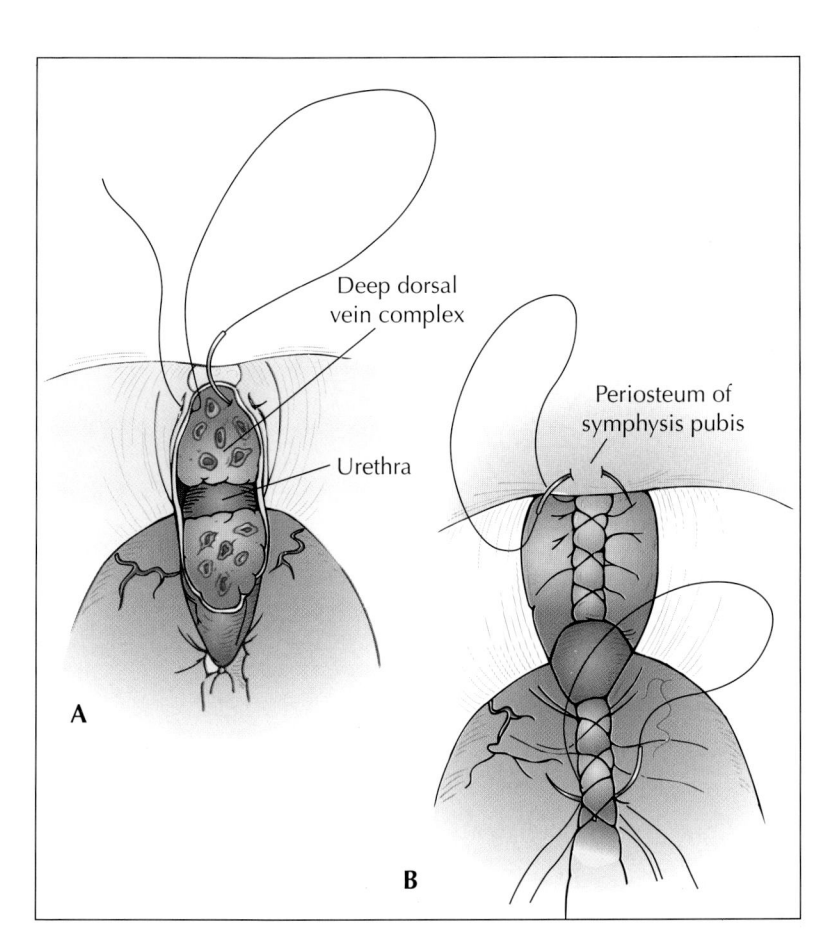

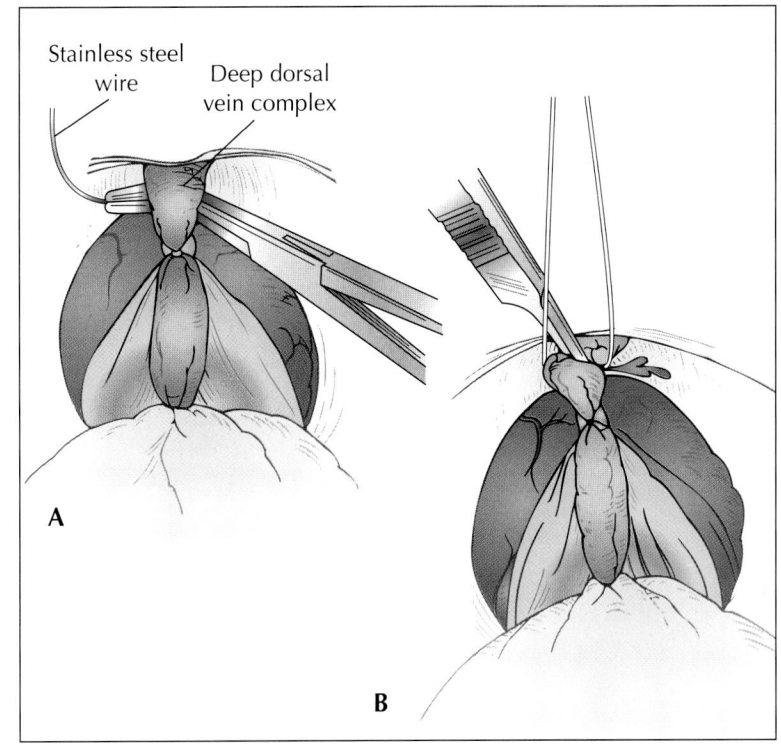

▶ **FIGURE 11-8.** Use of steel wire as a guide. Once the plane of dissection is established, a long-tipped, right-angled clamp is passed immediately superior to the urethra and a steel wire withdrawn to isolate the dorsal venous complex (**A**). With upward retraction on the wire and the prostate firmly pushed down with a sponge stick, the deep dorsal venous complex is sharply divided with a number 15 blade (**B**). Once completed, the bleeding is lessened by releasing the downward pressure on the prostate. With the surgeon standing adjacent to the patient's left thigh and facing cephalad, the dorsal venous complex is brought under control through apposition of the lateral pelvic fascia using a continuous vertical absorbable suture.

▶ **FIGURE 11-9.** Control of bleeding. Bleeding from the dorsal venous complex is controlled by apposing the lateral pelvic fascia with a continuous figure-of-eight absorbable polygalactin suture, sewn vertically (**A**), the last pass of which is brought through the periosteum of the pubis (**B**) to effectively compress the superficial dorsal veins in the anteroposterior plane and to fix the fascia to the periosteum, simulating the function of the puboprostatic ligaments. Back bleeding from the ventral prostate is controlled with a continuous hemostatic suture (**B**).

Nerve-sparing Radical Retropubic Prostatectomy

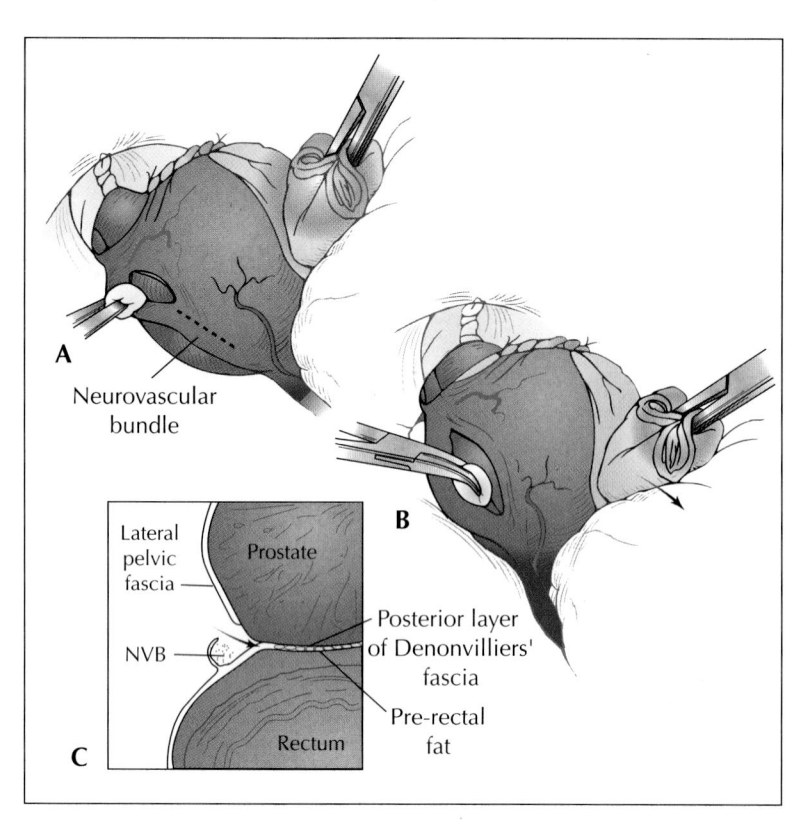

▶ **FIGURE 11-10.** Examination of each neurovascular bundle (NVB). Muscle bundles of the levator ani are stripped away from the apex of the prostate using scissors or bluntly with a peanut dissector to expose the prostatourethral region posterolaterally. By rotating the prostate with a sponge stick, the surgeon can examine the course of the NVBs in relation to the prostate and to any palpable tumor. Depending on the course of the NVB, a plane of division of the lateral pelvic fascia is chosen to assure a negative surgical margin while as much of the NVB is preserved as possible. Once the level of dissection is determined, the lateral pelvic fascia is sharply incised from the midprostate toward the apex (**A**). Using a peanut dissector, the correct plane is gently opened and extended distally to displace the NVB laterally (**B** and **C**).

Frequently, a shallow groove defines the superior margin of dissection for the preservation of each bundle and here the fascia is carefully divided from midprostate to the apex. Small vessels passing superiorly from the bundles are clipped parallel to the line of dissection and divided. Electrocautery must be avoided here to avoid damaging the neural elements.

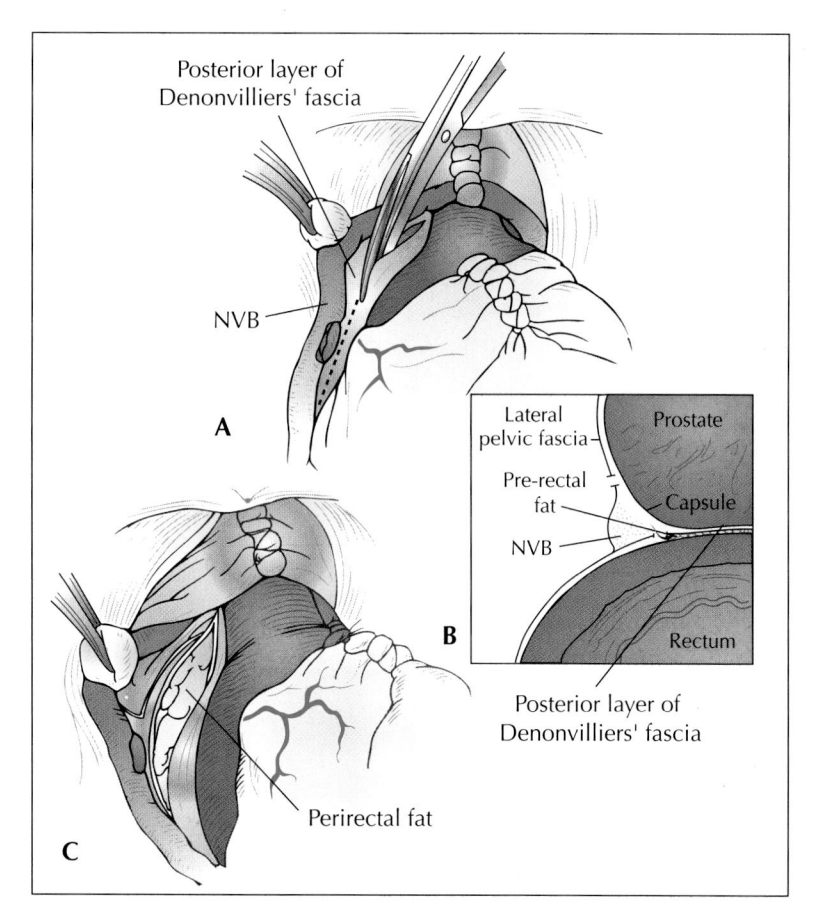

▶ **FIGURE 11-11.** Division of posterior layer of Denonvilliers' fascia. This layer can be punctured with closed scissors immediately lateral to the prostatourethral junction to expose perirectal fat. The plane of dissection is then developed using both a peanut dissector and scissors (**A** and **B**). Special attention is paid to continuing the posterolateral displacement of the neurovascular bundle (NVB) away from the urethra for a distance of almost 1 cm from the prostatourethral junction to lessen its risk of entrapment when the vesicourethral anastomosis is completed. If the tumor is palpably close to a neurovascular bundle (see Fig. 11-12), then the dissection is started further posterolaterally to include the bundles with the pathologic specimen.

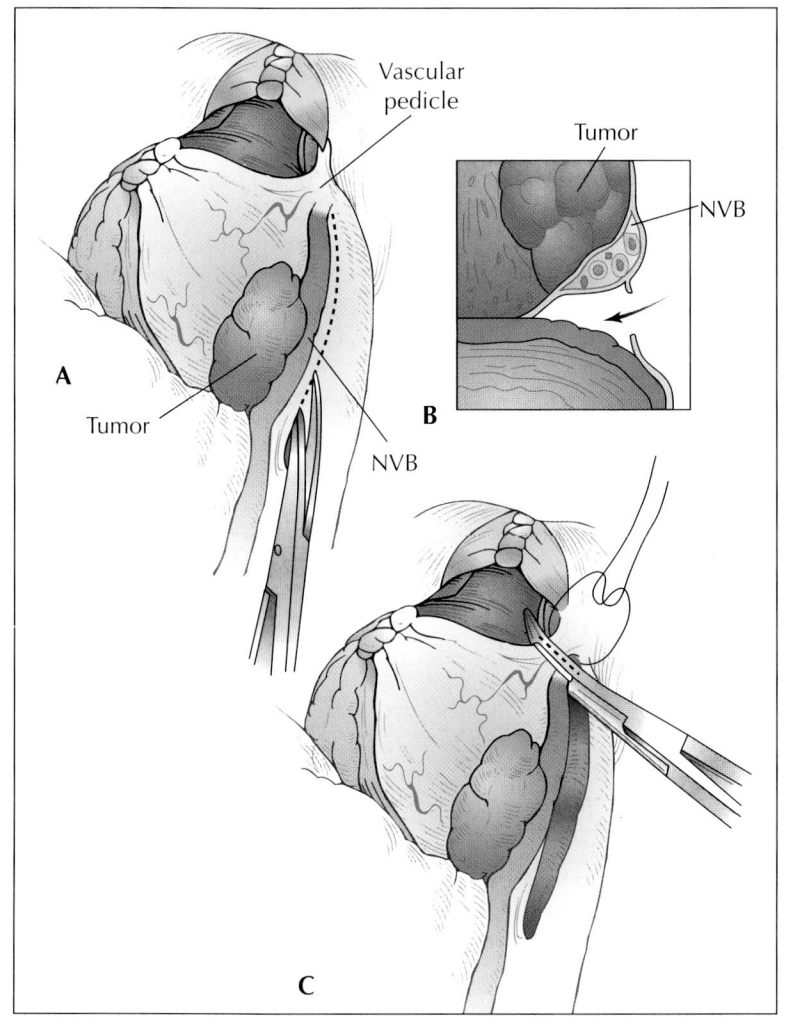

▶ **FIGURE 11-12.** Resection of one neurovascular bundle (NVB). Should the cancer lie close to an NVB, all or part of the bundle should be resected to assure a negative surgical margin. A plane of dissection is chosen laterally. If the entire bundle is to be resected, dissection begins over the lateral rectal wall, in the fat plane beneath the NVB (**A** and **B**). The incision is extended distally and the NVB is secured with clips or ties and divided distal to the apex of the prostate.

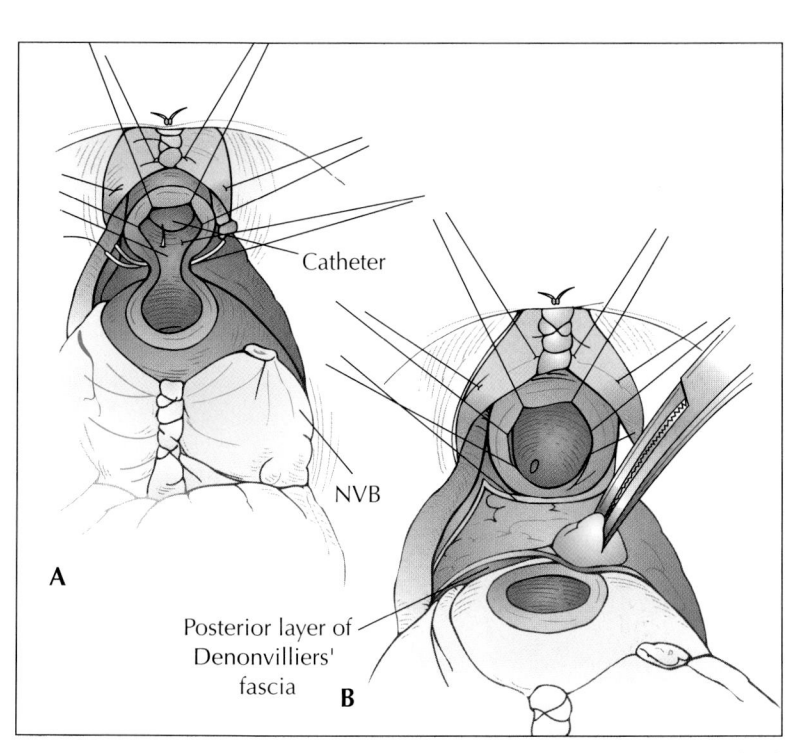

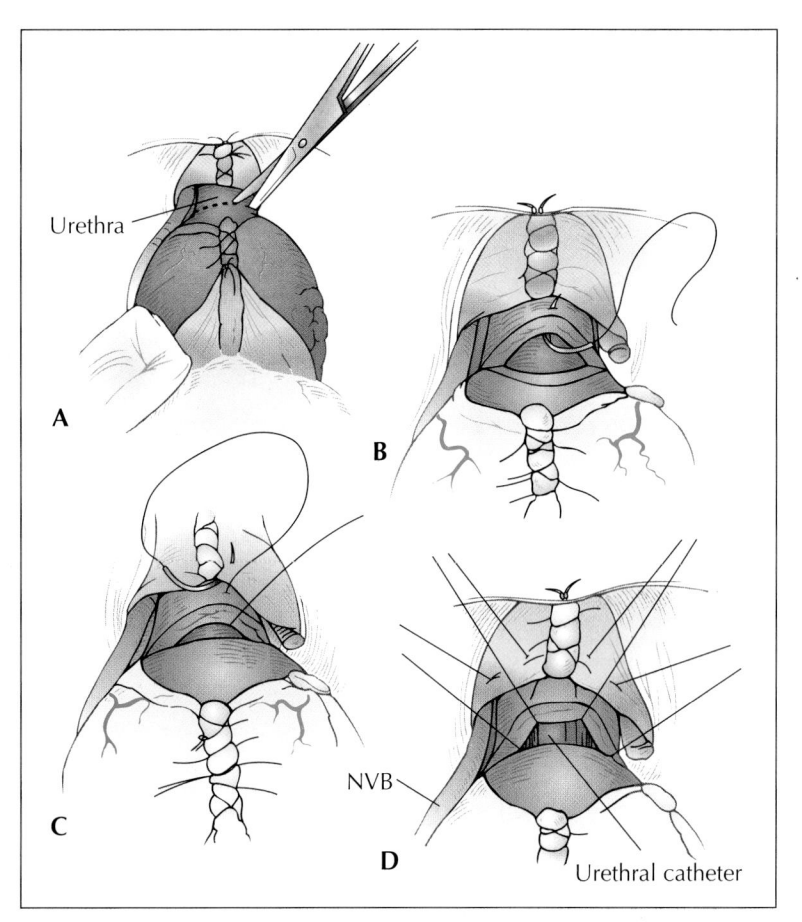

▶ **FIGURE 11-13.** Division of anterolateral urethra and placement of anastomotic sutures. The anterolateral urethra is divided 2 to 3 mm from the apex of the prostate (**A**) and four 2-0 monocryl sutures are placed at 1, 3, 11, and 9 o'clock. Each suture includes urethral mucosa (**B**) and, in a separate bite, a firm piece of lateral pelvic fascia (**C** and **D**). Additional security for each of these sutures is obtained by gathering a separate bite of several millimeters of the lateral pelvic fascia that had been sutured earlier to control the divided deep dorsal venous complex. The catheter is then pulled back to expose the entire urethra. Care is taken to ensure that the posterior apical prostatic tissue, often seen as a lip extending further posteriorly than its anterior counterpart, is fully resected with the specimen by careful blunt dissection with the peanut dissector.

▶ **FIGURE 11-14.** Completion of urethral division. Two posterior anastomotic sutures are placed at 5 and 7 o'clock to include the posterior layer of Denonvilliers' fascia (**A**). The needle on each of these two sutures is left on as a marking tag; the anterior four sutures will be sewn to the reconstructed bladder neck using a Mayo needle. The urethral division is completed and the incision is carried through the rectourethralis muscle to the fatty tissue anterior to the rectum. By dividing the posterior layer of Denonvilliers' fascia at the apex, the yellowish perirectal fat becomes visible and the correct plane of dissection can be confirmed. Sharp and blunt dissection is used to elevate the prostate together with the posterior layer of Denonvilliers' fascia, thus reducing the likelihood of a positive surgical margin [31].

Nerve-sparing Radical Retropubic Prostatectomy

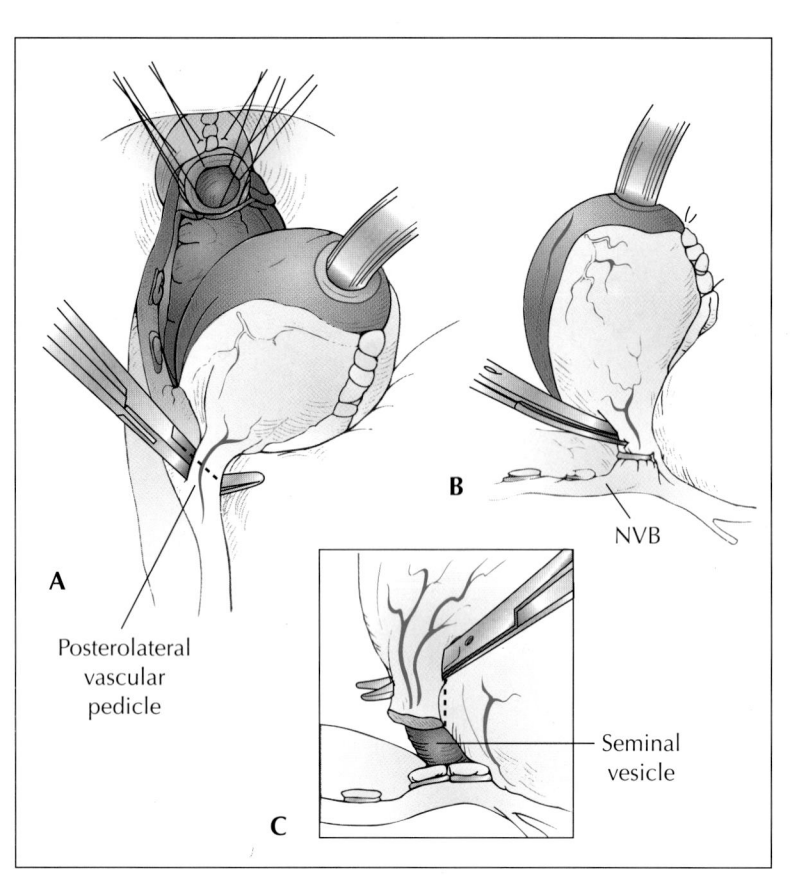

▶ **FIGURE 11-15.** Mobilization of the prostate. A new catheter is placed in the bladder to allow easy manipulation of the prostate, which is mobilized from its posterolateral attachments in a side-to-side fashion (**A**). Small vessels are controlled with clips placed parallel to the neurovascular bundle (NVB) (**B**). The posterolateral vascular pedicles of the prostate are identified with the aid of a right-angled clamp working in an up-and-down motion to separate tissue appropriate for clip ligation and division. In the posterior midline, the superficial layer of Denonvilliers' fascia is divided transversely at the level of the base of the prostate, entering the plane between the rectum and the seminal vesicles (**C**). This plane can then be widened with blunt finger dissection, but the rectovesical fascia should be left covering the resected seminal vesicles.

Once the apical half of the prostate is free, a separate catheter is placed in the bladder via the prostatic urethra and is used to retract the gland. The neurovascular bundles are dissected free as appropriate from the lateral margins of the prostate.

Systematic division of the lateral vascular pedicles is achieved without substantial blood loss using a right-angled clamp to isolate sections of this tissue for clip ligation and division. The surgeon needs to remain cognizant of the location of the neurovascular bundles during this dissection because they can be tented up and into the field secondary to ventral retraction of the prostate.

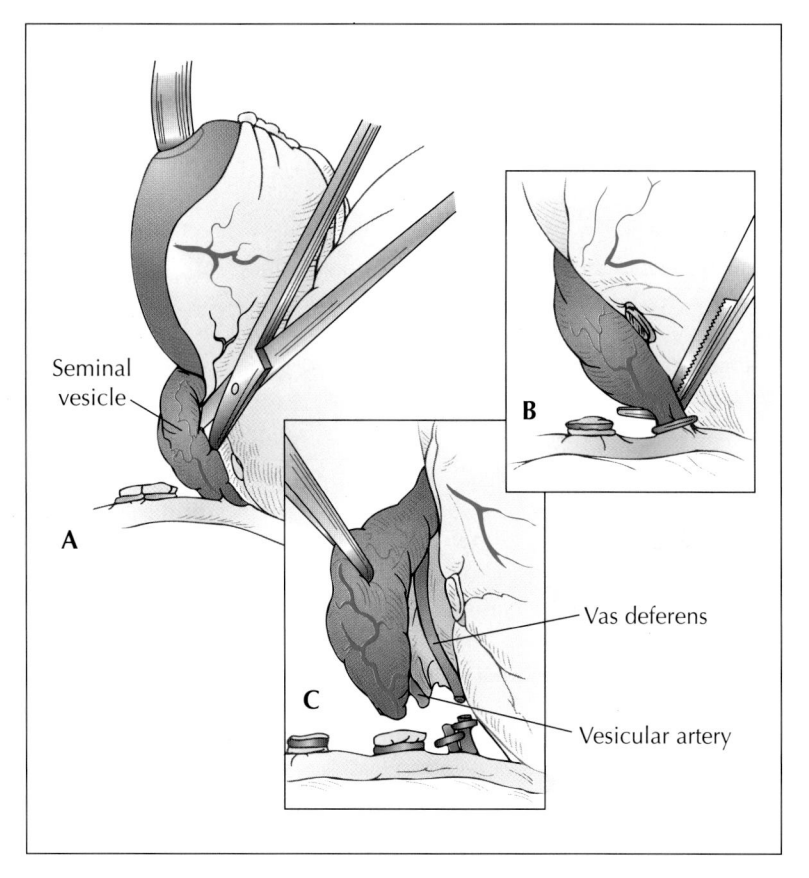

▶ **FIGURE 11-16.** Approach to the seminal vesicles. The seminal vesicles are typically approached laterally and the plane between the vesicles and the bladder developed with scissors and finger dissection (**A**). The major vascular supply to the seminal vesicles at this point lies anterior and lateral. When these are clipped and divided close to the wall of the vesicle, it is easier to identify the large artery that enters at the apex of the seminal vesicle (**B**). The ampullae of the vasa are clipped to include the vasal arteries, and divided (**C**).

II. The Prostate

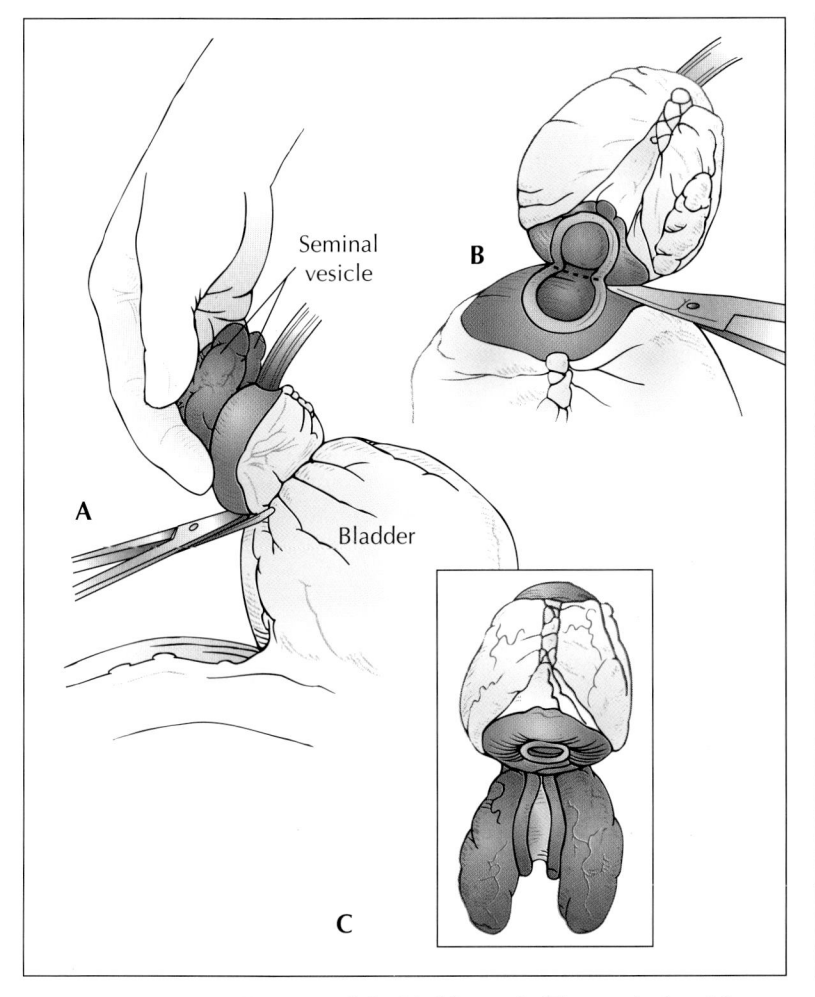

▶ **FIGURE 11-17.** Division of the bladder neck. The seminal vesicles and vasa are sharply dissected off of the posterior wall of the bladder. The small vessels from the bladder pedicles are controlled with clips or electrocautery (**A**). The bladder neck is then divided anteriorly, and the catheter balloon is removed through this incision (**B**). Care is taken to preserve as much bladder mucosa as practicable. The ureteral orifices are inspected for spontaneous efflux of urine prior to the complete removal of the specimen. The anterior bladder neck, as defined by the earlier suture placed to control the superficial dorsal venous complex, is divided with scissors. The posterior bladder neck is divided to preserve as much bladder mucosa as practicable, once the location of the trigone and ureteric orifices has been identified. However, the bladder neck should not be dissected out distally into the prostatic urethra, or the risks of a positive surgical margin will be substantially increased.

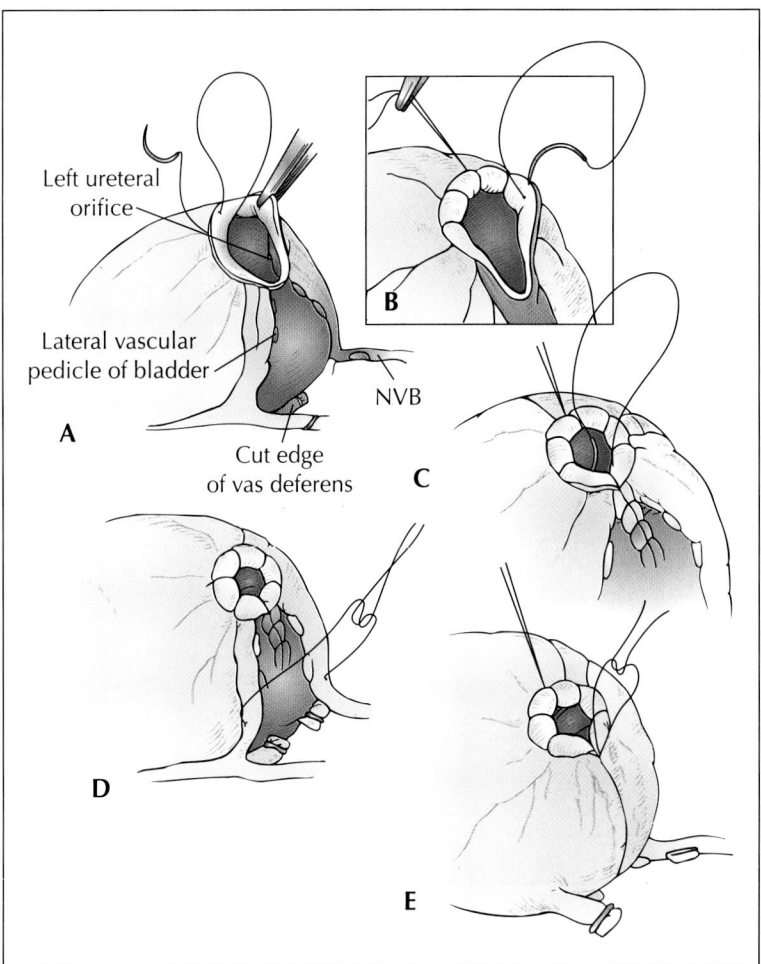

▶ **FIGURE 11-18.** Preparation of anterior bladder neck for anastomosis. The anterior bladder neck is prepared for the anastomosis by fully everting the mucosa anterolaterally with five vertical mattress sutures (**A** and **B**). The posterior bladder neck is closed in a "tennis racket" fashion with a continuous suture beginning at 6 o'clock and ending with a stitch that fully everts the bladder mucosa (**C** and **D**) providing an opening 8 to 10 mm (24 to 30F) in diameter. The lateral vascular pedicles of the bladder are reapproximated with a continuous suture (**D** and **E**) to secure hemostasis. The operative field is irrigated with 2 L of warmed sterile water. The exact size of the bladder neck is not critical to the attainment of postoperative continence. NVB—neurovascular bundle.

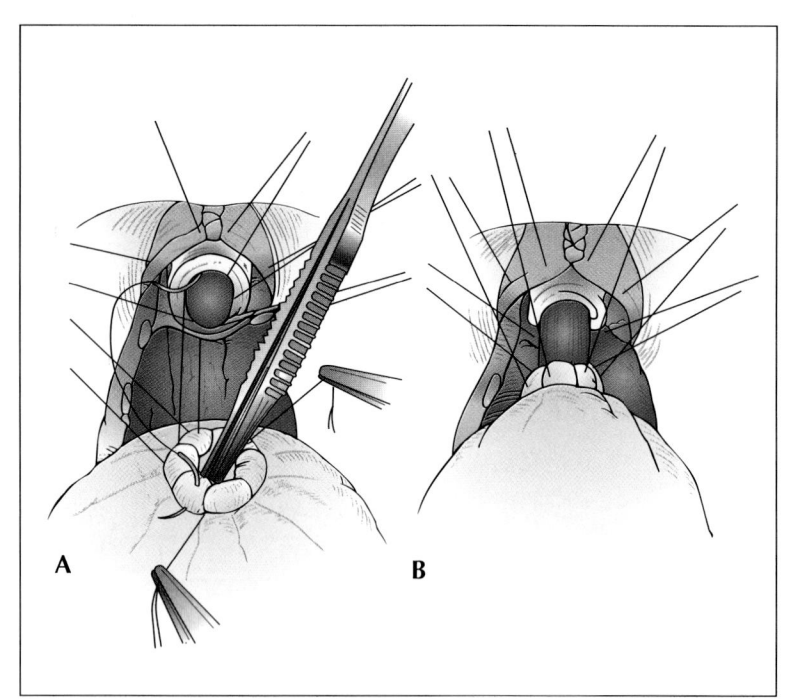

FIGURE 11-19. The four posterior anastomotic sutures previously placed in the urethra are positioned appropriately in the bladder neck with the needle entering and exiting through everted mucosa (**A**). The urethral catheter is placed in the bladder and the two anterior anastomotic sutures are secured before the catheter balloon is inflated with 15 cc. The operating table is taken out of the flex position to facilitate the advancement of the reconstructed bladder neck to the urethra. Firm traction on all six anastomotic sutures and on the catheter is important to facilitate apposition of the bladder neck to the urethra (**B**). As the sutures are tied, care is taken to exclude the preserved neurovascular bundles by gentle downward pressure applied with a sponge stick.

The bladder catheter is gently irrigated to provide a clear return and test the anastomosis for frank leakage. It is subsequently secured to the thigh without traction. Suction catheters are placed in each obturator fossa, and these are typically removed by postoperative day 3. The average hospital stay is 3 days. The patients are brought to the office for catheter removal, without a prior cystogram, on day 14.

COMPLICATIONS

Complications

Incontinence
Anastomatic stricture
Impotence

FIGURE 11-20. Complications. We believe that the early return of urinary control is dependent more on the functional length of the urethra than on the bladder neck configuration. Most patients experience adequate urinary control within weeks of catheter removal and 50% are completely dry or use one pad per day for minimal stress urinary incontinence (SUI) 6 weeks postoperatively [25]. By 12 months, 94% are continent, 5% have mild SUI, and 1% have troublesome or severe incontinence.

Patients receive advice regarding Kegel exercises. Although certainly it is our experience that these exercises are helpful in aiding timely urinary control, definitive proof of benefit has not been obtained.

The incidence of anastomatic stricture, previously a troublesome complication, has clearly been reduced as a result of vigorous bladder mucosal eversion and a water-tight mucosa-to-mucosa vesicourethral anastomosis. Among a total of 114 patients treated between November 1, 1993 and November 1, 1994 (minimum of 12 months follow-up), six (5%) have required urethral dilatation by a urologist in the office and four (3.5%) have required endoscopic division of anastomotic fibrous tissue. The onset of symptoms related to stricture typically occur in the first 12 months after the operation.

Regarding impotence, meticulous dissection of the neurovascular bundles away from the apex of the prostate and the adjacent urethra using sharp and blunt dissection early in the procedure has improved our potency rate significantly. This modification in surgical technique was instituted in November 1993, and the potency rate for men with a history of normal erections preoperatively and aged less than 60 years is currently 76% at 36 months. Older men and those with diminished potency before the operation are less likely to recur. Because there is often considerable delay in the return of postoperative potency, a penile prosthesis should not be considered before 2 years have elapsed. Rarely are there contraindications to the use of intracavernosal injection therapy or vacuum devices for the treatment of impotence in the early postoperative period (typically 6 weeks or longer postoperatively). Oral therapy with sildenafil (Viagra; Pfizer Inc., New York, NY) has been very effective unless both bundles are resected.

REFERENCES

1. Parker SL, Tong T, Bolden S, Wingo PA: Cancer Statistics, 1996. *CA Cancer J Clin* 1996, 46:5–27.
2. Franks LM: Latent carcinoma of the prostate. *J Pathol Bacteriol* 1954, 68:603–616.
3. McNeal JE: Origin and development of carcinoma in the prostate. *Cancer* 1969, 23:24–34.
4. Seidman H, Mushinski MH, Geib SK: Probabilities of eventually developing or dying of cancer - United States 1985. *CA Cancer J Clin* 1985; 35:36-56.
5. Scardino PT, Weaver R, Hudson MA: Early detection of prostate cancer. *Hum Pathol* 1992, 23:211–222.
6. Chodak GW, Thisted RA, Gerber GS, *et al.*: Results of conservative management of clinically localized prostate cancer. *N Engl J Med* 1994, 330:242–248.
7. Fleming C, Wasson JH, Albertsen PC, *et al.*: A decision analysis of alternative treatment strategies for clinically localized prostate cancer. *JAMA* 1993, 269:2650–2658.
8. Albertsen P, Fryback DG, Storer BE, *et al.*: Long-term survival after conservative treatment of clinically localized prostate cancer. *JAMA* 1995, 274:626–631.
9. Stamey TA, McNeal JE: Adenocarcinoma of the prostate. In *Campbell's Urology,* edn 6. Edited by Walsh PJ *et al.* Philadelphia: WB Saunders Company; 1992: 1159–1221.

10. Ohori M, Wheeler TM, Dunn JK, et al.: The pathologic features and prognosis of prostate cancers detectable with current diagnostic tests. *J Urol* 1994, 152:1714–1720.
11. Smith DS, Catalona WJ: The nature of prostate cancer detected through prostate specific antigen based screening. *J Urol* 1994, 152:1732–1736.
12. Epstein JI, Walsh PC, Carmichael M, Brendler CB: Pathologic and clinical findings to predict tumor extent of nonpalpable (stage T1c) prostate cancer. *JAMA* 1994, 271:368–374.
13. National Center for Health Statistics: *Vital Statistics of the United States, 1991 Life Tables.* Hyattsville, MD: US Department of Health and Human Services, National Center for Health Statistics; 1994.
14. Eastham JA, Scardino PT: Radical prostatectomy for clinical stage T1 and T2 prostate cancer. In *Comprehensive Textbook of Genitourinary Oncology.* Edited by Vogelzang NJ, Scardino PT, Shipley WU, Coffey DS. Baltimore: Williams & Wilkins; 1996:741–758.
15. Partin AW, Pound CR, Clemens JQ, et al.: Serum prostate specific antigen after anatomic radical prostatectomy: The Johns Hopkins experience after 10 years. *Urol Clin North Am* 1993, 20:713–725.
16. Catalona WJ, Smith DS: 5-year tumor recurrence rates after anatomical radical retropubic prostatectomy for prostate cancer. *J Urol* 1994, 152:1837–1842.
17. Catalona WJ: Surgical management of prostate cancer. *Cancer* 1995, 75:1903–1908.
18. Zincke H, Oesterling JE, Blute ML, et al.: Long-term (15 years) results after radical prostatectomy for clinically localized (stage T2c or lower) prostate cancer. *J Urol* 1994, 152:1850–1857.
19. Trapasso JG, deKernion JB, Smith RB, Dorey F: Incidence and significance of detectable levels of serum prostate specific antigen after radical prostatectomy. *J Urol* 1994, 152:1821–1825.
20. Reiner WG, Walsh PC: An anatomic approach to the surgical management of the dorsal vein and Santorini's plexus during radical retropubic prostatectomy. *J Urol* 1979, 121:198–200.
21. Goad JR, Scardino PT: Modifications in the technique of radical retropubic prostatectomy to minimize blood loss. *Atlas Urol Clin North Am* 1994, 2:65–80.
22. Leandri P, Rossignol G, Gautier J, Ramon J: Radical retropubic prostatectomy: morbidity and quality of life. Experience with 620 consecutive cases. *J Urol* 1992, 147:883–887.
23. Goad JR, Eastham JA, Fitzgerald KB, et al.: Radical retropubic prostatectomy: limited benefit of autologous blood donation. *J Urol* 1995, 154:2103–2109.
24. Eastham JA, Scardino PT, Yawn DH, et al.: Preoperative autologous blood donation in radical retropubic prostatectomy: a cost-effectiveness analysis. *Med Decis Making,* submitted.
25. Eastham JA, Kattan MW, Rogers E, et al.: Risk factors for urinary incontinence after radical retropubic prostatectomy. *J Urol,* submitted.
26. Fricker JP, Vergnes Y, Schach R, et al.: Low dose heparin versus low molecular weight heparin (Kabi 2165, Fragmin) in the prophylaxis of thromboembolic complications of abdominal oncological surgery. *Eur J Clin Invest* 1988, 18:561–567.
27. Cisek LJ, Walsh PC: Thromboembolic complications following radical retropubic prostatectomy: influence of external sequential pneumatic compression devices. *Urology* 1993, 42:406–408.
28. Bluestein DL, Bostwick DG, Bergstralh EJ, Oesterling JE: Eliminating the need for bilateral pelvic lymphadenectomy in select patients with prostate cancer. *J Urol* 1994, 151:1315–1320.
29. Kavoussi LR, Myers JA, Catalona WJ: Effect of temporary occlusion of hypogastric arteries on blood loss during radical retropubic prostatectomy. *J Urol* 1991, 146:362–365.
30. Peters CA, Walsh PC: Blood transfusion and anesthetic practices in radical retropubic prostatectomy. *J Urol* 1985, 134:81–83.
31. Rosen MA, Goldstone L, Lapin S, et al.: Frequency and location of extracapsular extension and positive surgical margins in radical prostatectomy specimens. *J Urol* 1992, 148:331–337.

External Beam Radiotherapy for Prostate Cancer

CANCEROUS DISEASE SECTION

Gregory M.M. Videtic, Edgar Ben-Josef & Arthur T. Porter

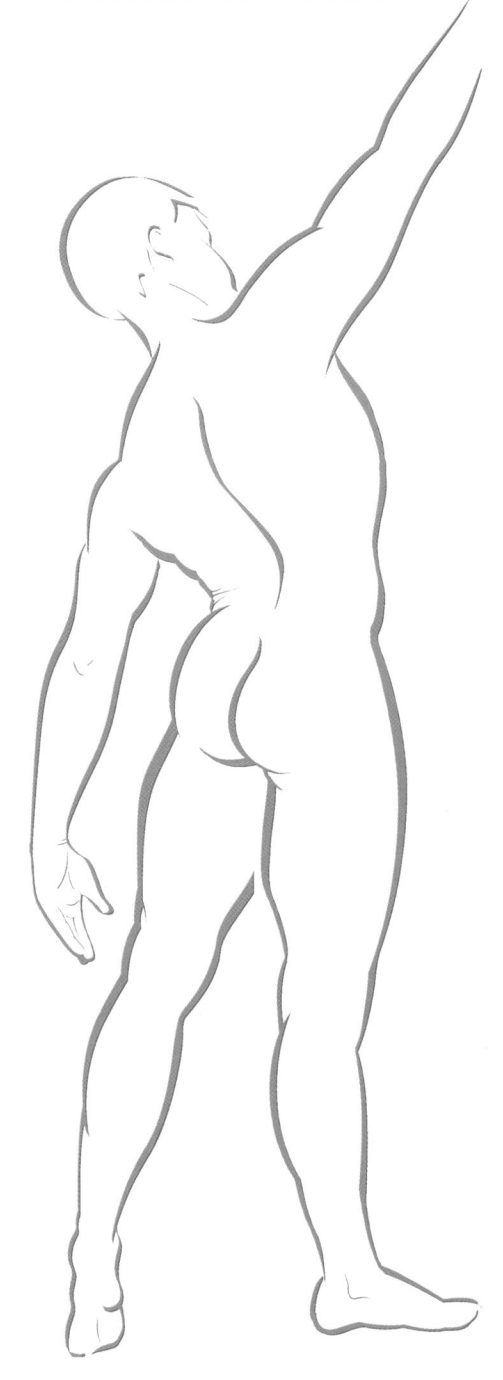

Controversies in treatment selection make decision-making for patients with prostate cancer one of the most challenging areas in contemporary oncology. External beam radiation therapy (EBRT) using photons is the one treatment modality that has applications at every stage in the natural history of carcinoma of the prostate. For early disease (*ie*, confined to the gland), it is considered a curative therapy that can eradicate organ-limited tumor with maximal preservation of adjacent normal tissues. It appears to be as effective as surgery regarding disease-free survival and overall survival, and is associated with a favorable side-effect profile when compared with resection [1]. Current randomized studies of early-stage disease are comparing its overall survival benefits to observation or surgery. Researchers are also looking at ways of escalating dose to the prostate while minimizing morbidity; these include combinations of EBRT with other forms of external radiation (*ie*, neutron beam) or with interstitial radioactive implants, and improvements in the technique of dose delivery (*eg*, three-dimensional conformal).

Along with hormonal manipulation, EBRT is used in the treatment of locally advanced prostate cancer, *ie*, tumor with either extension beyond the confines of the glandular capsule, into the seminal vesicles, or into regional structures [1]. As with early-stage disease, current EBRT trials involving dose and volume modifications, as well as radiation type, are being investigated in an attempt to improve the therapeutic yield. For those patients who have undergone surgical resection as the primary form of management for clinically staged, local disease, retrospective studies have identified an adjuvant role for EBRT; it provides improved local control for tumors with poor pathologic features (*eg*, positive margins, high grade, advanced pathologic tumor stage) [2]. Randomized studies are now looking at the impact of this treatment on overall survival for high-risk postoperative patients. Furthermore, EBRT has a role in salvaging patients who present with late local recurrences following surgery, whether detected on biochemical studies or physical examination. With respect to distant disease, prostate cancer spreads preferentially to bone and EBRT has a well-established role in the management of symptomatic osseous metastases. Short-course palliative EBRT generally provides quick and effective analgesic control [1].

Conventional EBRT treatment planning is essentially two-dimensional in nature, with fixed anatomic boundaries and orthogonal radiographic visualization techniques being used to define prostate treatment volumes. This necessitates wide normal tissue margins around the tumor so as to ensure adequate coverage of the disease. However, restrictions imposed by the tolerance of the normal tissues included in the radiation field limit the total dose that can be safely delivered, with consequent implications for local control. Recent advances in computer technology have made three-dimensional treatment planning possible. The major advantage of this process has been better definition of target volumes, facilitating delivery of higher doses of radiation while reducing early and late toxicities of the treatment for a given level of local control.

Prostate cancer is characterized by a potentially long natural history. This has had important implications in determining the optimal treatment regimen for a given stage of disease. This chapter, which reviews the therapeutic and technical aspects of EBRT in the current management of prostate cancer, reflects this need for outcomes assessment in clinical decision making.

IMPLICATIONS FOR EBRT REGARDING LOCAL ANATOMY AND PATTERNS OF DISEASE SPREAD

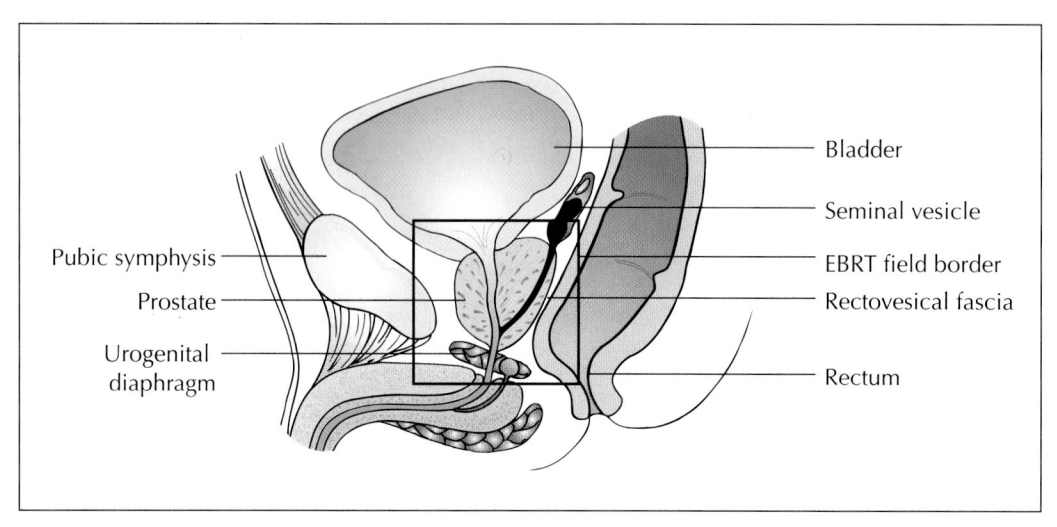

▶ **FIGURE 12-1.** View of the sagittal pelvis illustrating the anatomic relationships of the prostate to regional structures. Typical external beam radiotherapy (EBRT) field borders for treatment of early-stage prostate disease are shown. As illustrated, the prostate lies at the base of the urinary bladder, encompasses the male urethra, and rests on the urogenital diaphragm. Important anatomic relationships that come into consideration when planning EBRT treatment to the prostate include 1) the gland's proximity to the rectum from which it is separated by the rectovesical septum (Denonvilliers' fascia), 2) the size and orientation of the seminal vesicles with respect to the gland (typically, they pierce the posterosuperior aspect of the gland), 3) the relationship to the bladder neck, and 4) the relationship to the pubic symphysis. This understanding of local anatomy helps in delimiting the boundaries of the prostate because the gland cannot be visualized by conventional radiography and also allows predictions to be made as to the extent of treatment-related morbidity.

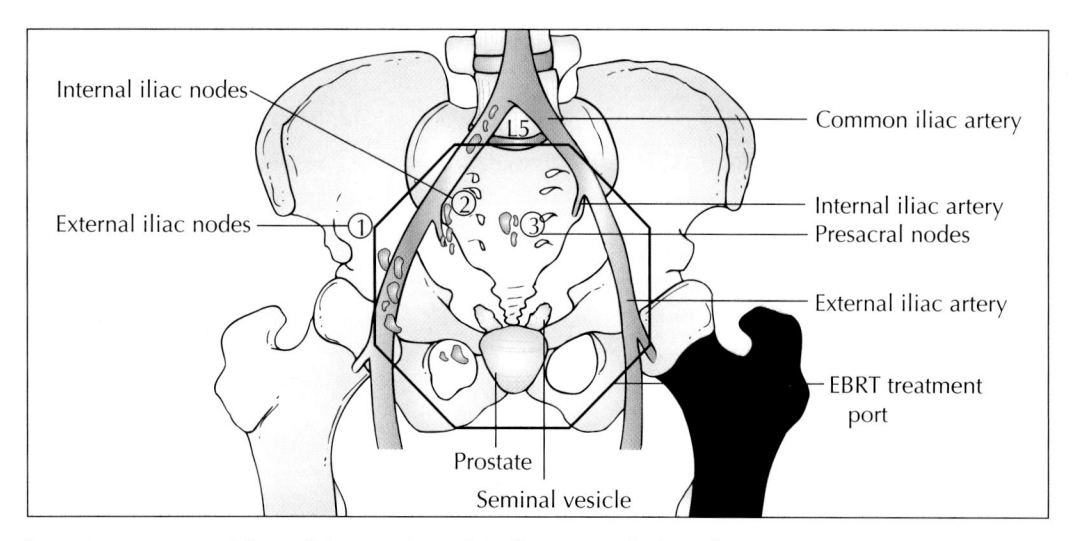

▶ **FIGURE 12-2.** View of the anterior pelvis illustrating the lymphatic drainage of the prostate, with a pelvic external beam radiotherapy (EBRT) field shown in outlining. Nodal metastases from the prostate first appear in periprostatic and obturator nodes. The lymphatic vessels ultimately terminate in the lymph nodes drained principally by the external and internal iliac nodal chains. Fewer than 10% of patients have involvement of presacral or presciatic nodes alone [1]. Enlarging treatment fields to include prostate nodes at risk potentially increases treatment-associated morbidity, particularly to the small intestine and bladder. The probability of pelvic lymph node involvement for any given prostate cancer is a reflection of tumor size (*ie*, stage) and grade (degree of differentiation) and can be correlated with PSA (prostate-specific antigen) levels. Controversy exists in the literature regarding the inclusion of pelvic nodes via large treatment portals when treating the prostate because a survival benefit from such an approach has not been unequivocally demonstrated.

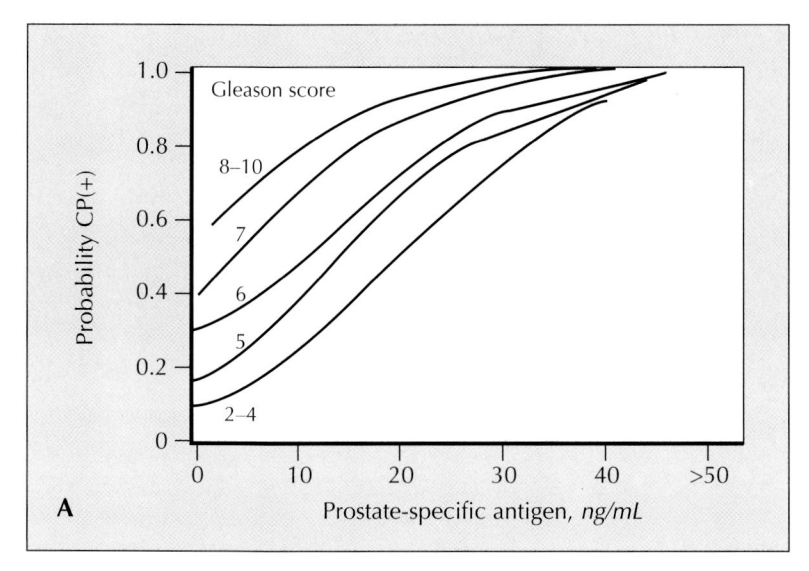

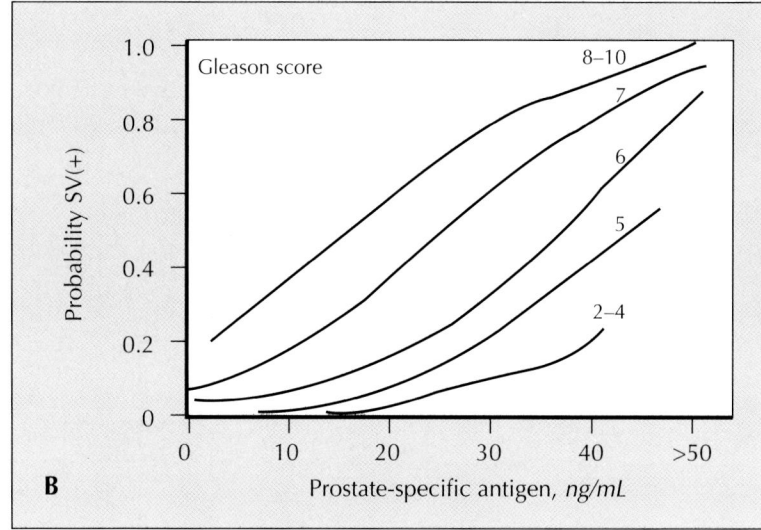

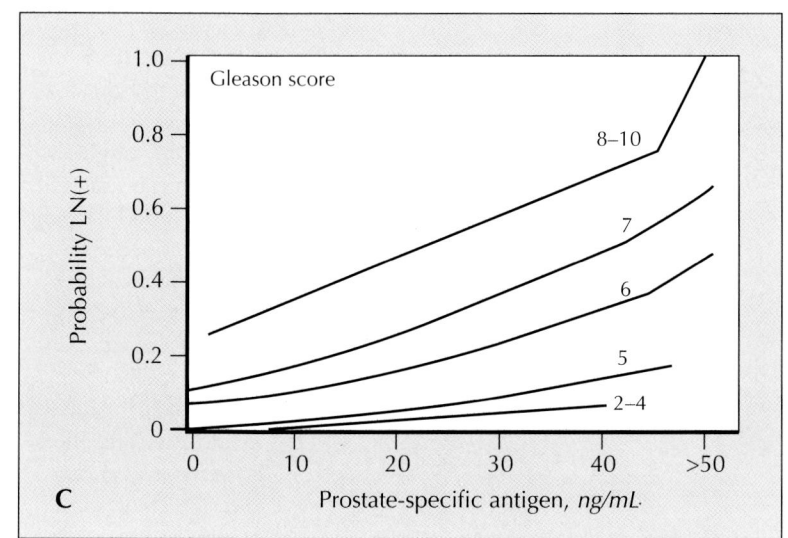

FIGURE 12-3. Probability of capsular penetration (CP+) (*panel A*), seminal vesicle involvement (SV+) (*panel B*), and lymph nodal involvement (LN+) (*panel C*) as a function of prostate-specific antigen (PSA) level and preoperative Gleason score. Extent of disease (*ie*, stage) is inadequately determined by clinical assessment alone, even when considering both physical examination and imaging studies. This has implications with respect to correct stage assignment and, ultimately, treatment selection. Predictions of the magnitude of local disease can now be made using PSA levels along with Gleason scores from biopsies, in conjunction with results of other investigations. Thus, a diagnosis of locally advanced disease (CP+; SV+) or unfavorable disease (on the basis of elevated PSA alone) would suggest external beam radiotherapy as the premier treatment modality along with antiandrogen therapy. (*Adapted from* Partin *et al.* [5].)

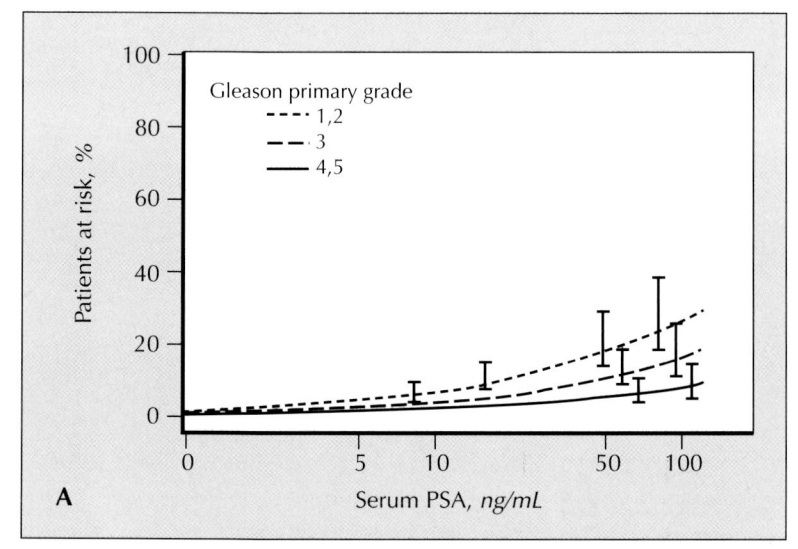

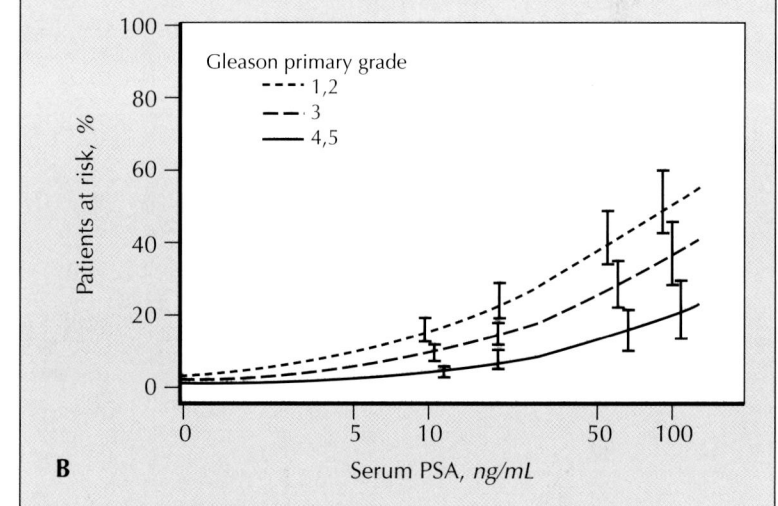

FIGURE 12-4. Risk of pelvic lymph node involvement for patients with clinical stage T1a to 2a (*panel A*), T2b to -c (*panel B*), and T3 (*panel C*) prostatic carcinoma correlated with pretherapy prostate-specific antigen (PSA) value and Gleason primary grade.

Vertical bars represent the 95% CIs for PSA values. Pelvic node status is an important predictor of prognosis and thus affects treatment selection. Pelvic lymphadenectomy studies have established that nodal metastases are a "marker" for distant disease. At 10 years of follow-up, node-positive patients have a greater than 85% chance of developing a distant metastasis when compared with node-negative patients (< 20%). Of interest, a single lymph node involved with disease is not a negative prognostic factor. Currently, the rate of nodal positivity appears to be decreasing and likely is a reflection of the earlier detection of prostate disease through PSA testing. In the context of known nodal metastases, studies show that treatment with EBRT alone would appear to be insufficient. Such patients require hormonal manipulation [1].

(Continued on next page)

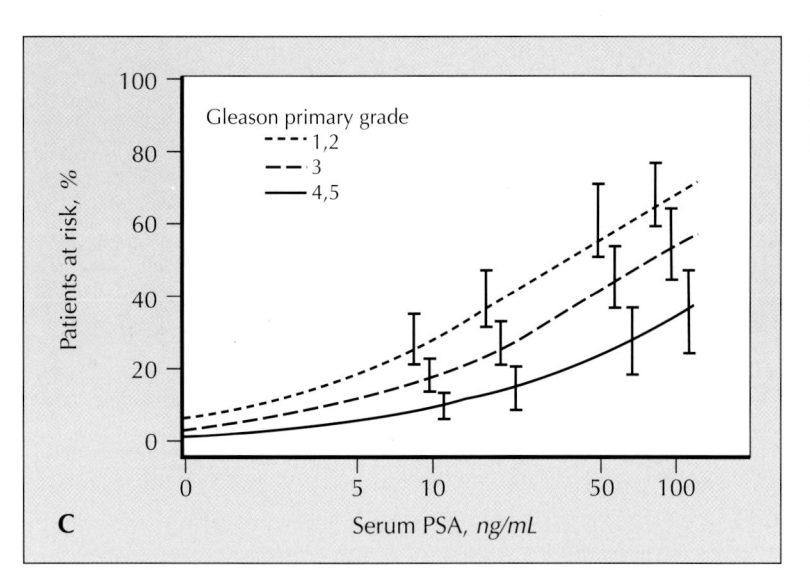

FIGURE 12-4. *(Continued)* Risk of pelvic lymph node involvement for patients with clinical stage T3 (*panel C*) prostatic carcinoma correlated with pretherapy PSA value and Gleason primary grade. (*From* Pisansky *et al.* [6]; with permission.)

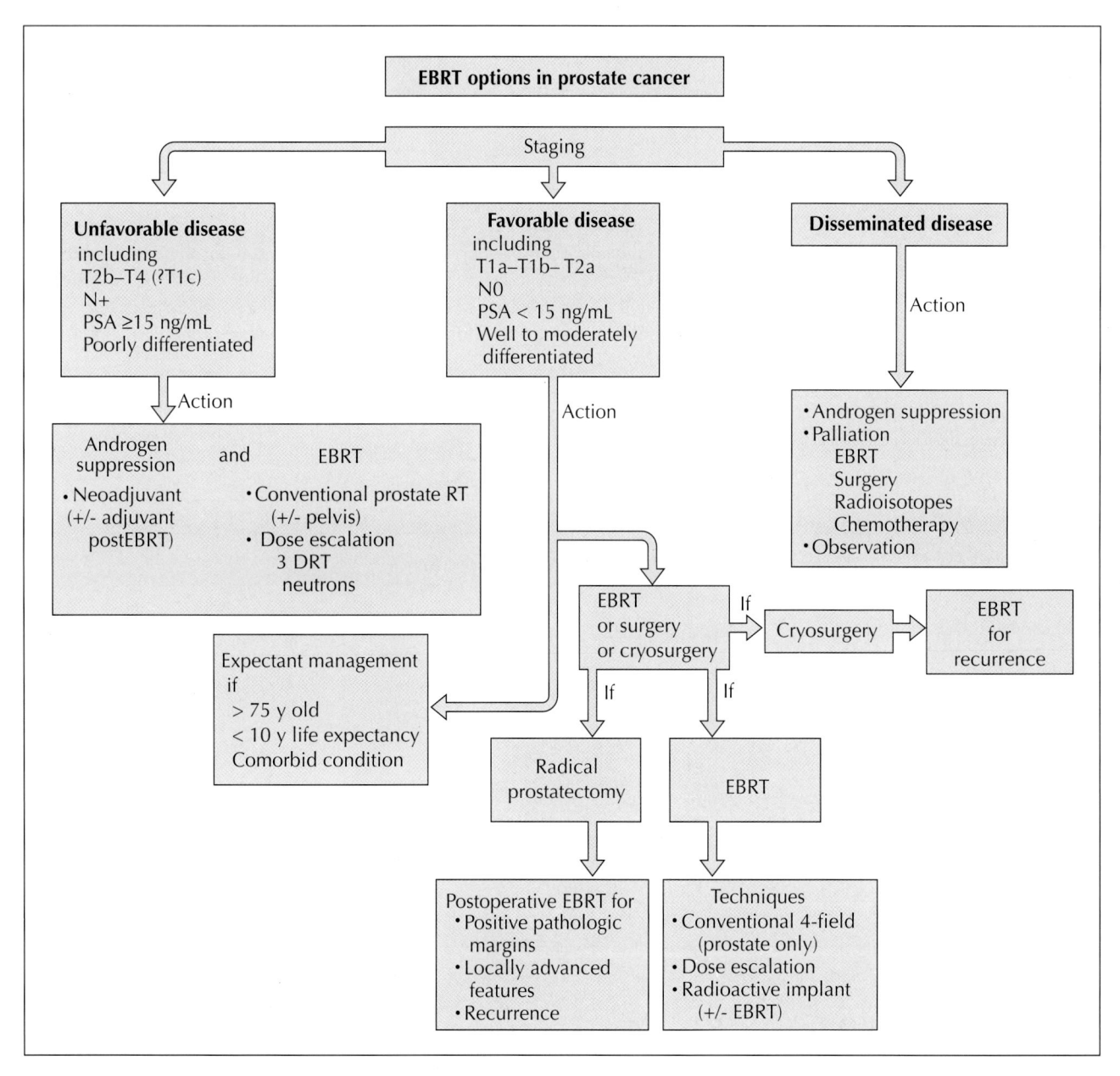

FIGURE 12-5. Standard treatment options for prostate cancer with emphasis on external beam radiotherapy (EBRT). Ideally, treatment decisions reflect the clinician's practice and the patient's desires. Selection of the optimal therapy for the individual patient involves consideration of treatment benefits and risks (in terms of quality and quantity of life) and the patient's overall health status. External beam radiotherapy (EBRT) has a role at every stage in the disease. N—lymph node; T—tumor.

II. The Prostate

12.4

CONVENTIONAL PHOTON EBRT

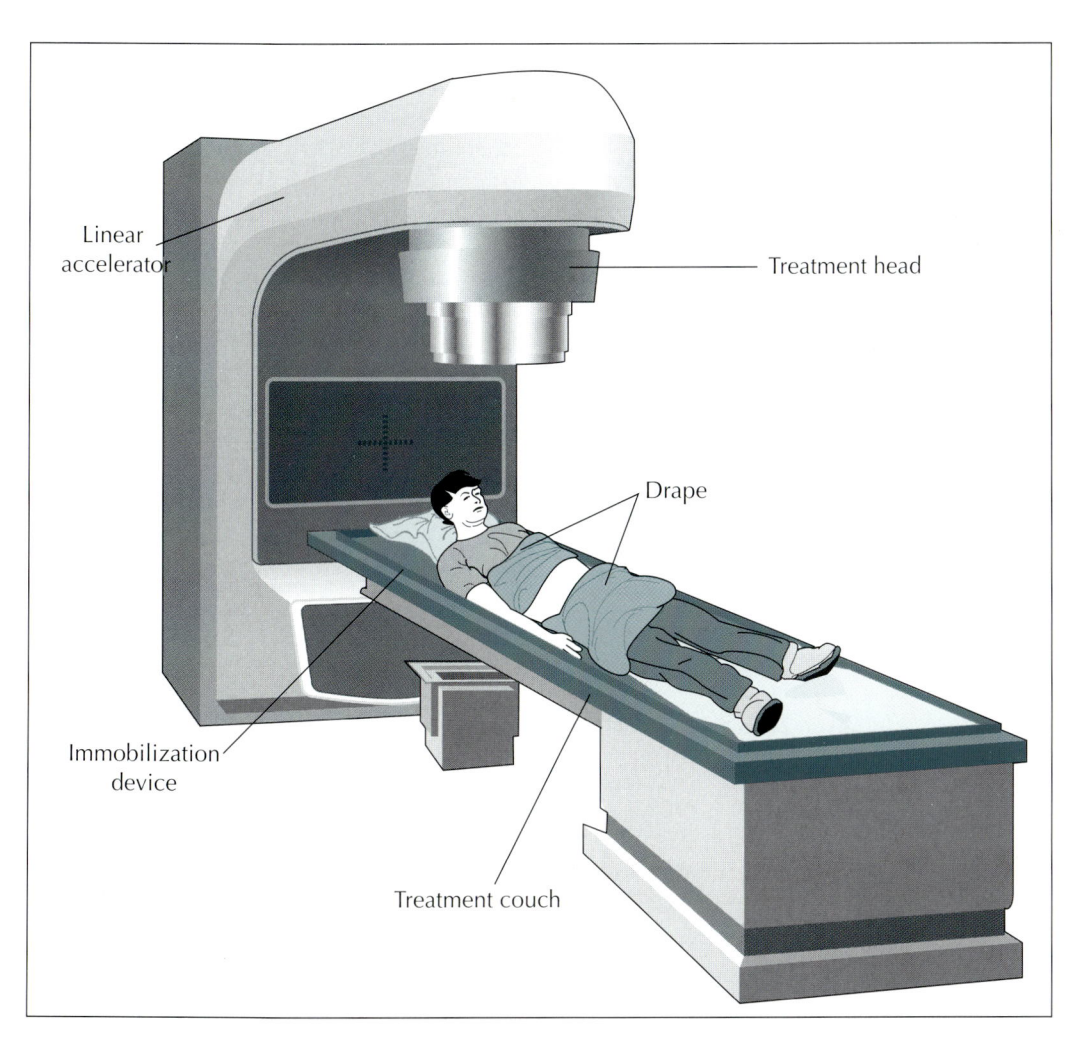

FIGURE 12-6. External beam radiotherapy (EBRT) set-up on a linear accelerator. Patients receiving EBRT for prostate cancer are best treated on linear accelerators that can generate high-energy photons (x-rays > 10 MeV). To limit day-to-day variations in positioning, an individually conformed immobilizing device (*eg*, Alpha cradle) maintains the patient in a set orientation. Reference points on the patient and the immobilizer are aligned with fixed, orthogonal laser-light points that are coordinated to the treatment unit. Typically, individuals are treated in the supine position; some clinicians treat prone because they believe that it may favor displacement of the prostate away from the anterior rectal wall (morbidity-sparing). Prostate treatment fields are "designed" at the time of simulation, which always precedes EBRT and constitutes the planning phase of treatment. These "simulated" fields are then replicated daily on the patient during treatment. Verification or "port" films are taken weekly to confirm the fiducial reproduction of the planned field set-up on the patient.

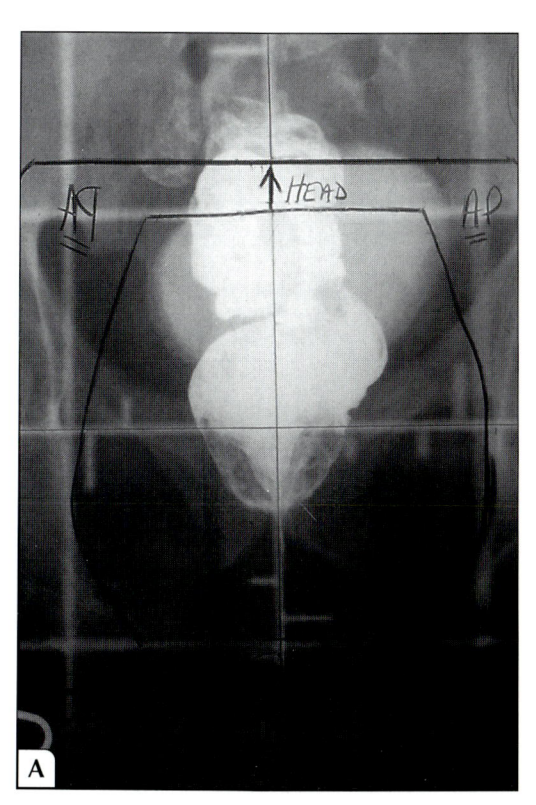

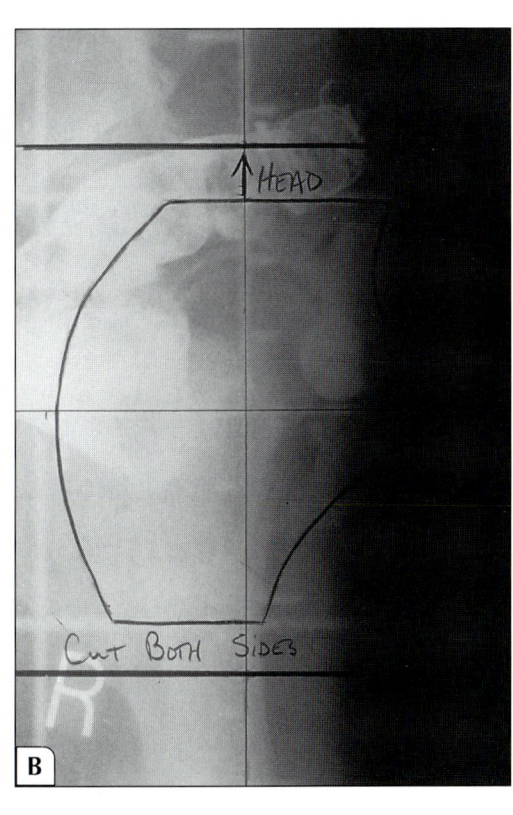

FIGURE 12-7. Orthogonal radiographic views of the prostate obtained at the time of treatment simulation. **A,** Anteroposterior. **B,** Right lateral. Prior to initiating external beam radiotherapy (EBRT), treatment planning is carried out using a simulator. This device replicates the orientation parameters and geometry of the treatment unit in every way without actually administering treatment. Anatomic structures are visualized and the prostate defined according to its relationship to local structures. The bladder, urethra, and rectum may be delineated using either radiographic contrast material or the placement of a temporary urinary catheter. Typically the prostate is treated using an arrangement of two sets of opposed fields (anteroposterior and posteroanterior; right and left laterals), also called four-field or "box" technique. Alternate field arrangements include rotational arc fields and, rarely, a three-field technique (anteroposterior; two laterals). Film records of planned treatment volumes are taken and shielding blocks are drawn onto these simulation films. These blocks (composed of lead or equivalent material) shield normal tissues from the treatment beam.

External Beam Radiotherapy for Prostate Cancer

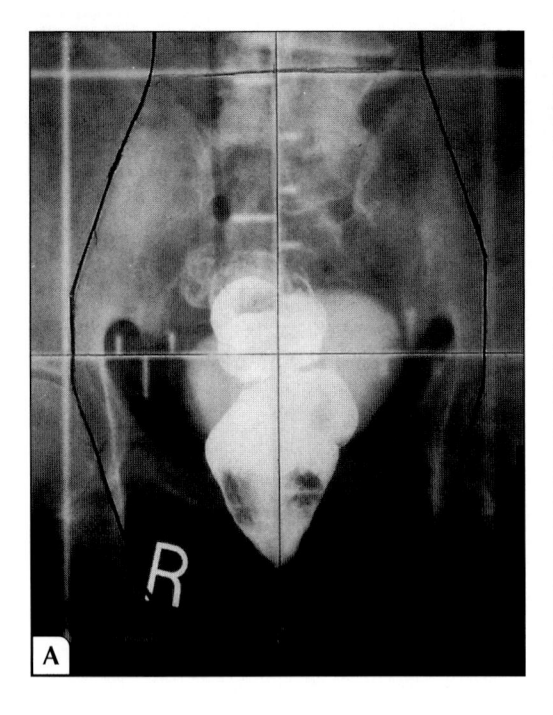

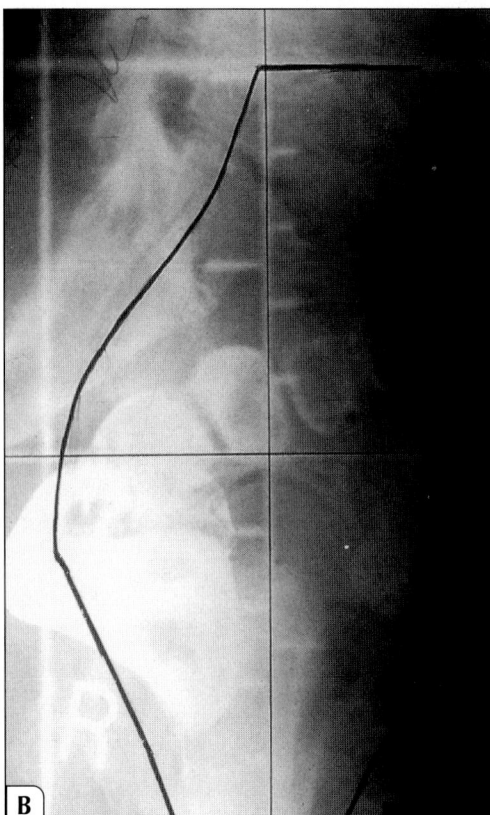

FIGURE 12-8. External beam radiotherapy (EBRT) fields for treatment of carcinoma of the prostate and pelvic nodes at risk. **A,** Anteroposterior. **B,** Right lateral. Controversy exists with respect to the volumes used when treating prostate cancer, especially when considering early stage disease. Typically, extended anteroposterior or lateral fields are used when including the pelvic lymph nodes in the field. Some prospective studies suggest that prophylactic pelvic nodal irradiation may have a survival benefit for T1 or T2 presentations [7]. Conversely, a randomized study conducted by the Radiation Therapy Oncology Group compared prostate irradiation with or without pelvic irradiation for T1b to T2 and N0M0 tumors and found no significant differences in local failure or survival [8].

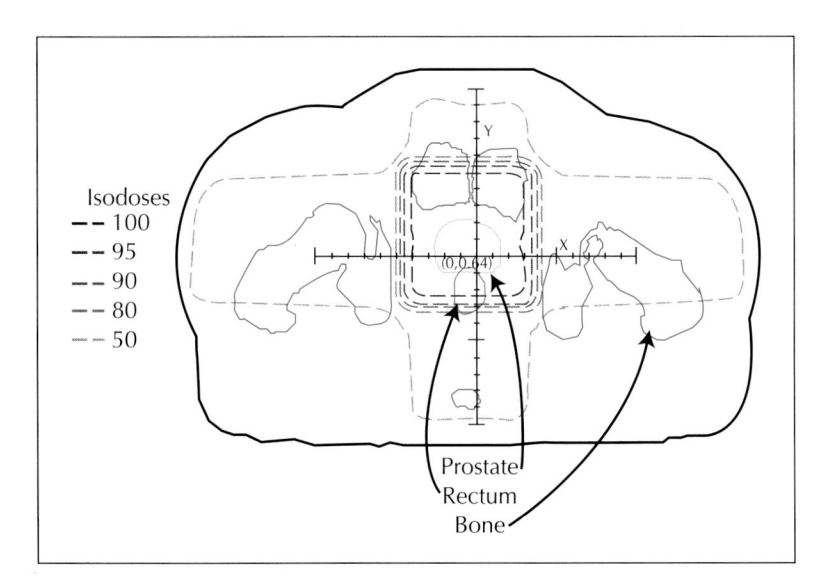

FIGURE 12-9. Isodose distributions for prostate, bladder, and rectum. The adequacy of delivering a prescribed dose to the volume of interest is paramount. For a given treatment volume to be treated with external beam radiotherapy (EBRT), a series of isodose curves can be generated. These curves represent points of equal dose (usually as percent-dose) in the volume of interest and reflect the way dose is absorbed in tissue along the track of the beams. For any given set of isodose curves, the distribution is a function of beam energy selected for treatment, the volume of the treatment portal, and the dimensions of the patient. Typically the goal is to encompass the tumor volume and tissues at risk by 100% of the prescribed dose. Dose distributions are usually plotted on a computer by a radiation dosimetrist using the field coordinates established at simulation. In conventional EBRT, a contour of the patient is taken along the central axis of the treatment field and correlated to a similar CT image. In this way, structures of interest such as the prostate, rectum, and seminal vesicles can then be matched to the isodose plan generated.

II. The Prostate

RESULTS OF EXTERNAL BEAM RADIOTHERAPY FOR PROSTATE CANCER

Results of Definitive Radiation Therapy for Prostate Cancer

Study	Stage	Patients, n	Overall Survival, %	Disease-Free Survival, %	Local Recurrence, %
Bagshaw et al. [12]	T1b	308	65	70	20
Hanks [13]	T1b	116	63	52	15
Perez et al. [14]	T1b	48	70	60	20
Bagshaw et al. [12]	T2	218	55	65	30
Hanks [13]	T2	415	46	34	29
Perez et al. [14]	T2	252	65	56	24
Bagshaw et al. [15]	T3	385	38	50	38
Hanks [13]	T3	296	32	26	30
Perez et al. [14]	T3	412	42	38	40

▶ FIGURE 12-10. Results of definitive radiation therapy for prostate cancer (selected studies with 10-year follow-up). Conventional oncology endpoints for assessing treatment effectiveness (*eg*, 5-year survival) have proved to be inadequate when considering patients treated for prostate cancer. Consequently, outcome measures based on longer survival intervals (*eg*, >10 years) have been judged more informative. More recently, other endpoints rather than death and clinical local failure have been estimated as more sensitive indicators of response. This has been particularly driven by the use of biochemical markers (*eg*, prostate-specific antigen [PSA]) for assessing treatment benefit. However, it remains unclear as to the value of such early detection [9]. In the cited selected studies, the data presented originates in the pre-PSA–guided era. Nonetheless, in comparing such results with the contemporaneous surgical literature, the American Urological Association Prostate Cancer Clinical Guidelines concluded that for early stage disease, EBRT and radical prostatectomy offer equivalent treatment benefits to patients with prostate cancer [10]. For locally advanced disease, the studies demonstrated that conventional EBRT alone can result in the long-term survival of only a minority of patients, thus necessitating alternative approaches for management of this stage [11].

Moderate and Severe Late Complications of Conventional (Nonconformal) EBRT for Prostate Cancer

		Genitourinary, %			Gastrointestinal, %				
Series	Patients, n	Hematuria/Cystitis	Stricture	Incontinence	Rectal	Small Intestine	Fistula, %	Other	Death, %
Stanford [16]	802	9.5*	9.5*	9.5*	4.4†	4.4†	0	1.7‡	0
RTOG [17]	453	4.4	5.1	0	3.3	0.4	0	0	0
Mallinckrodt [18]	577	2.9	4.5	0.1	5.9	2.0	0.5	3.6§	0.1
Johns Hopkins [19]	240	4.6	6.6	3.0	10.8	1.0	0	3.5‡	0
St. Francis [20]	251	5.0	6.0	0.4	10.0	1.6	0.4	0.8‡	0.4

*Includes all genitourinary complications.
†Includes all gastrointestinal complications.
‡Genital and leg edema.
§Pubic bone necrosis, genital and leg edema, subcutaneous fibrosis, and skin necrosis.

▶ FIGURE 12-11. Sequelae of conventional external beam radiotherapy (EBRT). Conventional EBRT is generally well tolerated, although a majority of patients will experience mild to moderate gastrointestinal, genitourinary, and skin symptoms. Gastrointestinal changes tend to be predominant. Side effects tend to develop in the latter part of a treatment course and usually resolve within weeks of ending irradiation. Persistent symptoms and late (> 3 months) complications are infrequent and likely associated with more profound parenchymal injury. The risk of late complications in conventional EBRT is associated with higher radiation doses (> 70 Gy), volume of normal tissues in the treatment field (*eg*, anterior rectal wall), and patient comorbidities. Sexual function after prostate irradiation has not been well studied; however, the literature suggests altered potency in up to 60 % of men. Unfortunately, most such studies do not account for the premorbid erectile status of the patients. RTOG—Radiation Therapy Oncology Group. (*Adapted from* Oesterling et al. [9].)

ADVANCES IN TREATMENT OF PROSTATE CANCER USING EXTERNAL BEAM RADIOTHERAPY

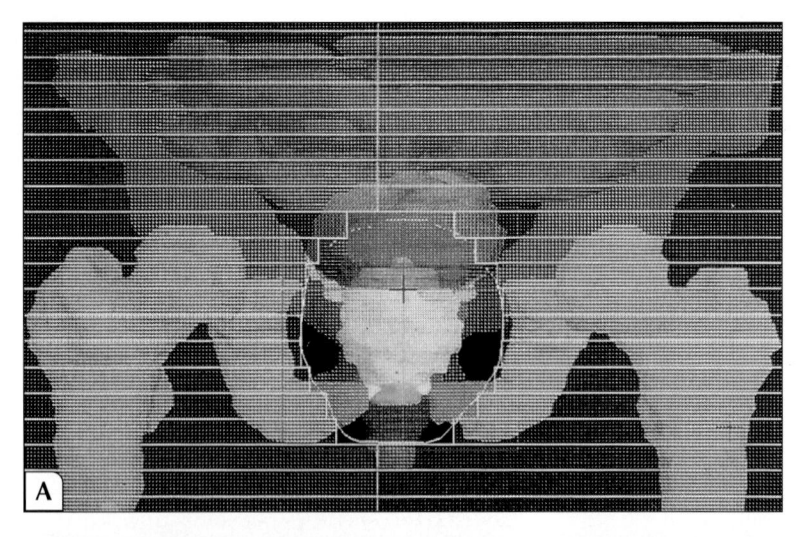

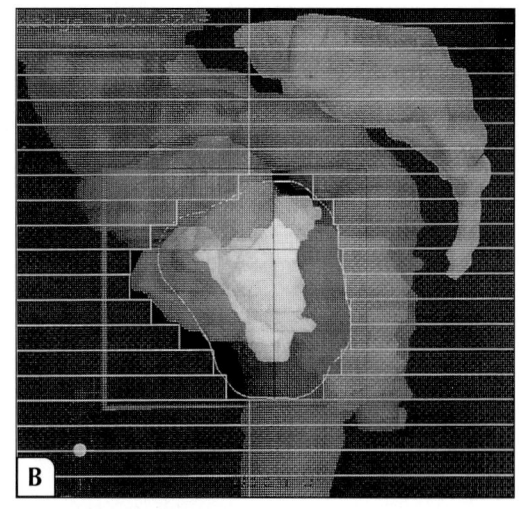

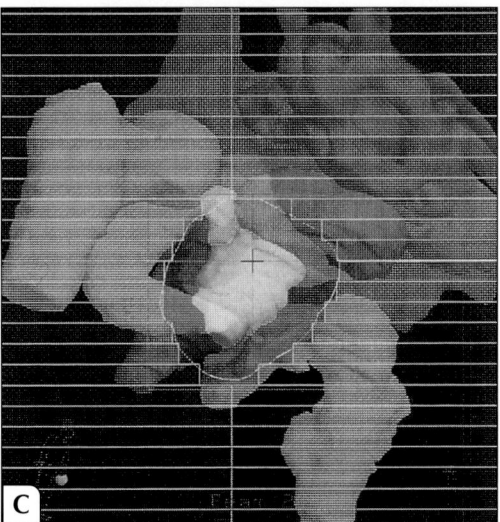

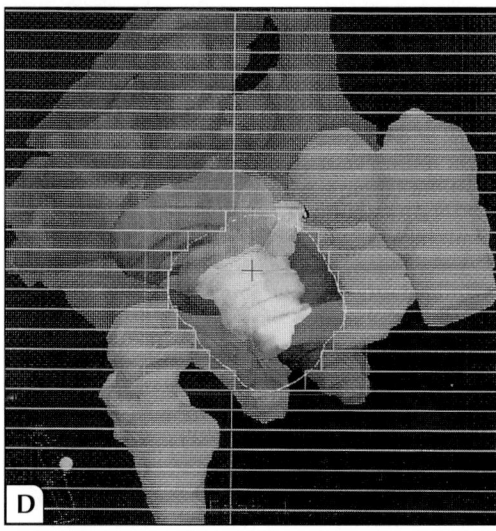

▶ **FIGURE 12-12.** Three-dimensional treatment planning (3DTP) of external beam radiotherapy for prostate cancer (beam shaping). Current studies have shown that 3DTP reduces the acute toxicity of radiotherapy. Data on late complications and disease control is still scarce. The figures show a beam's-eye-view reconstruction of the prostate, seminal vesicles, bladder, rectum, pelvic bones, and small intestine in an anteroposterior (*panel A*), lateral (*panel B*), right anterior inferosuperior oblique (*panel C*), and left anterior inferosuperior oblique (*panel D*) projections. The *solid white line* represents the edge of the fields that were designed to encompass the prostate gland with margins.

To generate these projections, the patient is scanned in the treatment position in an immobilization device (used throughout the treatment course to minimize movement and daily set-up errors), with radiopaque markers placed over localization points. The gross tumor volume (GTV) includes the tumor as visualized. The clinical target volume (CTV) includes the GTV plus the regions considered at risk for microscopic tumor spread. The planning target volume (PTV) includes the CTV plus an additional margin to allow for patient set-up errors and organ motion. The GTV and surrounding organs of interest are identified and their contours are entered on each CT slice on which they appear, using a tracking device. The isocenter is identified and the three-dimensional coordinates of its position are also entered. The PTV and the other organs of interest are reconstructed graphically in three dimensions. Their projection is displayed as seen from the beam's source (beam's-eye view), which enables the radiation oncologist to design beams that conform to the shape of the target.

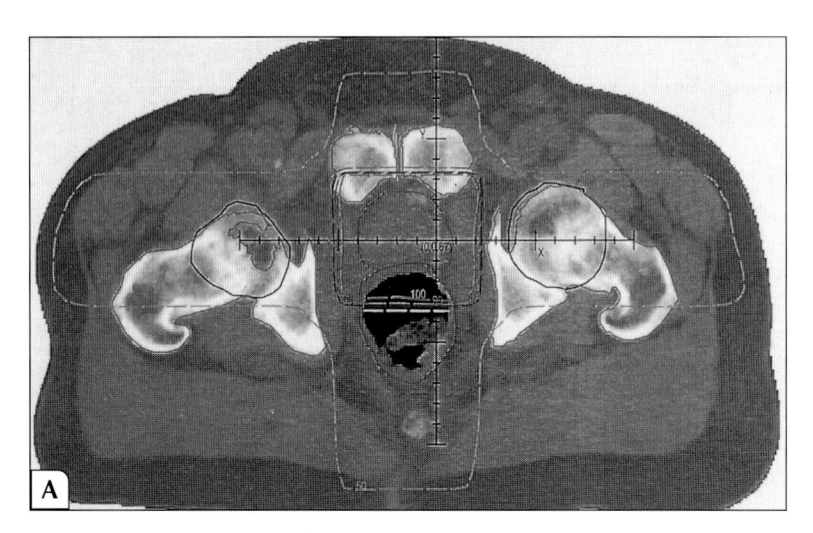

▶ **FIGURE 12-13.** Two-dimensional dose distribution and evaluation of plans. The dose distribution is computed for each field separately. Most plans involve the use of multiple fields of radiation. Once these fields are specified and weighted (each field is assigned its relative contribution to the total dose), dose computation can be carried out. The figure depicts dose distribution at the level of the central axis of a four-field "box" technique (*panel A*).

(Continued on next page)

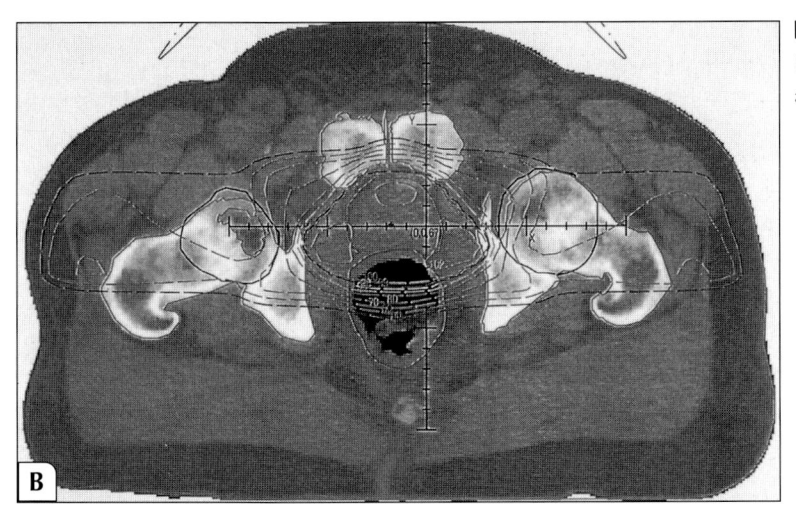

▶ **FIGURE 12-13.** *(Continued)* The figure depicts a nonaxial technique (*panel B*). The distribution of dose can be readily related to the relevant anatomy.

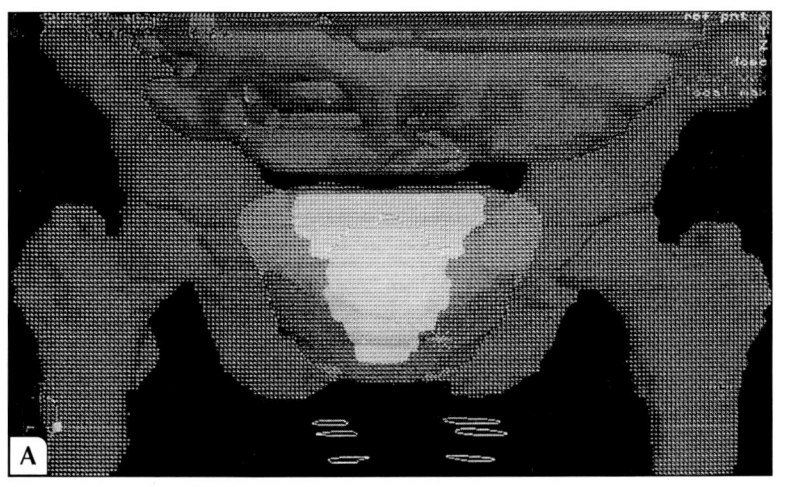

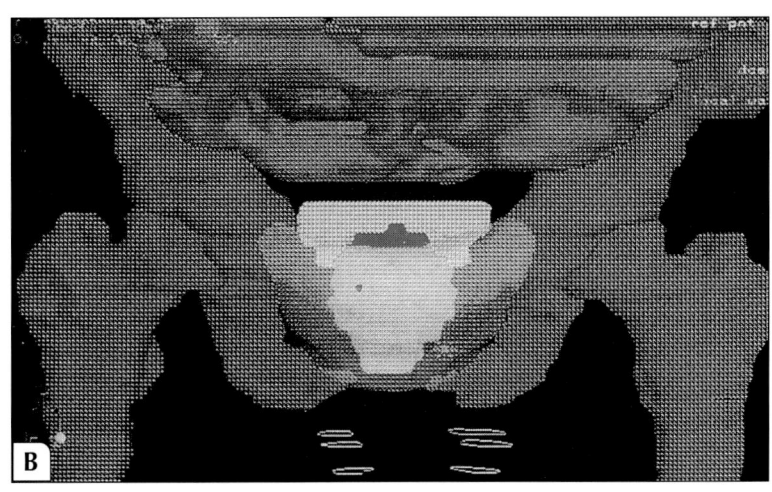

▶ **FIGURE 12-14.** Three-dimensional dose distribution and evaluation of plans. A unique feature of three-dimensional treatment planning systems is the ability to display the distribution of dose superimposed on any reconstructed axial, sagittal, coronal, or oblique plane. In addition, the distribution of dose can be viewed in three dimensions as isodose envelopes covering three-dimensional reconstructions of the target and adjacent organs. This figure depicts the distribution of dose viewed from an anteroposterior perspective. Note that while the 98% isodose envelope covers the target completely (*panel A*), the 100% isodose envelope leaves a region in the superior aspect of the gland uncovered (*panel B*). This tool allows easy identification of target regions that are underdosed or overdosed.

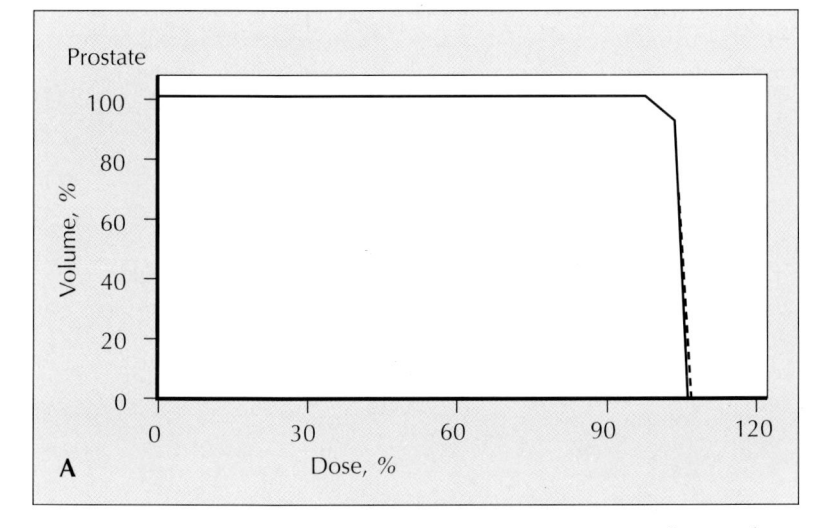

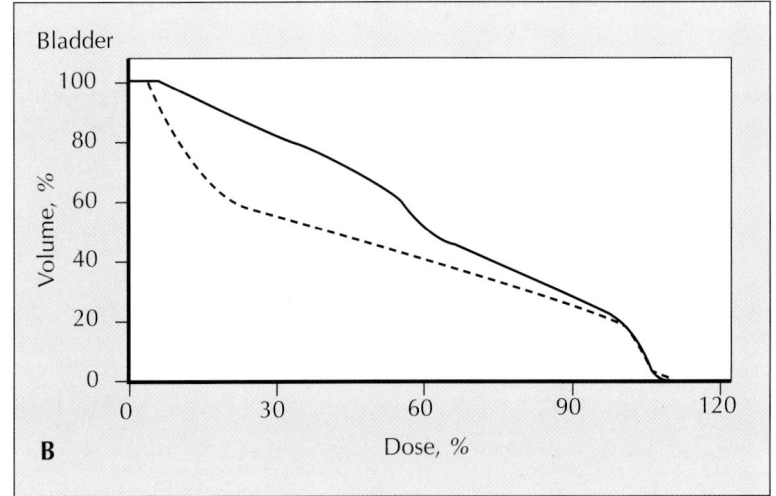

▶ **FIGURE 12-15.** Three-dimensional treatment planning of external beam radiotherapy (EBRT) for prostate cancer (dose-volume histograms [DVHs]). This histogram presents graphically the percentage of the total organ volume that receives at least a certain dose *D* (expressed as a percentage of the prescribed dose). A DVH of the target and all organs of interest are generated for each plan. This powerful tool allows quantitative comparison of different treatment plans and aids in selecting the best plan. The figure depicts DVH of the prostate (*panel A*), urinary bladder (*panel B*), and rectum (*panel C*) for two different plans.

(Continued on next page)

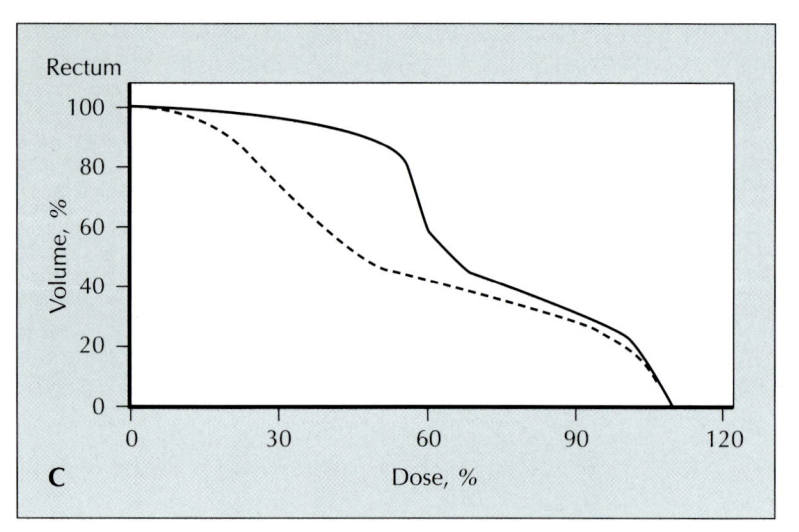

▶ **FIGURE 12-15.** *(Continued)* In plan 1 (*solid lines*), the dose is delivered to the prostate through four axial (coplanar) fields: anteroposterior, posteroanterior, and right and left laterals. This common field arrangement is also known as a four-field box technique. In plan 2 (*broken lines*), the anteroposterior and posteroanterior fields (which do not spare the rectum or bladder) have been replaced with right and left anterior inferosuperior oblique fields. The latter pair has two distinct advantages: 1) each field partially spares the bladder and rectum, and 2) the fields are nonaxial and therefore they overlap to a much lesser extent. Comparison of the DVHs reveals that whereas the coverage of the prostate remains unchanged, the volumes of bladder and rectum that receive the high doses are reduced in plan 2.

Prospective Randomized Trials of Androgen Suppression and Radiotherapy

		5-Year Biochemical DFS, %		5-Year Survival, %	
Series	Patients, n	Control Arm	Study Arm	Control Arm	Study Arm
RTOG 8610 [16]	471	15	36*	~60[†]	~60[†]
RTOG 8531 [20]	945	20	53*	71	75
MDA [21]	78	51[†]	66*[‡]	73	68
EORTC [22]	415	44	85*	58	78*

*Denotes statistically significant differences between the study and control arms.
[†]Estimated from a graph.
[‡]Clinical DFS; PSA data not available for analysis.

▶ **FIGURE 12-16.** Androgen deprivation and radiotherapy. Androgen deprivation has been combined with radiotherapy in an attempt to enhance prostate cancer cell kill. The table summarizes the results of four major prospective randomized clinical trials of this combination therapy. The Radiation Therapy Oncology Group (RTOG) trial 8610 randomly assigned 471 patients to radiotherapy alone or 4 months of androgen deprivation before and during radiotherapy. With a median follow-up time of 4.5 years, local control and disease-free survival were 54% versus 29% and 36% versus 15%, respectively [16]. The RTOG trial 8531 randomly assigned 945 patients to immediate therapy with luteinizing hormone–releasing hormone (LHRH) agonist or the same androgen suppression at time of relapse. Although local control and disease-free survival (DFS) were improved, there was no statistically significant impact on overall survival. In a subset analysis, patients with poorly differentiated tumors showed a significant survival advantage (66% vs 55%, $P = 0.03$). At the MD Anderson (MDA) Cancer Center, 78 patients with stage C prostate cancer were randomly assigned to receive radiotherapy with or without adjuvant estrogen. DFS in the adjuvant group was significantly higher than in the radiation-only group. At 5, 10, and 15 years, DFSs were 66%, 58%, 58%, and 51%, 46%, 37% in the adjuvant and control groups, respectively [21]. The benefit of early hormonal intervention was attributed to suppression of the emergence of distant metastases. Early estrogen administration was also associated with a trend toward higher local control, but the difference did not reach significance. The European Organization for Research and Treatment of Cancer (EORTC) conducted a multicenter prospectively randomized trial in patients with high-grade T1 to 2 or T3 to 4 prostate cancer. A total of 415 patients were randomly assigned to radiotherapy with or without 3 years of hormonal therapy. With a median follow-up time of 36 months, they reported a significant improvement in local control, disease-free survival, and, most importantly, a survival advantage (78% versus 56%) for those patients treated with hormones [22]. PSA—prostate-specific antigen.

Preliminary Results of Dose Escalation Trials

Series	Patients, n	Dose Level, Gy	Median Follow-Up, mo	Severe (Grade 3–4) Complications, %
MSKCC [23]	59	75.6	14	0
	21	81		0
FCCC [24]	136	71–73.99	36	1.8[‡]
	130	74–76.99		4.5[‡]
	19	77–79.99		12.3[‡]
WSU [25]	25	78*	20	0
	24	82.8[†]		0

*1.3 Gy twice daily.
[†]1.15 Gy twice daily.
[‡]Gastrointestinal complications.

FIGURE 12-17. Preliminary results of dose escalation trials. In recent years, along with the increase in use of prostate-specific antigen (PSA) in follow-up, it has become clear that standard treatment options for patients with locally advanced prostate cancer are suboptimal. Investigational efforts have focused on increasing the tumoricidal impact of therapy by increasing the physical dose, the biologic effective dose, or by combining radiotherapy with other tumoricidal treatments. The Patterns of Care study provided some evidence for a dose-response in prostate cancer [26]. Total doses in excess of 70 Gy were associated with an increase in local control. Unfortunately, such doses were also associated with an unacceptable complication rate. The underlying rationale for the phase I dose-escalation studies currently underway is that higher doses can be delivered safely using three-dimensional treatment planning. Higher doses are expected to improve local control. It is hoped that such an improvement will also translate into a survival advantage. This figure summarizes preliminary results of these studies at Memorial Sloan-Kettering Cancer Center (MSKCC), Fox Chase Cancer Center (FCCC), and Wayne State University (WSU). In general, the results are quite encouraging. With the exception of the results from FCCC, severe late complications appear to be lower than what has been reported with traditional treatment planning and conventional doses.

Prospective Randomized Trials of Neutron Radiotherapy for Locally Advanced Prostate Cancer

Series	Patients, n	Dose to Prostate	5-Year Local Control, %	5-Year Biochemical DFS, %	5-Year Survival, %
NTCWG 8523 [19]					
Control arm	85	70–70.2 Gy	78*	55*	73
Study arm	87	20.4 Ngy	89	83	68
RTOG 7704 [18]					
Control arm	36	70 Gy[†]	61*	NA	13*
Study arm	55	70 Gy[†]	81	NA	63

*Denotes statistically significant differences between the study and control arms.
[†]Photon equivalent dose. Patients were treated with a mixture of 40% neutrons and 60% photons. The daily neutron dose was adjusted at each institution, depending on the relative biologic effectiveness of the beam, so that equivalent biologic doses of neutron or photons were given each day.

FIGURE 12-18. Neutron radiotherapy for locally advanced prostate cancer. Fast neutrons are heavy subatomic particles with distinct radiobiologic advantages over photons. Cell kill with neutrons is less sensitive to the effects of tumor hypoxia (a major contributing factor to radioresistance), cell-cycle kinetics (cells in G_0 are relatively resistant to photons), and repair of sublethal damage. The Radiation Therapy Oncology Group (RTOG) conducted a prospective randomized trial (RTOG 7704) comparing a mixture of photons and neutron beams with photon radiotherapy in patients with locally advanced prostate cancer. At 8 years, the actuarial survival was 63% and 13% in the mixed beam and photon cohorts, respectively ($P = 0.001$). After correction for non-cancer–related deaths, there was still a significant advantage to the neutron–photon arm (82% vs 54%, $P = 0.02$). There was also a significant difference in local control (77% vs 31%, $P = 0.01$). In another trial, conducted by the Neutron Therapy Collaborative Working Group (NTCWG 8523), patients were randomly assigned to neutron or photon therapy. With a median follow-up of 68 months, there were significant differences in local control (87% vs 68%, $P = 0.01$), disease-free survival (83% vs 55%, $P < 0.001$), but not in survival [19]. A significant increase in severe morbidity was noted in the neutron arm; grade 4 complication occurred in 10 of 87 patients in the neutron group (including six colostomies), but in only one of 85 in the photon arm. Complications were mostly confined to institutions where neutron beam shaping was not available. With modern equipment and with the aid of three-dimensional treatment planning, neutron radiotherapy can be delivered without excessive complications [17]. DFS—disease-free survival; NA—not available.

EXTERNAL BEAM RADIOTHERAPY AFTER RADICAL PROSTATECTOMY

Ten-year Results of Adjuvant Irradiation for Postprostatectomy Patients at High Risk for Local Recurrence

Study	Radiotherapy*	Patients, n	Local Control	DFS, %	Overall Survival, %
Elias et al. [27]	+	31	97	61	81
	−	79	72	47	67
Anscher et al. [28]	+	46	92	55	62
	−	60	60	37	52
Shevlin et al. [29]	+	16	100	64	76
	−	57	72	56	80
Paulson et al. [30]	+	48	—	65	95
	−	116	—	80	55
Meier et al. [31]	+	19	94	68	61
	−	39	69	38	57

*Plus sign indicates with adjuvant radiation; minus sign indicates without adjuvant radiation.

▶ **FIGURE 12-19.** Selected series with 10-year results. This figure illustrates the role of adjuvant irradiation for postprostatectomy patients at high risk of local recurrence. Predictors of increased risk of local relapse after radical prostatectomy for localized carcinoma of the prostate include seminal vesicle invasion, poorly differentiated histology (Gleason score 8 through 10), or positive surgical margins. Postoperative external beam radiotherapy (EBRT) has been used as an adjuvant in these settings to increase local control. Whether the pelvic lymph nodes should be included with the prostate volumes to be irradiated in this setting remains controversial. Widespread use of prostate-specific antigen (PSA) testing in the follow-up of resected prostate cancer patients has also affected the timing and administration of adjuvant EBRT [11]. The impact of postoperative EBRT on overall survival has not been tested in a randomized fashion. The failure to demonstrate consistent survival benefits in nonrandomized studies may suggest that poor pathologic features found at surgery for this presentation are markers for distant disease and, therefore, adjuvant EBRT can have only a marginal benefit on survival. DFS—disease-free survival; OS—overall survival.

REFERENCES

1. Perez CA: Prostate. In *The Principles and Practice of Radiation Oncology.* Edited by Perez CA, Brady LW. Philadelphia: Lippincott-Raven Publishers; 1997:1583–1694.
2. Perez CA, Eisbruch A: Role of postradical prostatectomy irradiation in carcinoma of the prostate. *Semin Radiol Oncol* 1993, 3:198–209.
3. Netter FH: Pelvis and perineum. In *Atlas of Human Anatomy.* Summit, NJ: Ciba-Geigy Co.; 1989: 337–347.
4. Agur AHR: The perineum and pelvis. In *Grant's Atlas of Anatomy.* Baltimore: Williams & Wilkins, 1991:147–198.
5. Partin AW, Yoo J, Carter WH, et al.: The use of prostate specific antigen, clinical stage and Gleason score to predict pathological stage in men with localized prostate cancer. *J Urol* 1993, 150:110–114.
6. Pisansky TM, Zincke H, Sumer VJ, et al.: Correlation of pretherapy prostate cancer characteristics with histologic findings from pelvic lymphadenectomy specimens. *Int J Radiat Oncol Biol Phys* 1996, 34:33–39.
7. McGwan DG: The value of extended field radiation therapy in carcinoma of the prostate. *Int J Radiat Oncol Biol Phys* 1981, 7:1333–1339.
8. Asbell SO, Kroll JM, Pilepich MV, et al.: Elective pelvic irradiation in stage A2, B carcinoma of the prostate: analysis of RTOG 77-06. *Int J Radiat Oncol Biol Phys* 1988, 15:1307–1316.
9. Oesterling J, Fuks Z, Lee CT, et al.: Cancer of the prostate. In *Cancer: Principles and Practice of Oncology,* vol 1. Edited by DeVita VT, Hellman S, Rosenberg S. Philadelphia: Lippincott-Raven Publishers; 1997:1322–1386.
10. The American Urologial Association: *The American Urological Association Prostate Cancer Clinical Guidelines Panel Report on the Management of Clinically Localized Prostate Cancer.* Baltimore: American Urological Association; 1995.
11. Hartford AC, Zietman AL: Prostate cancer: who is best benefited by external beam radiation therapy? *Hematol Oncol Clin North Am* 1996, 10:595–610.
12. Bagshaw MA, Cox RS, Ramback JE: Radiation therapy for localized prostate cancer: justification by long term follow-up. *Urol Clin North Am* 1990, 17:787–802.
13. Hanks GE: Treatment for early stage prostate cancer: radiotherapy. In *Important Advances in Oncology.* Edited by Hellman S, DeVita V, Rosenberg S, et al. Philadelphia: JB Lippincott; 1993.
14. Perez CA, Lee H, Georgiou A, et al.: Technical and tumor-related factors affecting outcomes of definitive irradiation for localized carcinoma of the prostate. *Int J Radiat Biol Phys* 1993, 26:565–581.
15. Bagshaw MA, Cow RS, Ray GR: Status of radiation therapy of prostate cancer at Stanford University. *Monogr Natl Cancer Inst* 1988, 7:47–60.
16. Pilepich MV, Krall JM, al-Sarraf M, et al.: Androgen deprivation with radiation therapy compared with radiation therapy alone for locally advanced prostatic carcinoma: a randomized comparative trial of the Radiation Therapy Oncology Group. *Urology* 1995, 45:616–623.
17. Forman JD, Duclos M, Sharma R, et al.: Conformal mixed neutron and photon irradiation in localized and locally advanced prostate cancer: preliminary estimates of the therapeutic ratio. *Int J Radiat Oncol Biol Phys* 1996, 35:259–266.
18. Laramore GE, Krall JM, Thomas FJ, et al.: Fast neutron radiotherapy for locally advanced prostate cancer: final report of a RTOG randomized clinical trial. *Am J Clin Oncol* 1993, 16:164–167.
19. Russell KJ, Caplan RJ, Laramore GE, et al.: Photon versus fast neutron external beam radiotherapy in the treatment of locally advanced prostate cancer: results of a randomized prospective trial. *Int J Radiat Oncol Biol Phys* 1994, 28:47–54.
20. Pilepich MV, Caplan R, Byhardt RW, et al.: Phase III trial of androgen suppression using goserelin in unfavorable-prognosis carcinoma of the prostate treated with definitive radiotherapy: report of Radiation Therapy Oncology Group protocol 85-31. *J Clin Oncol* 1997, 15:1013–1021.
21. Zagars KG, Johnson DE, Von Eschenbach AC, Hussey DH: Adjuvant estrogen following radiation therapy for stage C adenocarcinoma of the prostate: long-term results of a prospective randomized study. *Int J Radiat Oncol Biol Phys* 1988, 14:1085–1091.
22. Bolla M, Gonzalez D, Warde P, et al.: Improved survival in patients with locally advanced prostate cancer treated with radiotherapy and goserelin. *N Engl J Med* 1997, 37:295–300.
23. Leibel SA, Zelefsky MJ, Kutcher GJ, et al.: Three-dimensional conformal radiation therapy in localized carcinoma of the prostate: interim report of a phase 1 dose-escalation study. *J Urol* 1994, 152:1792–1798.
24. Schultheiss TE, Lee R, Hunt M, et al.: Late GI and GU complications in the treatment of prostate cancer. *Int J Radiat Oncol Biol Phys* 1997, 37:3–11.

25. Forman JD, Duclos M, Shamsa F, et al.: Hyperfractionated conformal radiotherapy in locally advanced prostate cancer: results of a dose escalation study. *Int J Radiat Oncol Biol Phys* 1996, 34:655–662.

26. Hanks GE, Leibel SA, Krall JM, Kramer S: Patterns of care studies: dose-response observations for local control of adenocarcinoma of the prostate. *Int J Radiat Oncol Biol Phys* 1985, 11:153–157.

27. Elias S, Parker RG, Gallardo D, et al.: Adjuvant radiation therapy after radical prostatectomy for carcinoma of the prostate. *Am J Clin Oncol* 1997, 20:120–124.

28. Anscher MS, Robertson CN, Prosnitz LR: Adjuvant radiation therapy for pathologic stage T3/4 adenocarcinoma of the prostate: ten year update. *Int J Radiat Biol Phys* 1985, 33:37–43.

29. Shevlin BE, Mittal BB, Brand WN, et al.: The role of adjuvant irradiation following primary prostatectomy, based on histopathologic extent of tumor. *Int J Radiat Biol Phys* 1989, 16:1425–1430.

30. Paulson DF, Maul JW, Robertson JE, et al.: Post operative radiation therapy of the prostate for patients undergoing radical prostatectomy with positive margins, seminal vesicle involvement and/or penetration through the capsule. *J Urol* 1990, 143:1178–1182.

31. Meier R, Mark R, St Royal L, et al.: Postoperative radiation therapy after radical prostatectomy for prostate carcinoma. *Cancer* 1992, 70:1960–1966.

Interstitial Radiation Therapy

13
CANCEROUS DISEASE SECTION

William J. Ellis & John C. Blasko

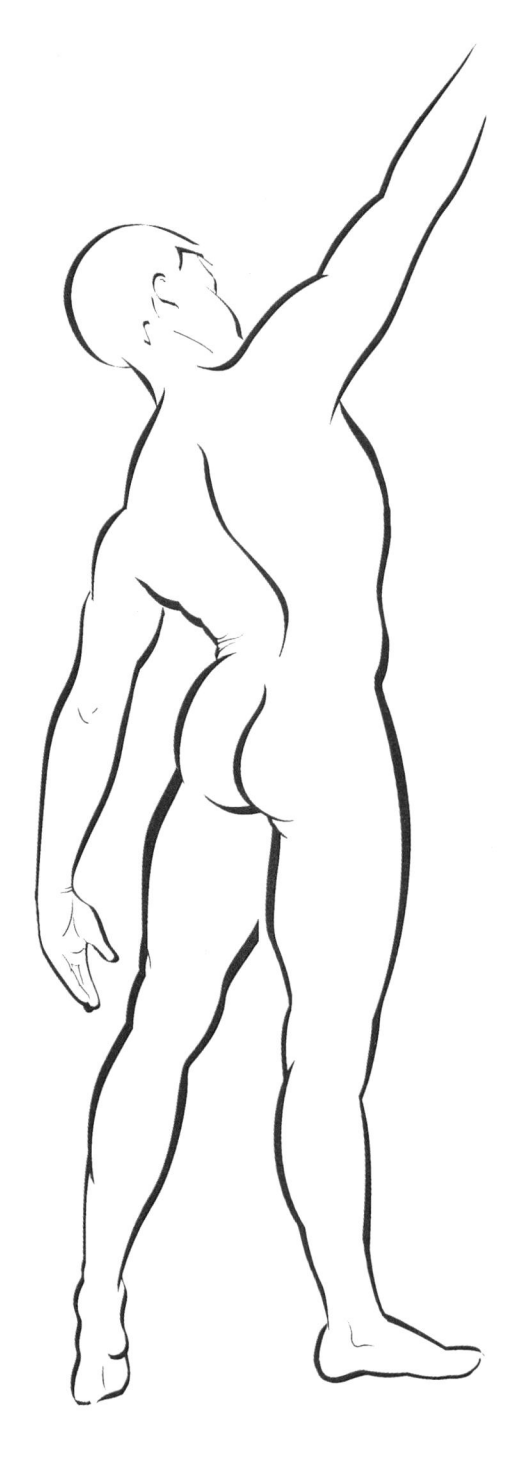

The open retropubic technique of prostate brachytherapy with permanent implants was popularized in the 1970s. However, because of poor long-term results and improvements in both external beam treatments and radical prostatectomy, the technique fell out of favor. After the introduction of transrectal prostate ultrasound in the 1980s, prostate brachytherapy was revived. With real-time ultrasonic guidance, seeds could be placed in a three-dimensional array with an accuracy far beyond that which could be obtained with the open technique.

In part due to the past experience with the open implant technique, acceptance of the closed implant procedure was initially slow. As follow-up data are now mature, long-term freedom of disease is approximating that of radical prostatectomy. The technique is now surging in popularity, as exemplified by the recent difficulties of manufacturers in keeping up with seed demand.

We believe a key to the development of a strong prostate brachytherapy program is a multidisciplinary team approach to brachytherapy. Combining the expertise of both a urologist and radiation oncologist in patient selection, implant technique, and management of posttreatment complications optimizes patient care. In addition, there are specific issues of physics, dosimetry, and nursing that are unique to prostate brachytherapy.

There are numerous variations on the technique of permanent prostate implants. These include fluoroscopic and CT guidance, CT-based planning, and intraoperative planning. The technique presented has evolved over the past decade, and we believe it optimizes both dosimetry and implantation. Variations of the technique are certainly acceptable based on staffing considerations, equipment availability, and local expertise.

Indications for Prostate Brachytherapy

Clinically localized prostate carcinoma
T1, T2, select T3
Life expectancy 10+ y
Negative metastatic evaluation in high-risk patients

FIGURE 13-1. Indications for prostate brachytherapy. The indications are similar to those for radical prostatectomy and include patients with clinically localized stage T1 and T2 tumors. In certain instances, patients with clinical stage T3 tumors would also be candidates for brachytherapy. As with any definitive therapy for prostate carcinoma, a minimum 10-year life expectancy is probably necessary for the patient to realize the benefits of definitive therapy.

Relative and Absolute Contraindications for Prostate Brachytherapy

Relative
  Large prostate
  High postvoid residual urine volume
  Severe voiding symptoms
  Previous definitive pelvic external beam radiation
  Previous prostate seed implantation
  Previous transurethral resection of the prostate
Absolute
  Metastatic disease
  Lack of a rectum

FIGURE 13-2. Relative and absolute contraindications for prostate brachytherapy. A large prostate can be technically difficult to implant due to pubic arch interference. Patients with large prostates are also more likely to develop urinary retention following implantation. Because of the potential for long-term urinary retention, we avoid implanting patients with high postvoid residual urine volumes or those with severe baseline voiding symptoms. Previous definitive external beam radiation or prostate seed implantation are considered relative contraindications to further treatment. In select cases, additional radiation can be delivered by seed implantation. However, the potential for complications, particularly incontinence, increases dramatically. Patients who have undergone previous transurethral resection of the prostate (TURP) also experience greater complications when they receive prostate seed implants. We believe the subset of patients who underwent TURP several years earlier and have at least 1 cm of prostate tissue around the central TURP defect may receive implants without undue risk of complications.

Although there are few absolute contraindications, in the setting of metastatic disease, there is little point to applying local definitive therapy. The lack of a rectum from previous prostatectomy is a technical contraindication to the prostate seed implant technique that we describe in this chapter.

PREOPERATIVE EVALUATION

Preoperative Evaluation: Tumor Evaluation

PSA level
Gleason score
Number of positive cores
Clinical stage
Bone scan (if indicated)
Pelvic lymph node dissection (if > 20% risk of nodal involvement and results would alter management)

FIGURE 13-3. Tumor evaluation. Our therapy recommendations are based on an assessment of the patient's prostate-specific antigen (PSA) level, Gleason score, the number of positive scores, and the clinical stage of the tumor. To exclude patients with metastatic disease, we generally perform a bone scan in patients with a PSA level greater than 10 ng/mL. We also recommend a staging pelvic lymph node dissection in those patients in whom the risk of nodal involvement is estimated to be greater than 20%. Nomograms and tables for calculating the risk of lymph node involvement are widely available.

Preoperative Evaluation: Voiding Parameters

American Urological Association symptom score
Peak urinary flow rate
Postvoid residual volume
Cystoscopy or pressure-flow urodynamics if significant bladder outlet obstruction is suspected

FIGURE 13-4. Voiding parameters. Symptoms of urinary frequency, urgency, and dysuria affect all patients to some degree postoperatively. Urinary retention is a more severe potential consequence of prostate brachytherapy, and efforts are made to identify those patients at risk for this complication. All patients are initially evaluated with an American Urological Association symptom score. In those patients with moderate to severe symptoms, we perform simple urodynamic studies consisting of a peak urinary flow rate and postvoid residual urine volume determinations. In symptomatic patients, treatment with hormonal downsizing of the prostate or α-blockade may be initiated prior to embarking on a brachytherapy treatment course. If significant bladder outlet obstruction is suspected, cystoscopy of pressure-flow urodynamic studies may be performed.

THERAPY SELECTION

Therapy Selection: Hormonal

Combined therapy administered a minimum of 3 mos
Provides approximately 40% decrease in prostate size
Large prostates with pubic arch interference
  Generally > 50 cc
Ideal size to implant: 20 to 40 cc
Small prostates (< 20 cc) difficult to implant
Used in some cases with large-volume disease, high-grade disease, or PSA level > 20 ng/mL

▶ **FIGURE 13-5.** Hormonal therapy. Neoadjuvant hormonal therapy is not our standard treatment. However, it is administered in many settings. The total androgen blockade administered for 3 months decreases the prostate size by roughly 40%. Patients with larger prostates and pubic arch interference are generally placed on hormonal therapy. The ideal prostate size for implantation is 20 to 40 cc. Large prostates (> 50 cc) are likely to have pubic arch interference, which places the patient at risk for urinary retention after implantation. Small prostates (< 20 cc) are difficult to implant because there is little tissue to hold the requisite number of seeds. In some patients with aggressive high-volume or high-grade tumors, hormonal therapy will be used in a neoadjuvant fashion for cancer control.

Therapy Selection: ^{103}Pd Versus ^{125}I

^{125}I half-life: 60 d
^{103}Pd half-life: 17 d
Theoretically, the choice is based on tumor-doubling times
No clear-cut clinical data to support one isotope over the other

▶ **FIGURE 13-6.** The isotopes ^{103}Pd and ^{125}I. These two isotopes are commonly used for prostate seed implantation. Theoretically, the high dose rate of ^{103}Pd results in a higher cell kill in those aggressive tumors with rapid doubling times. Conversely, the dose rate of ^{125}I may provide superior cell kill in those less aggressive tumors with long cell cycles. There is no clear-cut clinical evidence that supports the use of one isotope over the other. Many centers use one isotope for all cases.

Therapy Selection: Monotherapy Versus Boost

Monotherapy used for low-grade, low-stage disease
  Gleason score of 6 or less
  PSA level under 10 ng/mL
  T1c, T2a, and select T2b
EBRT plus implant used for others
Many cases are borderline and require clinical judgment for final determination

▶ **FIGURE 13-7.** Monotherapy versus boost. Monotherapy with brachytherapy alone will provide adequate dosimetry to the prostate with a margin of approximately 5 mm. For those tumors likely to be organ confined, with Gleason scores of 6 or less, prostate-specific antigen (PSA) values under 10 ng/mL, and in clinical T1c, T2a, and select T2b patients, monotherapy is our treatment of choice. However, those patients with high-grade tumors, bulky tumors, or a high likelihood of extensive extracapsular extension are generally treated with a combination of external beam radiation followed by a prostate seed implant boost to the prostate.

Frequently, one is faced with a case that appears to be a "borderline" situation. We may use additional findings in these cases. Factors that can increase the risk of extensive extracapsular disease include the presence of perineural invasion, a high number of positive biopsy cores, and prostate base involvement, which may indicate seminal vesicle involvement. In these patients, external beam therapy or androgen ablation may be indicated even if a strict interpretation of the algorithm would propose monotherapy. Similarly, a low-volume Gleason 7 tumor with a PSA level of less than 10 ng/mL may be adequately treated with monotherapy.

External Beam Treatment Protocol

Follows TRUS volume study
4500 cGy in 180-cGy fractions
Follow with implant boost 2–4 wks later

▶ **FIGURE 13-8.** External beam treatment protocol. In those patients in whom external beam treatment is planned, the protocol is as shown. A 2- to 4-week window is allowed between the external beam irradiation and the seed implant boost. This allows any mild proctitis that may develop after external beam irradiation to resolve. By giving external beam radiation prior to seed implantation, the patient receives the radiation sequentially. Other programs treat patients with seed implant first followed by external beam irradiation. With this type of protocol, patients simultaneously receive radiation from the implanted seeds, as well as the external radiation.

Interstitial Radiation Therapy

PROSTATE VOLUME STUDY

Purposes of the Prostate Volume Study

Simulates implant with images at 5-mm increments
Determines prostate size and shape
Can be used to determine pubic arch interference

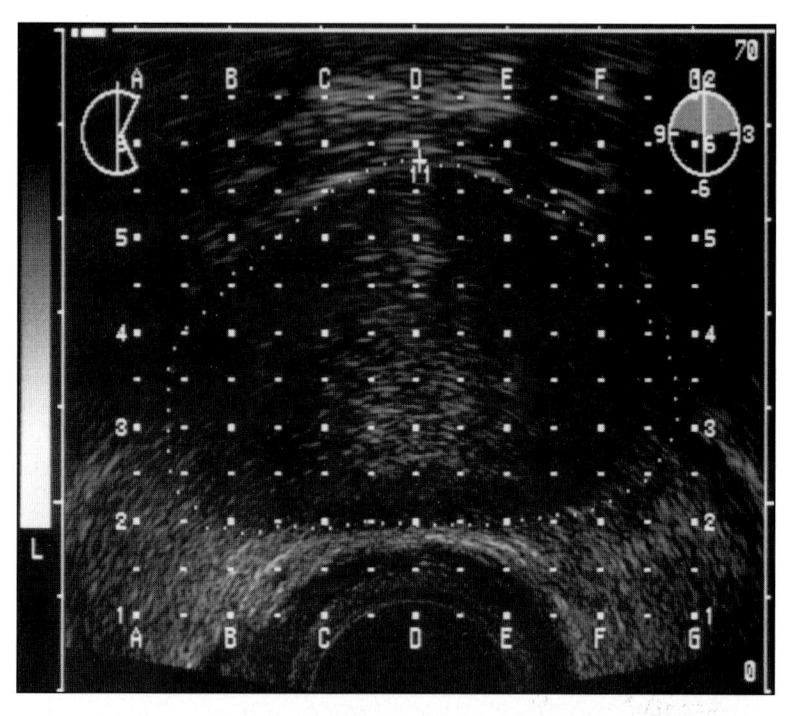

▶ **FIGURE 13-9.** Purposes of the prostate volume study. The prostate volume study serves several purposes. Most importantly the study simulates the implant and obtains the images that will be used by physicians for the treatment planning period. We believe that this preplanning allows dosimetry to account for variability in prostate shape. Intraoperative planning uses nomograms based on prostate size, but do not account for variability in prostate shape. The ultrasound determines prostate size, which is important to relate to the patient's voiding symptoms and gives an assessment of the patient's risk of urinary complications. Finally, the volume study can be used to image the pubic arch and determine the degree of pubic arch interference likely to be encountered.

▶ **FIGURE 13-10.** Transrectal prostate volume study. The first step in treatment planning is the transrectal ultrasound prostate volume study, which simulates the implant procedure. The patient is positioned in the lithotomy position exactly as he will be during the implantation. The transducer is positioned so that the prostate is aligned with the grid template as shown. The prostate is centered on the *D* row and the posterior margin of the prostate near the base is aligned with the *2* row in this example. Serial images are obtained from base to apex at 5-mm increments. The base plane comprises mainly the seminal vesicles, with a small area of prostate visible. The seminal vesicles often drop below the level of the posterior baseline. Near the apex the prostate generally rises off of the baseline. Additional images should be obtained for reference 5 mm beyond the prostate at the base and apex. This study also allows determination of prostate volume, which assesses candidacy for prostate brachytherapy.

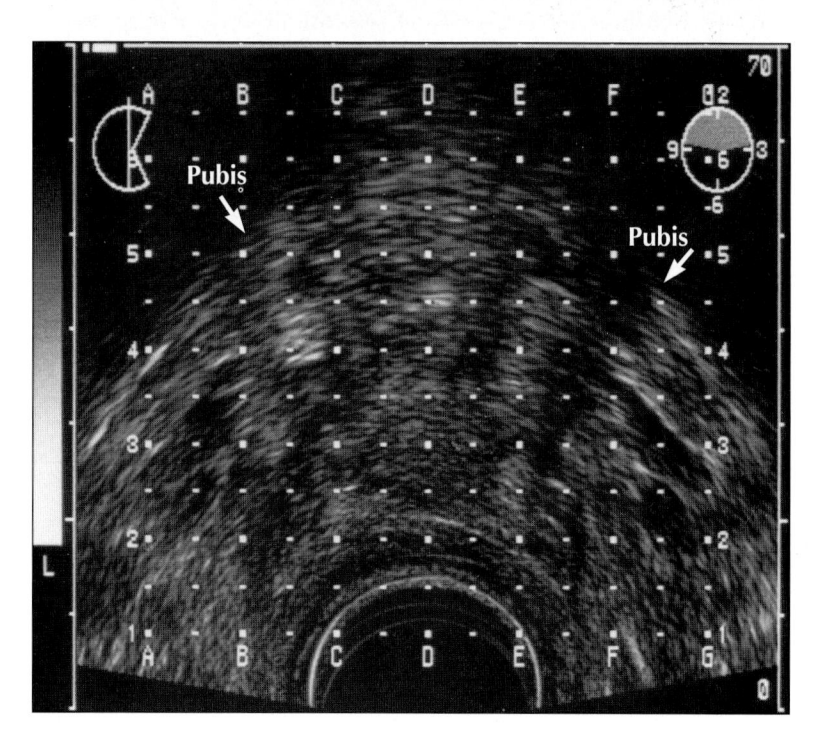

▶ **FIGURE 13-11.** Pubic arch interference assessment. Pubic arch interference can also be estimated by the treatment planning ultrasound. This image shows the inverted V of the pubic arch on transrectal ultrasound. Generally the arch is best imaged 1 to 2 cm cephalad to the prostatic apex. By comparing the grid coordinates of the pubic arch with those of the prostate, one can determine whether significant obstruction of the needle path exists.

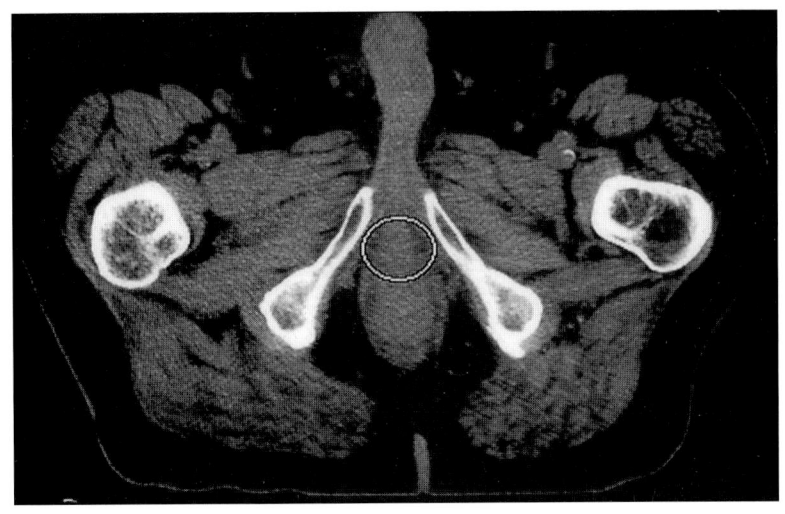

▶ **FIGURE 13-12.** An alternative mechanism of determining pubic arch interference by CT scanning. A pelvic CT is obtained with the knees elevated moderately. The prostate is outlined at its widest point and then superimposed on the image showing the pubic arch. If more than a third of the prostate area is obstructed by the pubic bone, then significant difficulty is likely to be encountered during the implantation of the anterolateral seeds. Because the knees are only moderately elevated during this procedure, there is less rotation of the prostate than with a full lithotomy position, resulting in an overestimation of the degree of pubic arch interference

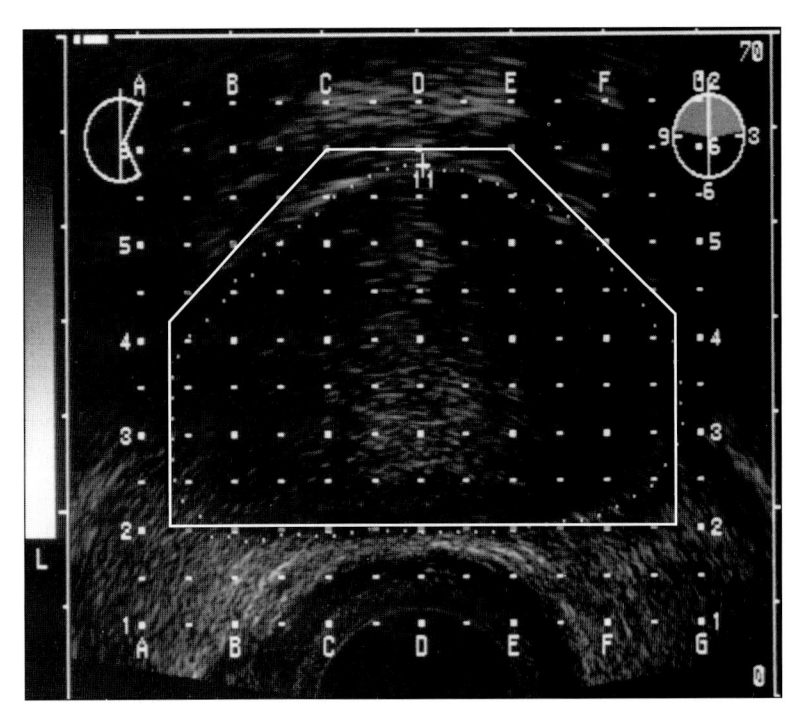

▶ **FIGURE 13-13.** Target volume. The target volume is determined at each level on the ultrasound study. We prefer to draw polygonal targets that are maintained for one to two levels. At the apex, where the prostate tapers to a smaller area, the targets are drawn with wider margins. A target is also drawn for at one level caudad to the prostate to account for potential prostate swelling and elongation.

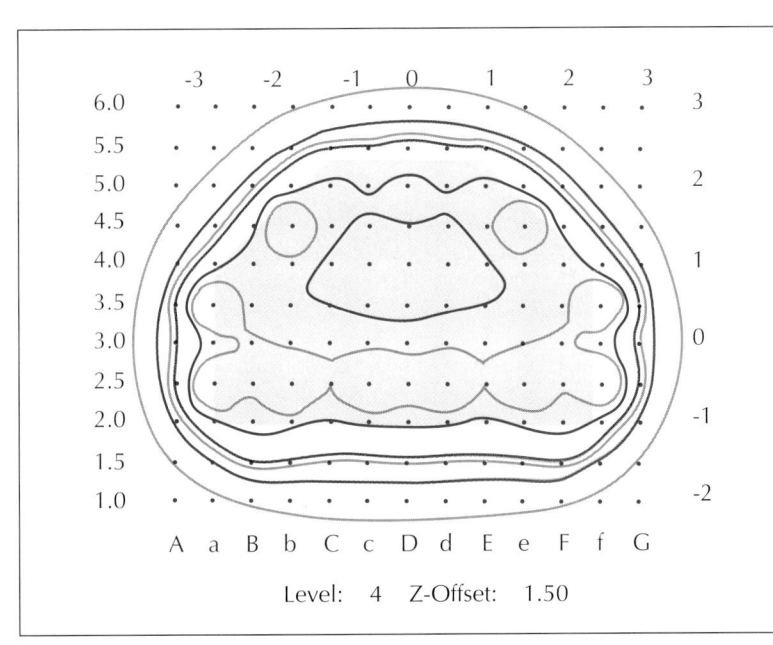

▶ **FIGURE 13-14.** The target volumes are digitized into commercially available software programs that reconstruct three-dimensional prostate images. The physicist and dosimetrist use these programs in conjunction with the radiation oncologist to determine the placement and the seeds. The pattern of seed placement can be varied to avoid structures such as the urethra or to minimize the potential for pubic arch interference. Several iterations of the plan may be developed before settling on a plan that optimizes dosimetry and minimizes potential technical difficulties or errors during the implantation. The resulting treatment plans show the coordinates of each needle to be used in the implant. The needles typically contain up to six seeds with interspersed spacers. Radiation doses to the urethra are decreased by a peripheral loading pattern and the use of "special" needles that contain additional spacers and relatively few seeds.

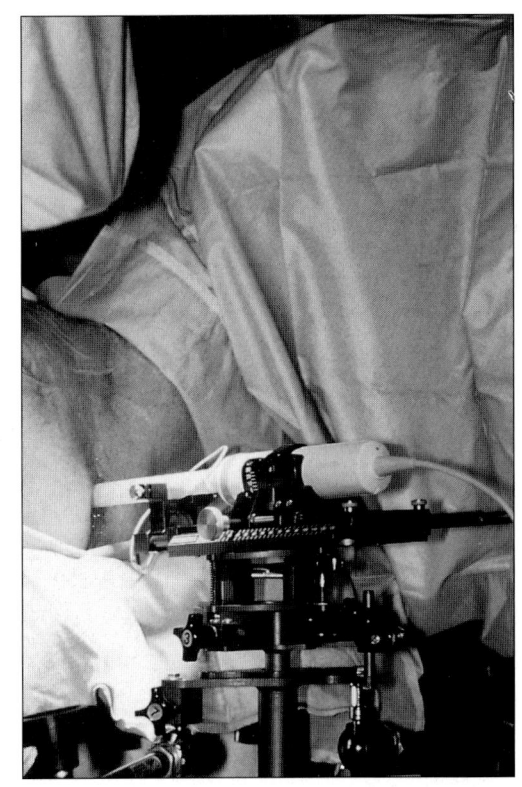

▶ **FIGURE 13-15.** Patient positioning during the implantation procedure. The patient is positioned in the full lithotomy position with the hips flexed 90°. The ultrasound transducer is placed in the rectum angled downward 10° to 15°. If the probe is fixed at a flat angle, then posterior seeds at or distal to the prostate apex will be too close to the rectum. If the probe angle is too steep, then the chance of encountering pubic arch interference is increased.

Interstitial Radiation Therapy

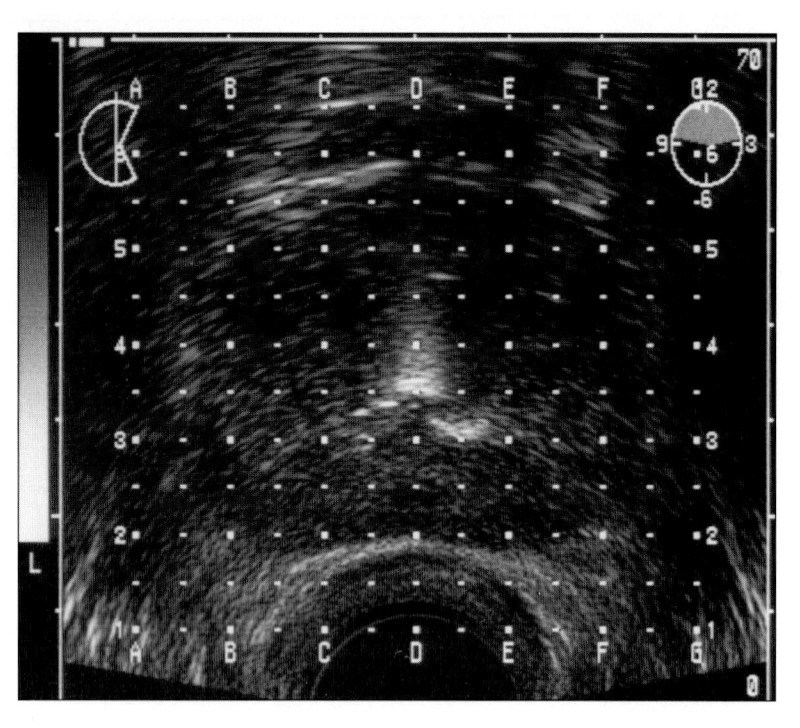

▶ **FIGURE 13-16.** Alignment of prostate with the grid as seen in the treatment plan. The base plan is determined and correlated with that in the treatment planning ultrasound. Instillation of aerated gel in the urethra just above D3.5 allows visualization of the urethra. The urethra is not necessarily centered on the grid. In asymmetric prostates, the lateral margins of the prostate should be centered. However, visualization of the urethra allows the operator to avoid intraurethral placement of seeds.

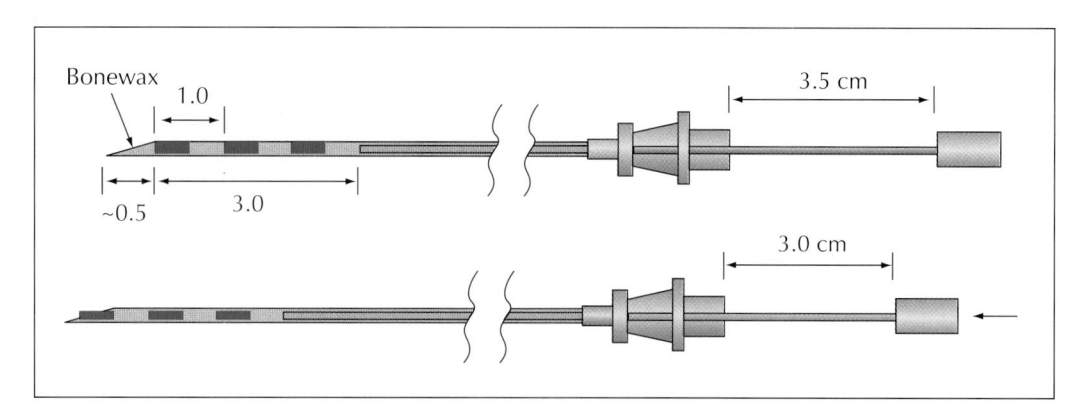

▶ **FIGURE 13-17.** A typical preloaded needle used in the treatment plan. The single tapered bevel of the needle allows steering of the needle as the needle will deviate in the direction of the bevel. Note that the 5-mm seeds are separated by a 5-mm spacer. The length of the seed and spacer combination will equal 1 cm. The protrusion of the stylet reflects the number of seeds and spacers plus several millimeters of bone wax at the tip of the needle. This bone wax should be extruded after the needle tip is positioned and before seed placement. Preloaded needles speed intraoperative seed placement, but require additional preparation time. Alternatively, the Mick applicator may be used to place the seeds individually.

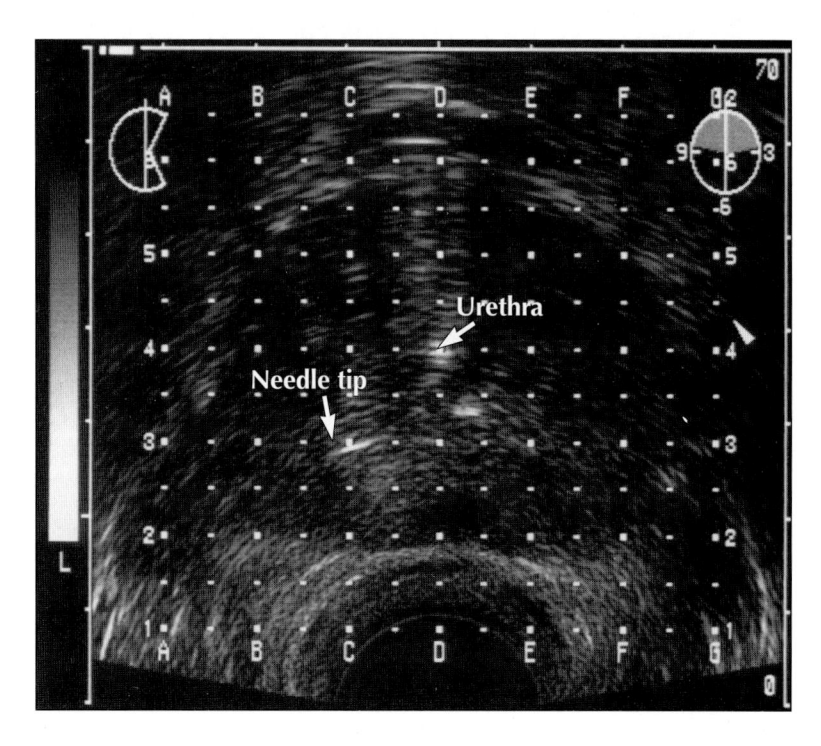

▶ **FIGURE 13-18.** Insertion of transducer. Prior to needle insertion the transducer is positioned at the appropriate level. Needle insertion is accomplished by placement of the needle in the appropriate coordinate of the template. The needle is sharply passed through the skin of the perineum. The needle will have a tendency to drift outward. Therefore, the bevel of the needle is directed toward the center of the prostate to counter this tendency. The prostate is surprisingly mobile and tends to push away from the needle. To prevent the seeds from being pushed back cephalad, the needle must be over-inserted, then pulled back until the tip of the needle is just visualized with the prostate in the neutral position. If the tip of the needle is in the plane of the ultrasound, the bevel will flash as the needle is rotated. In this example, the needle is visualized just above coordinate C3. Note the echogenic aerated gel identifying the urethra at D4 (*arrows*).

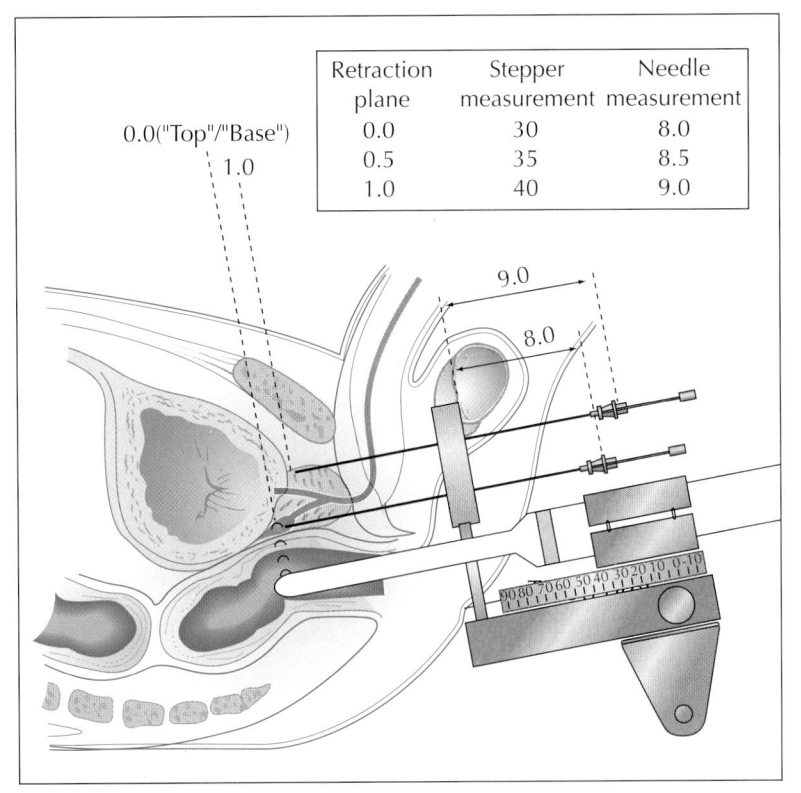

▶ **FIGURE 13-19.** Confirming the depth of insertion. The depth of insertion is confirmed by measuring the template to needle hub distance. This distance is established at the first needle placement. Once the measurement is known for one plane, the measurements for the other planes at 5-mm increments can easily be determined. A simple chart can be made by the nursing staff correlating the retraction plane with the predicted template to needle hub distance. These measurements are particularly helpful when the desired position is obscured by prostatic calculi, bleeding, or other interference. To properly locate the seeds the ultrasound is retracted several centimeters out of the plane of the interference. The needle is then aligned in the X and Y coordinates. The depth of insertion is determined by measurements rather than visually.

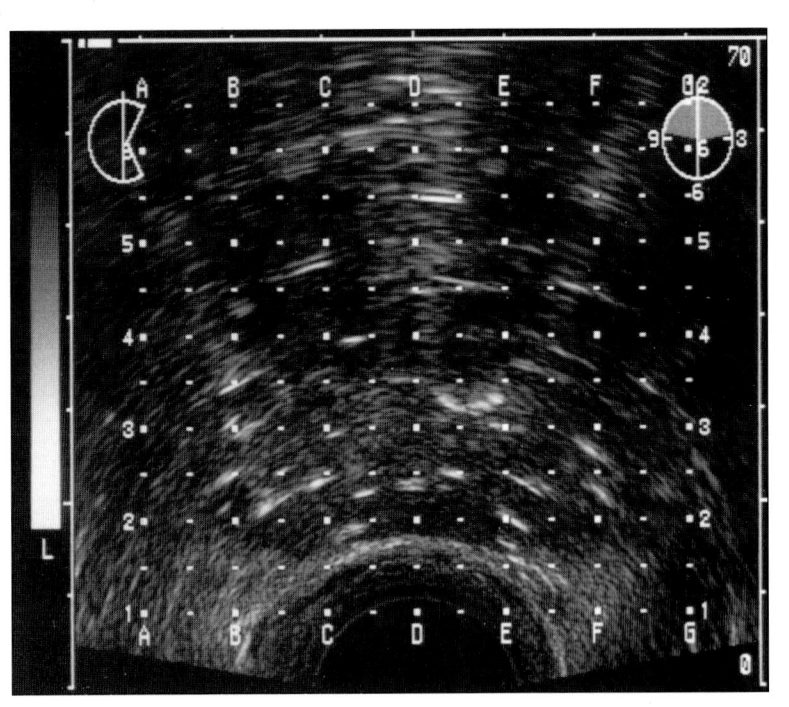

▶ **FIGURE 13-20.** Completed implant. The completed implant is viewed with ultrasound. Seeds appear as bright echogenic foci and may migrate several millimeters from their intended target. The implant is visualized from base to apex, taking note of any areas that appear to lack the planned number of seeds. The anteroposterior level for placement of "extra" seeds under fluoroscopic guidance is determined (usually the mid- to midposterior prostate).

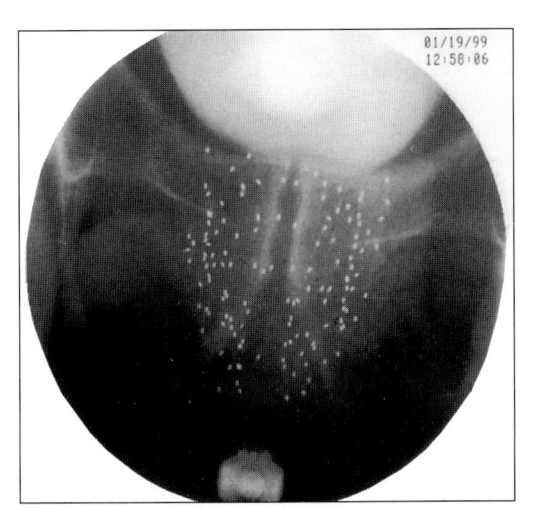

▶ **FIGURE 13-21.** Visualization of implant under fluoroscopic guidance. The implant is visualized fluoroscopically, and again any areas that appear to lack seeds are noted. Because of peripheral loading, the center of the gland is expected to appear relatively underimplanted. Particular attention is placed on areas of known cancer based on biopsy and digital rectal examination results. Under fluoroscopic guidance, additional seeds are placed in areas that appear relatively underimplanted. Because the fluoroscopic view gives only a two-dimensional view of seed placement, we rely on correlations from ultrasound imaging to guide the anterior-posterior seed placement.

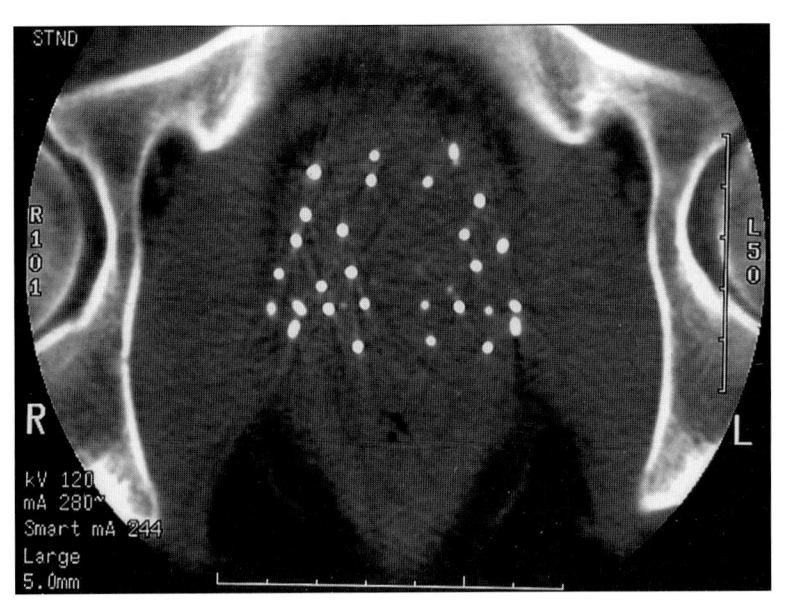

▶ **FIGURE 13-22.** Postimplantation CT scan. After the implant, a CT scan is obtained imaging the prostate at 5-mm intervals. These images are used for postimplant dosimetry determinations. The dosimetrists can use the same software used in the pretreatment planning to produce isodose curves. In addition, the percentage of the prostate receiving 100% of the prescribed radiation dose can be calculated with a dose-volume histogram.

Interstitial Radiation Therapy

RESULTS

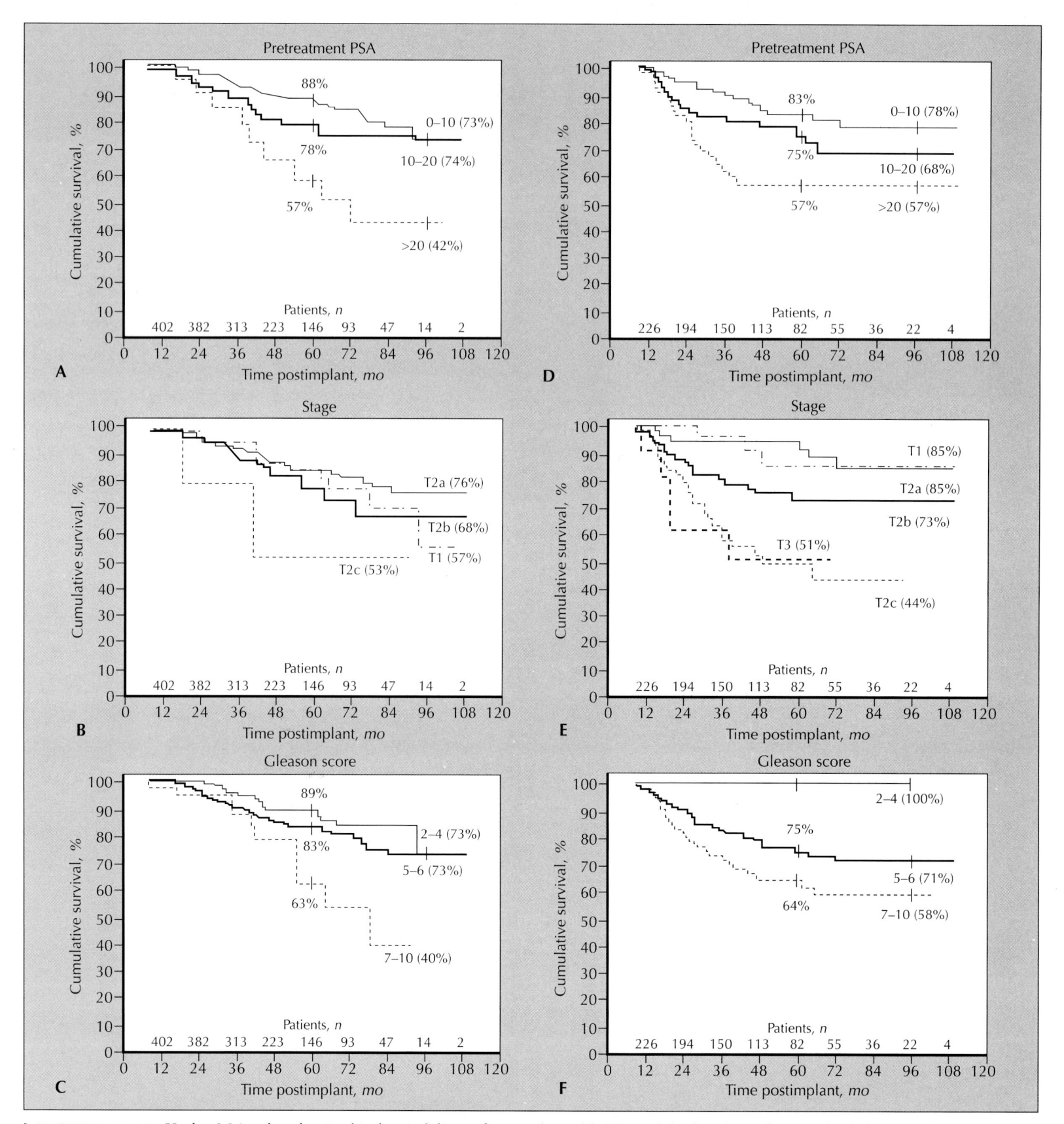

FIGURE 13-23. Kaplan-Meier plots showing biochemical disease-free survival. Here we define failure as either a serum prostate-specific antigen (PSA) level of greater than 1.0 ng/mL or three consecutive rises above the nadir PSA. Obviously, the definition of a successful treatment strongly influences the results reported. Three consecutive rises is the official definition of failure by the American Society of Therapeutic Radiation Oncologists (ASTRO). The time of failure is then backdated to the midpoint between the last stable PSA and the first elevated PSA. A level above 1.0 does not imply treatment failure in all patients, but a PSA nadir above 1.0 ng/mL is certainly a poor prognostic sign. The majority of patients in this study have been followed up for less than 5 years. Treatment failure correlates with tumor grade, stage, and initial PSA level, which are all known risk factors for disease progression. **A–C,** Monotherapy with ^{125}I and ^{103}Pd. **D–F,** Combination therapy using external beam radiotherapy plus ^{125}I and ^{103}Pd.

Complications

Hematuria (most patients)
Radiation urethritis/prostatitis (all patients)
Urinary obstruction/retention (10% to 20% transient retention)
Proctitis (10%)

▶ **FIGURE 13-24.** Sequela of prostate seed implantation. These include irritative and obstructive voiding symptoms, urinary retention, hematuria, and proctitis. The hematuria is limited to the first several days after the implant. Voiding dysfunction occurs in all patients to some degree following implantation. Initial symptoms are due to the trauma and contained bleeding associated with the implant. Later symptoms are related to radiation cystitis, urethritis, and prostatitis. Often these symptoms can be moderated with the use of α-blocking agents. Between 10% and 20% of men will undergo urinary retention following implantation, which usually resolves within 1 to 4 weeks. Urinary retention is generally treated with indwelling Foley catheterization or clean intermittent catheterization. Transurethral surgery for retention should be avoided because the irradiated prostate heals poorly, and superficial urethral necrosis may result. Proctitis is generally minimal and responds well to standard topical measures.

Cryoablation of Prostate Cancer

CANCEROUS DISEASE SECTION

Katsuto Shinohara & Peter R. Carroll

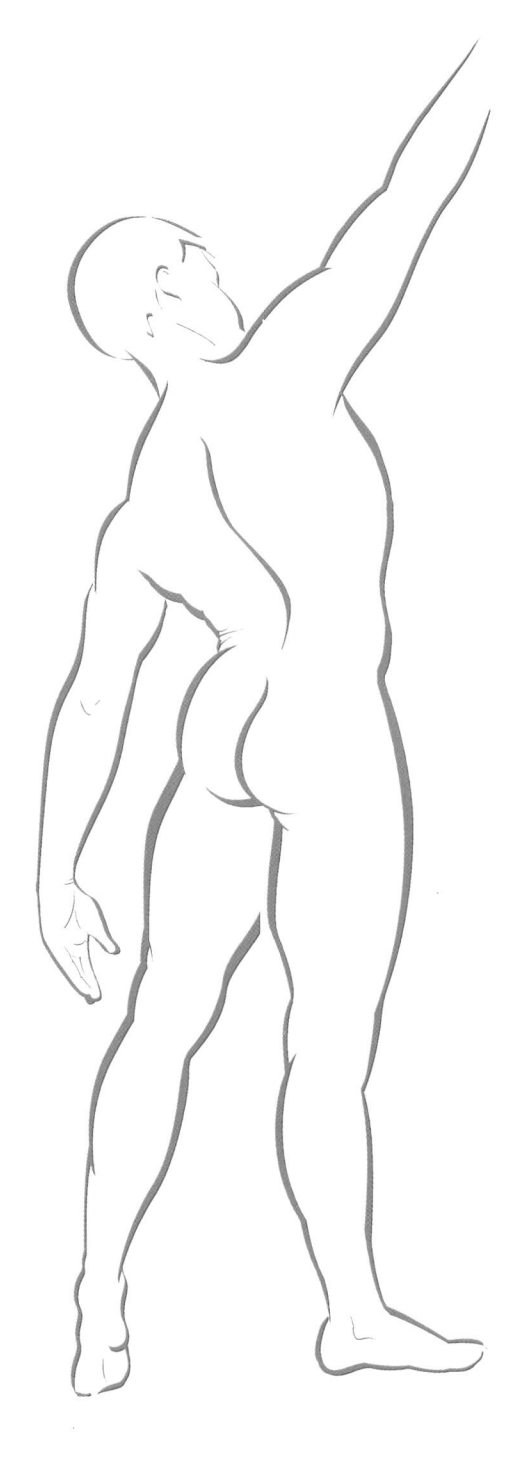

The incidence of prostate cancer has more than doubled since the late 1980s, and 184,500 new cases will be detected this year. This increase is largely due to increased use of prostate-specific antigen (PSA)-based screening, transrectal ultrasonography, and random biopsy of the prostate. The treatment of prostate cancer, however, remains controversial. No consensus has been established as to what constitutes appropriate treatment for any stage of disease, especially for localized cancers. Radical prostatectomy, radiation therapy, and watchful waiting all have been proposed, and their risks and benefits are frequently discussed. Radical prostatectomy has been criticized for its perceived high morbidity [1], whereas radiation therapy has been criticized for its uncertain efficacy [2]. Such criticisms of the conventional treatments have stimulated a search by patients and physicians for alternative treatments that may be both effective and associated with limited morbidity.

Cryosurgical ablation of the prostate was first attempted using an open technique, leading to high failure rates and significant side effects [3–6]. Improved percutaneous techniques, expertise in transrectal ultrasound, new cryotechnology, and better understanding of cryobiology have created a renewed interest in cryosurgical ablation of prostate cancer [7].

History of Cryosurgery for the Prostate Gland

Study (year)	Procedure
Gonder et al. [3] (1964)	Transurethral cryogenic prostatectomy for bladder outlet obstruction
Flocks et al. [4] (1969)	Transperineal open cryosurgery for prostate cancer
Reuter [5] (1972)	Transperineal trocar cryoablation for prostate cancer
Bonney et al. [6] (1982)	Transperineal open cryosurgery for prostate cancer follow-up results
Onik et al. [8] (1993)	Transperineal percutaneous ultrasound-guided cryoablation for prostate cancer

▶ **FIGURE 14-1.** Background. The first description of cryoablation of the prostate was published in 1966 [3]. Shortly thereafter, an attempt to destroy prostate cancer using a transperineally introduced probe was reported [5]. In 1969, urologists at the University of Iowa reported their experience with the transperineal approach [4]. Outcome, in terms of survival and recurrence, was related to stage and grade; about 41% of patients eventually had evidence of persistent or recurrent disease. Although the technique compared favorably with other treatment modalities with respect to survival, morbidity was significant. Urethral sloughing of tissue was common. Urethrorectal or urethrocutaneous fistulas developed in 13% of patients, bladder neck obstruction developed in 2.3%, and urinary incontinence developed in 6.5% [6]. This early experience was recently reviewed. Cancer recurrence was documented in 78.4% of the men, and 47.1% died of prostate cancer. Local recurrence was documented in at least 67% of those undergoing the procedure. Kaplan-Meier analyses demonstrated median progression-free and overall survival times of 34 and 75 months, respectively [7].

Despite the discouraging early results, enthusiasm for finding a minimally invasive alternative therapy for prostate cancer led to refinements in the technique of cryoablation. In 1991, Onik et al. [8] first reported the currently used technique of percutaneous transperineal ultrasound-guided cryoablation.

CRYOBIOLOGY

Mechanism of Cryogenic Tissue Ablation

Direct effect on cells
  Extracellular crystal formation leading to cellular dehydration
  pH change due to abnormal electrolyte concentration leading to denature of cellular proteins
  Thermal shock with damage to lipoproteins
  Mechanical cellular membrane disruption by intracellular crystallization
  Cellular swelling due to fluid shift during thawing
Vascular stasis due to thrombosis after freezing

▶ **FIGURE 14-2.** Biological mechanisms of tissue destruction. Cellular damage during freezing is the result of many mechanisms. Once the extracellular fluid reaches a tissue temperature of less than 0°C, it starts to crystallize. This increases the osmotic pressure of the unfrozen portion of the extracellular fluid compartment, leading to water shifting from the intracellular space to the extracellular space. As a result, cells become dehydrated. Cellular pH also changes, leading to denaturing of cellular proteins [9]. With further temperature drops, water in the intracellular space crystallizes. This mechanically breaks the cellular membrane. On thawing, extracellular fluid shifts back again into the intracellular space, leading to cellular bursting.

The blood vessels around the targeted tissue initially dilate after thawing. Hyperpermeability of the vessel wall occurs. After a few hours of this hyperemic state, microthrombi form on the damaged vessel wall, leading to ischemia of the tissue [10].

Tissue damage occurs, therefore, during both freezing and thawing. Both the duration and the number of freeze:thaw cycles are correlated with the extent of cell death. Once the tissue has reached a steady state of very low temperature, the duration of freezing appears to have little effect on tissue damage. It is known that repeating the freeze:thaw cycle creates a larger area of tissue damage, even though the low temperature achieved on each cycle is the same [11]. Cells that remain viable after the initial cycle are damaged on the second or third freeze:thaw cycle. The velocity of the temperature change also affects the extent of tissue damage. Faster freezing appears to cause more tissue damage than do slow temperature changes.

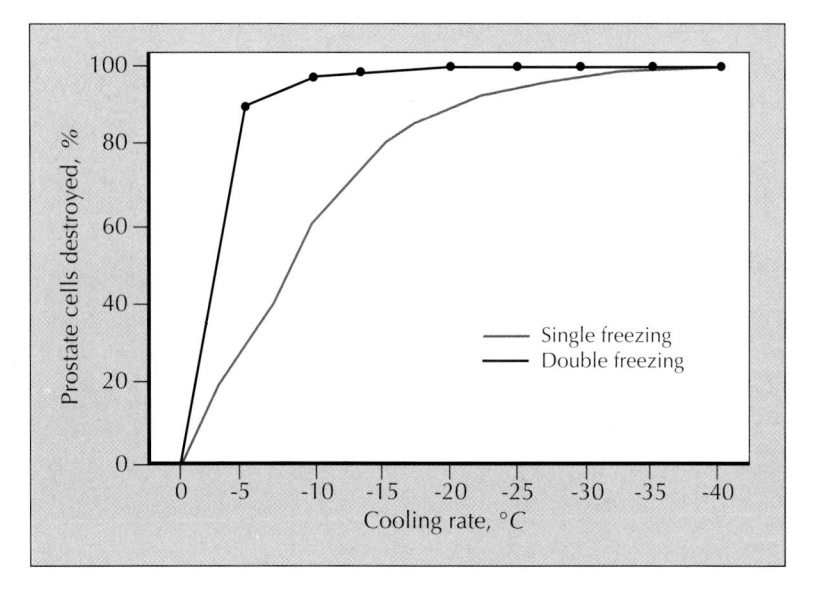

▶ **FIGURE 14-3.** Single freeze versus double freeze. Repeated freeze:thaw cycles create more extensive tissue damage than does a single cycle [11]. Tatsutani et al. [12] analyzed these effects in vitro using prostate cancer cell lines treated with various temperatures, speeds of freezing, and numbers of freeze:thaw cycles. They showed that cancer cells are not completely destroyed with a single freeze:thaw cycle to -40°C. However, cells are completely destroyed at -15°C if two freeze:thaw cycles are used [12]. (*Adapted from* Tatsutani et al. [12]; with permission.)

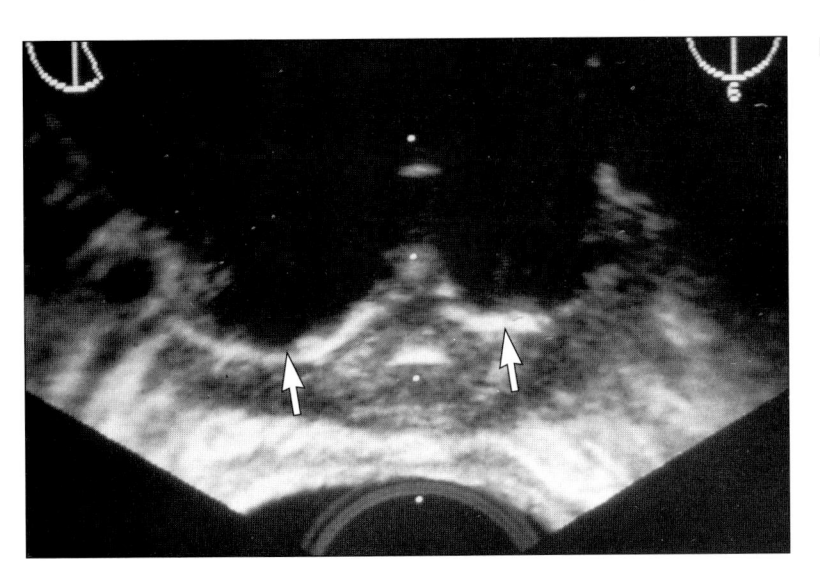

FIGURE 14-4. Ultrasound image of frozen tissue. In this transverse sectional transrectal ultrasound image of the prostate gland during cryosurgery, the edge of the ice ball is seen as a highly echogenic line with acoustic shadows behind it (*arrows*). Because the sound impedance drastically changes from the frozen tissue to the unfrozen tissue, most of the sound waves are reflected at the interface, creating the strong acoustic shadow. Beyond this interface, nothing can be monitored by ultrasound because of this artifact. The temperature at the leading edge of ice is approximately 0°C.

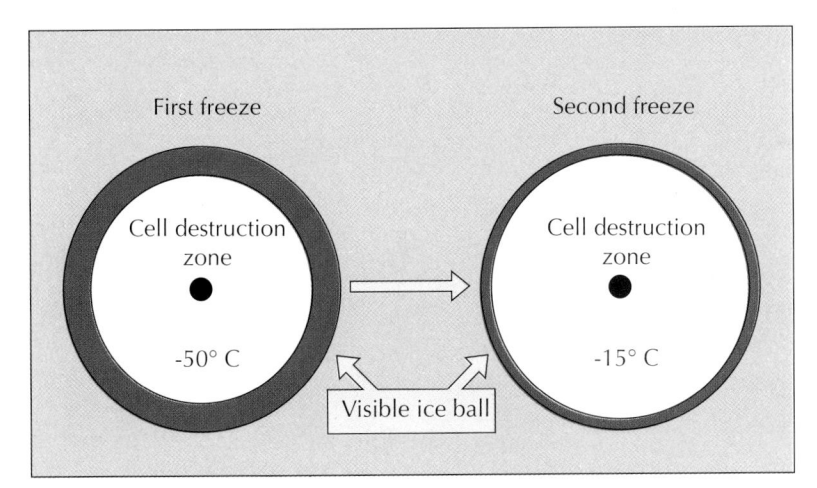

FIGURE 14-5. Frozen zone and tissue destruction zones. Complete cell death occurs in the area with temperature of -40°C or less, which is several millimeters inside the leading edge of the freezing zone (*left*). Therefore, completely covering the prostate with the ice ball does not guarantee complete cell death. It is necessary to extend the iceball beyond the edge of the prostate to ensure adequate tissue ablation at the edge of the prostate. On the second freeze:thaw cycle, the zone of tissue destruction comes closer to the edge of the iceball (*right*), based on the mechanism shown in Figure 14-1. Two freeze:thaw cycles are used routinely in areas of prostate cancer to ensure adequate tissue destruction.

EQUIPMENT

A. Currently Available Cryosurgical Devices for Use in the Prostate Gland

	Source of Freezing	Gas Recycle?	Cooling Temperature	Maximum Number of Probes
CMS	Liquid nitrogen	Yes	-195°C	5
Candela	Liquid nitrogen	No	-186°C	5
Endocare	Liquid argon	No	-130°C	8

FIGURE 14-6. Cryogenic equipment. **A** and **B**, Three cryosurgical devices for prostate cancer treatment are available in the United States. The Candela (Wayland, MA) system is a liquid nitrogen–based machine; the liquid nitrogen evaporates at the tip of the probe, leading to its cooling. Liquid nitrogen is not reused. The CMS (Rockville, MD) system uses ultracooled liquid nitrogen; the nitrogen is compressed and cooled to -206°C. At this temperature, liquid nitrogen becomes partly frozen (slush). This cools tissue down to approximately -185°C. Liquid nitrogen is reused in this system [13]. More recently developed is the Endocare (Irvine, CA) system, in which liquid argon is the source of freezing. The Candela and CMS systems can freeze up to five probes simultaneously; the Endocare system can freeze up to eight probes.

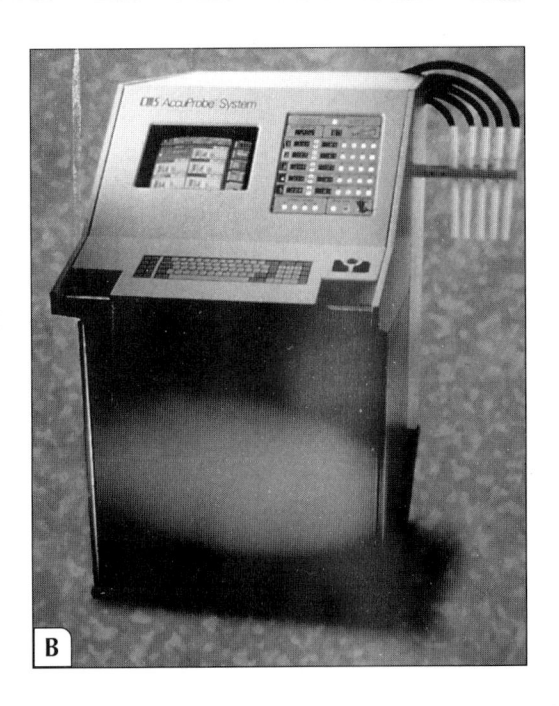

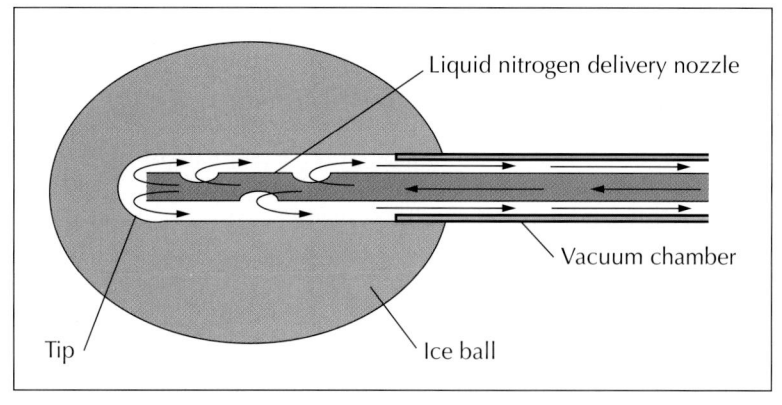

▶ **FIGURE 14-7.** Structure of the cryoprobe. The CMS cryoprobe is 3 mm in diameter and has a double lumen. Ultracooled liquid nitrogen is delivered through a thin lumen to the tip of the probe. Partially evaporated liquid nitrogen returns through the outer chamber, just underneath the surface of the probe. The shaft and base of the probe are insulated with a vacuum chamber to protect normal tissue from freezing.

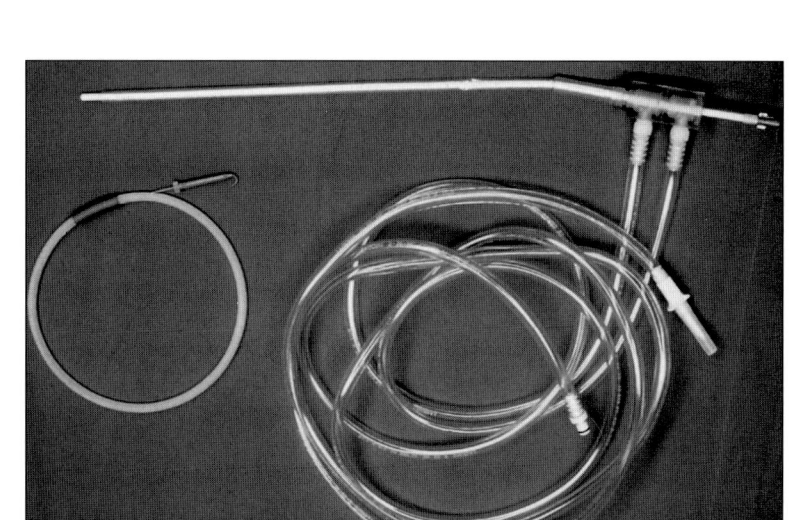

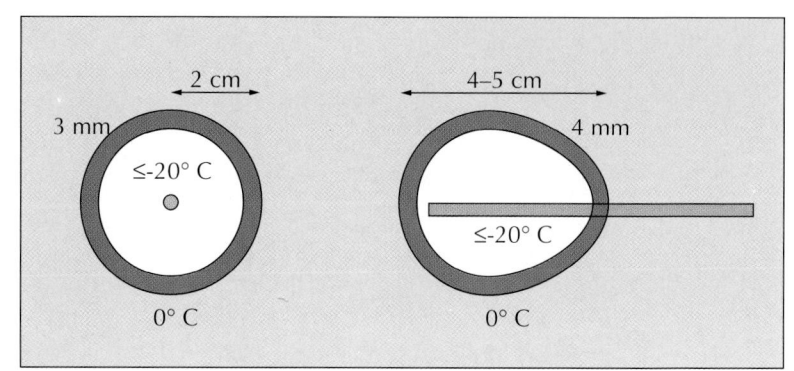

▶ **FIGURE 14-8.** Ice ball structure. An ideal cryosurgical device should create smoothly outlined and symmetrical ice formation around the probe. To destroy the tissue successfully, the temperature gradient around the probe should be steep, with a rapid temperature drop within a few millimeters of the surface. The probe temperature, therefore, should be very low. The iceball formed at the tip is elliptical in shape, with a maximal diameter of approximately 2 cm at the tip of the cryoprobe. The ice ball is about 4 to 5 cm in length [14].

▶ **FIGURE 14-9.** Urethral warmer. The urethral warmer is a flexible, double-lumen catheter through which warmed saline can be irrigated continuously at a high flow. The catheter surface is made of a thin membrane that conducts heat very well [15]. Use of an effective urethral warming device is essential to reduce the incidence of complications associated with cryoablation, such as tissue sloughing, stricture formation, and urinary incontinence.

PATIENT SELECTION

Conditions Suitable for Treatment With Cryoablation

Localized cancer confined within the gland (T1–2)
Localized cancer with extraprostatic extension (T3–4)
Local recurrence after radiation therapy
Local recurrence after radical prostatectomy
Local recurrence after cryoablation
Local tumor progression after hormone therapy

▶ **FIGURE 14-10.** Treatable prostate cancers. Cryoablation is associated with a very low operative risk. It usually can be done as an outpatient procedure, and no transfusion is required. This procedure has been used to treat not only localized disease, but also regionally extensive disease and cancers that have recurred after radiation and radical prostatectomy. Patients who have been treated previously with cryoablation and have had local recurrence of disease are candidates for repeat cryoablation. However, the patients most likely to respond favorably, showing low and stable posttreatment serum prostate-specific antigen (PSA) and negative biopsy, are those with localized prostate cancers.

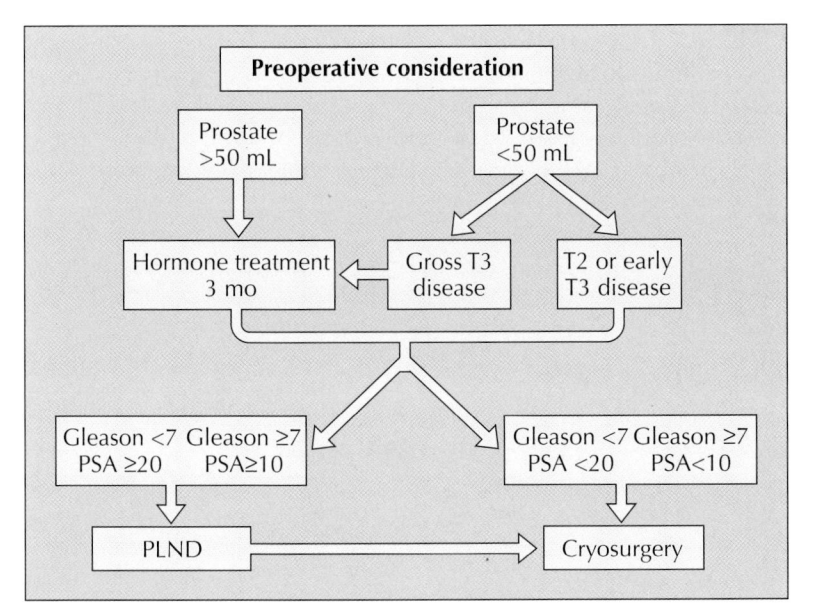

▶ **FIGURE 14-11.** Preoperative considerations. Patients with gross extracapsular extension or seminal vesicle invasion are treated with neoadjuvant hormone therapy to reduce the tumor volume and allow for easier inclusion within the iceball. If the prostate size is larger than 50 cm³, complete freezing of the prostate with a limited number of probes becomes difficult. In these patients, neoadjuvant hormone therapy also is indicated. Patients with a high likelihood of lymph node metastases (*ie*, Gleason grade ≥ 7 with prostate-specific antigen [PSA] over 10 or Gleason grade 6 or less but more than 20) are advised to undergo simultaneous pelvic lymph node dissection. This can be carried out through a small incision ("mini-lap") in the suprapubic area. Patients undergo light bowel preparation consisting of oral magnesium citrate the day before the procedure and a Fleet enema the morning of the procedure. PLND—pelvic lymph node dissection.

PROCEDURE

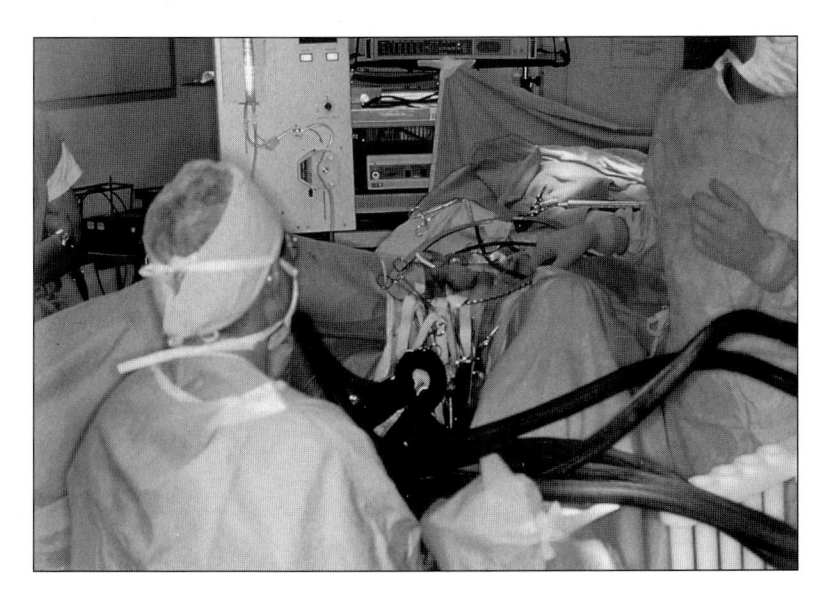

▶ **FIGURE 14-12.** Patient positioning. After induction of regional or general anesthesia, the patient is placed in the lithotomy position. A Foley catheter is inserted, and the bladder is distended with saline to prevent the intraperitoneal contents from being close to the freezing area. Before freezing, the Foley catheter is removed and replaced with the urethral warmer, and irrigation of the catheter with warm saline is begun. The cryoprobes are placed transperineally under ultrasound guidance.

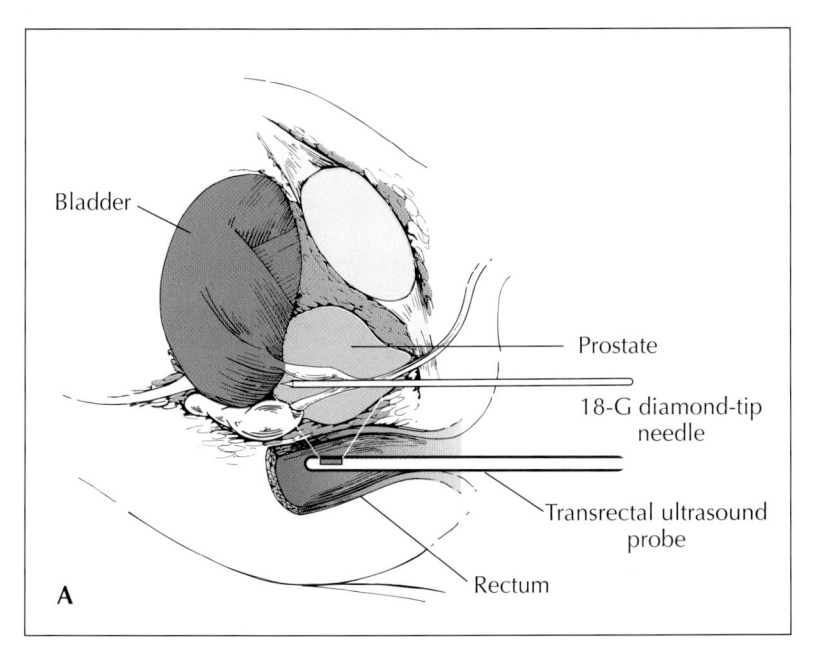

▶ **FIGURE 14-13.** Needle insertion. Using a perineal needle insertion guide, an 18-gauge, diamond-tipped, hollow-core needle is inserted into the prostate under ultrasound guidance (*panel A*).

(*Continued on next page*)

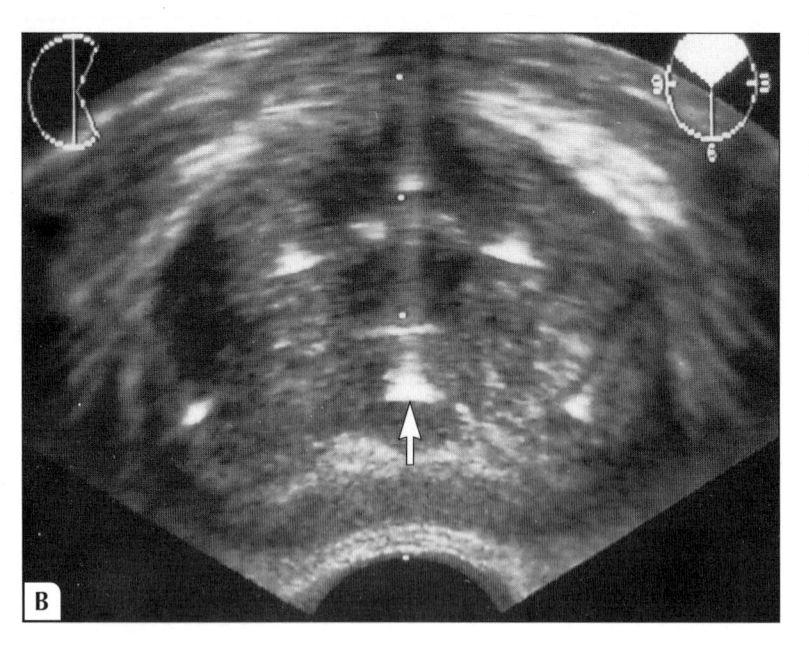

▶ **FIGURE 14-13.** (*Continued*) The needle locations are seen as bright dots on ultrasound imaging (*panel B, arrow*). The exact positioning of each needle and resulting probe is determined at this point. Each needle is advanced up to the desired location, usually up to the base of the prostate. Usually five to six needles are inserted, two anteromedially, two posterolaterally, and one or two posteriorly.

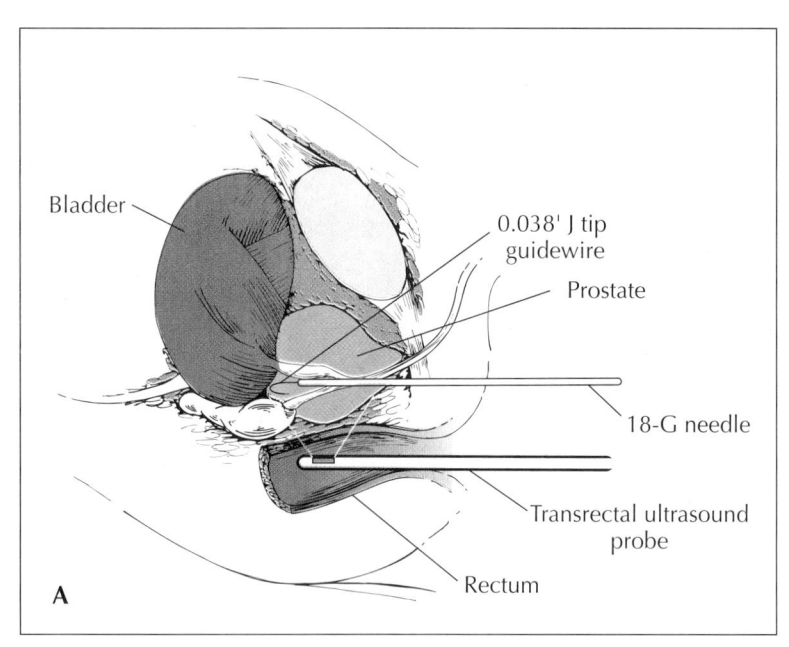

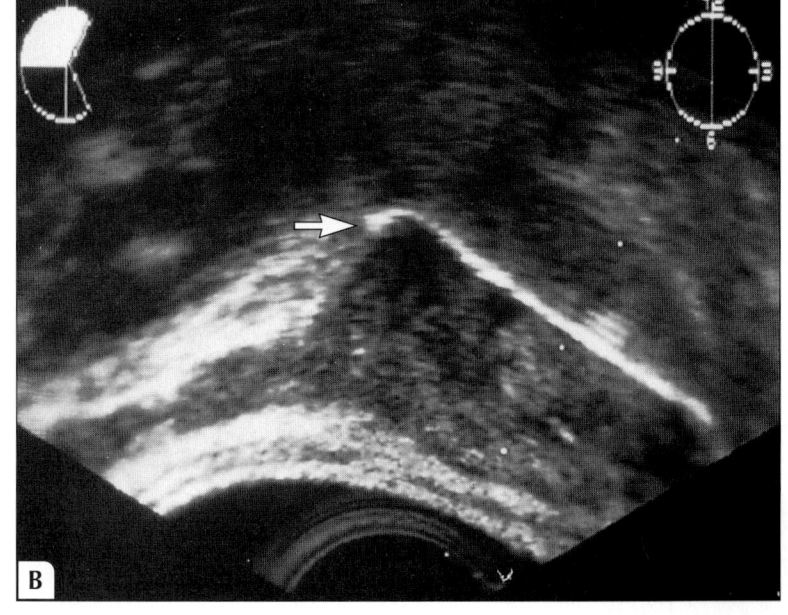

▶ **FIGURE 14-14.** J-guide wire placement. **A,** Once the needle is in position, a 0.038-in J-tipped guide wire is advanced through the needle to the proximal extent of the prostatic capsule. **B,** Sagittal view of the prostate gland shows the correct placement of the guide wire (*arrow*). The needle is removed after confirming that the guide wire is in position.

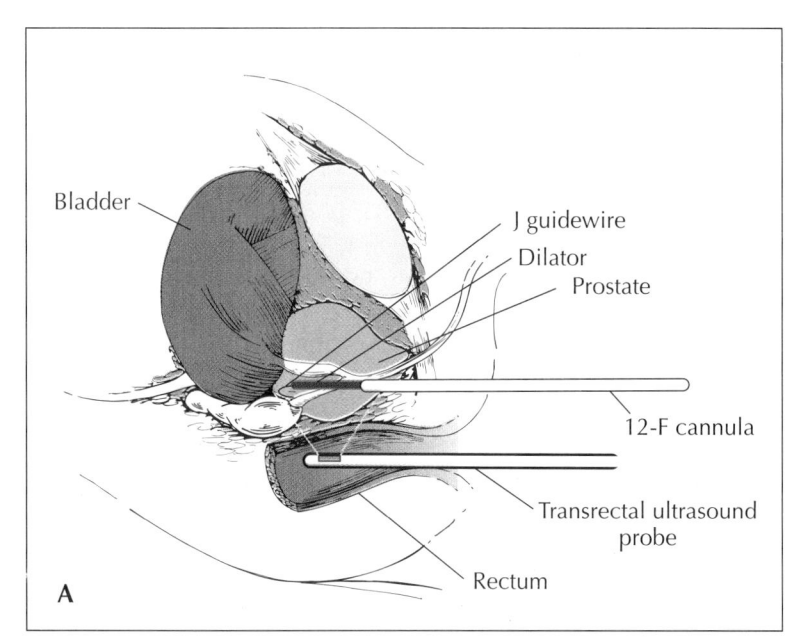

▶ **FIGURE 14-15.** Dilator and cannula placement. **A,** Dilators followed by 12-F cannulas are inserted into the prostate over the guide wires. The cannula is positioned against the proximal extent of the capsule, and both wire and dilator are removed.

(*Continued on next page*)

II. The Prostate

14.6

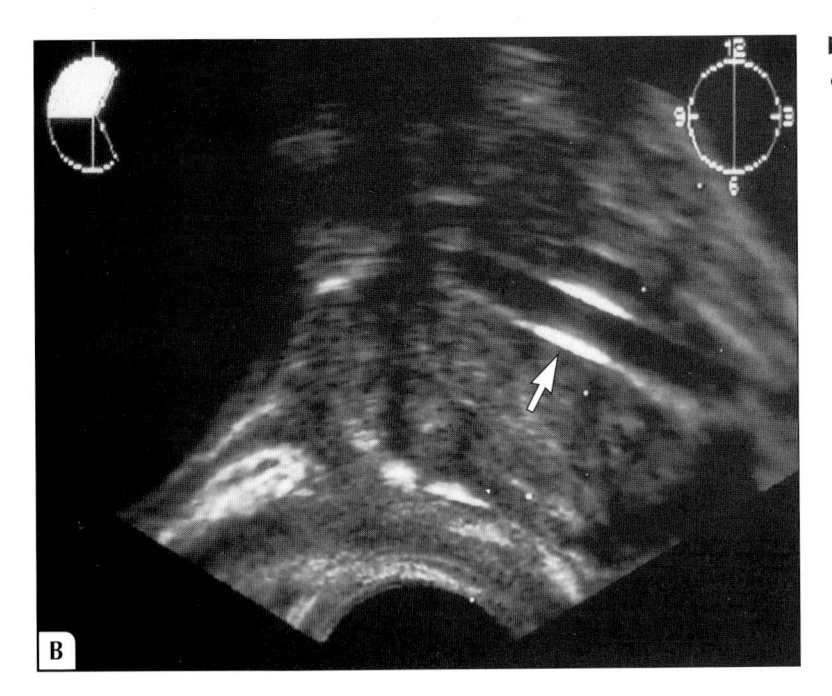

► **FIGURE 14-15.** (*Continued*) **B,** Sagittal view of the prostate confirming correct positioning of the cannula (*arrow*).

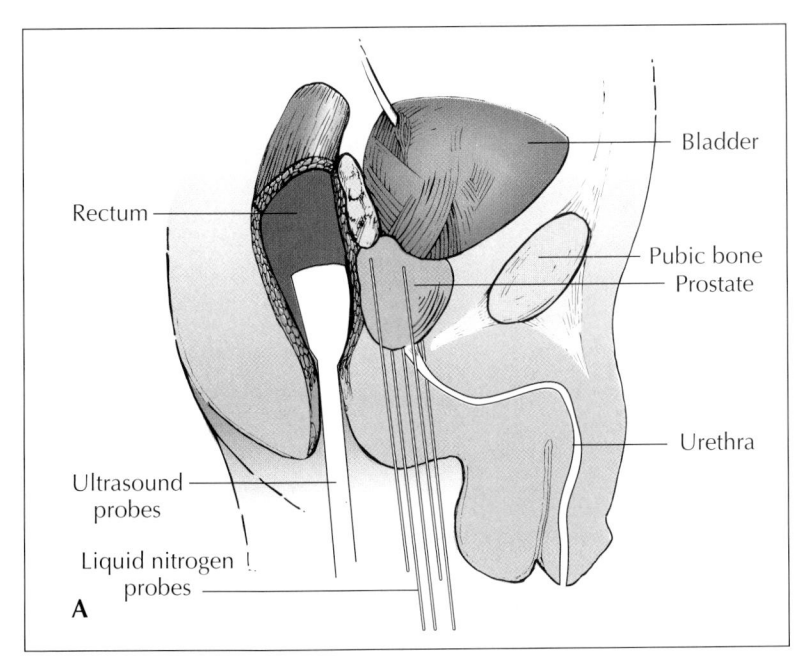

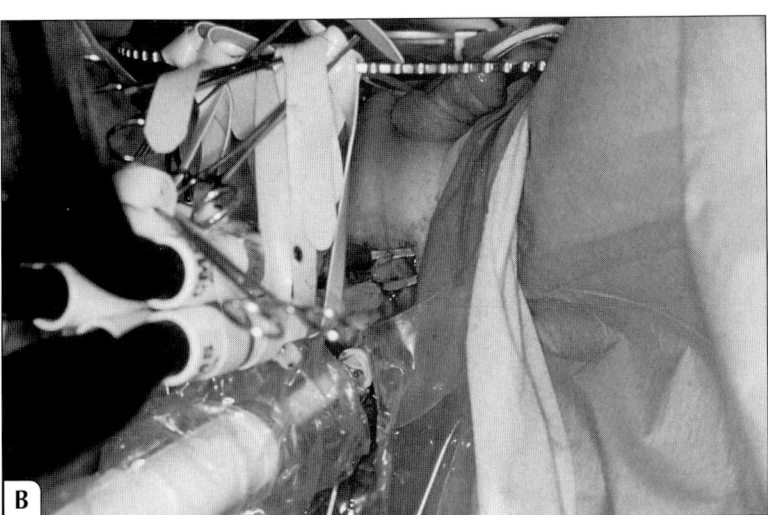

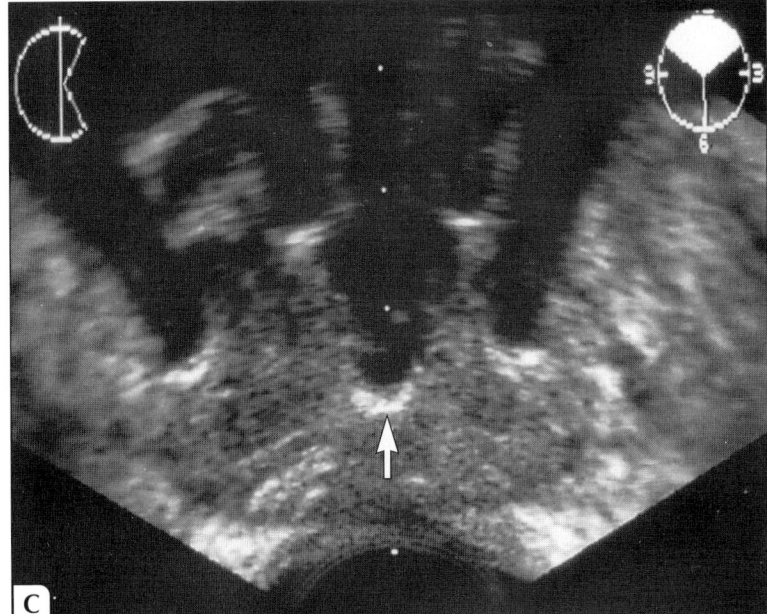

► **FIGURE 14-16.** Placement of cryoprobes. Before placement of the cryoprobes, the urethral warmer must be in position and irrigation with warm saline must be started. **A,** The cryoprobes are placed and the cannulas are retracted to expose the tip of the probe. **B,** Five probes are usually placed: two anteromedially and three posteriorly. Six to eight additional probes may be used to achieve more conformal freezing of the prostate gland. **C,** The probes are secured in position by freezing each probe to -70°C ("stick" temperature). This creates a small ice ball around the tip of the probe (*arrow*).

Cryoablation of Prostate Cancer

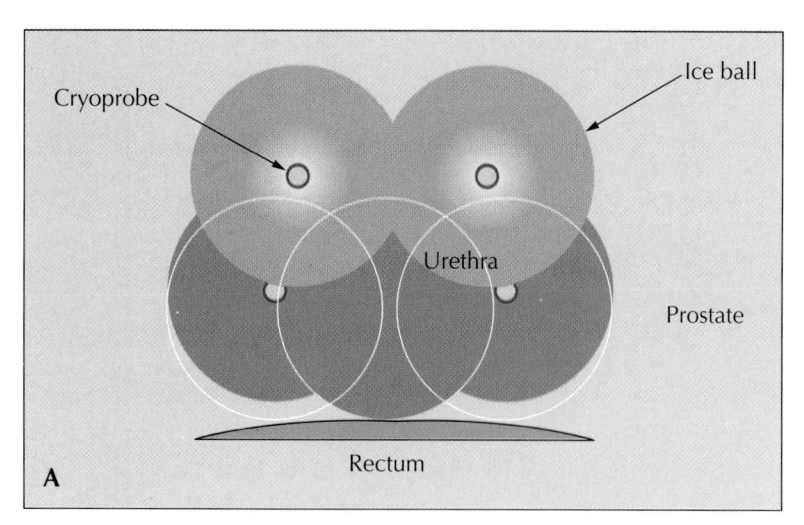

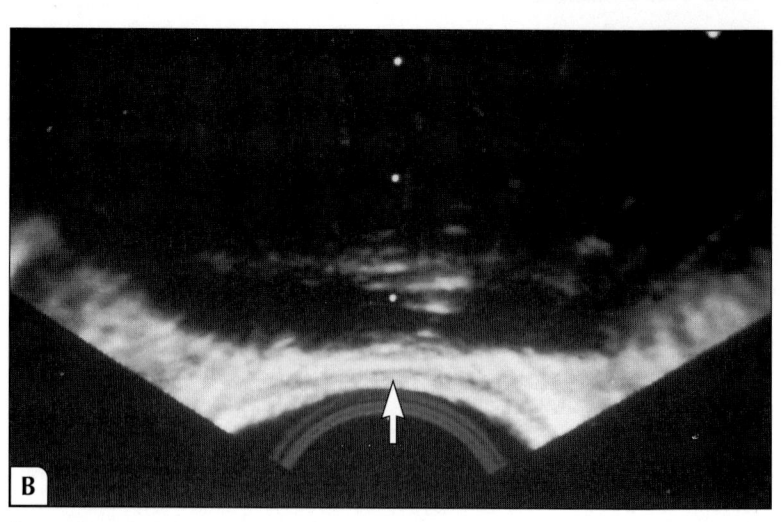

▶ **FIGURE 14-17.** Freezing from the anterior portion of the prostate gland. Liquid nitrogen is circulated through the anterior probes, and the resulting freezing zones or "iceballs" are monitored by ultrasound (*panel A*). Once ice is formed inside the prostate, everything anterior to the ice is hidden by the acoustic shadow (*arrow*). Therefore, the anterior probes must be activated first. The iceball is allowed to extend posteriorly and laterally. Once these have reached the desired positions (*panel B*), thawing is begun and the posterior probes are activated (*arrow*). The posterior iceballs are allowed to extend to the muscularis propria of the rectal wall. Freezing beyond this may result in damage to the rectum and development of a rectourethral fistula.

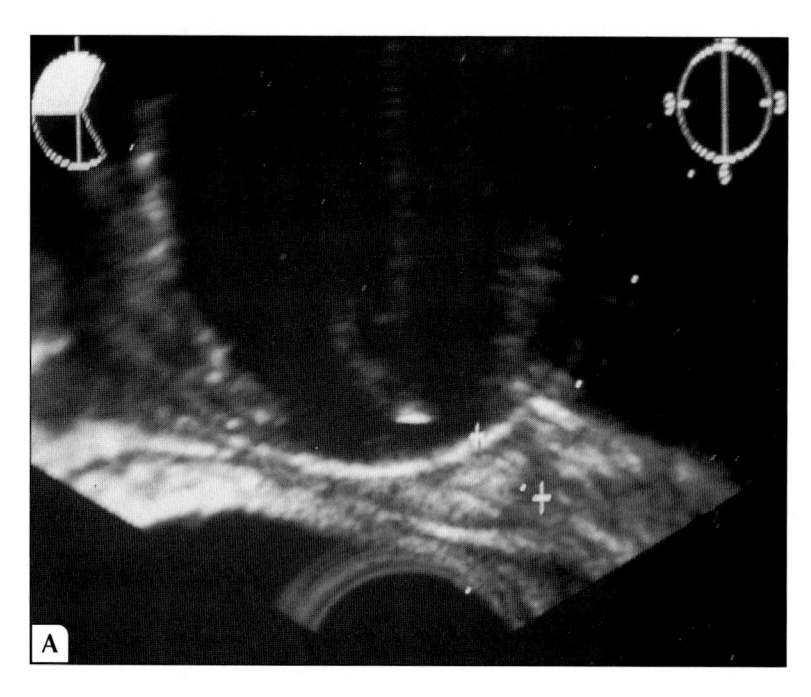

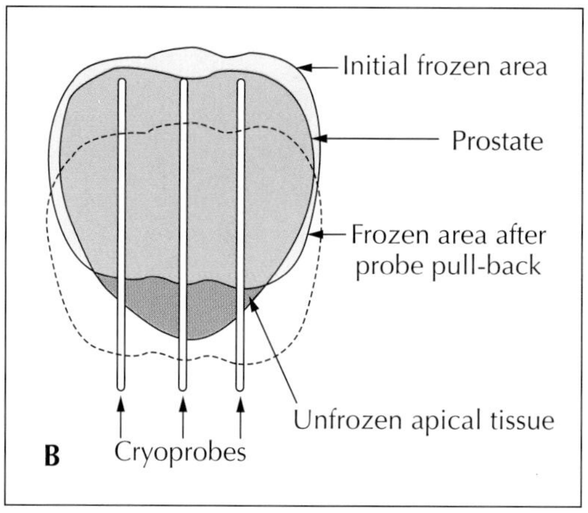

▶ **FIGURE 14-18.** Unfrozen apical tissue. Most surgeons routinely perform two freeze:thaw cycles. If the iceball does not extend adequately to the apex of the prostate (*panel A*), the cryoprobes are pulled backwards into the apex and additional freezing is carried out (*panel B*). The use of two freeze:thaw cycles is more likely to result in complete cancer ablation than is the use of a single cycle, as stated previously.

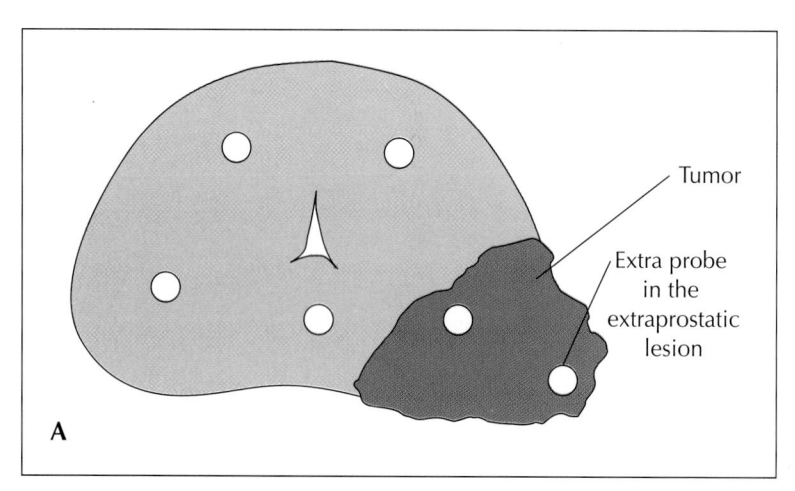

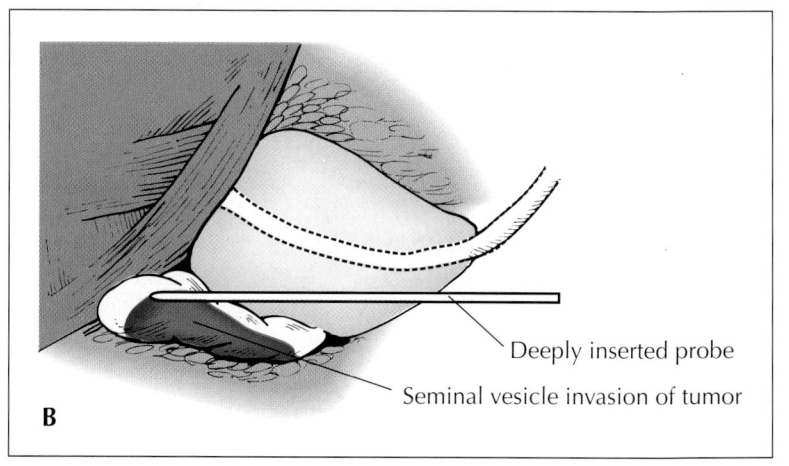

▶ **FIGURE 14-19.** Freezing of extraprostatic lesions. To ensure adequate treatment of cancer, the iceball often is allowed to extend 2 to 4 mm laterally into the periprostatic tissues, 6 mm beyond the apex and into the muscularis propria of the rectum posteriorly. In areas of extracapsular cancer extension, greater propagation of the freeze zone is permitted laterally. If necessary, an additional probe may be placed in such areas (*panel A*). When seminal vesicle invasion is present, probes must be placed deep into the seminal vesicles (*panel B*).

II. The Prostate

COMPLICATIONS

Complications Associated With Cryoablation of the Prostate Gland

	Incidence of Complications, %	
	Mixed Cases	**Radiation Failure**
Tissue slough	15.4	22
Urinary retention	2.9–23.0	27.0–40.9
Stricture	4.0–7.0	5.1–33.0
Incontinence	2.0–8.5	10.3–95.5
Impotence	20–84	100
Pelvic or rectal pain	0–5	8.0–40.9
Penile numbness	0.5–10.0	22
Rectourethral fistula	0–4	0–11
Hydronephrosis	0	0–36.4

FIGURE 14-20. Complications associated with prostate cryosurgery. Various complications have been reported after cryoablation of the prostate. These complications are caused mainly by freezing of the normal surrounding tissue, such as the urethra, sphincter, pelvic musculature, rectum, and ureter. These complications usually are not apparent initially, but are noted 2 to 3 weeks after the procedure. Common complications include tissue sloughing, pelvic pain, and impotence. Rectourethral fistulas are rare.

Patients treated after radiation therapy have significantly higher numbers of complications and morbidity than do those who have not had such previous treatment. Lee *et al.* [16] reported that incidences of rectourethral fistula and total incontinence after cryosurgery were 0.33% for patients who had not received radiation, but were 8.7% for those patients who had been treated previously with radiation [16]. (*Data from* Lee *et al.* [14], Lee *et al.* [16], Bahn *et al.* [18], Patel *et al.* [19], Miller *et al.* [20], Coogan and McKiel [21], Bales *et al.* [22], Weider *et al.* [23], Shirohara *et al.* [24], and Pisters *et al.* [25].)

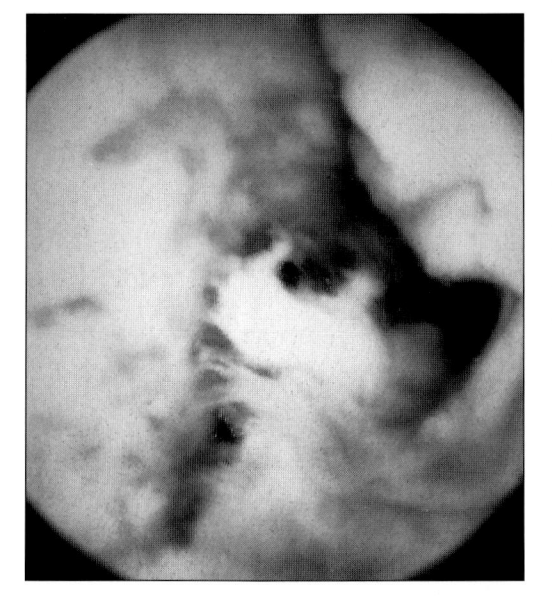

FIGURE 14-21. Tissue sloughing requiring transurethral resection. Formerly, one of the more common complications of cryosurgery was tissue sloughing, caused by inadequate urethral protection from freezing and, possibly, infection of the frozen tissue. Cystoscopy revealed soft necrotic prostatic tissue occluding the prostatic urethra. Tissue slough often was associated with urinary tract infection. Infection of the sloughed tissue was not always symptomatic. Transurethral resection often was necessary to remove the obstructing sloughed tissue. Formation of both strictures and stones occurred as a result of urethral damage in some patients. There was a significant relationship between the incidence of tissue sloughing and the type of urethral warmer used (see Fig. 14-8). The incidence of this complication has decreased significantly as a result of routine use of an effective urethral warmer and the practice of leaving a urethral catheter in place after the procedure for 2 or 3 weeks.

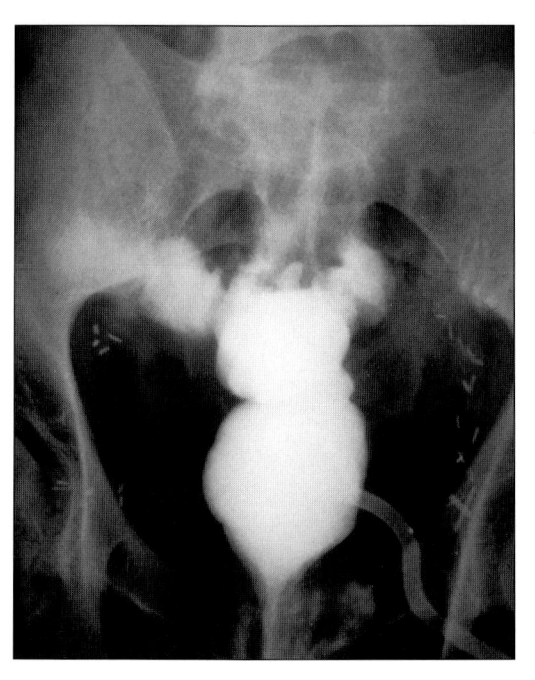

FIGURE 14-22. Rectourethral fistula formation. Rectourethral fistulas are rare, but the complication is difficult to treat when it occurs. Fistulas are more likely to develop in patients who have received radiation. Patients with this complication report watery stools consistent with leakage of urine into the rectum. A cystogram or CT scan confirms the diagnosis and location of the fistula. This voiding cystogram shows radiocontrast medium leaking into the rectum and sigmoid colon. Conservative treatment with a Foley catheter or a suprapubic catheter rarely results in complete healing of the fistula, although it should be performed initially. The tissue around the fistula is necrotic, and at least 6 months of tissue healing is necessary before operative repair of the fistula can be done. During this period, diversion of urine using a catheter is advisable. Both transperineal and transrectal approaches to repair have been used with high success rates.

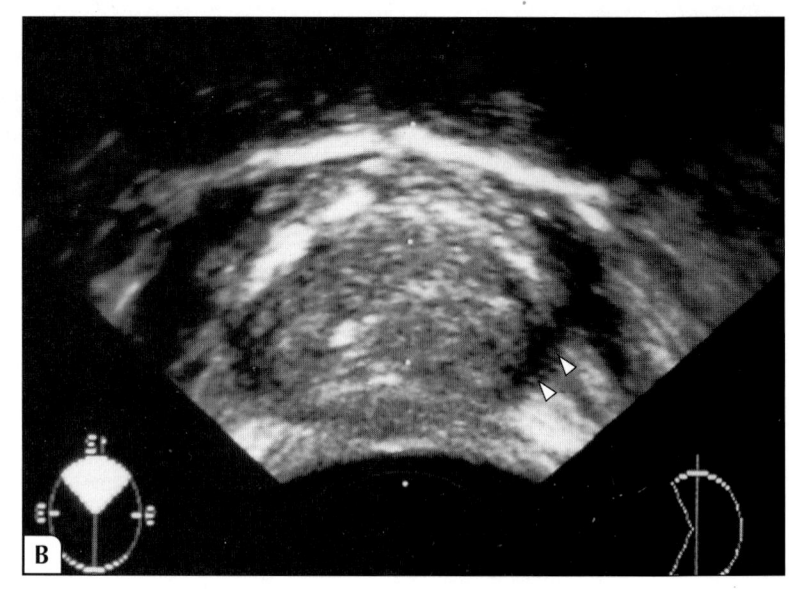

TUMOR CONTROL

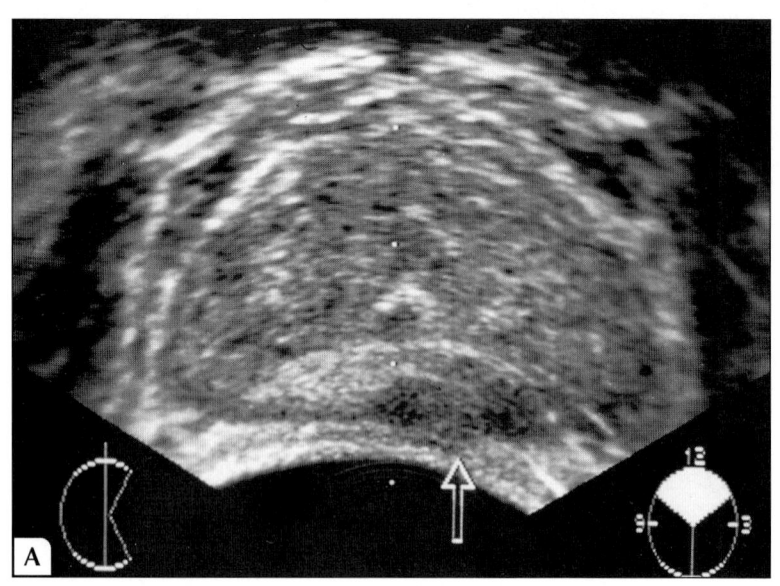

FIGURE 14-23. Transrectal ultrasound images of before and after treatment. **A,** Transverse, transrectal ultrasound view of a localized prostate cancer before cryoablation. A hypoechoic area representing the cancer is seen in the left peripheral zone (*arrow*). Six months after cryoablation, the prostate is significantly smaller with rather heterogeneous echogenicity and lack of delineation of the internal anatomy. **B,** The prostate boundary is obscured because of complete freezing of the gland up to and including the prostatic capsule (*arrowheads*). The hypoechoic area seen on preoperative ultrasonography is no longer visible.

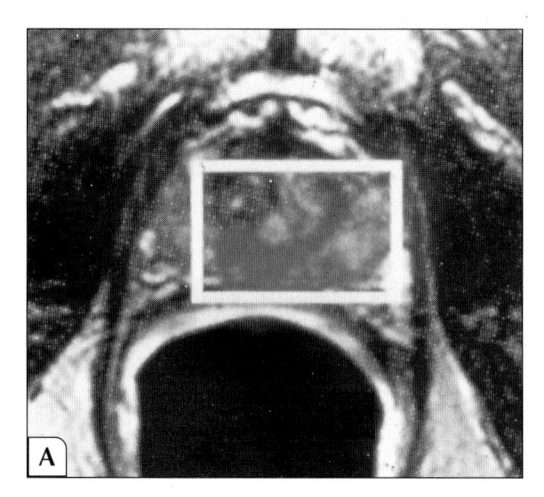

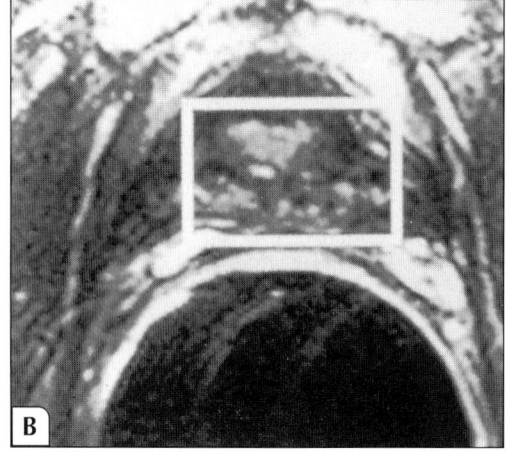

FIGURE 14-24. *(See Color Plate)* Magnetic resonance imaging and spectroscopy after cryoablation of the prostate. Cancer tissue has higher choline and lower citrate levels than does benign prostate tissue. Magnetic resonance spectroscopy of the prostate performed preoperatively shows tissue with abnormal choline: citrate signal ratios corresponding with a biopsy-proven prostate cancer (*red area in panel A*). After successful cryosurgery, all signals in the prostate disappear, indicating total necrosis of the gland (*panel B*) [17].

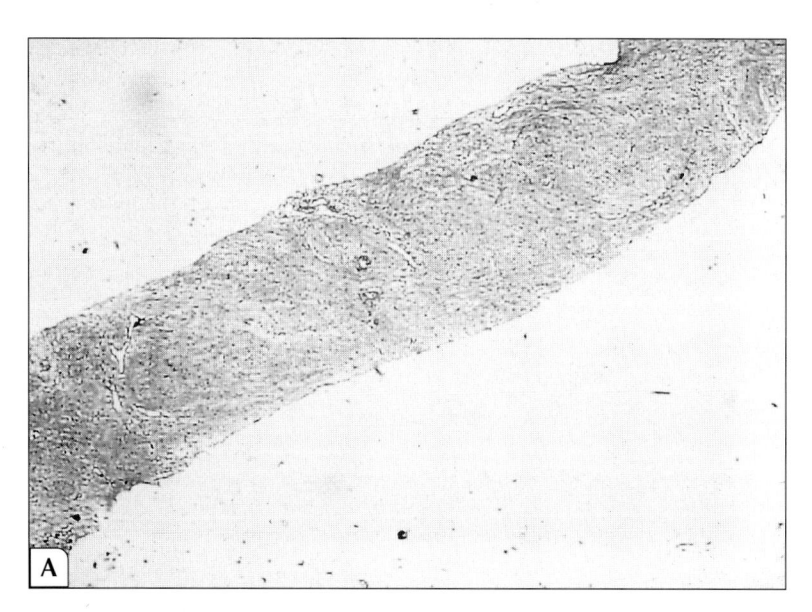

FIGURE 14-25. Biopsy of the prostate after cryoablation. **A,** Biopsy of the prostate reveals fibrous stroma tissue with complete disappearance of glandular tissue.

(*Continued on next page*)

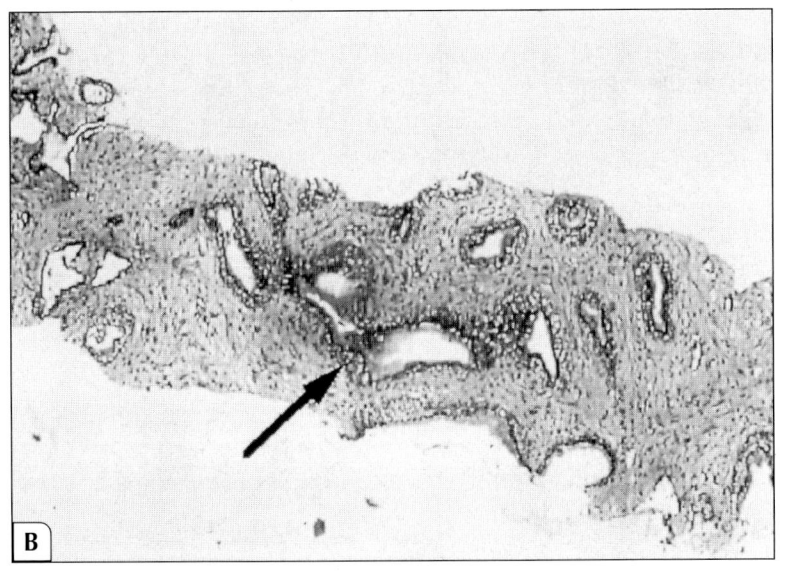

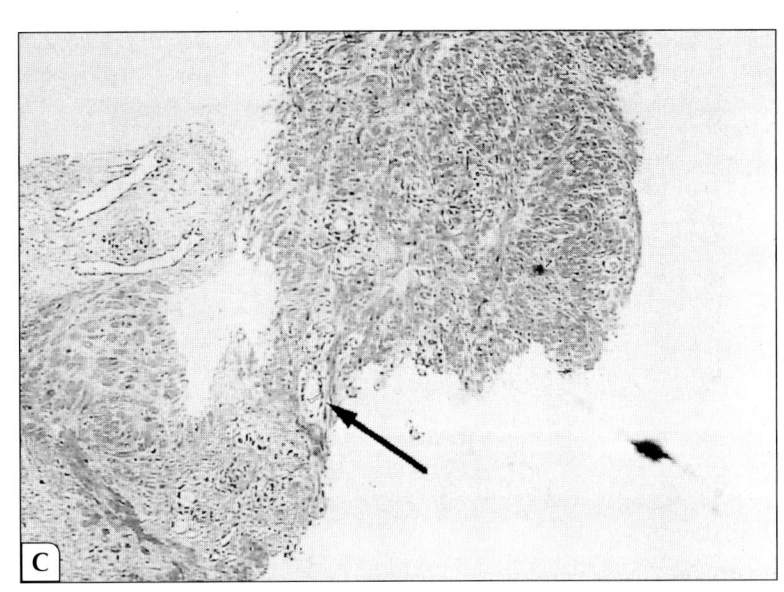

FIGURE 14-25. (*Continued*) **B**, Occasional glandular structures (*arrow*) can be seen. These glands may represent either residual prostate tissue around the urethra or regrowth of prostatic duct epithelium in the area of treatment (basal cell hyperplasia). **C**, Residual cancer (*arrow*) is seen more commonly in the apex of the prostate and in the seminal vesicles (see Fig. 14-27). Residual cancer may be found in the periurethral region and around large vessels, where temperatures may be higher than in the surrounding tissues.

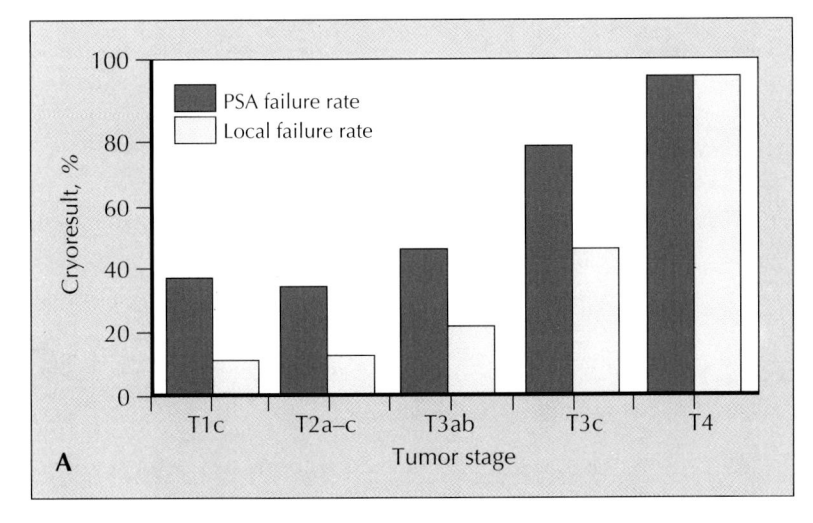

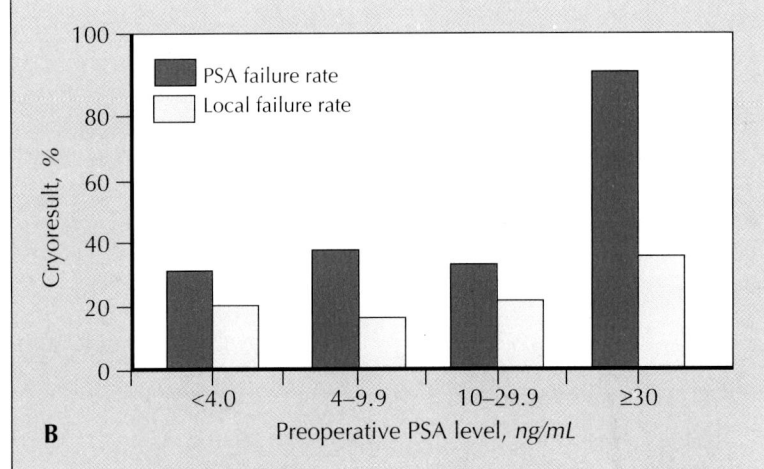

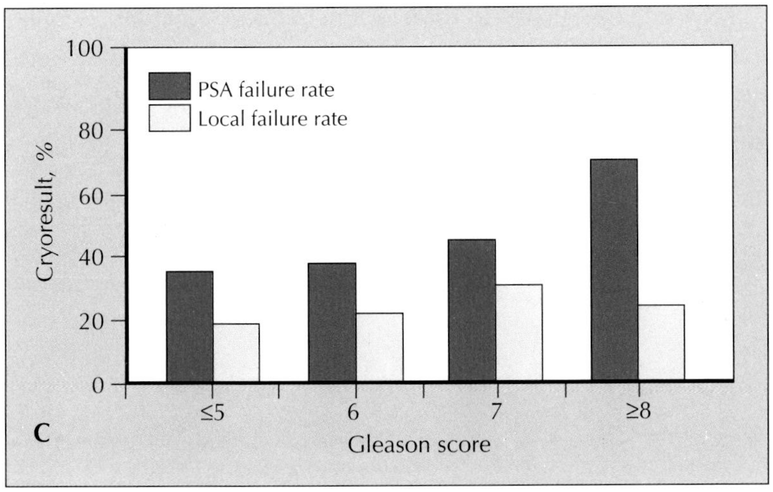

FIGURE 14-26. Tumor stage and cryotherapy results. Results of cryosurgery at the University of California at San Francisco (UCSF) based on biochemical prostate-specific antigen (PSA) and biopsy-proven local failure. **A**, Tumor stage and cryotherapy results. **B**, Preoperative PSA and cryotherapy results. **C**, Gleason grade and cryotherapy results. At UCSF, cryoablation often has been applied to treat high-stage disease. More than 60% of the patients treated at UCSF have had T3 or higher stage disease. Overall, biochemical and biopsy failure rates were 47% and 24%, respectively. Fifty-four percent of the patients achieved undetectable PSA totals (<0.1 ng/mL), and such patients have had the lowest failure rates. Stages T1 and T2 disease, serum PSA less than 20 ng/mL, and cancers of Gleason grade lower than 8 are associated with favorable results [18].

Cryoablation of Prostate Cancer

14.11

Location of Residual Cancer After Cryoablation

	Preoperative Number of Cancers	Postoperative Number of Cancers	Residual Disease, %
Apex	42	4	9.5
Mid-prostate	49	2	4.1
Base	55	0	0.0
Seminal vesicle	16	7	43.8

FIGURE 14-27. Correlation between tumor location and local recurrence. Cancers at the apex or in the seminal vesicle are more likely to recur than are those confined to the midgland or base. Careful and complete cryoablation of tissue in cancers located at the apex and seminal vesicles is important. Preoperative careful mapping of the tumor location by multiple biopsies, including the biopsies of seminal vesicles, is essential for treatment planning.

Published Results of Cryosurgery

Study (year)	Patients, n	Local Recurrence, %	Biochemical Failure, %
Miller et al. [20] (1994)*	62	21	49
Coogan and McKiel [21] (1995)	95	17	14
Bales et al. [22] (1995)*	23	14	67
Weider et al. [23] (1995)	83	13	Not available
Shinohara et al. [27] (1997)	110	24	47
Lee et al. [16] (1997)	347	19.8	Not available
Pisters et al. [25] (1997)*	150	23	69
Long et al. [26] (1988)	145	16	41

*Salvage cryotherapy only.

FIGURE 14-28. Published results of cryoablation. The reported local failure rate after prostate cryoablation varies between 13% and 24%. Results correlate with stage and grade and the length of follow-up. Biochemical failure after cryoablation is not clearly defined, and the definition varies among series. The biochemical failure rate has been reported to range between 14% and 69%. Undetectable serum prostate-specific antigen (PSA) levels (*ie*, < 0.2 ng/mL) after cryosurgery are achieved in 33% to 58% of patients.

CONCLUSIONS

Although early results with cryosurgery are promising in terms of cancer control, long-term follow-up is lacking. The best results with cryosurgery are achieved in patients with organ-confined disease—the same patients who would be expected to do well with radical prostatectomy or radiation therapy. Although the procedure is associated with a limited, but still important, risk of complications, the likelihood of complications has been reduced by the use of an effective urethral warmer and increased experience with the technique. Further refinements in technique, equipment, and patient selection, and further follow-up of previously treated patients are required to better define the role of this procedure in the treatment of localized prostate cancer.

REFERENCES

1. Fowler FJ Jr, Barry MJ, Lu-Yao G, et al.: Patient reported complications and follow-up treatment after radical prostatectomy. The National Medicare Experience: 1988–1990. *Urology* 1993, 42:622–629.
2. Fleming C, Wasson JH, Albertsen PC, et al.: A decision analysis of alternative treatment strategies for clinically localized prostate cancer. *JAMA* 1993, 269:2850.
3. Gonder M, Soanes W, Shulman S: Cryosurgical treatment of the prostate. *Invest Urol* 1966, 3:372–378.
4. Flocks RH, Nelson CMK, Boatman DL: Perineal cryosurgery for prostatic carcinoma. *J Urol* 1972, 108:933–935.
5. Reuter HJ: Endoscopic cryosurgery of prostate and bladder tumors. *J Urol* 1972, 107:389–393.
6. Bonney WW, Fallon B, Gerber WL, et al.: Cryosurgery in prostatic cancer survival. *Urology* 1982, 19:37–42.
7. Porter M, Ahaghotu C, Loening S, See W: Disease-free and overall survival after cryosurgical monotherapy for clinical stages B and C carcinoma of the prostate: a 20-year followup. *J Urol* 1997, 158:1466–1469.
8. Onik GM, Cohen JK, Reyes GD, et al.: Transrectal ultrasound-guided percutaneous radical cryosurgical ablation of the prostate. *Cancer* 1993, 72:1291–1299.
9. Mazur P: Cryobiology: the freezing of biological systems. *Science* 1970, 168:939–949.
10. Ablin RJ: *Handbook of Cryosurgery.* New York: Mercel Dekker; 1980: 15–68.
11. Gage AA: Experimental cryogenic injury of the palate: observations pertinent to cryosurgical destruction of tumors. *Cryobiology* 1978, 15:415–425.
12. Tatsutani K, Rubinsky B, Onik G, Dahiya R: Effect of thermal variables on frozen human primary prostatic adenocarcinoma cells. *Urology* 1996, 1996, 48:441–447.

13. Chang Z, Finkelstein J, Ma H, *et al.*: Development of a high performance multi-probe cryosurgical device. *Biomed Instrum Technol* 1994, 28:383–390.
14. Lee F, Bahn DK, McHugh TA, *et al.*: US-guided percutaneous cryoablation of prostate cancer. *Radiology* 1994, 192:769–776.
15. Cohen JK, Miller RJ, Shuman BA: Urethral warming catheter for use during cryoablation of the prostate. *Urology* 1995, 45:861–864.
16. Lee F, Bahn DK, McHugh TA, *et al.*: Cryosurgery of prostate cancer: use of adjuvant hormonal therapy and temperature monitoring. A one-year follow-up. *Anticancer Res* 1997, 17:1511–1516.
17. Parivar F, Hricak H, Shinohara K, *et al.*: Detection of locally recurrent prostate cancer after cryosurgery: evaluation by transrectal ultrasound, magnetic resonance imaging, and three-dimensional proton magnetic resonance spectroscopy. *Urology* 1996, 48:594–599.
18. Bahn DK, Lee F, Solomon MH, *et al.*: Prostate cancer: US-guided percutaneous cryoablation. *Radiology* 1995, 194:551–556.
19. Patel BG, Parsons CL, Bidair M, Schmidt JD: Cryoablation for carcinoma of the prostate. *J Surg Oncol* 1996, 63:256–264.
20. Miller RJ, Cohen JK, Shuman B, Merlotti LA: Percutaneous, transperineal cryosurgery of the prostate as salvage therapy for post radiation recurrence of adenocarcinoma. *Cancer* 1994, 77:1510–1514.
21. Coogan CL, McKiel CF: Percutaneous cryoablation of the prostate: preliminary results after 95 procedures. *J Urol* 1995, 154:1813–1817.
22. Bales GT, Williams MJ, Sinner M, *et al.*: Short term outcomes after cryosurgical ablation of the prostate in men with recurrent prostate carcinoma following radiation therapy. *Urology* 1995, 46:676–680.
23. Weider J, Schmidt J, Casola G, *et al.*: Transrectal ultrasound-guided transperineal cryoablation in the treatment of prostate carcinoma: preliminary results. *J Urol* 1995, 154:435–441.
24. Shinohara K, Connolly JA, Presti JC Jr, *et al.*: Cryosurgical treatment of localized prostate cancer (stages T1 to T4): preliminary results. *J Urol* 1996, 156:115–120.
25. Pisters LL, von Eschenbach AC, Scott SM, *et al.*: The efficacy and complications of salvage cryotherapy of the prostate. *J Urol* 1997, 157:921–925.
26. Long JP, Fallick ML, LaRock DR, Rand W: Preliminary outcomes following cryosurgical ablation of the prostate in patients with clinically localized prostate carcinoma. *J Urol* 1998, 159:477–484.
27. Shinohara K, Rhee B, Presti JC, Carroll PR: Cryosurgical ablation of prostate cancer: pattern of cancer recurrence. *J Urol* 1997, 158:2206–2210.

Management of Metastatic Prostate Cancer

15
CANCEROUS DISEASE SECTION

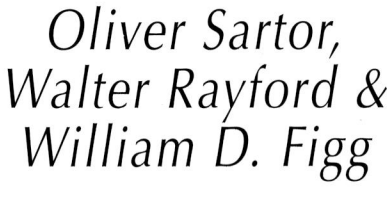

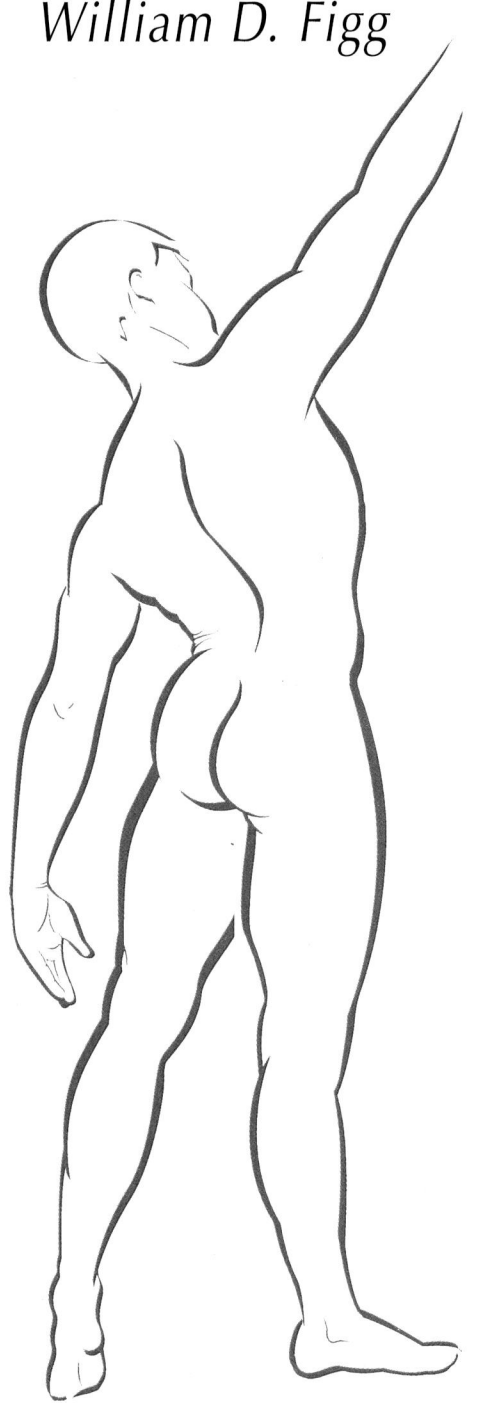

*Oliver Sartor,
Walter Rayford &
William D. Figg*

Management of metastatic prostate cancer depends on a variety of factors, including accurate diagnosis, staging, and treatment planning. Although the definition of metastatic prostate cancer has been formalized in several well accepted staging systems, newer concepts are constantly challenging our thinking. Whereas in the past, metastatic prostate cancer was typically defined in terms of a positive bone scan, today metastatic disease may be suspected because of marked elevations in prostate-specific antigen (PSA) or an increased uptake on a radiolabeled monoclonal antibody scan.

Once the diagnosis and staging of metastatic prostate cancer have been established, treatment planning can commence. Despite the many advances in staging and detection of cancer, treatment of hormonally sensitive metastatic prostate cancer has changed relatively little since the pioneering observations of Huggins and Hodges [1] over half a century ago. Androgen deprivation remains the cornerstone of therapy, but today many more options are available to reach that goal. During the 1960s, controlled clinical trials helped to determine the appropriate doses of estrogens [2]. During the 1970s, discovery of the hypothalamic control of pituitary secretion of luteinizing hormone (LH) led to the development of potent luteinizing hormone–releasing hormone (LHRH) agonists [3], which enabled patients to have androgen deprivation without the side effects of estrogens or surgical removal of the testicles. During the 1980s, combined androgen blockade (a combination of testicular androgen suppression and adrenal androgen blockade), was introduced with great hopes [4]. After almost two decades of study, however, most investigators agree that the clinical benefits of combined androgen blockade are not as great as had been originally anticipated [5]. Newer approaches to hormonal therapies focus on improving quality of life and decreasing the side effects associated with traditional hormonal approaches. Potency-sparing therapies [6] and intermittent administration of hormones [7] are claimed to have certain advantages, but prospective randomized clinical trials have yet to prove that these approaches are as effective as conventional therapies.

One recurring problem has yet to be solved. Nearly all men with metastatic prostate cancer eventually fail hormonal therapy and die with hormone-refractory prostate cancer. No peer-reviewed publication has ever shown that treatment of hormone-refractory disease can prolong survival. Despite the obvious shortcomings of current therapies for hormone-refractory metastatic prostate cancer, advances in palliative management have been made, and a variety of experimental approaches are now being evaluated in clinical trials.

This chapter reviews the staging and management of metastatic prostate cancer. Both hormone-sensitive and hormone-refractory disease are discussed, with particular emphasis on state of the art concepts and management techniques.

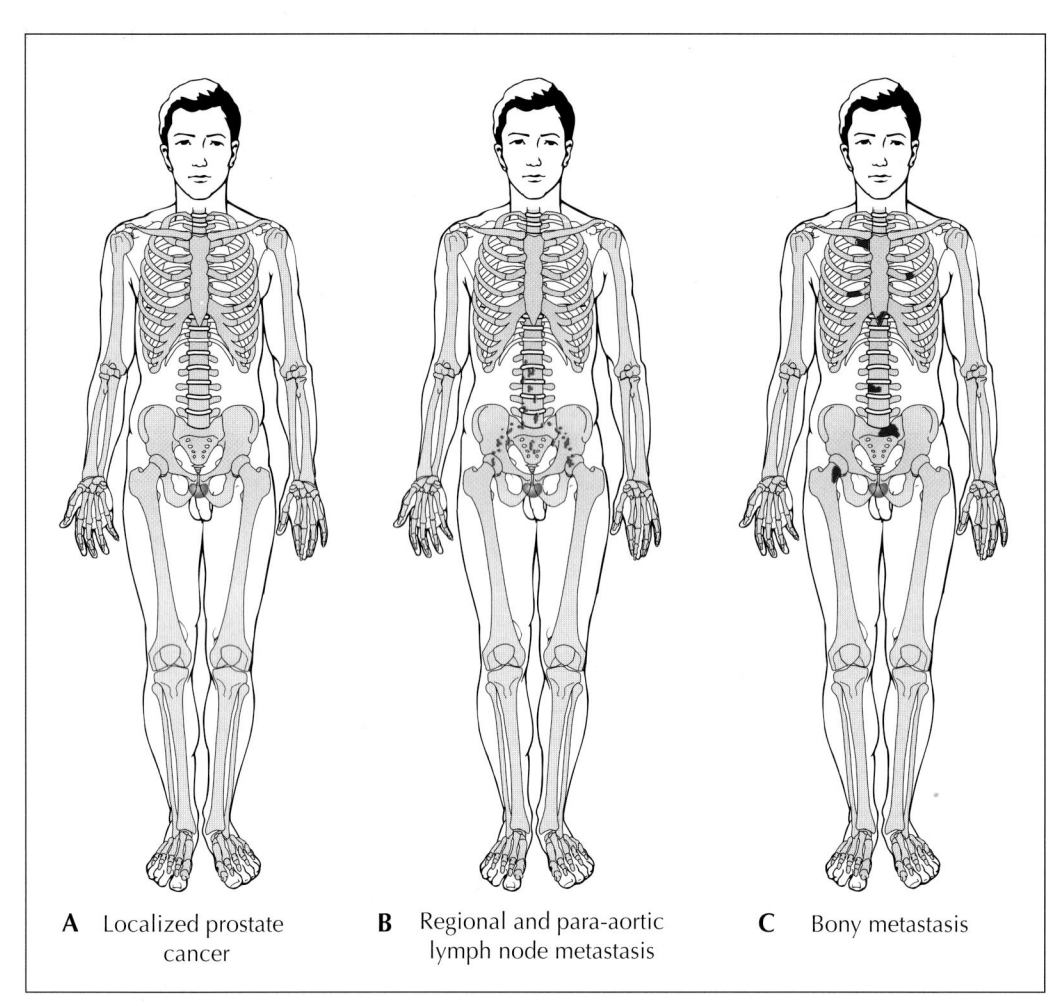

FIGURE 15-1. Typical regions of metastatic disease. **A,** Localized prostate cancer. **B,** Regional and para-aortic lymph node metastases. **C,** Bony metastases. The optimal management strategy of prostate cancer relies on the sensitive and specific detection of locoregional and distant metastatic disease. The most common sites of distant metastasis of prostate cancer identified in pathologic studies are regional lymph nodes and bone; lung and liver metastases also can be detected [8]. Identification of distant soft tissue metastases traditionally has relied on radiographic imaging with CT or magnetic resonance imaging. Bone scans are the preferred methodology for detecting lesions in the bone. More contemporary radiographic imaging now includes radioimmunoscintigraphy. Prostate-specific antigen (PSA)-producing cells can be detected with great sensitivity by molecular methodologies that use the polymerase chain reaction (PCR). Local definitive therapies are doomed to failure, however, for patients with metastatic disease, and some form of systemic therapy is required for optimal patient treatment.

A Localized prostate cancer

B Regional and para-aortic lymph node metastasis

C Bony metastasis

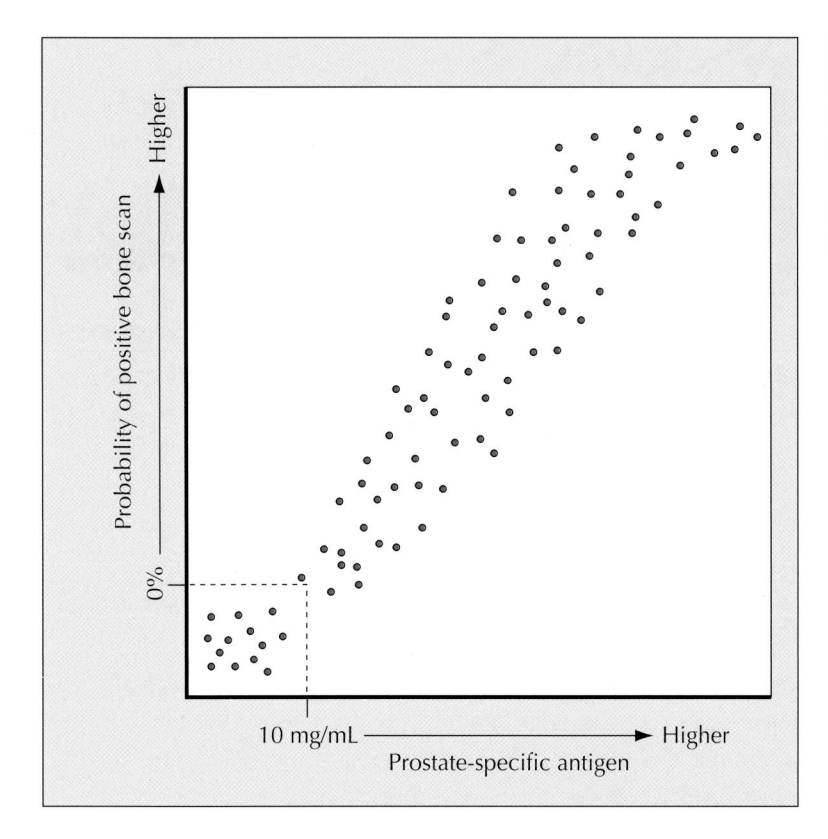

FIGURE 15-2. The probability of positive bone scans can be predicted by serum prostate-specific antigen (PSA). Contemporary techniques of PSA determination have greatly reduced the need for bone scans in patients diagnosed with clinically localized prostate cancer. If the serum PSA is less than 10 ng/mL, the probability of detecting bony metastases by bone scan is remote [9]. Furthermore, a bone scan is not recommended in the post–radical prostatectomy patient with an undetectable PSA level [10].

II. The Prostate

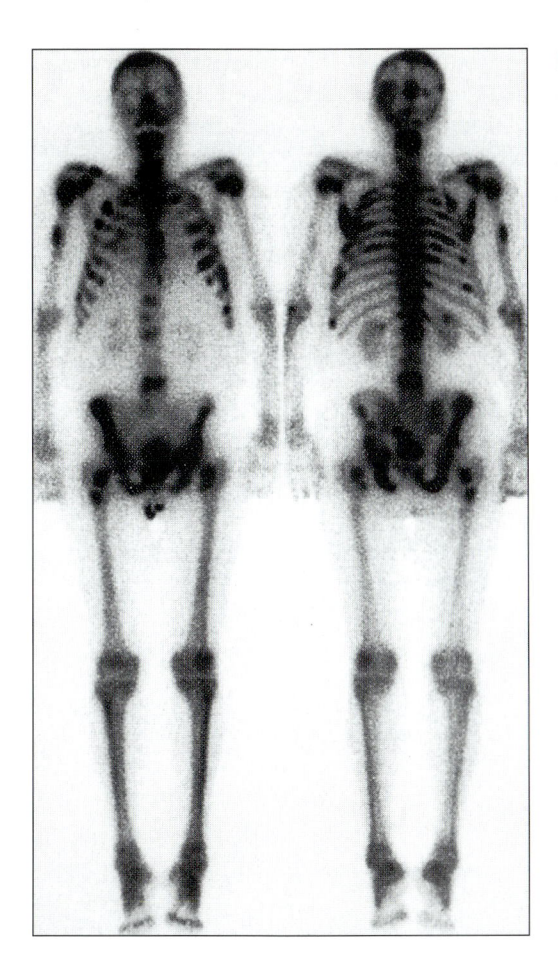

▶ **FIGURE 15-3.** The radioscintigraphic bone scan is the most sensitive imaging technique to detect metastases to bone. These lesions typically appear as asymmetric areas of increased tracer uptake, particularly in the axial skeleton. The advantages of bone scintigraphy are its overall high sensitivity and ability to evaluate the entire skeletal system at a relatively low cost. Bone scans, however, are limited by the nonspecific nature of the information they provide. Increased uptake can be associated with a number of nonmalignant lesions, such as trauma, arthritis, and Paget's disease. (*From* Manyak [11]; with permission.)

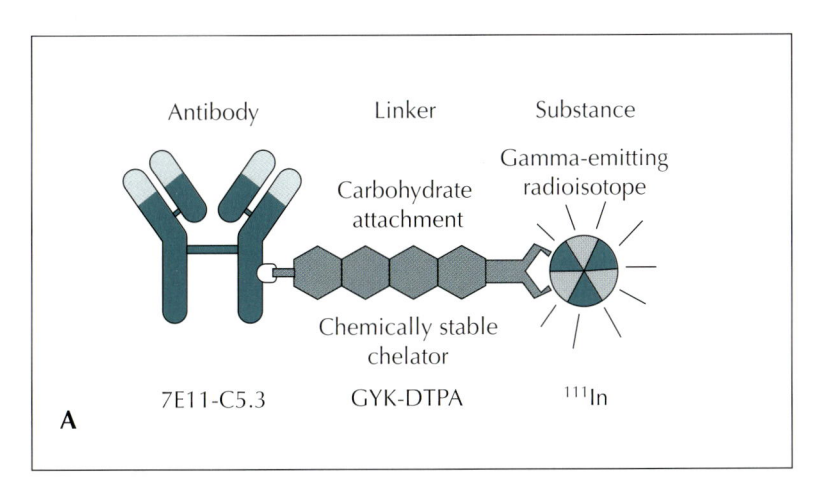

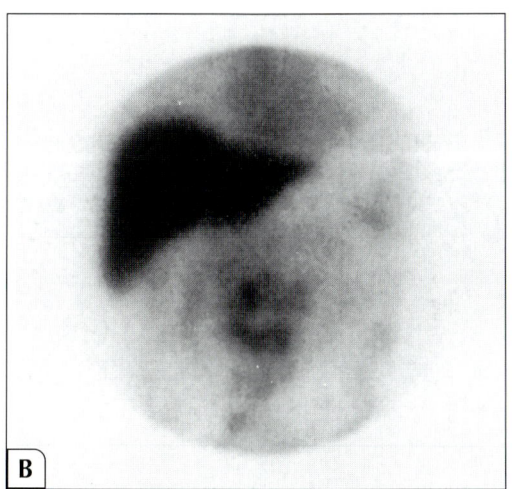

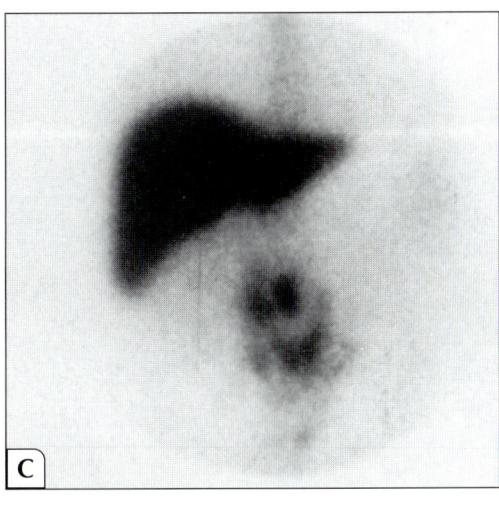

▶ **FIGURE 15-4.** **A,** Product formulation of a radiolabeled monoclonal antibody for detection of prostate cancer. **B** and **C,** Images of metastatic disease obtained using capromab pendetide. Although CT and magnetic resonance imaging (MRI) scans are well accepted in staging patients with a variety of malignancies, studies in prostate cancer patients indicate that these methodologies have very poor sensitivity for the detection of early metastatic prostate cancer. Recently the Food and Drug Administration (FDA) has approved for use a radiolabeled monoclonal antibody to the prostate-specific membrane antigen (PSMA). This radiolabeled antibody (^{111}In-labeled capromab pendetide) can be used to image prostate cancer soft tissue metastases in a much more sensitive manner than is possible using traditional radiographic tests [12,13]. Unfortunately, the test is somewhat cumbersome to administer, requiring a period of 3 to 4 days, and both false-positive and false-negative results are obtained in about 30% of cases. (*Panels B and C from* Manyak [11]; with permission.)

Management of Metastatic Prostate Cancer

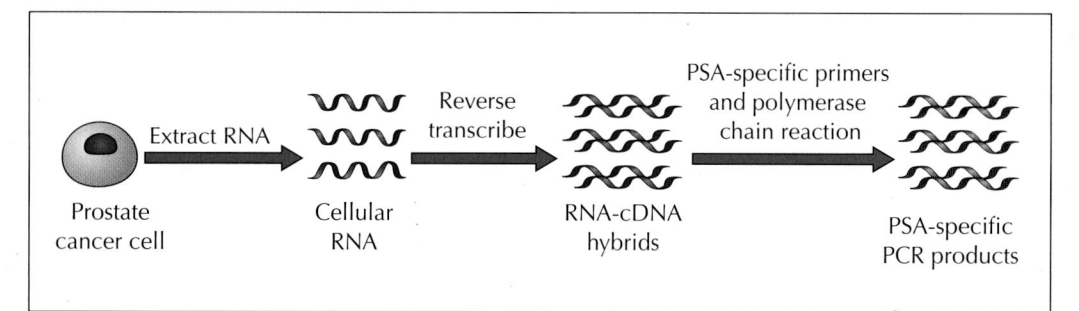

◗ **FIGURE 15-5.** Detection of prostate-specific antigen (PSA)-producing cells by reverse transcription polymerase chain reaction (RT-PCR). This method potentially can detect one PSA-producing cell in a background of 10,000,000 non–PSA-producing cells. RT-PCR has been used to detect PSA-producing cells in several sources, including the bloodstream, the bone marrow, and the lymph nodes [14–16]. Messenger RNA is purified from a cellular source and reverse transcribed, and then PSA-specific message is amplified using specific primers and the polymerase chain reaction. The clinical validity of observations related to RT-PCR still must be confirmed in multicenter trials. Controversy continues to surround this new and sensitive staging methodology, particularly with reference to the clinical relevance of detecting PSA-specific mRNA in the blood stream. A variety of other potential prostate-specific messenger RNAs (*eg*, prostate-specific membrane antigen) also can be detected by RT-PCR methodologies.

◗ **FIGURE 15-7.** Conversion of testosterone to dihydrotestosterone is catalyzed via 5α-reductase enzymes. Although testosterone is the most potent androgen secreted by the testicles, testosterone is converted to an even more potent androgen, dihydrotestosterone, in selected tissues by enzymes known as 5α-reductase. These enzymes exist in two isoforms (types I and II), and in the adult are expressed in a variety of tissues, particularly the prostate and skin. Inhibition of type II 5α-reductase activity by finasteride decreases serum prostate-specific antigen (PSA) and can decrease prostate gland size. Inhibitors of types I and II enzymes are being evaluated in clinical trials as anticancer agents.

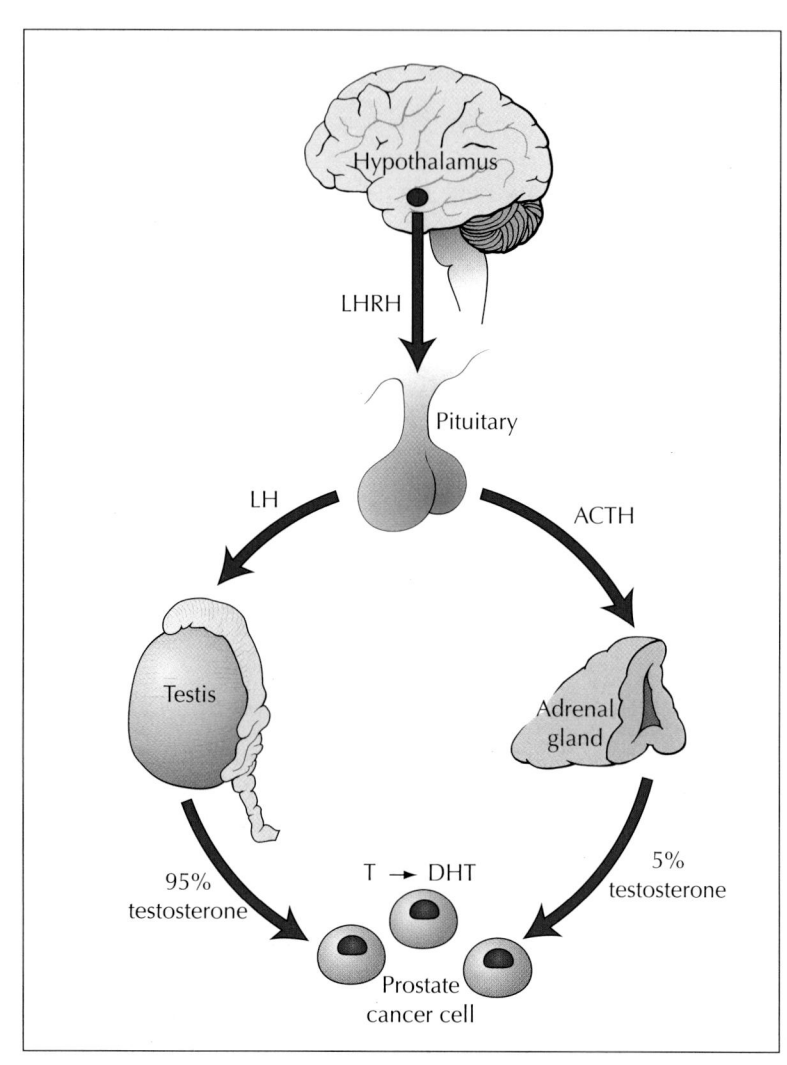

◗ **FIGURE 15-6.** Sources of androgen production. Control of androgen secretion is relatively well understood. Luteinizing hormone–releasing hormone (LHRH) is secreted into the hypophyseal portal system and circulates to the pituitary, where it stimulates the release of luteinizing hormone (LH) from gonadotrophs. LH binds to specific receptors on testicular Leydig cells, resulting in the production and secretion of testosterone into the bloodstream. This pathway accounts for approximately 95% of circulating testosterone. The remaining 5% is derived from the adrenal cortex, which is under the control of pituitary adrenocorticotropic hormone (ACTH).

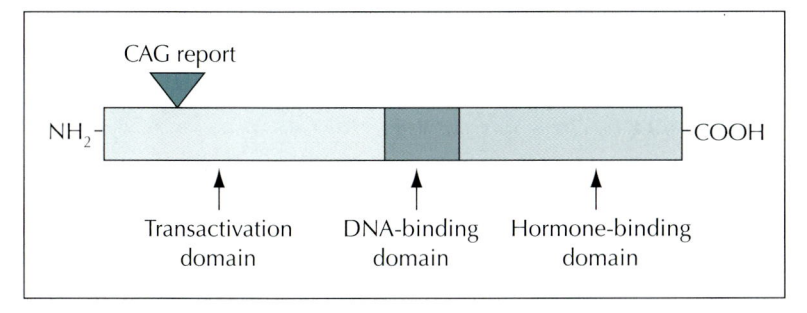

FIGURE 15-8. Androgenic actions are mediated by a ligand-dependent transcriptional regulator, the androgen receptor. The androgen receptor is a member of a steroid hormone receptor superfamily that includes progesterone, estrogen, and glucocorticoid receptors [17]. Three distinct domains characterize this protein: 1) a DNA-binding domain flanked by 2) an aminoterminal transactivation domain, and 3) a carboxy-terminal hormone-binding domain. The transactivation domain contains a variable number of glutamine repeats (encoded by CAG repeats). Binding of androgen to the androgen receptor results in DNA-receptor binding via specific DNA sequence recognized by the DNA binding domain of the androgen receptor [18]. This gene expression, in turn, regulates growth and differentiation of a variety of androgen-dependent tissues, including the prostate.

HORMONAL THERAPY

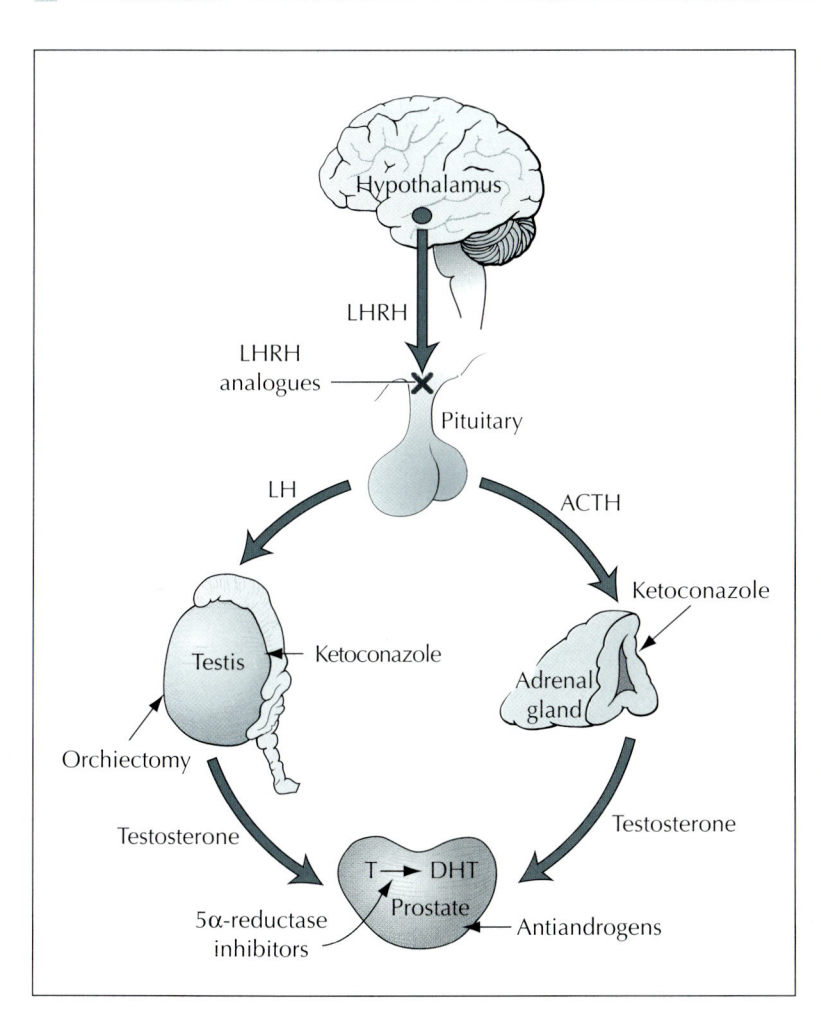

FIGURE 15-9. Blockade of androgen action can be achieved via many routes. Understanding the hormonal control mechanisms underlying prostatic cancer growth has given physicians multiple potential targets for therapeutic intervention. The gold standard for eliminating gonadal androgen secretion is bilateral orchiectomy, a procedure pioneered over 50 years ago for the treatment of prostate cancer [1]. Within hours of surgical castration, 95% reduction in serum testosterone levels is achieved.

The luteinizing hormone–releasing hormone (LHRH) analogues currently approved by the Food and Drug Administration in the United States potently bind and stimulate the LHRH receptors on the pituitary. This agonist activity initially results in a marked increase in luteinizing hormone (LH) and testosterone secretion, followed by a paradoxic decline to castrate levels after 2 to 4 weeks. Current LHRH agonists, such as leuprolide and goserelin acetate, are available in depot formulations capable of inhibiting testosterone secretion for 3 to 4 months per injection [19]. Estrogens such as diethylstilbestrol (DES) have been used in the treatment of prostate cancer for decades. DES is no longer manufactured in the United States. DES acts as a potent inhibitor of LH secretion [20], thereby indirectly lowering testosterone secretion.

Antiandrogens block the effects of androgens by acting as antagonists at the androgen receptor. Both steroidal (cyproterone acetate) and non-steroidal (flutamide, bicalutamide, and nilutamide) antiandrogens have been used in the treatment of prostate cancer. These agents inhibit the effects of androgens on the pituitary as well as prostatic tissue. Administration of antiandrogens is associated with an increase in circulating testosterone [21]. A variety of agents can inhibit adrenal androgen secretion. The agents most commonly used in patients with prostate cancer are ketoconazole and aminoglutethimide. Ketoconazole also dramatically inhibits testicular androgen secretion and can be used to achieve castration levels of testosterone within 24 to 48 hours [22].

Toxicities of Hormonal Therapies

	Decreased Libido	Decreased Potency	Gynecomastia	Edema	Hot Flashes	Fatigue
Orchiectomy	++++	++++	++	+	++++	++
LHRH	++++	++++	++	+	++++	++
Estrogens	++++	++++	++++	+++	+	++
Anti-androgens	++	++	+++	+	++	++

Plus signs *indicate degree of toxicity.*

▶ **FIGURE 15-10.** Toxicities of hormonal therapies. Although hormonal therapies are well tolerated as compared with most other cancer treatments, significant side effects are associated with traditional hormonal therapies. Particularly distressing to many men is the loss of sexual function (both libido and potency). Some men have considerable psychologic difficulty undergoing surgical orchiectomy; most choose to receive alternative therapies if given a choice. Long-term effects of hormonal therapies can include hot flashes, muscle mass loss, fatigue, and anemia [23]. If estrogens are used, gynecomastia, thromboembolisms, and fluid retention can be significant problems in addition to the toxicities of androgen deprivation. Antiandrogen monotherapy, or antiandrogens combined with a 5α-reductase inhibitor, are associated with a lower incidence of potency problems than is traditional hormonal therapy. LHRH—luteinizing hormone–releasing hormone.

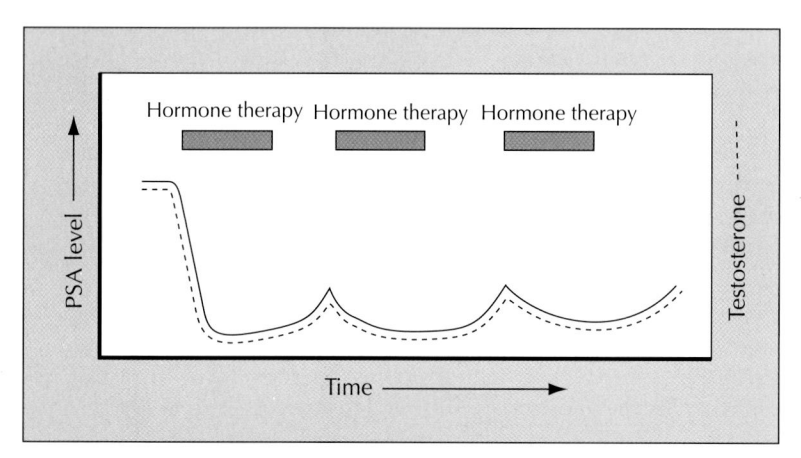

▶ **FIGURE 15-11.** Intermittent androgen deprivation. The concept of intermittent rather than continuous androgen suppression recently has been advanced. In animal studies, some data suggest that intermittent hormonal therapy delays onset of the hormone-refractory state [24]. In addition, men often prefer to have periods off hormonal therapy when their sexual function can return to normal. Although many variants of intermittent therapy have been reported, most monitor levels of prostate-specific antigen (PSA) closely and allow PSA changes to drive subsequent treatment decisions [25]. No randomized studies comparing intermittent with continuous hormonal therapies have been published, so definitive conclusions cannot yet be drawn.

Experimental Forms of Hormone Therapy

LHRH antagonists
  PPI-149
Dual 5α-reductase inhibitors
  LY320236
  FK143
  FCE 28260
  GG 745

▶ **FIGURE 15-12.** Experimental hormonal therapy. Orchiectomy, antiandrogens, estrogens, and luteinizing hormone–releasing hormone (LHRH) agonists are well described in the prostate cancer literature. Newer forms of hormonal therapy are being developed. These experimental forms of hormonal therapy include novel 5α-reductase inhibitors and LHRH antagonists. The 5α-reductase inhibitors block conversion of testosterone to the more potent dihydrotestorone. Two types of 5α-reductase inhibitors exist: types I and II enzymes. Although the type II inhibitors such as finasteride are clearly inadequate to treat prostate cancer patients, compounds that inhibit both types I and II enzymes are under active investigation [26]. The advantages of an LHRH antagonist over an LHRH agonist primarily relate to the fact that no tumor flare would be expected with an antagonist. Furthermore, because small increases in testosterone are documented in many patients after each LHRH agonist injection, use of LHRH antagonists would have the potential advantage of avoiding these effects.

Selected Combinations of Hormonal Therapy

LHRH analogues + anti-androgens
Anti-androgens + 5α-reductase inhibitors
Ketoconazole + glucocorticoids

▶ **FIGURE 15-13.** Selected combinations of hormonal therapy. Combinations of hormonal therapy have been carefully evaluated over the past several decades. Combined androgen blockade, which consists of testicular deprivation therapy combined with an antiandrogen, has certain theoretical advantages over hormonal monotherapy. Although some prospective randomized trials using combinations of luteinizing hormone–releasing hormone (LHRH) analogues and antiandrogens are reported to have positive effects in terms of patient survival [28], meta-analysis of all trials demonstrate that the effects are relatively minor [5]. Combinations of orchiectomy and antiandrogens also have been evaluated in prospective controlled trials, but recently presented results do not indicate an advantage of combined approaches [29].

Antiandrogens such as flutamide have been combined with 5α-reductase inhibitors such as finasteride in an effort to diminish the traditional side effects of hormonal therapy for prostate cancer [29]. This combination is associated with less impairment of potency than LHRH analogues or orchiectomy. Efficacy has not been shown to be equivalent in controlled clinical trials, however.

Evaluating Treatment Outcomes in Patients With Metastatic Prostate Cancer

Host factors	Measures of tumor growth
Survival	Bone scan lesions
Tumor-specific survival	Bidimensional measures
Pain	CT scan
Anorexia	MRI scan
Weight loss	Physical examination
Analgesic consumption	Tumor markers
Performance status	PSA
Quality of life	Prostatic acid phosphatase

FIGURE 15-14. Evaluating treatment outcomes in patients with metastatic prostate cancer. The efficacy of any treatment can be measured only by use of standardized and generally recognized endpoints. Commonly evaluated endpoints include both host-specific and tumor-specific effects as well as treatment-associated toxicities. In patients with advanced prostate cancer, *host-oriented* endpoints include survival, tumor-specific survival, pain, anorexia, weight loss, analgesic consumption, performance status, and quality of life. Some of these endpoints have been formally defined by various validated tools. Tumor-specific endpoints include radiographic changes, physical findings, and biopsy findings, as well as a variety of markers either directly reflective (*eg*, prostate-specific antigen [PSA] or prostatic acid phosphatase) or indirectly reflective (*eg*, alkaline phosphatase or hemoglobin) of tumor activity. Each of these endpoints can be statistically evaluated in terms of absolute change, duration of change, or duration without progression (progression-free survival). Most physicians agree that host-specific factors are most helpful in evaluating the efficacy of therapies.

Results of Early Hormonal Treatment

Survival	↑
Pathologic fractures	↓
Ureteral obstruction	↓
Spinal cord compression	↓
Bladder outlet obstruction	↓

FIGURE 15-15. Early hormonal treatment has improved survival and decreased morbidity in a controlled randomized trial [30]. Despite the general agreement that hormonal therapies are the best currently available treatments for patients with metastatic prostate cancer, significant controversies remain as to when these therapies are best initiated. As with many areas of prostate cancer, controversies exist because of a paucity of prospective trials comparing various treatment options.

Recent data from the UK's Medical Research Council group [31] provide valuable insight into the effects of immediate versus deferred treatment for advanced prostate cancer. In this study, patients were randomized to receive treatment either immediately at the time that the disease was diagnosed, or at the time of "clinically significant progression." Findings from this study indicated a statistically significant survival advantage for patients treated with immediate hormonal therapy. Subset analysis revealed that this advantage was confined to those patients with TxNxM0 (nonmetastatic) disease. These results imply that once a patient is diagnosed with stage M1 disease, it is too late for immediate therapy to confer a survival advantage. Potential advantages to immediate versus delayed hormonal therapy were not confined to survival. Pathologic fractures, ureteral obstruction, spinal cord compression, and surgical interventions for bladder outlet obstruction were statistically increased in those patients receiving deferred therapy.

HORMONE-REFRACTORY PROSTATE CANCER

Criteria for Diagnosis of Hormone-refractory Prostate Cancer

Castrate levels of testosterone
Progressive disease
  PSA level
  Bone scan
  Soft tissue disease
  Symptoms

FIGURE 15-16. Criteria for the diagnosis of hormone-refractory prostate cancer. The definition of hormone-refractory disease has changed dramatically as our ability to monitor the effects of therapy and the progression of prostate cancer has become more precise. Before the era of radioimmunoassay, definitions of hormone-refractory disease did not include the measurement of testosterone levels. Today, many physicians believe that testosterone must be suppressed below castrate levels before patients can be labeled as "hormone refractory." Most importantly, application of different criteria can dramatically change the population of patients in question. Traditional criteria for "hormone-refractory" disease have revolved around the onset of new symptoms or new lesions using radiologic imaging tests. More recently, increases in prostate-specific antigen (PSA) levels have become accepted by many investigators as an appropriate endpoint. The precise definition of an "increasing" PSA also is subject to controversy [31]. Some investigators suggest that any confirmed rise in PSA should constitute progression. Others have used minimal values for PSA increases (>10 ng/mL), whereas still others have preferred to use defined percentage increases over prior PSA nadirs (*eg*, 50% increase over nadir values).

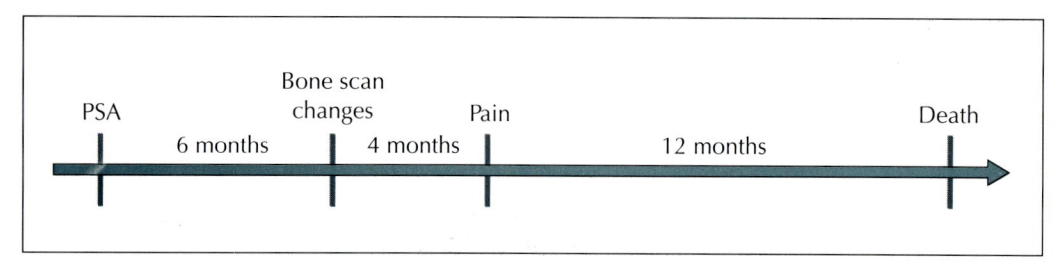

FIGURE 15-17. Natural history of hormone-refractory prostate cancer. As the natural history of hormone-refractory prostate cancer has become better understood, it is generally agreed that prostate-specific antigen (PSA) rises typically precede progression on bone scans and that progression on bone scans typically precede changes in pain. Studies of patients with stage D2 disease indicate that PSA rises precede bone scan changes by approximately 6 months and that bone scan changes will precede pain by approximately 4 months [33]. For patients with pain, average life expectancy is less than 1 year. When reading the literature regarding hormone-refractory prostate cancer, it is essential to carefully ascertain the definition of hormone-refractory disease used in each particular study to assess the therapeutic results reported.

Treatment Options for Hormone-refractory Prostate Cancer

Withdrawal therapies
Secondary hormonal therapies
Radiation therapies
Chemotherapy
Experimental therapies

FIGURE 15-18. Treatment options for hormone-refractory prostate cancer. The treatment options for hormone-refractory prostate cancer can be roughly divided into withdrawal therapies, hormonal therapies, irradiation, chemotherapy, and experimental approaches. Withdrawal therapies have been described in recent years and can influence both patient care and clinical trial results. Some patients who fail initial hormonal therapy with standard approaches (*eg*, luteinizing hormone–releasing hormone [LHRH] analogues, orchiectomy) can have subjective and objective responses to secondary hormonal manipulation. Radiation therapy for advanced prostate cancer can be delivered by either external beam or intravenous methods.

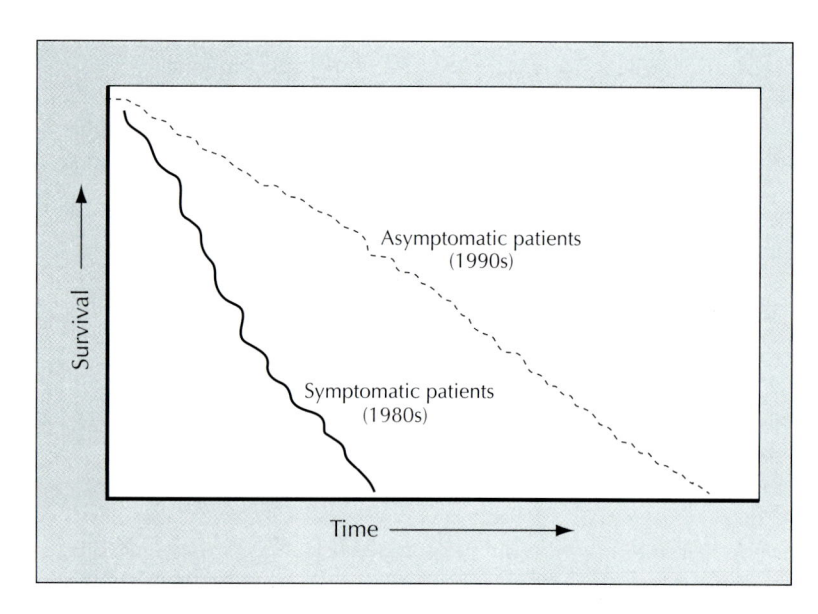

FIGURE 15-19. Survival with hormone-refractory prostate cancer. Survival of patients with hormone-refractory prostate cancer has become progressively longer, but no peer-reviewed trial or randomized prospective trial has yet shown a survival advantage of one treatment over another. The survival of patients in various trials has depended primarily on the type of patients enrolled in that trial rather than the therapy used. Trials conducted more recently have shown longer survival as compared with older trials, but this may be due to detection of rising prostate-specific antigen (PSA) values, rather than symptoms, in patients enrolled on hormone-refractory protocols.

Withdrawal Responses in Hormone-refractory Prostate Cancer

Anti-androgens
 Flutamide
 Bicalutamide
 Nilutamide
Estrogens
Megestrol acetate
Estramustine
Retinoids
TNP-470

FIGURE 15-20. Withdrawal responses in hormone-refractory prostate cancer. Certain patients may benefit from withdrawal of a therapeutic agent as well as its administration. Withdrawal responses have been recognized in recent years, initially with antiandrogens [34,35]. Currently, all agents (except one) described as having withdrawal activity in prostate cancer are known to interact with steroid receptors. Agents with reported withdrawal activity include the antiandrogens (flutamide, bicalutamide, and nilutamide), estrogens [36], megestrol acetate [37], estramustine [38], and an antiangiogenic agent TNP470 [39]. The mechanism of withdrawal activities is still debated. The most commonly cited hypothesis involves the development of mutant receptors that recognize antiandrogens as receptor agonists rather than antagonists.

II. The Prostate

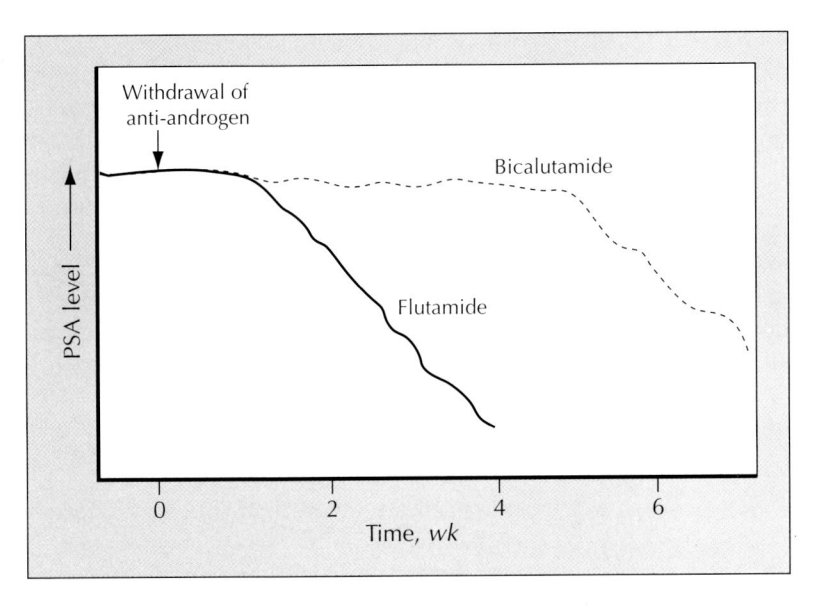

FIGURE 15-21. Kinetics of withdrawal responses vary by agent. Although withdrawal activity has now been described for all antiandrogens, clinically significant differences have been noted between these compounds [40]. For instance, withdrawal responses to flutamide are typically noted within 2 weeks after discontinuation of the agent, whereas bicalutamide withdrawal responses are typically delayed until 6 to 8 weeks after the agent is discontinued. The differences in the kinetics of the withdrawal responses may be related to differences between agents in functional half-life; bicalutamide has a serum half-life of approximately 6 days, whereas flutamide has a half-life of approximately 6 hours.

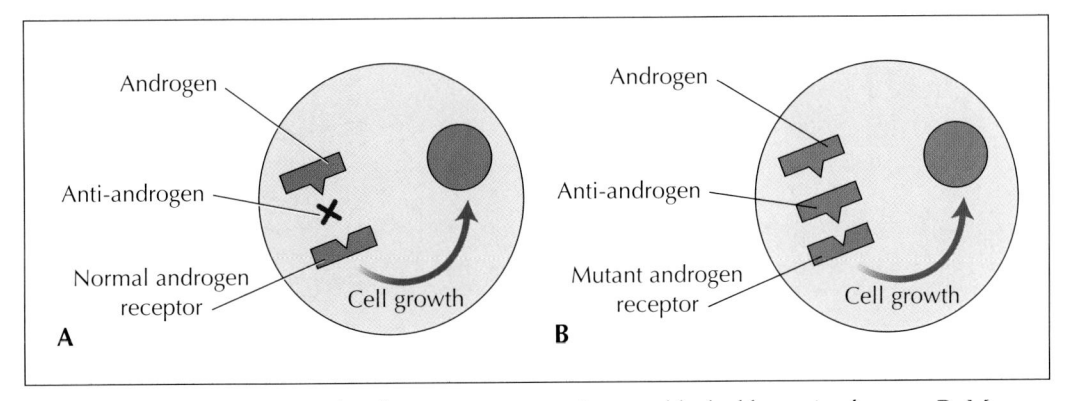

FIGURE 15-22. **A,** Normal androgen receptors actions are blocked by antiandrogens. **B,** Mutant androgen receptor actions can be activated by antiandrogens. Although the clinical significance of mutant androgen receptors is debated, most investigators agree that mutants can be detected in selected patients with prostate cancer [41]. Most of the controversy surrounding these findings has concerned the frequency, location, and significance of these mutations. Because the androgen receptor gene is X-linked, there is only one allele per cell. Thus, any genetic changes in these sequences would not be opposed by the action of a normal gene expressed on another chromosome. The potential importance of mutations is magnified in comparison with genes expressed from two alleles, therefore.

The first androgen receptor mutation described in patient-derived material was sequenced from a cell line termed LNCaP. This cell line contains a point mutation within the hormone-binding domain of the androgen receptor [42]. The functional significance of mutations in the hormone-binding domain was notable: receptors bearing a selected mutation recognized a variety of ligands in a promiscuous manner. Instead of receptor activation being triggered by androgens and blocked by antiandrogens, mutant receptor activation can be triggered by a variety of compounds including antiandrogens, estrogens, and progesterone. Clinical observations indicate that antitumor responses after withdrawal of antiandrogens may be linked to the presence of selective mutations in the hormone-binding domain of the androgen receptors expressed in sufficient quantities in patients with hormone-refractory prostate cancer.

Hormonal Treatments for Hormone-refractory Prostate Cancer

Anti-androgens
  Flutamide
  Bicalutamide
  Nilutamide
Glucocorticoids
  Prednisone
  Dexamethasone
  Hydrocortisone
Estrogens
  Diethylstilbestrol
  Estramustine (other activities reported)
Progesterones
  Megestrol acetate
Adrenal suppressives
  Ketoconazole
  Aminoglutethimide

FIGURE 15-23. Hormonal treatments for hormone-refractory prostate cancer. Antiandrogens [43], glucocorticoids [44], adrenal suppressive agents such as ketoconazole [45], megestrol acetate [46], estrogens [47], and estramustine [48] are all known to interact with hormonal receptors, and all have some activity in patients with hormone-refractory prostate cancer. The duration of responses typically is limited to 2 to 4 months. The described activity of these hormonal agents in patients with hormone-refractory disease clearly underlines the ambiguity of the current nomenclature describing this disease.

Management of Metastatic Prostate Cancer

Radioisotopes in Treatment of Hormone-refractory Prostate Cancer

Product	Half-life, d	Decay	Energy (β-MeV) max
^{89}Sr	50.5	β$^-$	1.46
^{153}Sm	1.9	β$^-$, γ	0.81
^{32}P	13.6	β$^-$	1.71
^{186}Re	3.8	β$^-$, γ	1.07

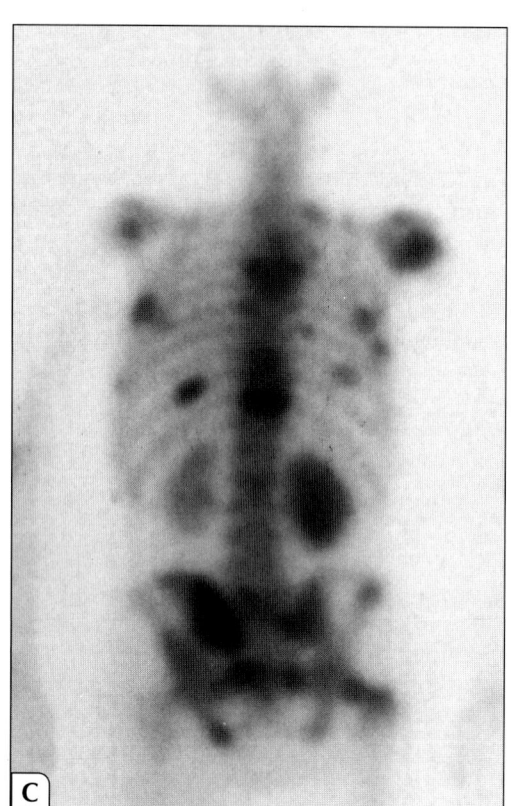

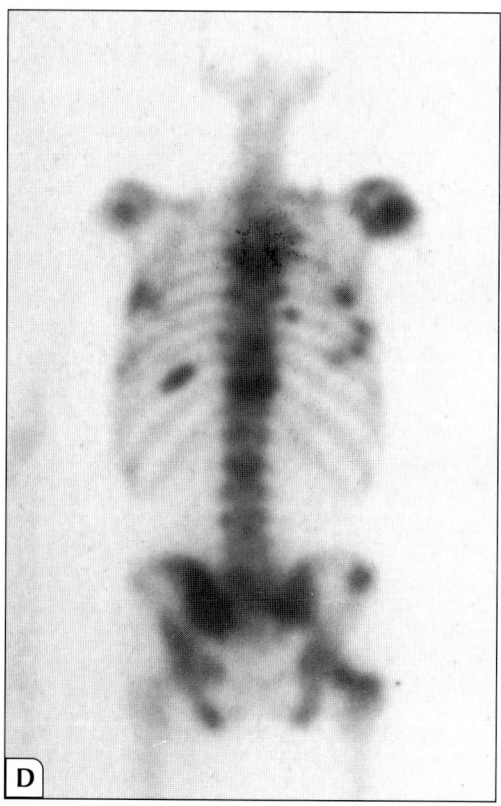

▶ **FIGURE 15-24.** Radioisotopes in the treatment of hormone-refractory prostate cancer. Radiation therapies have long been known to provide effective palliation for patients with advanced prostate cancer. Although external beam radiation has been the radiation treatment of choice, newer data suggest that intravenously administered radioisotopes might also have significant therapeutic efficacy, particularly in patients with painful bony metastasis. Radioactive phosphorus (^{32}P) has long been available, but several other therapeutic bone-seeking radioisotopes have been introduced in recent years, including ^{89}Sr and ^{153}Sm. A physical comparison of these isotopes demonstrates significant differences in physical half-life and particle energy.

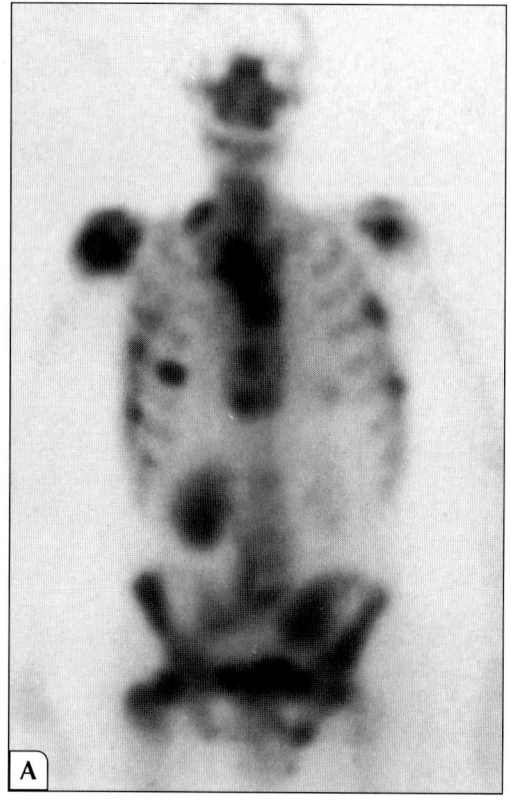

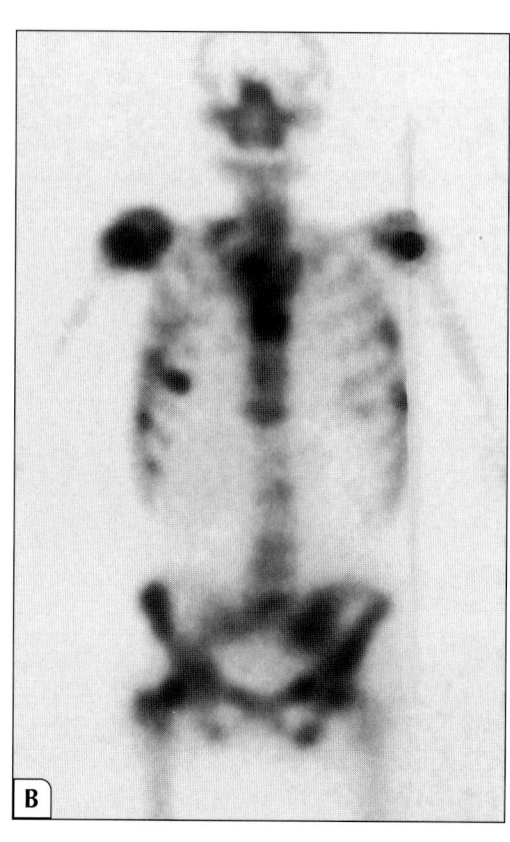

▶ **FIGURE 15-25.** Imaging and treatment with a single injection can be accomplished with ^{153}Sm-EDTMP. Because ^{153}Sm is both a β- and γ-emitting isotope, both imaging and treatment can be accomplished with a single agent. No difference in imaging between conventional bone scans (*panels A and C*) and ^{153}Sm-EDTMP (*panels B and D*) can be readily distinguished.

II. The Prostate

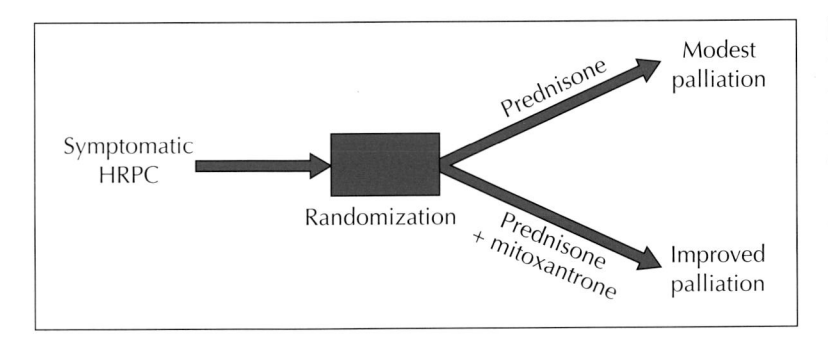

FIGURE 15-26. Mitoxantrone in the treatment of hormone-refractory prostate cancer. Although chemotherapy has not been perceived traditionally as an active modality in patients with prostate cancer, recent data from prospective randomized trials indicate that mitoxantrone plus low-dose prednisone is superior to low-dose prednisone alone in achieving pain relief in symptomatic patients with metastatic hormone-refractory prostate cancer. Data published by Tannock *et al.* [44] indicate that the percentage of patients achieving pain relief or having declines in analgesic consumption is substantially higher in patients receiving mitoxantrone. HRPC—hormone-refractory prostate cancer.

Estramustine-based Chemotherapy

Combination	PSA Decline > 50%
Estramustine + vinblastine	61%
Estramustine + UP-16	52%
Estramustine + paclitaxel	52%
Estramustine + docetaxel	62%

FIGURE 15-27. Estramustine-based chemotherapy. Estramustine-based chemotherapies have been evaluated in phase I and II trials in patients with advanced prostate cancer.

Estramustine, an agent with both hormonal and chemotherapeutic properties, has been combined with a variety of chemotherapeutic agents that inhibit microtubule formation. In vitro studies indicate the possibility of synergism with these combinations. Phase I and II clinical trials with potentially interesting activity have been reported with estramustine plus vinblastine [49], estramustine plus VP-16 [50], estramustine plus paclitaxel [51], and estramustine plus docetaxel [52].

Endogenous Angiogenic Stimulators and Inhibitors

Endogenous angiogenic stimulators
  Fibroblast growth factors
  Angiogenesis
  Transforming growth factors (α and β)
  Platelet-derived growth factor
  Angiotropin
  Vascular-endothelial growth factor
Endogenous angiogenic inhibitors
  Angiostatin
  Endostatin
  Platelet factor-4
  Glucocorticoids
  Interferons (α and β)
  Thrombospondin-1

FIGURE 15-28. Endogenous angiogenic and antiangiogenic factors regulate new blood vessel formation. Tumor angiogenesis is the formation of new blood vessels within a malignancy. Tumor cells stimulate the proliferation of endothelial cells and new capillaries, allowing enlargement of the tumor mass via increased nutritional supply to the cells. This stimulation appears to be a result of change in the balance between endogenous inhibitors and inducers [53]. Inhibition of this phenomenon as a potential therapeutic modality has been the goal of much work. Inhibition of tumor recruitment of new blood vessels probably would isolate a tumor to a local primary site and limit its growth to only a few millimeters in diameter.

Inhibitors of Angiogenesis

TNP-470
Carboxyamidotriazole
Thalidomide
Pentosan polysulfate
Interferon-α
Vitamin D_3 analogues
Endostatin
Angiostatin

FIGURE 15-29. Inhibitors of angiogenesis currently are in various drug development phases. A variety of antiangiogenic factors (*eg*, TNP-470, carboxyamidotriazole, thalidomide, pentosan polysulfate, interferons, and vitamin D analogues) are being evaluated in clinical trials. Endogenous inhibitors such as endostatin and angiostatin have received considerable recent interest because of their effectiveness in animal models [54,55]. Endostatin is a 20-kD C-terminal fragment of collagen XVIII. Angiostatin is a 38-kD fragment of plasminogen.

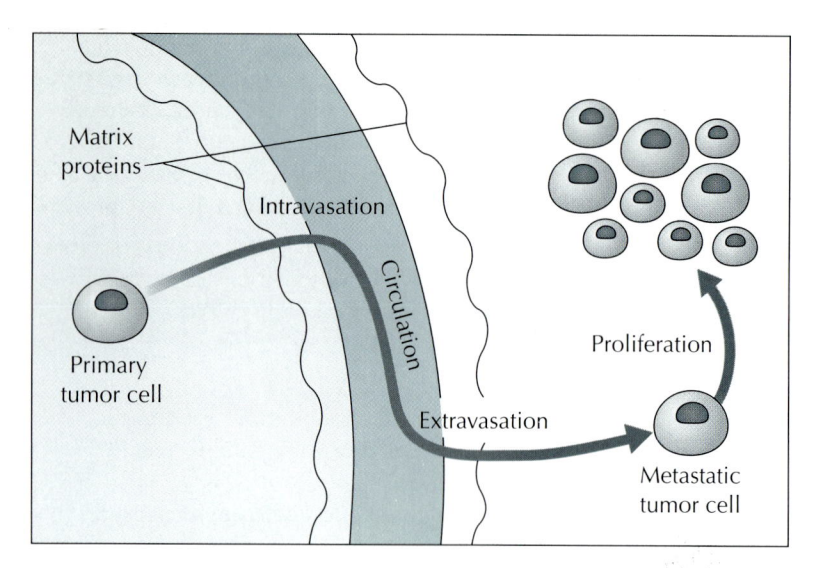

FIGURE 15-30. The complexity of tumor metastasis. Remodeling of the extracellular matrix is a physiologic function necessary for metastasis and tumor growth. The metastatic process is complex and involves several steps: access to the blood vessels (intravasation), circulation, extravasation, and proliferation at distant sites. Inhibition of any one of these steps could result in stabilization of the tumor.

Matrix Metalloproteinases and Tissue Inhibitors of Metalloproteinases

Matrix metalloproteinases
 Collagenases (MMP-1)
 Gelatinases (MMP-2 and -9)
 Stromelysins (MMP-3)
 Matilysins (MMP-7)
Tissue inhibitors of metalloproteinases
 TIMP-1
 TIMP-2
 TIMP-3
 TIMP-4

FIGURE 15-31. Imbalances between matrix metalloproteinases (MMPS) and MMP inhibitors (tissue inhibitors of metalloproteinases [TIMPs]) promote tumor growth and metastasis. The destruction of extracellular matrixes is postulated to occur when local concentrations of MMP exceed those of TIMPs [56]. A number of MMPs have been identified. These can be divided roughly into four subgroups: interstitial collagenases, gelatinases, stromelysins, and membrane-type MMPs [57]. The physiologic role for each of these enzymes is not completely understood, but MMP2 and MMP9 appear to be important in the growth of a tumor. Both of these enzymes are expressed in prostate cancer cells, as well as other tumor types.

A. Antimetastatic Agents

Batimistat	AG3340
Marimistat	CGS-27023A
Ilomastat	COL-3

FIGURE 15-32. Several antimetastatic agents are in development as therapeutic agents. **A**, Scientists have accelerated the discovery of a variety of agents with antimetastatic activity [58], in particular those agents with matrix metalloproteinase activity (*ie*, batimastat, marimistat, AG3340, CGS-27023A, and COL-3). **B**, Tumor cells, in order to metastasize, must invade blood vessels (intravasation), circulate in the blood stream, and exit the vessels (extravasation). Matrix metalloproteinases are key to both entry and exit from the vessels.

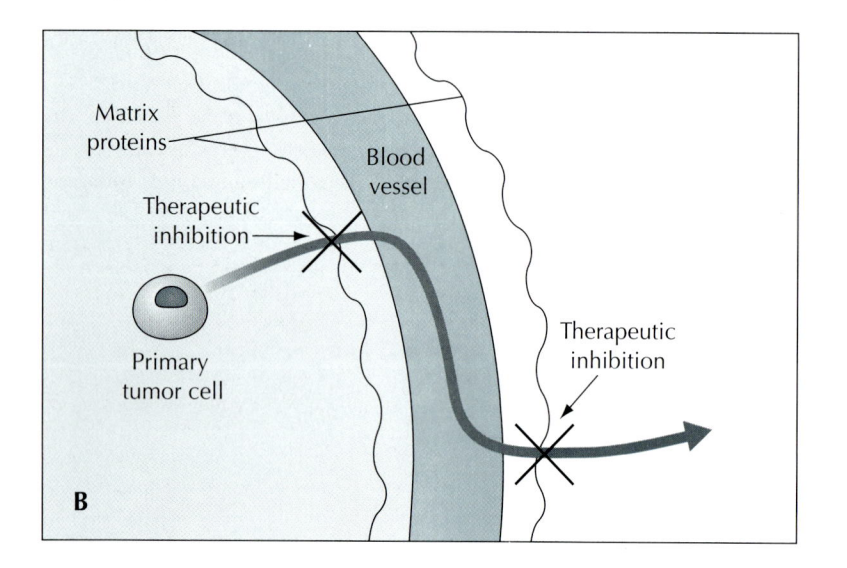

REFERENCES

1. Huggins C, Hodges CV: Studies on prostatic cancer: I. The effect of castration of estrogen and of androgen injection on serum phosphatases in metastatic carcinoma of the prostate. *Cancer Res* 1941, 1:293–297.
2. Veteran's Administration Cooperative Urological Research Group: Carcinoma of the prostate (treatment comparisons). *J Urol* 1997, 98:516–522.
3. Auclair C, Kelly PA, Coy DH, et al: Potent inhibitory activity of [D-Leu-6, des-Gly-NH2] LHRH ethylarnide on LH/hCG and prolactin testicular receptor levels in the rat. *Endocrinology* 1977, 101:1890–1893.
4. Labrie F, Dupont A, Belanger A, et al.: New approach in the treatment of prostate cancer: complete instead of partial withdrawal of androgens. *Prostate* 1983, 4:579–594.
5. Prostate Cancer Trialists' Collaborative Group: Maximum androgen blockade in advanced prostate cancer: an overview of 22 randomised trials with 3283 deaths in 5710 patients. *Lancet* 1995, 346:265–269.
6. Brufsky A, Fontaine R, Berlane K, et al.: Finasteride and flutamide as potency sparing androgen-ablative therapy for advanced adenocarcinoma of the prostate. *Urology* 1997, 49:913–920.
7. Higano CS: Intermittent androgen suppression with leuprolide and flutamide for prostate cancer: a pilot study. *Urology* 1996, 48:800–804.
8. Franks LM: The spread of prostate carcinoma. *J Pathol* 1956, 72:603–611.
9. Lee CT, Oesterling JE: Using prostate-specific antigen to eliminate the staging radionuclide bone scan. *Urol Clin North Am* 1997, 24:389–394.
10. Terris MK, Klonecke AS, McDougall IR, Stamey TA: Utilization of bone scans in conjunction with prostate specific antigen levels in the surveillance for recurrence of adenocarcinoma after radical prostatectomy. *J Nucl Med* 1991, 32:1713–1718.
11. Manyak M: Advances in Imaging Prostate Cancer. In *Advances in Prostate Cancer* 1997, 1:5–7.
12. Kahn D, Williams RD, Manyak MJ, et al.: 111-Indium-Capromab pendetide in the evaluation of patients with residual or recurrent prostate cancer after radical prostatectomy. *J Urol* 1998, 159:2040–2047.
13. Maguire RT: 111-In Capromab pendetide (Prostascint) for presurgical staging of patients with prostate cancer. *J Nucl Med* 1995, 29:108–113.
14. Moreno JG, Croce CM, Fischer R, et al.: Detection of hematogenous micrometastases in patients with prostate cancer. *Cancer Res* 1992, 52:6110–6112.
15. Deguchi T, Doi T, Ehara H, et al.: Detection of micrometastatic prostate cancer cells in lymph nodes by reverse transcriptase-polymerase chain reaction. *Cancer Res* 1993, 53:5350–5354.
16. Wood DP Jr, Bankes ER, Humphreys S, et al.: Identification of bone marrow micrometastases in patients with prostate cancer. *Cancer* 1994, 74:2533–2540.
17. Chang C, Kokontis J, Liao S: Molecular cloning of the human and rat complementary DNA encoding androgen receptors. *Science* 1988, 240:324–326.
18. Beato M: Gene regulation by steroid hormones. *Cell* 1989, 56:335–344.
19. Sharifi R, Knoll LD, Smith J, Kramolowsky E: Leuprolide acetate (30 mg depot every 4 months) in the treatment of advanced prostate cancer. *Urology* 1998, 51:271–276.
20. Shupnik MA, Schreihofer DA: Molecular aspects of steroid hormone action in the male reproductive axis. *J Androl* 1997, 18:341–344.
21. Soloway MS, Matzkin H: Antiandrogenic agents as monotherapy in advanced prostate carcinoma. *Cancer* 1993, 71:1083–1088.
22. Bamberger MH, Lowe FC: Ketoconazole in initial management and treatment of metastatic prostate cancer to spine. *Urology* 1988, 32:301–303.
23. Strum SB, McDermed JE, Scholz MC, et al.: Anaemia associated with androgen deprivation in patients with prostate cancer receiving combined hormone-blockade. *Br J Urol* 1997, 79:933–941.
24. Sato N, Gleave ME, Bruchovsky N, et al.: Intermittent androgen suppression delays progression to androgen independent regulation of prostate specific antigen gene in the LNCaP prostate tumor model. *J Steroid Biochem Mol Biol* 1996, 58:139–146.
25. Oliver RT: Intermittent androgen deprivation after PSA complete response as a strategy to reduce induction of hormone resistant prostate cancer. *Urology* 1997, 49:79–82.
26. Kojo H, Nakayama O, Hirosumi J, et al.: Novel steroid 5 alpha-reductase inhibitor FK143: its dual inhibition against the two isozymes and its effects on the transcription of the isozyme genes. *Mol Pharmacol* 1995, 48:401–406.
27. Presti JC Jr, Fair WR, Andriole GL, et al.: Multi-center, randomized, double-blind placebo-controlled study to investigate the effect of finasteride (MK-906) on stage D prostate cancer. *J Urol* 1992, 148:1201–1204.
28. Crawford ED, Eisenberger MA, McLeod DG, et al.: A controlled trial of leuprolide with and without flutamide in prostatic carcinoma. *N Engl J Med* 1989, 321:419–424.
29. Eisenberger MA, Blumenstein BA, Crawford ED, et al.: Bilateral orchiectomy with or without flutamide for metastatic prostate cancer. *N Engl J Med* 1998, 339:1036–1042.
30. Fleshner NE, Fair WR: Anti-androgenic effects of combination-finasteride plus flutamide in patients with prostatic carcinoma. *Br J Urol* 1996, 78:907–910.
31. The Medical Research Council Prostate Cancer Working Party Investigators Group: Immediate versus deferred treatment for advanced prostatic cancer: initial results of the Medical Research Council Trial. *Br J Urol* 1997, 79:235–246.
32. Dawson NA: Apples and oranges: building a consensus for standardized eligibility criteria and end points in prostate cancer clinical trials. *J Clin Oncol* 1998, 16:3398–3405.
33. Newling DWW, Denis L, Vermeylen K, for the European Organization for Research and Treatment of Cancer-Genitourinary Group: Orchiectomy versus goserelin and flutamide in the treatment of newly diagnosed metastatic prostate cancer. *Cancer* 1993, 72:3793–3798.
34. Scher HI, Kelly WK: The flutamide withdrawal syndrome: its impact on clinical trials in hormone-refractory prostate cancer. *J Clin Oncol* 1993, 11:1566–1572.
35. Figg WD, Sartor O, Cooper MR, et al.: Prostate specific antigen decline following the discontinuation of flutamide in patients with stage D2 prostate cancer. *Am J Med* 1995, 98:412–414.
36. Bissada NK, Kaczmarek AT: Complete remission of hormone refractory adenocarcinoma of the prostate in response to withdrawal of diethylstilbestrol. *J Urol* 1995, 153:1944–1945.
37. Dawson NA, McLeod DG: Dramatic prostate specific antigen decrease in response to discontinuation of megestrol acetate in advanced prostate cancer: expansion of the antiandrogen withdrawal syndrome. *J Urol* 1995, 153:1946–1947.
38. Nishiyama T, Terunuma M: Prostate specific antigen and prostate acid phosphatase declines after estramustine phosphate withdrawal: a case report. *Int J Urol* 1994, 1:355–356.
39. Sartor O: Prostate-specific antigen changes before and after administration of an angiogenesis inhibitor. *Oncology Reports* 1995, 2:1101–1102.
40. Schellhammer PF, Venner P, Haas GP, et al.: Prostate specific antigen decreases after withdrawal of antiandrogen therapy with bicalutamide or flutamide in patients receiving combined androgen blockade. *J Urol* 1997, 157:1731–1735.
41. Taplin ME, Bubley GJ, Shuster TD, et al.: Androgen receptor mutations in metastatic androgen independent prostate cancer. *N Engl J Med* 1995, 332:1393–1398.
42. Veldscholte J, Ris-Stalpers C, Kuipper GGJM, et al.: A mutation in the ligand binding domain of the androgen receptor of human LNCaP cells affects steroid binding characteristics and response to antiandrogens. *Biochem Biophys Res Commun* 1990, 173:534–540.
43. Fowler JE Jr: Endocrine therapy for localized prostate cancer. *Uro Ann* 1996, 10:57–77.
44. Tannock IF, Osoba D, Stockler MR, et al.: Chemotherapy with mitoxantrone plus prednisone or prednisone alone for symptomatic hormone-resistant prostate cancer: a Canadian randomized trial with palliative end points. *J Clin Oncol* 1996, 14:1756–1764.
45. Small EJ, Baron AD, Fippin L, Apodaca D: Ketoconazole retains activity in advanced prostate cancer patients with progression despite flutamide withdrawal. *J Urol* 1997, 157:1204–1207.
46. Osbom JL, Smith DC, Trump DL: Megestrol acetate in the treatment of hormone refractory prostate cancer. *Am J Clin Oncol* 1997, 20:308–310.
47. Smith DC, Redman BG, Flaherty LE, et al.: A phase II trial of oral diethylstilbestrol as a second line hormonal agent in patients with advanced prostate cancer. *Urology* 1998, 52:257–260.
48. Walzer Y, Oswalt J, Soloway MS: Estramustine phosphate-hormone, chemotherapeutic agent, or both? *Urology* 1984, 24:53–58.
49. Hudes GH, Greenberg R, Krigel R, et al.: Phase II study of estramustine and vinblastine, two microtubule inhibitors, in hormone refractory prostate cancer. *J Clin Oncol* 1992, 10:1754–1761.
50. Pienta KJ, Redman B, Hussain M, et al.: Phase II evaluation of oral estramustine and oral etoposide in hormone-refractory adenocarcinoma of the prostate. *J Clin Oncol* 1994, 12:2005–2012.

51. Hudes GR, Nathan F, Khater C, *et al.*: Phase II trial of 96-hour paclitaxel plus oral estramustine phosphate in metastatic hormone-refractory prostate cancer. *J Clin Oncol* 1997, 15:3156–3163.
52. Petrylak DP, Shelton G, Judge T, *et al.*: Phase I trial of docetaxel and estramustine in androgen-insensitive prostate cancer [abstract]. *Proc Soc Am Soc Clin Oncol* 1997, 16:A1103.
53. Folkinan J, D'Amore PA: Blood vessel formation: what is its molecular basis? *Cell* 1996, 87:1153–1155.
54. O'Reilly MS, Boehm T, Shing Y, *et al.*: Endostatin: an endogenous inhibitor of angiogenesis and tumor growth. *Cell* 1997, 88:277–285.
55. Zetter BR: Angiogenesis and tumor metastasis. *Ann Rev Med* 1998, 49:407–424.
56. Chambers AF, Matrisian LM: Changing views of the role of matrix metalloproteinases in metastasis. *J Natl Cancer Inst* 1997, 89:1260–1270.
57. Duffy MJ, McCarthy K: Matrix metalloproteinases in cancer: prognostic markers and targets for therapy. *Int J Oncol* 1998, 12:1343–1348.
58. Denis LJ, Verweij J: Matrix metalloproteinase inhibitors: present achievements and future prospects. *Invest New Drugs* 1997, 15:175–185.

INDEX

A

Ablation, transurethral needle, 4.16-4.23 *See also* Transurethral needle ablation
Abrams-Griffith nomogram, in bladder outlet obstruction, 2.8
Actin, in benign prostatic hyperplasia, 1.8
Acute prostatitis, 7.3-7.4, 7.9
Adenocarcinoma, prostatic *See* Prostate cancer
Adenoma, laser prostatectomy for, 5.7
  surgical resection of, 6.12
Adrenal androgens, in hypothalamic-gonadal axis, 3.3
α-Adrenergic blockade, in benign prostatic hyperplasia, 1.7
Adrenoreceptors, in benign prostatic hyperplasia, 1.7, 3.8
Age, lower urinary tract symptoms and, 2.1
  prostate-specific antigen and, 8.5
Agency for Health Care Policy and Research, on benign prostatic hyperplasia, 3.1, 6.3
American Cancer Society, on prostate cancer, 8.16
American Society of Therapeutic Radiation Oncologists, treatment failure defined by, 13.8
American Urological Association score, in benign prostatic hyperplasia, 2.1, 2.3, 3.1, 6.2
  in prostate cancer, 13.2
  in prostatitis, 7.8
Aminoglutethimide, in prostate cancer, 15.5, 15.9
Anastomotic stricture, after radical retropubic prostatectomy, 11.10
Androgen receptors, in metastatic prostate cancer, 15.5, 15.9
Androgen suppression, in prostate cancer, 15.1, 15.5-15.6
Androgen withdrawal therapy, neoadjuvant, 10.11
  radiotherapy and, 12.10, 13.3
Androgens *See also* Testosterone
  in benign prostatic hyperplasia, 1.4-1.5
  in hypothalamic-gonadal axis, 3.3
  in metastatic prostate cancer, 15.4-15.5
Anesthesia, in benign prostatic hyperplasia, 1.3
  for radical retropubic prostatectomy, 11.2
Angiogenesis inhibitors, in hormone-refractory prostate cancer, 15.11
Antennae, in transurethral microwave thermotherapy, 4.9
Antiandrogens, in benign prostatic hyperplasia, 3.4, 3.7
  in prostate cancer, 15.5-15.6, 15.9
Antimicrobial agents, in bacterial prostatitis, 7.5
  before prostatectomy, 11.2
Argon, in cryoablation, 14.3
Aromatase inhibitors, in benign prostatic hyperplasia, 3.7
Asymptomatic inflammatory prostatitis, 7.9
Autologous blood banking, for prostatectomy, 10.2, 11.2

B

Bacterial prostatitis, 7.2, 7.4-7.5, 7.9
Bacteriuria, in prostatitis, 7.4-7.5, 7.9

Balloon dilation, in benign prostatic hyperplasia, 6.8
Baltimore Longitudinal Study of Aging, benign prostatic hyperplasia in, 1.2
Benign prostatic hyperplasia, anatomic features of, 1.2
  cystourethroscopy in, 2.14
  definitions in, 1.2-1.3
  diagnosis of, 2.1-2.2, 2.14-2.16
  epidemiology of, 1.1
  impact index of, 6.2
  medical management of, 3.1-3.14
    α-blocker therapy in, 3.8-3.11, 6.8
    combination therapy in, 3.11
    endocrine therapy in, 3.3-3.7
    patient selection for, 3.2
    phytotherapy in, 3.12
    timeline for, 3.14
    trends in, 3.2, 3.13
  minimally invasive treatment of, 4.1-4.23
    laser prostatectomy in, 5.1-5.9
    microwave hyperthermia in, 4.4-4.5
    needle ablation in, 4.16-4.23
    principles of thermal, 4.1-4.4
    transurethral microwave, 4.6-4.13
    ultrasound in, 4.13-4.15
  natural history of, 3.2
  pathophysiology of, 1.1-1.10
    adrenoreceptors in, 1.7
    biologic progression in, 1.3
    bladder dysfunction in, 1.8-1.10
    cellular stress study in, 1.8
    classic view of, 1.4
    clinical progression in, 1.2
    force generation of prostate tissue in, 1.6-1.7
    histologic features in, 1.2
    Northern blot analysis in, 1.9
    prostate size and, 1.3-1.4
    5α-reductase in, 1.4-1.5
    smooth muscle in, 1.8-1.10
    stromal hyperplasia in, 1.6
    testosterone in, 1.5
  placebo effect in studies of, 3.2
  prevalence of, 3.1, 3.13
  prostate-specific antigen levels in, 8.4
  prostatism *versus*, 2.1
  radiologic imaging in, 2.10-2.13
  surgical anatomy of, 6.5, 6.7
  surgical treatment of, 6.1-6.13
    indications for, 6.1

Benign prostatic hyperplasia, anatomic features of, *(continued)*
    instruments in, 6.5
    open prostatectomy in, 6.10-6.11
    outcomes in, 6.8-6.9
    patient positioning for, 6.4
    prostatectomy as, 3.2
    retropubic prostatectomy in, 6.12-6.13
    transurethral incision in, 6.9
    transurethral resection in, 6.1-6.8
  symptoms of, 3.2
    index of, 6.2
    lower urinary tract, 2.1-2.16
    as quality-of-life issue, 2.2
  symptoms similar to, 2.3
  treatment algorithm for, 3.13, 6.3-6.4
  urodynamic evaluation of, 2.4-2.10
Biopsy, in benign prostatic hyperplasia, 1.10
  in prostate cancer, 8.4, 8.12-8.14
    after cryoablation, 14.10-14.11
Bladder, diverticulum of, 2.13
  dysfunction of, benign prostatic hyperplasia, 1.2-1.3, 1.8-1.10, 2.2-2.4
  herniation of, 2.12
  in lower urinary tract symptom evaluation, 2.14
  outlet obstruction of *See* Bladder outlet obstruction
  in prostatitis, 7.4
  trabeculated, 1.10
Bladder compliance, cystometry in evaluation of, 2.5
Bladder neck, in radical prostatectomy, 10.8-10.9, 11.9
Bladder outlet obstruction, benign prostatic hyperplasia and, 1.2, 1.8-1.10, 2.1-2.15, 3.1
  cystourethroscopy in, 2.11, 2.14
  diagnosis of, 2.1-2.16
  endoscopy of, 1.10
  Northern blot analysis in, 1.9
  radiologic imaging in, 2.10-2.13
  surgical treatment for, 6.1
  urodynamic evaluation of, 2.4-2.10
  in prostatitis, 7.2
  renal function and, 2.4
α-Blocker therapy, in benign prostatic hyperplasia, 3.8-3.11
  adverse effects of, 3.7, 3.11
  cardiovascular effects of, 3.10
  outcome of, 6.8
Blood banking, for prostatectomy, 10.2, 11.2
Blood flow, in normal and tumor tissue, 4.2
Blood pressure, α-blocker therapy and, 3.10-3.11
Blood type screening, for prostatectomy, 10.2, 11.2
Bone scanning, in prostate cancer, metastatic, 15.2-15.3
  staging of, 8.8
Bougie-á-boules, for prostate resection, 6.5
Brachytherapy *See also* Interstitial radiotherapy
  in prostate cancer, 13.1

C

Cancer, metastatic prostate *See* Metastatic prostate cancer
  prostate *See* Prostate cancer
Candela system, in cryoablation, 14.3
Carcinoma, prostatic *See* Prostate cancer
Cardiovascular effects, of α-blocker therapy, 3.10-3.11
Catheters, in cryoablation, 14.4-14.5, 14.9
  in radical retropubic prostatectomy, 11.8, 11.10
  in transurethral microwave thermotherapy, 4.9
  in transurethral needle ablation, 4.17
Cell death, cold-induced, 14.2-14.3
  heat-induced, 4.2
Cellular stress study, in benign prostatic hyperplasia, 1.8
Central nervous system, in benign prostatic hyperplasia, 1.7, 2.1
Chemotherapy, in hormone-refractory prostate cancer, 15.11-15.12
Chronic pelvic pain syndrome, in prostatitis, 7.8-7.9
Chronic prostatitis, 7.3, 7.5, 7.9
CMS system, in cryoablation, 14.3
Coagulation necrosis, in laser prostatectomy, 5.1-5.4, 5.7-5.8
Comorbidity, in benign prostatic hyperplasia, 2.2
  in prostate cancer treatment decisions, 9.4
Computed tomography, in interstitial radiotherapy, 13.5, 13.7
  in prostate cancer staging, 8.9
Conventional photon external beam radiotherapy, 12.5-12.6
Corticotropin, in hypothalamic-gonadal axis, 3.3
Cryoablation of prostate cancer, 14.1-14.12
  complications of, 14.9
  cryobiology in, 14.2-14.3
  equipment in, 14.3-14.4
  history of, 14.1-14.2
  patient positioning in, 14.5
  patient selection in, 14.4-14.5
  procedure for, 14.5-14.8
  tumor control with, 14.10-14.12
Cryobiology, in cryoablation, 14.2-14.3
Cryoprobes, in cryoablation, 14.4, 14.7
Cystitis, after radiotherapy, 12.7
Cystometry, in lower urinary tract symptom evaluation, 2.5
Cystoscopes, in laser prostatectomy, 5.4, 5.8
Cystourethrography, in lower urinary tract symptom evaluation, 2.10-2.13
Cystourethroscopy, in lower urinary tract symptom evaluation, 2.14-2.15

D

Decongestants, in benign prostatic hyperplasia, 1.3
Denonvilliers' fascia, in radical retropubic prostatectomy, 11.6-11.8
Detrusor muscle, in benign prostatic hyperplasia, 1.7-1.8, 2.1-2.5
  after transurethral needle ablation, 4.20
  surgery *versus* needle ablation in, 4.22
  in lower urinary tract symptom evaluation, 2.3-2.5, 2.7-2.8
  radiologic imaging in, 2.10-2.13
Diarrhea, from hormonal therapy, 3.7

Diet, before prostatectomy, 11.2
Diethylstilbestrol, in prostate cancer, 15.5
Digital rectal examination, in prostate cancer, 8.3-8.4
    staging of, 8.7-8.8
Dihydrotestosterone, in benign prostatic hyperplasia, 1.4-1.5, 3.4-3.5
  in finasteride mechanism of action, 3.4
  in metastatic prostate cancer, 15.3
Diverticulum, bladder, 2.13
Dizziness, from α-blocker therapy, 3.11
Dogs, benign prostatic hyperplasia in, 1.2
Doppler transrectal ultrasound, in prostate cancer, 8.6
  in transurethral microwave thermotherapy, 4.8
Doxazosin, in benign prostatic hyperplasia, 1.7, 3.10
Drugs, lower urinary tract effects of, 2.1, 2.3

E

Ejaculatory dysfunction, from transurethral microwave thermotherapy, 4.11
Endocare system, in cryoablation, 14.3
Endocrine therapy *See also* specific hormones
  in benign prostatic hyperplasia, 3.3-3.7
Endocrinopathy, lower urinary tract symptoms of, 2.3
Endoscopy, in benign prostatic hyperplasia, 1.10
  in lower urinary tract symptom evaluation, 2.14
Endothelin, in prostatic smooth muscle contraction, 1.7
Energy transmission, principles of radiofrequency, 4.16
  in transurethral microwave thermotherapy, 4.9
Enzymes, in benign prostatic hyperplasia, 1.4-1.5
  in metastatic prostate cancer, 15.4, 15.6
Epithelial cells, in benign prostatic hyperplasia, 1.2, 1.5-1.6
Erectile dysfunction, after benign prostatic hyperplasia treatment, 6.8
  after cryoablation, 14.12
  after hormonal therapy, 3.7
  after radical retropubic prostatectomy, 11.10
  after radiotherapy, 12.7
  after transurethral microwave thermotherapy, 4.11
  from hormonal therapy, 15.6
Escherichia coli, prostatitis from, 7.2, 7.5
Estradiol, prostatic volume and, 3.7
Estramustine, in hormone-refractory prostate cancer, 15.11
Estriol, prostatic volume and, 3.7
Estrogens, in benign prostatic hyperplasia, 3.7
  in prostate cancer, 15.5-15.6, 15.9
European Organization for Research and Treatment of Cancer, trial of, 12.10
Expressed prostatic secretion leukocytes, in prostatitis, 7.4
External beam radiotherapy, advances in, 12.8-12.11
  after radical prostatectomy, 12.12
  androgen suppression and, 12.10
  conventional photon, 12.5-12.6
  in hormone-refractory prostate cancer, 15.10
  indications for, 12.1
  interstitial radiotherapy and, 13.3
  patterns of disease spread and, 12.2-12.4
  results of, 12.7
  treatment options in, 12.4
  treatment planning in, 12.1-12.2, 12.8-12.9
Extracellular matrix, in benign prostatic hyperplasia, 1.6

F

Fertility, prostatitis and, 7.6, 7.9
Fiber discharge, temperature and, 4.2-4.3
Finasteride, in benign prostatic hyperplasia, 1.3-1.5, 3.5-3.7, 3.11
  outcome of, 6.8
  mechanism of action of, 1.5, 3.4
  in metastatic prostate cancer, 15.6
Fistula formation, from cryoablation, 14.9
Fluoroscopy, in interstitial radiotherapy, 13.7
  in voiding profilometry, 2.9-2.10
Force generation of prostate tissue, in benign prostatic hyperplasia, 1.6-1.7
Fourth International Consultation on Benign Prostatic Hyperplasia, on hyperthermia, 4.5
Freezing, therapeutic, 14.1-14.12 *See also* Cryoablation of prostate cancer
Frequencies, wave, biologic effects of, 4.3

G

Galvanocautery, in benign prostatic hyperplasia, 4.1
Gastrointestinal disorders, after radiotherapy, 12.7
General anesthesia, for radical retropubic prostatectomy, 11.2
Gleason grading system, in prostate cancer staging, 8.7, 8.10-8.15, 12.3-12.4
  cryoablation results and, 14.11
Glucocorticoids, in prostate cancer, 15.9
Granulomatous prostatitis, 7.3
Growth factors, in benign prostatic hyperplasia, 1.5-1.6
Gynecomastia, from hormonal therapy, 3.4, 15.6

H

Headache, from α-blocker therapy, 3.11
Heat therapy, in benign prostatic hyperplasia, 4.1-4.23 *See also* specific techniques; Thermal therapy
Hematuria, after interstitial radiotherapy, 13.9
  after radiotherapy, 12.7
  from transurethral microwave thermotherapy, 4.11
Hemospermia, from transurethral microwave thermotherapy, 4.11
Hemostasis, in radical retropubic prostatectomy, 11.5, 11.9
Herniation, bladder, 2.12
High-intensity focused ultrasound, in benign prostatic hyperplasia, 4.13-4.15
  in cancer therapy, 4.15
Histology, in benign prostatic hyperplasia, 1.2
  in prostate cancer, 8.12-8.14
  in prostatitis, 7.2-7.4

Holmium:yttrium-aluminum-garnet laser prostatectomy, in benign prostatic hyperplasia, 5.1, 5.6-5.7
Hormonal therapy See also specific hormones
  in benign prostatic hyperplasia, 3.3-3.7
    adverse effects of, 3.7
  in prostate cancer, metastatic, 15.1, 15.5-15.7
    neoadjuvant, 10.11, 12.10, 13.3, 14.5
Hormone-refractory prostate cancer, 15.1, 15.7-15.12
  natural history of, 15.8
  prostate-specific antigen levels in, 15.7
  survival in, 15.8
  treatment of, chemotherapy in, 15.11-15.12
    hormonal therapy in, 15.9
    options in, 15.8
    radioisotopes in, 15.9
    withdrawal responses in, 15.8-15.9
Hot flashes, from hormonal therapy, 15.6
Hot water perfusion of the urethra, in benign prostatic hyperplasia, 4.1
Ho:YAG laser resection of the prostate, in benign prostatic hyperplasia, 5.6-5.7
Hydrolysis, myosin in, 1.9
Hyperplasia, benign prostatic See Benign prostatic hyperplasia
Hyperthermia, defined, 4.2
  microwave, in benign prostatic hyperplasia, 4.4-4.5
Hypotension, from α-blocker therapy, 3.10-3.11
Hypothalamic-gonadal axis, anatomy of, 3.3

I
Ice balls, in cryoablation, 14.4, 14.7-14.8
Immunoscintigraphy, in prostate cancer staging, 8.10
Implantation, prostate seed, in interstitial radiotherapy, 13.1-13.9
Impotence See Erectile dysfunction
Incontinence See Urinary incontinence
Index of coexistent disease, in prostate cancer treatment decisions, 9.4
Infection, prostatitis from, 7.2, 7.4-7.5, 7.9
Infertility, in prostatitis, 7.6, 7.9
Inflammation, prostatic See Prostatitis
Inguinal hernia, bladder dysfunction in, 2.12
Insomnia, lower urinary tract symptoms of, 2.3
International Prostate Symptom Score, 6.2
  in benign prostatic hyperplasia, 2.1, 4.20
Interstitial laser prostatectomy, in benign prostatic hyperplasia, 5.7-5.9
Interstitial radiotherapy, complications of, 13.9
  contraindications to, 13.2
  indications for, 13.1-13.2
  preoperative evaluation in, 13.2
  prostate volume study in, 13.4-13.7
  results of, 13.8
  therapy selection in, 13.3
  treatment failure in, 13.8
Interstitial thermometry, in experimental benign prostatic hyperplasia, 4.4

Isodoses, in external beam radiotherapy, 12.6, 12.9
Isoenzymes, 5α-reductase, in benign prostatic hyperplasia, 1.4-1.5

K
Kaplan-Meier plot, of disease-free cancer survival, 13.8
Kegel exercise, in incontinence treatment, 11.10
Ketoconazole, in prostate cancer, 15.5, 15.9
Kitner dissector, for radical retropubic prostatectomy, 11.4

L
Laboratory testing, in benign prostatic hyperplasia, 2.2
Laser fibers, in prostatectomy, 5.8
Laser prostatectomy in benign prostatic hyperplasia, 5.1-5.9
  complications of, 5.5
  Ho:YAG, 5.5-5.7
  interstitial, 5.7-5.9
  Nd:YAG, 5.3-5.5
  results of, 5.5
  ultrasound-guided, 5.2
Lasers, tissue effects of, 5.2
Lauer forceps, in radical perineal prostatectomy, 10.6-10.7
Leukocytes, in prostatitis, 7.4, 7.6-7.7
Libido, hormonal therapy as inhibitor of, 3.4, 3.7
Liquid gases, in cryoablation, 14.3-14.4, 14.8
Lithotomy position, for cryoablation, 14.5
  for interstitial radiotherapy, 13.5
  for prostate resection, 6.4
  for radical perineal prostatectomy, 10.3
Lower urinary tract symptoms, in benign prostatic hyperplasia, 2.1-2.16
  See also Benign prostatic hyperplasia
  incidence of, 4.1
  possible causes of, 2.2, 2.14-2.16
Lowsley retractor, in radical perineal prostatectomy, 10.3, 10.5, 10.8
Luteinizing hormone, in hypothalamic-gonadal axis, 3.3
  in prostate cancer, 15.1, 15.4-15.5
Luteinizing hormone-releasing hormone, in hypothalamic-gonadal axis, 3.3
  in metastatic prostate cancer, 15.3, 15.5-15.6
Luteinizing hormone-releasing hormone agonists, in benign prostatic hyperplasia, 3.3, 3.7
Lymph nodes, in pelvic anatomy, 12.2
  in prostate cancer, dissection of, 10.1, 11.2-11.3, 14.5
    metastatic patterns in, 12.2-12.4, 15.2
    radiotherapy of, 12.6
Lymphocytes, in benign prostatic hyperplasia, 1.6-1.7

M
Magnetic resonance imaging, after cryoablation, 14.10
  in prostate cancer staging, 8.9
Major histocompatibility complex, in bladder obstruction
Malignant cells, effects of heat on, 4.2
  vasodilation and, 4.2

Malignant disease, prostatic *See* Prostate cancer
Markov models, in prostate cancer treatment decisions, 9.2, 9.5
Meares-Stamey prostatitis definition, 7.4
Medical Research Council, on prostate cancer treatment, 15.7
Metalloproteinases, in tumor growth, 15.12
Metastatic prostate cancer, management of, 15.1-15.12
    androgen mechanism and, 15.4-15.5
    bone scans in, 15.2-15.3
    hormonal therapy in, 15-5-15.7
    hormone-refractory, 15.7-15.12
    monoclonal antibodies in, 15.3
    polymerase chain reaction in, 15.4
    principles of, 15.1
    prostate-specific antigen in, 15.2, 15.4
  scanning for detection of, 8.8, 8.10
  sites of, 8.3, 15.2
Microwave energy, tissue penetration depth and, 4.4
Microwave hyperthermia, in benign prostatic hyperplasia, 4.4-4.5
    experimental, 4.4
    ineffectiveness of, 4.5
Microwave thermotherapy, transurethral, 4.6-4.13 *See also* Transurethral microwave thermotherapy
Micturitional urethral pressure profilometry, in bladder outlet obstruction, 2.9-2.10
Mitoxantrone, in hormone-refractory prostate cancer, 15.11
Monoclonal antibodies in prostate cancer, metastatic, 15.3
  staging of, 8.10
Mortality, from prostate cancer, 11.1
Muscle, detrusor *See* Detrusor muscle
  effects of vasodilation in, 4.2
  frequency dependence of penetration of, 4.4
Mutagenicity, of phenoxybenzamine, 3.9
Myosin, in benign prostatic hyperplasia, 1.6, 1.8-1.9
  structure of, 1.9

N
National Institute of Diabetes and Digestive and Kidney Diseases, on prostatitis, 7.8-7.9
Nd:YAG free-beam laser prostatectomy, in benign prostatic hyperplasia, 5.3-5.5
Necrosis, coagulation, in laser prostatectomy, 5.1-5.4, 5.7-5.8
  from transurethral microwave thermotherapy, 4.7
Needle ablation, transurethral, 4.16-4.23 *See also* Transurethral needle ablation
Neoadjuvant hormonal therapy in prostate cancer, 10.11
  cryoablation and, 14.5
  interstitial radiotherapy and, 13.3
Neodymium:yttrium-aluminum-garnet laser prostatectomy, in benign prostatic hyperplasia, 5.3-5.5
Neoplasia, prostatic intraepithelial, in prostate cancer, 8.12-8.13
Nerve-sparing surgery, radical perineal prostatectomy as, 10.1-10.2
  radical retropubic prostatectomy as, 11.1-11.10

Nesbit technique, for prostatic resection, 6.5-6.7
Neuropathy, lower urinary tract symptoms of, 2.1-2.2
Neurovascular bundle, in radical retropubic prostatectomy, 11.6-11.7
Nitric oxide pathway, in prostatic smooth muscle contraction, 1.7
Nitrogen, in cryoablation, 14.3-14.4, 14.8
Nomograms, in prostate cancer treatment decisions, 9.5-9.7
Norephinephrine, in prostatic smooth muscle contraction, 1.7
Northern blot analysis, in bladder obstruction, 1.9

O
Obstruction, bladder outlet *See* Bladder outlet obstruction
O'Connor drape, in radical perineal prostatectomy, 10.4
O'Connor sheath, in prostatic resection, 6.6
Open prostatectomy, in benign prostatic hyperplasia, 6.10-6.11
    outcome of, 6.8
Orchiectomy in prostate cancer, hormonal effects of, 15.5-15.6

P
Pain, in prostatitis, 7.6-7.8
  skin temperature and, 4.3
Pain perception, skin temperature and, 4.3
Partin nomograms, in prostate cancer treatment decisions, 9.5-9.6
Passive urethral resistance relation, in bladder outlet obstruction, 2.7-2.9
Peanut dissector, for radical retropubic prostatectomy, 11.4, 11.6-11.7
Pelvic anatomy, 12.2
Pelvic floor tension myalgia, in prostatitis, 7.6
Penetration, frequency-dependent depth of tissue, 4.4
Penfield dissector, in radical perineal prostatectomy, 10.6
Perineal prostatectomy, radical, 10.1-10.11 *See also* Radical perineal prostatectomy
Pharmacotherapy, lower urinary tract effects of, 2.1, 2.3
Phenoxybenzamine, in benign prostatic hyperplasia, 3.9
Photon external beam radiotherapy, conventional, 12.5-12.6
Physical examination, in benign prostatic hyperplasia, 2.1
  digital rectal, in prostate cancer, 8.2-8.4, 8.7
Phytosterols, in benign prostatic hyperplasia, 3.12
Phytotherapy, in benign prostatic hyperplasia, 3.12
  defined, 3.12
Piezoceramic transducer, in high-intensity focused ultrasound, 4.13
Polymerase chain reaction, in metastatic prostate cancer, 15.2, 15.4
Postvoid dribble, causes of, 2.12
  retrograde urethrography in, 2.12
Prazosin, in benign prostatic hyperplasia, 3.9
Pressure-flow studies, in benign prostatic hyperplasia, surgery *versus* needle ablation in, 4.22
  in lower urinary tract symptom evaluation, 2.6-2.8
    other studies *versus*, 2.13
ProstaScint scanning, in prostate cancer staging, 8.10
Proctitis, after interstitial radiotherapy, 13.9
Profilometry, in bladder outlet obstruction, 2.9-2.10

Progesterones, in prostate cancer, 15.9
Proscar Long-term Efficacy and Safety Study, benign prostatic hyperplasia in, 1.3-1.4
Prostate, adenoma of *See* Adenoma
 anatomy of, 8.2, 12.2
 benign hyperplasia of *See* Benign prostatic hyperplasia
 cancer of *See* Prostate cancer
 effect of heat on, 4.2
 histology of normal, 7.2
 possible disorders of, 7.1
 rectal palpation of, 8.2
 resection of *See also* Prostatectomy
  transurethral, 6.1-6.8
 surgical anatomy of, 8.2
 transurethral incision of, 6.9
 volume changes in benign prostatic hyperplasia of, 1.3
Prostate cancer, clinical overview of, 8.1-8.16
 early detection of, 8.3-8.6
  as controversial, 8.3
 high-intensity focused ultrasound in, 4.15
 hormone-refractory, 15.7-15.12 *See also* Hormone-refractory prostate cancer
 incidence of, 14.1
 localized, cryoablation in, 14.1-14.12
  radical perineal prostatectomy in, 10.1-10.11
  radical retropubic prostatectomy in, 11.1-11.10
  treatment decisions in, 9.1-9.7
 lower urinary tract symptoms of, 2.3
 metastatic, 15.1-15.12 *See also* Metastatic prostate cancer
 mortality in, 8.16
 nonpalpable, 8.16
 pathologic considerations in, 8.12-8.14
 patterns of spread in, 12.3-12.4
 prevalence of, 3.7, 11.1
 prostate-specific antigen screening for, 3.7
 recurrent, after radical perineal prostatectomy, 10.11
  nomograms for, 9.7
 sites of, 8.2-8.3
 staging of, 8.7-8.12
  treatment decisions and, 9.5-9.7
 survival in, radiotherapy and, 12.7
 treatment of, cryoablation in, 14.1-14.12
  decision variables in, 9.1-9.7
  external beam radiotherapy in, 12.1-12.12
  interstitial radiotherapy in, 13.1-13.9
  options in, 12.4
  radical perineal prostatectomy in, 10.1-10.11
  radical retropubic prostatectomy in, 11.1-11.10
Prostate seed implantation, in interstitial radiotherapy, 13.1-13.9
Prostate volume study, in interstitial radiotherapy, 13.4-13.7
Prostatectomy, in benign prostatic hyperplasia, decline in, 3.2
 laser, 5.1-5.9 *See also* Laser prostatectomy
 open technique for, 6.10-6.11
 retropubic technique for, 6.12-6.13
 external beam radiotherapy after, 12.12
 radical perineal, 10.1-10.11 *See also* Radical perineal prostatectomy
 radical retropubic, 11.1-11.10 *See also* Radical retropubic prostatectomy
Prostate-specific antigen, in benign prostatic hyperplasia, 8.4
 finasteride and, 3.7
 in prostate cancer, 8.3-8.5, 8.15-8.16, 14.1
  cryoablation results and, 14.11
  in disease-free survival statistics, 13.8
  hormone-refractory, 15.7
  metastatic, 15.2, 15.4
  neoadjuvant androgen withdrawal therapy and, 10.11
  postoperative values of, 11.1
  staging of, 8.7-8.9, 8.11-8.12, 12.3-12.4
  treatment decisions in, 9.5-9.7
Prostate-specific membrane antigen, in prostate cancer, metastatic, 15.3
 staging of, 8.10
Prostatic calculi, voiding cystourethrogram of, 2.11
Prostatic desiccation, in benign prostatic hyperplasia, 4.1
Prostatic hyperplasia, benign *See* Benign prostatic hyperplasia
Prostatic intraepithelial neoplasia, in prostate cancer, 8.12-8.13
Prostatic reflux, voiding cystourethrogram of, 2.11
Prostatic tissue necrosis, from transurethral microwave thermotherapy, 4.7
Prostatism, in benign prostatic hyperplasia, 2.1-2.16 *See also* Benign prostatic hyperplasia
 silent, 1.3
Prostatitis, 7.1-7.9
 acute, 7.3-7.4, 7.9
 after interstitial radiotherapy, 13.9
 asymptomatic, 7.9
 bacterial, 7.4-7.5
 chronic, 7.3, 7.5, 7.9
 definitions of, 7.4-7.8
 fertility and, 7.6
 granulomatous, 7.3
 histopathologic criteria for, 7.2-7.4
 prostatodynia in, 7.6
 symptoms of, 2.2-2.3, 7.6-7.7, 7.9
Prostatodynia, in prostatitis, 7.6
Prostatron device, in transurethral microwave thermotherapy, 4.8-4.12
Pseudohermaphroditism, transrectal ultrasound in, 3.4
Psychiatric disorders, lower urinary tract symptoms of, 2.3
Psychologic factors, in prostatitis, 7.6, 7.8
Pubic arch interference assessment, in interstitial radiotherapy, 13.4-13.5

Q

Quality of life, in prostate cancer treatment decisions, 9.2-9.3
Quality of life score, in benign prostatic hyperplasia, surgery *versus* needle ablation in, 4.20
Quality-adjusted survival, in prostate cancer treatment decisions, 9.3

R

Race, prostate-specific antigen and, 8.5
Radiation Therapy Oncology Group, trial of, 12.10
Radiative heating, tissue penetration depth in, 4.4
Radical perineal prostatectomy, 10.1-10.11
　complications of, 10.9
　indications for, 10.1-10.2
　modifications of, 10.10
　patient positioning for, 10.3
　postoperative care in, 10.2
　preoperative considerations in, 10.2
　　neoadjuvant therapy as, 10.11
　　radical retropubic prostatectomy *versus*, 10.10
　recurrent disease after, 10.11
　results of, 10.9-10.10
　technique for, 10-3-10.9
Radical prostatectomy, external beam radiotherapy after, 12.12
Radical retropubic prostatectomy, 11.1-11.10
　complications of, 11.10
　indications for, 11.1
　patient positioning for, 11.2-11.3
　preoperative considerations in, 11.2
　technique for, 11.3-11.10
Radiofrequency energy, principles of, 4.16
Radioisotopes, in hormone-refractory prostate cancer, 15.10
Radiologic imaging, in lower urinary tract symptom evaluation, 2.10-2.13, 2.15
　in prostate cancer staging, 8.7-8.10
Radioscintigraphic bone scanning, in metastatic prostate cancer, 15.3
Radiotherapy, cryoablation after, 14.9
　external beam, 12.1-12.12 *See also* External beam radiotherapy
　in hormone-refractory prostate cancer, 15.10
　interstitial, 13.1-13.9 *See also* Interstitial radiotherapy
α-Receptors, in benign prostatic hyperplasia, 1.7
Rectal examination, in benign prostatic hyperplasia, 2.1
　in prostate cancer, 8.3-8.4, 8.7
　prostatic anatomy and, 8.2
Rectourethral fistula formation, from cryoablation, 14.9
5α-Reductase, 1.4-1.5, 15.4, 15.6
5α-Reductase deficiency syndrome, 1.4
Renal function, bladder outlet obstruction and, 2.4
Resectoscope, in transurethral prostatectomy, 6.1, 6.5
Retrograde urethrography, in lower urinary tract symptom evaluation, 2.12
Retropubic prostatectomy, in benign prostatic hyperplasia, 6.12-6.13
　radical, 11.1-11.10 *See also* Radical retropubic prostatectomy

S

Saw palmetto berry, in benign prostatic hyperplasia, 3.12
Scintigraphy, in metastatic prostate cancer, 15.3
Sculley scissors, in radical perineal prostatectomy, 10.5
Seminal fluid, in prostatitis, 7.6-7.7
Seminal vesicles, in radical retropubic prostatectomy, 11.8-11.9

Serenoa repens, in benign prostatic hyperplasia, 3.12
Sexual dysfunction, in benign prostatic hyperplasia, 6.8
　from α-blocker therapy, 3.11
　from hormonal therapy, 3.7, 15.6
Sexual function, after radical perineal prostatectomy, 10.1-10.2
Silent prostatism, defined, 1.3
Skin, effects of vasodilation in, 4.2
　pain and temperature of, 4.3
Smooth muscle, in benign prostatic hyperplasia, 1.6, 1.8-1.10
　prostatic, adrenoreceptors and, 3.8
Sonablate ultrasound device, in benign prostatic hyperplasia, 4.14
Spectroscopy, after cryoablation, 14.10
Sperm, in prostatitis, 7.6-7.7
Staging of prostate cancer, 8.7-8.12
　cryoablation results and, 14.11
　treatment decisions and, 9.5-9.7
Steroid receptors, in benign prostatic hyperplasia, 1.5
Stricture, after radiotherapy, 12.7
Stroma, prostatic, 1.6, 8.2
Stromal cells, in benign prostatic hyperplasia, 1.2, 1.5-1.6
Surgery, in benign prostatic hyperplasia, 6.1-6.13
　finasteride and, 1.4, 3.6
　open prostatectomy in, 6.10-6.11
　retropubic prostatectomy in, 6.12-6.13
　transurethral incision in, 6.9
　transurethral resection in, 6.1-6.8
　in treatment trends, 3.13
　nerve-sparing, radical perineal prostatectomy as, 10.1-10.11
　　radical retropubic prostatectomy as, 11.1-11.10
　in prostate cancer, radical perineal prostatectomy as, 10.1-10.11
　　radical retropubic prostatectomy as, 11.1-11.10

T

Tamsulosin, in benign prostatic hyperplasia, 3.10
Target volume, in interstitial radiotherapy, 13.5
TARGIS device, in transurethral microwave thermotherapy, 4.7-4.10, 4.13
Temperature *See also* specific techniques; Thermal therapy
　in cryoablation, 14.2-14.3
　effect on prostate of, 4.2
　in laser prostatectomy, 5.1
　pain and, 4.3
　radiofrequency and, 4.16
　ultrasound and, 4.13
Terazosin, in benign prostatic hyperplasia, 3.9, 3.11
Testosterone, in benign prostatic hyperplasia, 1.4-1.5, 1.8
　in finasteride mechanism of action, 3.4
　in hypothalamic-gonadal axis, 3.3
　in metastatic prostate cancer, 15.3
　prostatic volume and, 3.7
Thermal therapy, in benign prostatic hyperplasia, 4.1-4.23
　high-intensity focused ultrasound in, 4.13-4.15

Thermal therapy, in benign prostatic hyperplasia, *(continued)*
  microwave hyperthermia in, 4.4-4.5
  principles of, 4.1-4.4
  transurethral microwave thermotherapy in, 4.6-4.13
  transurethral needle ablation in, 4.16-4.23
Thermometry, in experimental benign prostatic hyperplasia, 4.4
Thromboembolism, preoperative prophylaxis against, 11.2
Time tradeoff technique, in prostate cancer treatment decisions, 9.3
Tissue necrosis, from transurethral microwave thermotherapy, 4.7
Tissue sloughing, from cryoablation, 14.9, 14.12
TNM staging system in prostate cancer, 8.7, 8.11-8.12
  cryoablation results and, 14.11
  treatment decisions and, 9.5-9.7
Trabeculated bladder, biopsy of, 1.10
Transducers, in high-intensity focused ultrasound, 4.13-4.14
  in interstitial radiotherapy, 13.6
Transrectal high-intensity focused ultrasound, in benign prostatic hyperplasia, 4.14
Transrectal microwave hyperthermia, in benign prostatic hyperplasia, 4.4-4.5
Transrectal prostate volume study, in interstitial radiotherapy, 13.4
Transrectal ultrasound, in cryoablation, 14.10
  in prostate cancer, 8.3, 8.6
    prostate volume study in, 13.5
    staging of, 8.9
Transurethral incision of the prostate, in benign prostatic hyperplasia, 6.9
  outcome of, 6.8-6.9
  in prostatodynia, 7.6
Transurethral microwave hyperthermia, in benign prostatic hyperplasia, 4.5
Transurethral microwave thermotherapy, in benign prostatic hyperplasia, 4.6-4.13
  adverse effects of, 4.11
  assessment of, 4.7-4.8
  equipment in, 4.8-4.10
  failure of, 4.11
  hyperthermia *versus*, 4.6
  results of, 4.10-4.13
  surgery *versus*, 4.12
Transurethral needle ablation, in benign prostatic hyperplasia, 4.16-4.23
  adverse events in, 4.23
  equipment in, 4.17
  imaging in, 4.18-4.19
  principles of, 4.16
  procedure for, 4.18
  results of, 4.19-4.20
  surgery *versus*, 4.20-4.23
Transurethral resection of the prostate, in benign prostatic hyperplasia, 6.1-6.8
  adverse events in, 4.23
  needle *versus*, 4.20-4.23
  outcome of, 6.8-6.9
  as standard care, 4.1

  thermotherapy *versus*, 4.12
  interstitial radiotherapy and, 13.2
  in prostatodynia, 7.6
  risks of, 4.1
Transurethral ultrasound, in benign prostatic hyperplasia, laser prostatectomy guided by, 5.2
  other therapy *versus*, 4.20
Trendelenburg position, for radical retropubic prostatectomy, 11.2-11.3
Trigone, in radical perineal prostatectomy, 10.8
Tuberculosis, prostatitis in, 7.3
Tumors *See also* Adenoma; Prostate cancer
  cryoablation in control of, 14.10-14.12
  effects of heat on, 4.2
  metastasis of, 15.12
  preoperative evaluation of, 13.2
  vasodilation and, 4.2
Turner Warwick retractor, for radical retropubic prostatectomy, 11.3

U

Ultrasound, in benign prostatic hyperplasia, high-intensity focused technique in, 4.13-4.15
  laser prostatectomy guided by, 5.2
  other therapy *versus*, 4.20
  in cryoablation, 14.3, 14.10
  transrectal, in prostate cancer, 8.3, 8.6, 8.9
  in transurethral microwave thermotherapy, 4.8
Ureteral reflux, radiologic imaging in, 2.12
Urethra, in radical prostatectomy, 10.7, 10.9, 11.7
Urethral heating, in benign prostatic hyperplasia, 4.6
Urethral resistance factor, in bladder outlet obstruction, 2.8
Urethral stricture, in radical perineal prostatectomy, 10.9
Urethral warmer, in cryoablation, 14.4-14.5
Urethritis, after interstitial radiotherapy, 13.9
Urethrography, retrograde, in lower urinary tract symptom evaluation, 2.12
Urinary disorders, in benign prostatic hyperplasia, 6.2
  surgical treatment for, 6.1
  in prostatitis, 7.4, 7.6
Urinary flow, in benign prostatic hyperplasia, after microwave thermotherapy, 4.10
  after transurethral needle ablation, 4.19
  surgery *versus* needle ablation in, 4.20
  in lower urinary tract symptom evaluation, 2.4
  in preoperative evaluation, 13.2
Urinary incontinence, after benign prostatic hyperplasia treatment, 6.8
  after cryoablation, 14.12
  after radical prostatectomy, 10.9, 11.10
  after radiotherapy, 12.7
Urinary retention, after interstitial radiotherapy, 13.9
  in benign prostatic hyperplasia, 1.3, 3.2
    after thermotherapy, 4.11
    α-blocker therapy for, 3.13
    finasteride for, 1.4, 3.6, 3.13

surgical treatment for, 6.1
 in prostate cancer, after cryoablation, 14.12
  preoperative evaluation of, 13.2
Urinary tract symptoms, in benign prostatic hyperplasia, 2.1-2.16
 of prostatitis from infection, 7.2, 7.4-7.5, 7.9
Urodynamic evaluation, of lower urinary tract symptoms, 2.1-2.2, 2.4-2.10
  indications for, 2.15-2.16
other studies *versus*, 2.13
Uroflowmetry, in lower urinary tract symptom evaluation, 2.4, 2.15
Urowave device, in transurethral microwave thermotherapy, 4.8-4.10

V

Vascularity, heat susceptibility and, 4.2
Vasodilation, in normal tissue *versus* tumor, 4.2

Venn diagram, of lower urinary tract symptoms, 2.2
Vesicourethral dysfunction, benign prostatic hyperplasia and, 2.2-2.4
Veterans Affairs Cooperative Study, of benign prostatic hyperplasia, 3.11
Videourodynamics, in lower urinary tract symptom evaluation, 2.10-2.11, 2.15
Visual analog scale, in transurethral microwave thermotherapy, 4.13
Voiding cystourethrography, in lower urinary tract symptom evaluation, 2.10-2.13
Voiding parameters, in preoperative evaluation, 13.2
Voiding profilometry, in bladder outlet obstruction, 2.9-2.10

W

Watts factor, in bladder outlet obstruction, 2.8
Wave frequencies, biologic effects of, 4.3
Whitmore-Jewett staging system, in prostate cancer, 8.7

COLOR PLATES

FIGURE 1-13.

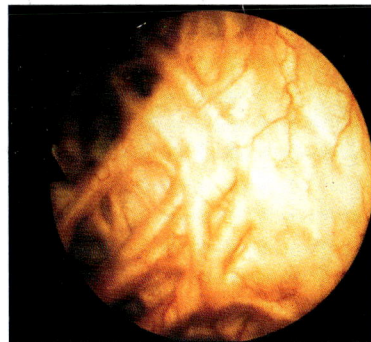

FIGURE 1-31.

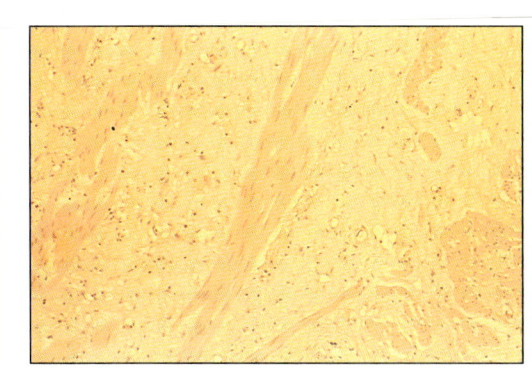

FIGURE 1-32.

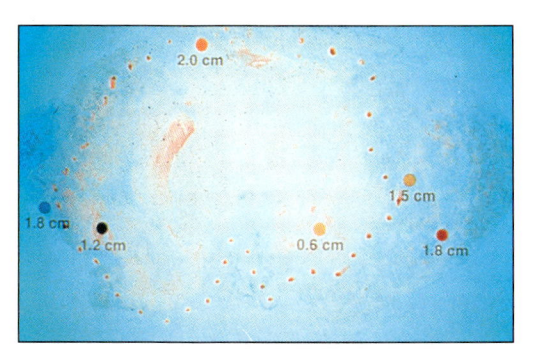

FIGURE 4-14.

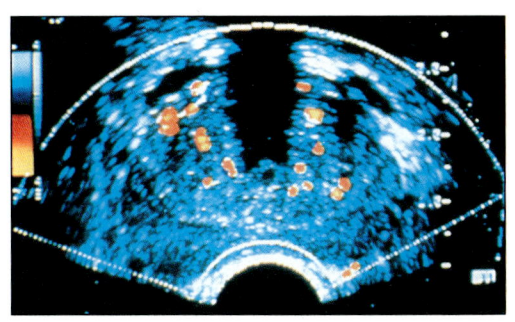

FIGURE 4-16A.

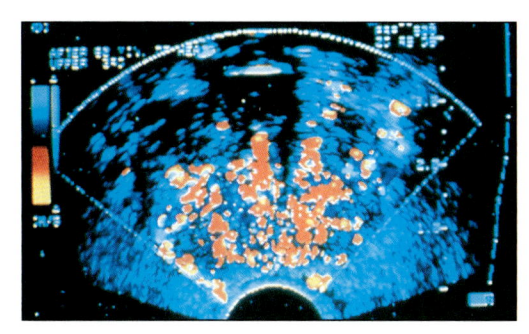

FIGURE 4-16B.

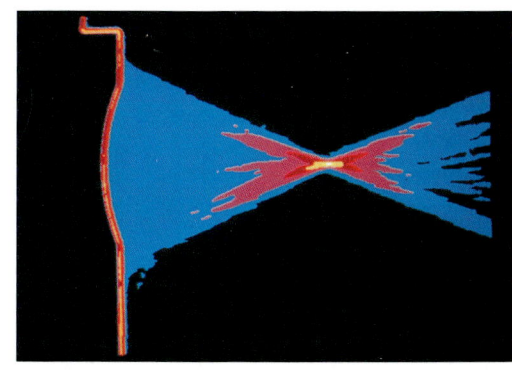

FIGURE 4-28.

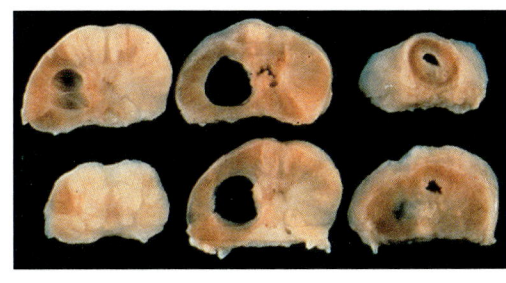

FIGURE 4-32.

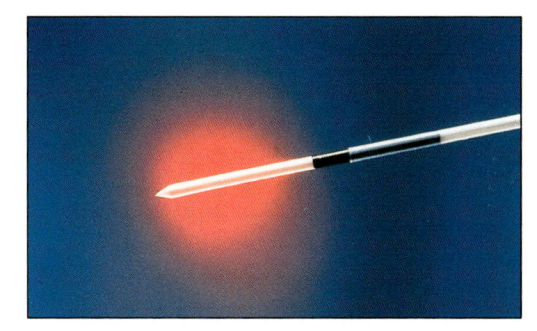

FIGURE 5-15B.

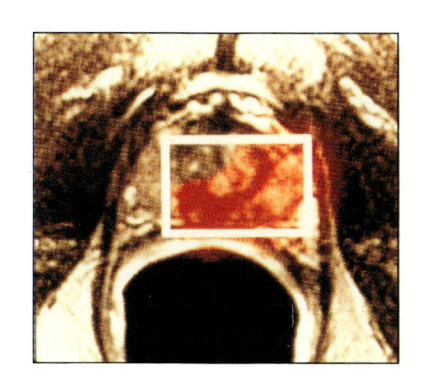

FIGURE 14-24A.